# MATERIA MEDICA OF AYURVEDA

*Todarananda-Ayurveda Saukhyam Series No.6*

# MATERIA MEDICA OF AYURVEDA

## BASED ON AYURVEDA SAUKHYAM OF TOḌARĀNANDA

VAIDYA BHAGWAN DASH
D.A.M.S., H.P.A., M.A., Ph. D.
Deputy Adviser (Ayurveda)
Ministry of Health &
Family Welfare
New Delhi

VAIDYA LALITESH KASHYAP
B.I.M.S.
Senior Physician (Ayurveda)
Central Govt. Health Scheme
Directorate General of Health Services,
New Delhi

CONCEPT PUBLISHING COMPANY, NEW DELHI-59

ISBN 81-7022-024-6 (Set)
ISBN 81-7022-020-3

First Published 1980
Reprinted 1987, 1994, 2000



Vaidya Bhagwan **Dash** (*b.* 1934- )
Vaidya (Miss) Lalitesh **Kashyap** (*b.* 1939- )

*Printed and Published by*
Ashok Kumar Mittal
**Concept Publishing Company**
A/15-16, Commercial Block, Mohan Garden
New Delhi-110059 (India)

*Phones:* 5648039, 5649024
*Fax:* 091–(11)–5648053

*Email:* publishing@conceptpub.com

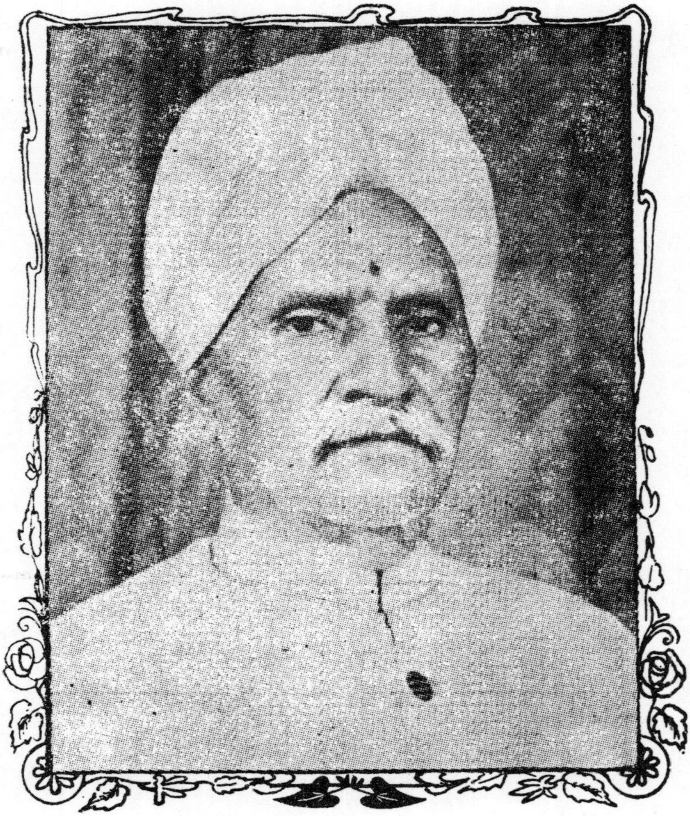

*Dedicated to the memory*
*of*

Late PANDIT RAM PRASAD SHARMA
(Ex-Rajavaidya of Patiala)
in
Grateful acknowledgement of his
erudite scholarship and unwearied
services for the revival and
development of Ayurveda

# FOREWORD

Though several important works on Ayurveda have been published till now, there is a large number of works which are still in the manuscript stage in libraries and could not see the light. The name of some of these works we know by coming across them in commentaries and compilations. The reason is mostly economic because the texts which are included in the prospectus are studied in institutions and get priority in publication while others lag behind. The result is that to-day teachers and students are not acquainted with even the names of such texts what of going through them.

*Toḍarānanda* is a work named on Rājā Toḍaramalla, a minister of Mughal Emperor Akbar (16th Cent. A.D.). This is an encyclopaedic work having *Ayurveda Saukhya* as a component. *Ayurveda Saukhya* too is a voluminous work dealing with several aspects of Ayurveda. The present volume deals with the portion of Materia Medica which is generally known as *Nighaṇṭu*.

In 1972, when I was editing the *Mādhava Dravyaguṇa*, I had the opportunity to see a manuscript of the *Ayurveda Saukhya*. I was surprised to find that it followed Mādhava's *Dravyaguṇa* faithfully in the context of *Nighaṇṭu* portion though the author did not mention the name of *Mādhava* or its work anywhere. It is also to be noted that though in other portions, source books are quoted explicitly, in *Nighaṭṇu* portion it is conspicuously absent. Hence, it cannot be said definitely what was the source of this portion.

It is almost certain that Mādhava's *Dravyaguṇa* was quite earlier than the *Āyurveda Saukhya* because of its having been quoted by medieval authors and commentators like Sarvānanda (12th Cent. A.D.) and Vopadeva (13th Cent. A.D.). As regards Bhāva Miśra, he happened to be in 16th Cent. A.D. and thus may be contemporary to the work *Āyurveda Saukhya.* The verses of the Bhāva Prakāśa found in the *Āyurveda Saukhya* lead us to think that either these verses are later interpolations (particularly if they are not found in majority of the MSS.) or Bhāva Miśra himself might be associated with this work. A number of expert scholars of Banaras were engaged by Rājā Toḍaramalla for this encyclopaedic work, and it is not improbable if Bhāva Miśra, a resident of Magadha (Gayā) adjoining Kashi and a renowned expert of *Dravya guṇa* himself participated in this great task. It is to be noted that Bhāva Miśra, apart from the *Bhāva Prakāśa Nighaṇṭu,* also composed another *Nighaṇṭu* entitled *Guṇa ratna mālā.* Without close association, it becomes difficult to explain such situations. The possibility of a common source of both the authors, as proposed by the editor, is also not improbable.

Vaidya Bhagwan Dash, the editor of this work, is well-known for his devotion to enriching the literature of Ayurveda and also to making it intelligible to the outer world. He has done this job with great labour and deserves congratulations not only of myself but of the entire circle of intellectuals interested in the study of Ayurveda. I hope, he will be able to bring out other remaining volumes so as to present a total picture of the work.

Banaras Hindu University,
VARANASI

20th September 1979

P.V. SHARMA
Professor and
Head of the Department of
Dravyaguna,
Institute of Medical Sciences

# PREFACE

There has been an increasing interest in the utilisation of the traditional systems of medicine for promotive, preventive and curative health services in many countries of the world. Ayurveda is perhaps the oldest traditional system of medicine in India catering at present to the medical needs of a large section of both the urban and rural population of this country. This system of medicine has also caught the attention of medical practioners in the West. The Materia Medica of ayurveda represents a rich storehouse of knowledge of drugs based on centuries of experience. Scientists, research workers, physicians and students interested in ayurveda, often experience great difficulty in obtaining authentic works on the subject with a translation in a language generally understood by them. To cater to this long felt need, we are happy to present here the Materia Medica of Ayurveda by Rājā Toḍaramalla with its English translation along with critical notes.

Toḍaramalla hailed from Oudh in Uttar Pradesh, India. He was the *dewan* (Minister) under the great Moghul Emperor Akbar who ruled during the sixteenth century A.D. The emperor was well known for his secular outlook. Toḍaramalla, in spite of his unquestioned loyalty to this Muslim emperor, was a staunch follower of Hinduism. It was apparent to him that Hindu culture in India was in a decadent state and at a low ebb. Quite apart from religion, even sciences like astrology and medicine had fallen into disrepute. Very little original work, if any, was being done in these areas of knowledge and even the extant texts on various subjects were falling into disuse. Such of them as were available had been mutilated and subjected to unauthorised interpolations with the accretion of superstitious ideas through the centuries.

In his mission to revive and revitalise Hindu culture both in the religious and secular fields, he took the help of several eminent Sanskrit scholars of Varanasi and composed encyclopaedic works on 23 different subjects by collecting material from authentic texts which were then available. To this, the added knowledge and experiences of the experts in the subject were incorporated. Most of the original texts which were then utilised for the composition of these works are no more extant and those which have survived the vicissitudes of time are now in a mutilated form with several unauthorised and erratic interpolations. It is in this context, therefore, that today Toḍarmalla's work has gained considerable importance, and it is for the first time that the Materia Medica portion of his encyclopaedic work on ayurveda is being brought under print. The series of works on 23 topics of Hindu culture composed under the auspices of Rājā Toḍaramalla is called *Toḍarānanda* which means "the delight of Toḍaramalla". The term *saukhyaṁ* meaning "happiness" is suffixed to the name of each text on a particular topic. Thus the text on ayurveda is called *Ayurveda Saukhyaṁ*. This *Ayurveda Saukhyaṁ* comprises several chapters each one of which is called *harṣa* meaning "pleasure".

In the beginning of each *harṣa*, *maṅgalācaraṇa* or the auspicious invocation in the form of a prayer to God is furnished. The colophons at the end of each chapter indicate the contents and chapter number, among others. These invocations and colophons are missing in some manuscripts.

Calligraphic errors have not left this monumental work untouched. Six different manuscripts collected from various libraries of India and Nepal were utilised for the collation and editing of this work. Some of these manuscripts are incomplete. But in others which appeared at first to be complete, some chapter numbers have been arranged and named differently. Some chapters have also been omitted in some of these manuscripts. Therefore, while editing, it was felt desirable to serialise and renumber all these chapters making up a total of 97. This was a delicate job to perform because at the end of the chapters, in some manuscripts, the colophons are missing. For the preparation of this work on Materia Medica, ten chapters of *Ayurveda Saukhyaṁ* have been utilised. On the basis of the remaining chapters, it is contemplated to prepare separate volumes on different topics shortly and these texts will be in the hands of scholars gradually and in stages.

*Ayurveda Saukhyaṁ* deals with various topics of ayurveda including fundamental principles, anatomy, physiology, hygiene and public health, examination of patients, diagnosis, prognosis and treatment of diseases, iatro-chemistry and materia medica. Materia Medica and allied topics are found scattered in ten different chapters of this work. The eighth chapter deals with the properties of drugs. This chapter is available in five out of the six manuscripts consulted. In one manuscript, however, this chapter is left incomplete.

This eighth chapter *inter alia* deals with some extraneous topics like *vamana* (emetic therapy) and *virecana* (purgation therapy). These topics, along with other allied topics, like *snehana* (oleation therapy), *svedana* (fomentation therapy), *nirūha* and *anuvāsana* (medicated enema), *nasya* (inhalation therapy) and *rakta mokṣaṇa* (blood letting) are described in detail in the 85th to 88th chapters of the edited text. It is proposed to bring out a separate volume on these topics, which taken together, are called *pañcakarma* therapy. These extraneous topics, therefore, are excluded from this work. This 8th chapter of the original text is divided into 29 chapters in the present work—one chapter dealing exclusively with one group of items.

The 12th chapter of the original text deals with the description of various groups of drugs collected from classics like *Suśruta Saṁhitā*. This chapter is, therefore, included in the 30th chapter of the present work. This chapter is available in three manuscripts.

The last eight chapters of the original text deal with mostly the *nighaṇṭus* or synonyms of drugs and the method of preparation of some food items. Details of these chapters are given overleaf :

| Chapter Nos. given in the manuscripts | Chapter Nos. in the edited text | Chapter Nos. in the present work | The number of manuscripts in which these chapters are available |
|---|---|---|---|
| 84 | 90 | 31 | 4 |
| 85 | 91 | 32 | 2 |
| 86 | 92 | 33 | 3 |
| 87 | 93 | 34 | 3 |
| 88 | 94 | 35 | 3 |
| 89 | 95 | 36 | 3 |
| 90 | 96 | 37 | 3 |
| 91 | 97 | 38 | 3 |

There are of course, separate texts on the synonyms of drugs of ayurveda. But most of the extant ayurvedic works on materia medica invariably provide synonyms of drugs along with their properties. It is keeping in view this tradition of ayurveda, and also in order to make the present work more useful to research workers, physicians and students that these eight chapters have been included here.

All the manuscripts procured for the editing of this work were full of grammatical and syntactical errors. Some of these mistakes were common to all the manuscripts. Even the arrangement of topics in these manuscripts varied considerably. Many terms and suffixes used in this work do not stand correct according to the tradition of Pāṇini's grammar. The readers will find some such terms even in the present publication. It is likely that these mistakes were there in the original texts from where references were collected and the scholars who did the job did not think it proper to make any change. The other possibility is that these errors were introduced by subsequent calligraphers.

There are some orthographical peculiarities in all the manuscripts of this work. In several places *ṇa* has been used in the places of *na*, *sa* in the place of *śa* and *ṣa*, *ba* in place of *va*, *kha* in the place of *ṣa*, *ja* in the place of *ya*, *ra* in the place of *la*, *gha* in the place of *dha* and *vice versa.* In several places the consonants after *ra* are duplicated.

While editing this work, the variant readings (which include some grammatical errors also) are given at the end of each chapter under Notes and References and the original manuscripts are referred to as *ādarśa pustikā.* Some topics given in this work are also available in other extant ayurvedic works. The variant readings in these texts are given at the end and these extant texts are referred to as *ākara.* Some portions of the manuscripts were so corrupt and incomplete that we did not think it proper to include them in the main text. In view of their significance from the materia medica point of view, they are given in the "Notes and References" at the end of the chapters.

In the manuscripts some texts are originally referred to by name from where the information was collected by the scholars. The readings in these texts bear a striking resemblance to those of *Mādhava dravyaguṇa* and *Bhāva prakāśa.* The former has been edited by Prof. P.V. Sharma and published by Chawkhamba Vidya Bhawan, Varanasi in 1973. References to these works are conspicuous by their absence in the original manuscripts. However, to facilitate research and study on this subject, these references are provided in the present work in square brackets [ ]. Since the names of these texts are not described in the original manuscripts, it is very difficult to determine as to who borrowed from whom. It is also very likely that both have borrowed their texts from a third source which has since become extinct.

While providing the English translation of the text, we have been very conscious of avoiding mistranslation. Where equivalent English words are not available, in the English text, the Sanskrit words have been transliterated as such and printed in italics. The glossary appended to this work provides a brief explanation of such terms. The nearest English equivalents of many such technical terms are given in parentheses in the English text itself.

The botanical names of most of the medicinal plants are given in parentheses against the Sanskrit names of drugs in the side-headings. Similarly, the English equivalents of animals, metals, minerals, etc., are provided. Wherever there is any controversy regarding the correct indentification of a drug, the botanical or English names have not been provided, lest the reader should be misguided.

One manuscript of this work was procured from a private individual of Varanasi. Some scholars had attempted a Hindi translation of this work. From the language and the paper, it appears that this attempt was not of recent origin. In some places, this Hindi translation has been consulted to decide upon the exact reading of the text.

**Acknowledgements**

Authors are exceedingly grateful to Pandit Shiv Sharma, President of the Central Council of Indian Medicine for supplying two manuscripts of this work from the collections of his illustrious father Vaidya Rama Prasad Sharma, who was the Raja Vaidya (Physician to the ruler) of Patiala. Greateful thanks are also due to the curators of the Abhilekhalaya, Kathmandu, the Royal Asiatic Society and Sanskrit College both at Calcutta for providing calligraphic/photostat copies of the manuscripts of this work available with them.

For the preparation of this work, Subhash Gupta, Kanchan Gupta and Sharada Gupta have provided considerable assistance. The authors are extremely thankful to them.

A publication of this kind may not be a commercially viable proposition. It must, therefore be said to the credit of the publishers that they have brought it out in a spirit of dedication solely with the aim of propagating this unique science of medicine in the service of the suffering humanity.

BHAGWAN DASH

LALITESH KASHYAP

# CONTENTS

kharāhvā [114], dhānyaka [115-117], jambīra [117], bhaṅgā [118], surabhi [119], tumburu [120], varvarī [120-121], kṛṣṇa gandhā [121], śigru [122], madhu śigru [122], varuṇa [123], pāribhadra [123], bilva [124], pāṭalā [124], kāśmarī [125], vahni mantha [125], eraṇḍa [126], trikaṇṭaka [126], kaṇṭakārikā [127], bṛhatī [127], pṛśni parṇī [128], sthirā [128], jīṅginī [129], balā [130], mahā balā [130], nāga balā [131], aśva gandhā [131], māṣa parṇī [132], mudga parṇī [132], ṛddhi [132], vṛddhi [133], kākolī [133-134], medā [134-135], jīvaka [135-136], ṛṣabhaka [135-136], aṣṭa varga [136-137], viśālā [137], sārivā [138], gavādanī [138], anantā [139], gundrā [139], lodhra [140], sāvara lodhra [140], madhuka [141], prapauṇḍarīka [142], mañjiṣṭhā [142[, lākṣā [143], muśalī [143-144], śatāvarī [144-146], pārtha [146], asthi saṁhāra [147], mārkava [147], droṇa puṣpīkā [148], giri karṇikā [148], vṛścikālī [149], dugdhikā [149-150] ahiṁsrā [150], sudarśanā [150], bhārgī [151], guñjā [151], jayantī [151], sairīya [151], prasāriṇī [152], kokilākṣa [152], kulāhala [152], dhuttūra [153], halinī [154], karavīra [154], āvartakī [154], kośātakī [155], jyotīṣmatī [155], brāhmī [156], vacā [156], kukkurunda [157], śaṅkha puṣpī [157], haṁsa pādī [158], muṇḍī [158-159], mālatī [159], mukula [160], nāga damanī [160], śirīṣa [161], sikthaka [161], āphūka [162-163], dūrvā, [163] niśā [164], dārvī [165], avalguja [165-166], prapunnāḍa [166], karañja [167], kiṁśuka [167], ariṣṭa [167], viḍaṅga [168], āsphotā [168], tiniśā [168], asana [169], śiṁśapā [169], dhātakī [169], kadara [169], apāmārga [170], sinduvāra [170], lajjālu [170-171], vaṁśa [171], rohitaka [172], vṛhaddāra [172], tagara [173], kauntī [173], śrīvāsa [174-175], sarala [174-175], bola [174-175], kunduru [174-175], granthi parṇa [174-175], turuṣka [174-175], silhaka [174-175], spṛkkā [174-175], gundrā [174-175], sarja [174-175], murā [174-175], nakha [174-175], rālā [176], candana [177-179], pataṅga [179], padmaka [180], sevya [180], kuṁkuma [181], kastūrī [181], aguru [182], sura dāru [182], kattṛṇa [183], kuṣṭha [183], śaṭī [184], kaṅkola [184], jātī phala [185], jāti kośa [185], karpūra [186-189], rāsṇā [189-190], elā [190-191], lavaṅga [191], latā kastūrikā [192], kaṭphala [192], madana [193], śatāhvā [194], phalinī [195], gandha priyaṅgu [195], hapuṣā [196], rāṣṇā [197], pauṣkara [197], śṛṅgī [198], varāṅga [198-199], nāga kesara [199], patraka [200], tālisa patra [200-201], vaṁśa rocanā [201], tugākṣīrī [202], vāsaka [202-203],

## INDO-ROMANIC EQUIVALENTS OF DEVNĀGARĪ

| | | | | | | | |
|---|---|---|---|---|---|---|---|
| अ | a | क | ka | ण | ṇa | व | va |
| आ | ā | ख | kha | त | ta | श | śa |
| इ | i | ग | ga | थ | tha | ष | ṣa |
| ई | ī | घ | gha | द | da | स | sa |
| उ | u | ङ | ṅa | ध | dha | ह | ha |
| ऊ | ū | च | ca | न | na | | |
| ऋ | ṛ | छ | cha | प | pa | | |
| ॠ | ṛ | ज | ja | फ | pha | | |
| ए | e | झ | jha | ब | ba | | |
| ऐ | ai | ञ | ña | भ | bha | | |
| ओ | o | ट | ṭa | म | ma | | |
| औ | au | ठ | ṭha | य | ya | | |
| अं | ṁ | ड | ḍa | र | ra | | |
| अः | ḥ | ढ | ḍha | ल | la | | |

# INTRODUCTION

The history of the materia medica of ayurveda is as old as the Vedas. The *Ṛk Veda* (prior to 4500 B.C.), which is the oldest repository of human knowledge, has described about 67 plants. Other Vedas, namely, *Sāman*, *Yajus* and *Atharvan* are also replete with references to various aspects of ayurveda, including the description of drugs and their therapeutic effects. Medicinal plants are also described in the *saṁhitā*, *upaniṣat* and *purāṇa* texts.

Ayurveda is an *upaveda* or subsidiary text of the *Atharva veda* and it has the following specialised branches ;

(1) *Kāya cikitsā* or Internal medicine ;
(2) *Śalya tantra* or Surgery ;
(3) *Śālākya tantra* or the treatment of diseases of head and neck ;
(4) *Agada tantra* or Toxicology ;
(5) *Bhūta vidyā* or the management of seizures by evil spirits and other mental disorders ;
(6) *Bāla tantra* or Paediatrics ;
(7) *Rasāyana tantra* or Geriatrics including Rejuvenation therapy ; and
(8) *Vājikaraṇa tantra* or Science of Aphrodisiacs.

Classics were composed on each of these specialised branches. In some classics, all these branches of ayurveda were put together. Prior to the seventh century B.C., many ayurvedic classics were composed. The important ones, among them, are *Caraka saṁhitā*, *Suśruta saṁhitā*, *Bhela saṁhitā*, *Kāśyapa saṁhitā* and *Hārīta saṁhitā*. Most of these texts are not available in their original form now. *Caraka saṁhitā*, which was originally composed by Agniveśa and was called *Agniveśa sāṁhitā*, was subsequently redacted by Caraka. Even this redacted version is not available in its entirety now. Out of 120 chapters, about 41 chapters were missing and were subsequently added by a fourth century scholar named Dṛḍhabala. *Suśruta saṁhitā* was also redacted by Nāgārjuna. The remaining three texts are not available in their complete form. *Hārīta saṁhitā*, which is available now, appears to be different from the original one. Subsequently, two texts of Vāgbhaṭa, namely, *Aṣṭāṅga hṛdaya* and *Aṣṭāṅga saṁgraha* were added to this series of classics and both these works are available in their complete form. In all these important ayurvedic classics, separate chapters are provided for the description of drugs and their therapeutic properties. The fundamental principles dealing with the concept of drug composition and drug action are also described in these texts. *Dravya guṇa* or materia medica, as a separate text, came into existence much later.

The advent of Buddhism in India brought considerable change in the practice of ayurveda. Surgery, the performance of which is invariably associated with pain, was treated as a form of *hiṁsā* or violence, and therefore, its practice was banned. To compensate this loss, and to alleviate the sufferings of ailing humanity, more drugs were added during this period to ayurvedic materia medica. Prior to this period, metals and minerals were no doubt used for therapeutic purposes. But their use was in a crude form and they were sparingly used. Buddhist scholars added considerably to the metals and minerals in ayurvedic materia medica, inasmuch as *Rasa śāstra* or Iatro-chemistry, formed a specialised branch and many authentic texts were composed on this subject. Thus, the loss by discarding the practice of surgery was well compensated by the addition of iatro-chemistry to the materia medica of ayurveda during this period.

Some of the Buddhist rulers, like Aśoka, established several herb-gardens, so that people could get drugs conveniently for the treatment of their diseases. Buddhist monks were encouraged to learn ayurveda and practise it, which was considered to be the most convenient and popular method of spreading the teachings of their Preceptor. Thus, through Buddhism, ayurveda spread to Śrī Laṅkā, Nepal, Tibet, Mongolia, the Buriyat Republic of Soviet Russia, China, Korea, Japan and other South-East Asian countries. Ayurvedic texts, including texts on materia medica, were translated into the languages of these countries and these are still available in translated form even though some of their originals have become extinct in the country of their origin. Based upon the fundamental principles of ayurveda, some local herbs, diet and drinks were included in the traditional medicine of the respective countries. The materia medica of ayurveda was thus enriched.

India was severally invaded by outsiders like the Greeks, the Saks and the Hoons. When these people came into contact with the rich tradition of India, especially the medical science, they carried back with them medicines and doctors. Indian doctors who went with them, translated ayurvedic texts into their languages. The new drugs which were specially used in those places were incorporated into the ayurvedic pharmacopoeiá. Such repeated exchanges of scholars enriched ayurveda and its materia medica. Through commercial channels ayurvedic drugs and spices were exported to these countries and they were held in high esteem there.

Several universities were established during this period for imparting theoretical and practical training in different religious and secular subjects. Taxila and Nalanda were the two such universities which attracted not only intellectuals, from different parts of this country but many from abroad. In Taxila, there was a medical faculty with Ātreya as its Chairman. In Buddhist literature, there are many interesting stories and anecdotes about the activities of these universities, their scholars and faculty members. One such anecdote is related to Jīvaka who was three times crowned as the King of Physicians because of his proficiency in the art of healing. He was an expert in paediatrics and brain surgery. It was the practice at that time for candidates desirous of admission to the faculty in the university to appear for a test before the Dvārapāla or the gate-keeper. Jīvaka and several other princes had to face these tests before being considered for admission to the medical faculty. They were asked to go to the nearby forests and collect as many plants as possible, which did not possess any medicinal property. By the evening candidates returned with several plants which they considered to be free from medicinal properties. Jīvaka did not return for several days and, when he did, he was empty handed. On a query from the gate-keeper, Jīvaka replied, "I could not find any plant, or for that matter anything which does not have medicinal value." He alone was selected for admission to the medical faculty. This was the status of knowledge of the candidates for the medical faculty at that time. This was the time when the knowledge of materia medica became highly developed.

As has been mentioned before, Buddhism was partially responsible for the arrest of development in some branches of ayurveda. Foreigners who ruled over India brought with them medicines and medical men from their own countries and patronised them. The practice of ayurveda, thus, lost the support and patronage of the rulers. Apart from foreign invasions, during the medieval period, the ruling states in this sub-continent itself were engaged in fighting amongst themselves. The spread of Buddhism was so rapid among the masses of India and abroad that the intellectuals of the country were terribly afraid for their own existence. While their rulers were engaged in political battles, these intellectuals quarrelled among themselves in the name of religion. During this process, many libraries were burnt. Quite apart from any original thinking, the scholars could not preserve even the books which had already been composed prior to this period. The practice of ayurveda was despised. It was considered sinful to touch a dead body or a woman giving birth to a child. Thus, the practice of obstetrics, anatomical dissections and surgery went out of the hands of the physicians. Examination of urine and stool was considered unclean. Pulse examination by touching the patient was frowned upon. Thus, the practitioners of ayurveda became outcastes. The profession did not attract intellectuals. Specialised branches disappeared from the scene. What remained were only a few medicines for a few diseases and these were practised by people of low intellectual calibre.

Because of the arrest of the progress, many superstitious interpolations and redactions crept into the medical texts. Even these texts were not readily available Such was the state of affair during the sixteenth century A.D. which moved Rājā Toḍaramalla to salvage the remanants of these sciences from the then available mutilated texts by incorporating the knowledge and experience of the scholars of that time. In this encyclopaedic work different topics of ayurveda are described in 97 chapters. Out of these, only ten selected chapters have been utilised for preparation of the present work on materia medica.

**Literature on Ayurvedic materia medica**

The oldest text on the materia medica of ayurveda now extant is the *Rasa vaiśeṣika* of Nāgārjuna (fifth century A.D.). It deals, among others, with various concepts of drug composition and drug action. During the medieval period, the *Aṣṭāṅga nighaṇṭu* was composed by one Vāhaṭācārya. This work describes the synonyms of drugs belonging to various groups or *gaṇas* of *Aṣṭāṅga saṁgraha*. This Vāhaṭācārya seems to be different from Vāgbhaṭa, the author of *Aṣṭāṅga hṛdaya* and *Aṣṭāṅga saṁgraha.* This seems to be the work done during the eighth century A.D..

The *Paryāya ratnamālā* of Mādhava (9th century A.D.) describes the synonyms of different groups of drugs. *Dhanvantari nighaṇṭu* is perhaps the most popular text where the properties of different groups of drugs are described along with their synonyms. This work was composed prior to the thirteenth century A.D. *Nighaṇṭu śeṣa* was composed by a Jain scholar namely Hemacandra in twelfth century A.D. It contains the synonyms of different types of plants. *Śoḍhala nighaṇṭu* is another important work on the materia medica of ayurveda next to *Dhanvantari nighaṭu.* It was composed during the twelfth century A.D. *Madanapāla nighaṇṭu* composed by Madana pāla in 1374 A.D. describes the properties of different types of drugs. *Kaiyadeva nighaṇṭu* written by Kaiyadeva, describes the properties of 9 groups of drugs. It was composed during A.D. 1450. Bhāva miśra composed an encyclopaedic work called *Bhāva prakāśa* during the sixteenth century A.D. It has a separate section on the description of drugs and their synonyms. Besides, several texts on *rasa śāstra* were composed during this period. In these texts the properties of metals and minerals and a few vegetable as well as animal products are also described.

These texts on the materia medica of ayurveda were composed prior to the composition of *Āyurveda Saukhyaṁ* of Toḍarānanda. Many verses of *Āyurveda Saukhyaṁ* are also available in the *Bhāva-prakāśa*, *Āyurveda prakāśa* and *Mādhava nighaṇṭu*, even though these names are not quoted by the author. A cursory glance through the text of *Āyurveda Saukhyaṁ* of Toḍaramalla indicates that the author has taken care to indicate the name of the text or the author from where material has been compiled. *Mādhava nighaṇṭu*, *Āyurveda prakāśa* and *Bhāva prakāśa* were already composed when *Āyurveda Saukhyaṁ* was under preparation. Either these works were not considered important enough to be cited as references or they were not available to the scholars who compiled the text of *Āyurveda Saukhyaṁ*. The identity of the texts between these works namely, *Āyurveda Saukhyaṁ* on the one hand, and *Mādhava nighaṇṭu*, *Āyurveda prakāśa* and *Bhāva prakāśa* on the other, indicates that all of them might have collected their textual material from another work which has since gone extinct.

The classification of drugs, food and drinks in these texts vary from each other. The system of classification followed by *Mādhava nighaṇṭu* is closer to the classification followed in *Ayurveda Saukhyaṁ*.

**Basic Concepts regarding the Creation of the universe**

Ayurveda has drawn its basic concepts from the different philosophical systems of ancient India. The *Sāṁkya-Pātañjala* system and the *Nyāya-Vaiśeṣika* system have considerably influenced the physical, physico-chemical, physiological and pharmocological theories of ayurveda. *Sāṁkya-Pātañjala* system accounts for the creation of the universe and composition of matter on the principles of cosmic evolution. The *Nyāya vaiśeṣika* system lays down the methodology of scientific studies and elaborates the concepts of mechanics, physics and chemistry.

The manifested world, according to the *Sāṁkya* is an evolution of the unmanifested *Prakṛti* or primordial matter stuff, which is conceived as formless and undifferentiated, limitless and ubiquitous, indestructible and undecaying, ungrounded and uncontrolled as well as without beginning and without end. This unity of *Prakṛti* is a mere abstraction. It is in reality an undifferentiated manifold and indeterminate infinite continuum of three attributes called (1) the *sattva* (2) the *rajas* and (3) the *tamas*. The *sattva* attribute is the medium of reflection of intelligence. The *rajas* represents the energy which creates a tendency for work by overcoming resistance. The *tamas* is the mass or inertia where the effects of *rajas* and *sattva* in the form of energy and conscience respectively are manifested.

These three *guṇas* or attributes are interdependant. The *rajas*, in combination with the *sattva*, helps in the creation of the sensory and motor faculties including the mental faculty. The *rajas*, in combination with *tamas*, gives rise to the five categories of *tanmātrās* which are also known as subtle *bhūtas*. These *tanmātrās* are in the form of quanta of different types of energy, which, by different types of of permutation and combination, gives rise to different categories of material. All these quanta of energy are present in all the types of matter. Therefore, there is nothing like a pure substance consisting of only one type of energy. It is at this stage that the energy is transformed into matter with undifferentiable distinction.

These unmanifested *tanmātrās* and the manifested *mahābhūtas* are of five types namely, *pṛthvī*, *ap*, *tejas*, *vāyu* and *ākāśa*. Since there is nothing like a pure substance, as has already been explained, the substance of a drug is called *pārthiva*, *āpya*, *taijasa*, *vāyavīya* or *ākāśīya*, depending upon the predominance of the *tanmātrās* of *pṛthvī*, *ap*, *tejas*, *vāyu* and *ākāśa* respectively in its composition.

According to *Nyāya-Vaiśeṣika* system, there are nine *dravyas* or categories of matter. They are the five *mahā bhūtas*, namely, *pṛthvī*, *ap*, *tejas*, *vāyu* and *ākāśa* and *dik* (direction or space), *kāla* (time), *ātman* (soul) and *manas* (mind). It is significant to note here that the time and space are considered in *Nyāya-Vvaiśeṣika* as two different categories of matter. Similarly, *ātman* and *manas* are also considered as matter. Thus, according to *Nyāya-Vaiśeṣika*, the entire universe, including the time, space, soul and mind is of nine categories. Depending upon their attributes all the basic atoms of modern physics and chemistry can be classified into these five categories of *mahā bhūtas*. If these items are to be explained according to the *Sāṁkya-Pātañjala* system then each one of these atoms is a conglomeration of five categories of energy or *tanmātrās*, having a mass in the form of *pṛthvī*, cohesion or gravitation in the form of *ap*, heat or light in the form of *tejas*, motion in the form of *vāyu* and intermittant space in the form of *ākāśa tanmātrā*. Thus, the *Nyāya-Vaiśeṣika* concept of matter begins from where the *Sāṁkhya-Pāṭañjala* concept of matter ends. There is a subtle difference between these two concepts.

These *mahābhūtas* are present both in drugs and in human bodies, in a particular proportion. The human body grows during young age, gains stability during adulthood and gets decayed or reduced during the old age. During all these stages of human life, these *mahābhūtas* remain in a particular proportion in a state of equilibrium in the human body. During the different stages of life, because of the activities of life force represented in the form of the action of *agni* or enzymes, there is a natural consequence of these *mahābhūtas* being consumed for the manifestation of energy and heat. This natural loss is replenished and the normal growth and maintenance of stability are achieved by the supplementation of these *mahābhūtas* through intrinsic and extrinsic sources i.e., food, drinks, senses, air, light and mental activities.

If there is any change in this equilibrium of *mahābhūtas* in the human body, it results in disease and decay. To correct this state of imbalancement, the patients are given different types of drugs, food, drinks and regimens which help in the maintenance of this state of equilibrium. This, in brief, is the concept on the basis of which a drug is selected for the treatment of a disease. But it is very difficult to ascertain the nature of the *mahābhūtas* which have undergone changes in the body. It is also difficult to ascertain the quantum of *mahābhūta* present in a particular drug, diet or regimen. That is why, for all practical purposes, this theoretical concept in ayurveda has further been simplified with a view to enable the physician to determine with ease and convenience the nature of disturbance in the body and the type of drug, diet and regimen required for a healthy person and a patient.

**Composition of Human body**

The five *mahābhūtas* which enter into the composition of the human body are classified into three categories, namely (1) *doṣas*, (2) the *dhātus* and (3) the *malas*. *Doṣas* govern the physiological and physico-chemical activities of the body and these are three in number, namely (1) *vāyu*, (2) *pitta* and (3) *kapha*. (These are often mistranslated as wind, bile and phlegm respectively). *Vāyu* is responsible for all the movements and sensations, including motor actions inside the body. *Pitta* is responsible for all physio-chemical activities of the body in the form of metabolism, production of heat and energy. *Kapha* is the substance which maintains compactness or cohesiveness in the body by providing the fluid matrix to it. These *doṣas* are dominated by different *mahābhūtas* as per the table given below :—

| *Doṣa* | *Dominating mahābhūta* |
|---|---|
| 1. *Vāyu* | *Vāyu* and *ākāśa mahābhūtas* |
| 2. *Pitta* | *Tejas mahābhūta* |
| 3. *Kapha* | *Pṛthvī* and *ap mahābhūtas.* |

These *doṣas*, namely, *vāyu*, *pitta* and *kapha*, are further divided into five categories each. Their locations and functions are described in detail in ayurvedic classics. Diseases that are produced by the aggravation or diminution of *doṣas* are also described in ayurvedic texts. From these signs and symptoms manifested in the human body, the physician can judge the type of *mahābhūta* that has gone astray resulting in the manifestation of the disease and this helps the physician to select a particular drug.

The *dhātus* are the basic tissue elements of the body. They are seven in number, namely, (1) *rasa* or chyle or plasma, (2) *rakta* or the red-blood corpuscles, (3) *māṁsa* or muscle tissue, (4) *medas* or the fat tissue, (5) *asthi* or bone tissue, (6) *majjā* or the bone marrow and (7) *śukra* and *rajas* or the sperm and ovum which are responsible for procreation.

These *dhātus* or basic tissue elements remain in a particular proportion in the human body and any change in their equilibrium leads to disease and decay. Their functions are described in detail in ayurvedic classics. Diseases are produced only when the *doṣas* interact with these *dhātus* and this happens only when there is disturbance in their equilibrium.

These seven *dhātus* are also composed of five *mahābhūtas*. However, *pṛthvī mahābhūta* predominates in muscle and fat tissues; *jala mahābhūta* predominates in lymph, chyle and other fluid tissue elements; the hemoglobin fraction of the blood is primarily composed of *tejas mahābhūta*; bones are composed of *vāyu mahābhūta* and the pores inside the body are dominated by *ākaśa mahābhūta*.

If there is any change in the equilibrium of these *dhātus* certain signs and symptoms are manifested in the body which are described in detail in ayurvedic classics. From these signs and symptoms, the physician can ascertain the *mahābhautic* requirement of the body for the correction of the disease, and drugs are selected accordingly.

The *malas* or the waste products are primarily of three categories, namely, (1) the stool, (2) the urine and (3) the sweat. These are required to be eliminated regularly. The catabolic products of the body in the form of unwanted *mahābhūtas* are eliminated through them. If these are not eliminated in the required quantity, then this results in disease and decay, and various signs and symptoms are manifested in the body. From these signs and symptoms, the physician can ascertain the exact *mahābhautic* requirement of the body and select a drug or recipe for correcting the disease.

Thus, the physician can ascertain the exact position of the *mahābhūtas* in the body from certain external signs and symptoms.

**Drug Composition**

Depending upon the predominance of *mahābhūtas*, drugs

are classified into five categories details of which are given in the table below :

| Predominance of *mahābhūta* in the drug. | Attributes and actions of the drug. |
|---|---|
| (1) | (2) |
| *Pṛthvi* | Substances that are heavy, tough, hard, stable, non-slimy, dense, gross and abounding in the quality of smell are dominated by *pṛthvī*; they promote plumpness and stability. |
| *Ap* | Substances that are liquid, unctuous, cold, dull, soft, slimy and abounding in the qualities of taste are dominated by *ap* or *jala*; they promote stickiness, unctuousness, compactness, moistness and happiness. |
| *Tejas* | Substances that are hot, sharp, subtle, light, ununctuous, non-slimy and abounding in the qualities of vision are dominated by *tejas*; they promote combustion, metabolism, lustre, radiance and colour. |
| *Vāyu* | Substances that are light, cold, ununctuous, rough, non-slimy, subtle and abounding in the qualities of touch are dominated by *vāyu*; they promote roughness, aversion, movement, non-sliminess and lightness. |

| (1) | (2) |
|---|---|
| *Ākāśa* | Substances that are soft, light, subtle, smooth and dominated by the qualities of sound are dominated by *ākāśa*; they promote softness, porosity and lightness. |

From the above description alone, it becomes difficult at times to select a particular drug, diet, drink or regimen for the treatment of a particular disease. To facilitate the understanding of the *mahābhautic* composition of a drug and to ascertain its exact action on the human body, drugs are classified into six categories on the basis of their tastes; into 20 categories on the basis of their *guṇas* or attributes; into eight or two categories on the basis of their *vīrya* or potency and into three categories on the basis of their *vipāka* or the taste that emerges after digestion. In ayurvedic texts, the actions of different groups of drugs on the above lines are described in detail. From these tastes (*rasas*), attributes (*guṇas*), potency (*vīrya*) and the taste that emerges after digestion (*vipāka*), one can determine the *mahābhautic* composition of the drug. The dominating *mahā bhūtas* in drugs of different tastes are given in the table below :

| *Taste* | *Predominating mahā bhūtas* |
|---|---|
| 1. Sweet | *Pṛthvi* and *ap* |
| 2. Sour | *Ap* and *tejas* |
| 3. Saline | *Pṛthvī* and *tejas* |
| 4. Pungent | *Vāyu* and *tejas* |
| 5. Bitter | *Vāyu* and *ākāśa* |
| 6. Astringent | *Vāyu* and *pṛthvī*. |

*Mahābhautic* predominance for the manifestation of twenty *guṇas* or attributes is given in the table below :

| *Guṇa* | *Predominating mahā bhūtas* |
|---|---|
| 1. *Guru* (heavy) | *Pṛthvī* and *ap* |
| 2. *Laghu* (light) | *Tejas*, *vāyu* & *ākāśa* |

| | |
|---|---|
| 3. *Śita* (cold) | *Ap* |
| 4. *Uṣṇa* (hot) | *Tejas* |
| 5. *Snigdha* (unctuous) | *Ap* |
| 6. *Rūkṣa* (ununctuous) | *Pṛthvī, tejas* and *vāyu* |
| 7. *Manda* (dull) | *Pṛthvī* and *ap* |
| 8. *Tīkṣṇa* (sharp) | *Tejas* |
| 9. *Sthira* (stable) | *Pṛthvī.* |
| 10. *Sara* (fluid) | *Vāyu* and *ap* |
| 11. *Mṛdu* (soft) | *Ap* and *ākāśa* |
| 12. *Kaṭhina* (hard) | *Pṛthvī* |
| 13. *Viśada* (non-slimy) | *Pṛthvī, tejas, vāyu* and *ākāśa* |
| 14. *Picchila* (slimy) | *Ap* |
| 15. *Slakṣṇa* (smooth) | *Tejas* |
| 16. *Khara* (rough) | *Vāyu* |
| 17. *Sūkṣma* (subtle) | *Tejas, vāyu* and *ākāśa* |
| 18. *Sthūla* (gross) | *Pṛthvī* |
| 19. *Sāndra* (dense) | *Pṛthvī* |
| 20. *Drava* (liquid) | *Ap* |

About *vīrya* or potency, there are two different views. One group of scholars hold *uṣṇa* (hot) and *śita* (cold) to be the two types of *vīryas*. Regarding their *mahābhautic* composition *uṣṇa dravyas* are dominated by *tejas mahā bhūta* and *śita dravyas* are dominated by *ap* and *pṛthvī mahā bhūtas*. Another group of scholars hold eight attributes as *vīryas* and their *mahā bhautic* composition is given below :

| *Vīrya* | *Predominating mahā bhūtas* |
|---|---|
| 1. *Śīta* | *Pṛthvī* and *ap* |
| 2. *Uṣṇa* | *Tejas* |
| 3. *Snigdha* | *Jala* |
| 4. *Rūkṣa* | *Vāyu* |
| 5. *Guru* | *Pṛthvī* and *ap* |
| 6. *Laghu* | *Tejas, vāyu* and *ākāśa* |
| 7. *Manda* | *Ap* |
| 8. *Tīkṣṇa* | *Tejas* |

*Vipāka* or the taste of a drug after digestion, is of three types, namely, *madhura* (sweet), *amla* (sour) and *kaṭu* (pungent).

The *mahābhautic* composition of these *vipākas* is determined according to those of the respective tastes.

The action of some drugs cannot be explained according to their *rasa* (taste), *guṇa* (attribute), *vīrya* (potency) and *vipāka* (taste that emerges after digestion). It is because the *mahā bhūtas* which take part in the manifestation of *rasa*, *guṇa* etc., do not actually take part in producing the therapeutic action of the drug. They manifest their action only when the drug is administered to the patient and this is called *prabhāva* or specific action.

It will be seen from the above that a drug, diet or drink, for a healthy person or a patient to prevent and cure a disease, is not selected empirically but on the basis of a rational theory. In the ayurvedic texts on materia medica, in respect of each drug, such rational explanations are not provided because such details were not found necessary. None the less, these rational explanations are always kept in view before deciding upon the therapeutic effect of a drug. On the basis of accumulated experience and the repeated observations through centuries, these actions are determined. A physician or a research worker is supposed to have prior comprehension of the rationality of these actions on the basis of *paribhāṣā* that is described in the fundamental concepts.

**Mechanism of Drug Action**

Before closing this topic, it will be necessary to explain some basic differences in the mechanism of drug action between ayurveda and the modern allopathic system of medicine. Ayurveda, like other systems of traditional medicine, has its unique features. It lays more emphasis on the promotion of positive health and prevention of diseases. The existence of organisms and their role in the causation of several infective diseases in the body have been recognised and elaborated. But for the prevention and cure of such diseases, the drugs and therapies prescribed in ayurvedic classics and administered by ayurvedic physicians do not aim at only killing these organisms. Some of these medicines might have bacteriostatic or bactericidal effects. But most of them do not act in this way. In ayurveda, more emphasis is laid upon the "field" than the "seed". If the field is barren then the seed, howsoever potent it may be, will not germinate. Similarly, howsoever potent the germ or the bacteria may be, they will not be able to produce disease in the human body unless the tissues of the body are fertile (vitiated) enough to accept them and help in their growth and multiplication. Killing these germs by administering medicine would not solve the problem permanently. It may give instant relief, and perhaps the body resistance during this period will be developed enough as a reaction to the infection by these germs which may result in the prevention of their further attacks. Man cannot live in an absolutely germ-free atmosphere even though he can minimise it. The only thing that can be done safely is to keep the tissues of the body barren and unreceptive towards these germs. Once the body is afflicted, the tissues should be so conditioned by drugs, diet and other regimen that these germs or bacteria, by whatsoever name we may call them, will find the atmosphere hostile towards their survival, multiplication and growth. All medicines and therapies including preventive measures prescribed in ayurveda aim at conditioning the tissues and not killing the invading organisms.

Allopathic drugs which are employed specially for killing organisms may produce the same or a similar effect on the tissues of the body. When they are given in a dose sufficient to kill the invading organisms, they may simultaneously kill the friendly organisms in the body as well, and may impair the normal functioning of the tissues. Thus, they produce side or toxic effects while curing the disease. Ayurvedic medicines, on the other hand, while conditioning the tissues of the body against the organisms, nourish and rejuvenate them. Thus, when the disease is cured, the individual gets many side benefits. It is because of this that all ayurvedic medicines are tonics.

Except for a few modern drugs, e.g. minerals and vitamins, all others are meant exclusively for patients. All ayurvedic drugs, on the other hand, can be given to both patients and healthy individuals simultaneously—in patients they cure diseases and in healthly individuals they prevent disease and promote positive health. To illustrate the point: *vāsā* (*Adhatoda vasica* Nees) is very often prescribed by ayurvedic physicians to a patient suffering from bronchitis, laryngitis, pharyngitis and even tuberculosis. May be, some fractions of this drug have properties to kill some of the organisms causing these ailments. But that is not the primary consideration which motivates the physician to prescribe this drug. These organisms thrive and multiply to produce a disease in the respiratory tract and throat only when the local tissue elements are afflicted with excessive *kapha doṣa*. *Vāsā* counteracts this aggravated *kapha doṣa*, and helps in the maintenance of its state of equilibrium in the body by which the organisms become incapable of producing these ailments.

In ayurveda the treatment prescribed does not aim at correcting the afflicted part alone. In the process of manifestation of the disease several organs are involved. The disease takes its origin from a particular place. It moves through a particular channel and then gets manifested in a particular organ. Therefore, the treatment always aims at correcting the site of origin, the channels of circulation along with the site of manifestation of the disease—all together. Take for example, the treatment of bronchial asthma which in ayurvedic parlance is known as *tamaka śvāsa*. The breathing difficulty in the disease is caused by the spasm of the bronchi, and to relieve it, antispasmodic drugs are generally prescribed in modern medicine. But the aim of the ayurvedic treatment of this disease is different. May be, some ayurvedic drugs used against this disease have this antispasmodic effect which can be demonstrated even in animals under experiment. But most of the drugs which are used in this treatment will not produce any anti-spasmodic effect and a pharmacologist will be at a loss and reject them as useless in the treatment of bronchial asthma. A clinician, on the other hand, will appreciate its effects on his patients even though he may not be able to explain their effects in terms of modern physiological and pathological concepts. This disease takes its origin from the stomach and small intestine. The primary aim of the ayurvedic physician is to correct these two organs either by giving emetic therapy, or by giving such medicines which will keep the bowels clean. *Harītakī* (*Terminalia chebula* Retz.) along with other medicines is useful in correcting these two organs of the body, and therefore, all preparations indicated for the treatment of bronchial asthma invariably contain *harītakī* and other drugs having identical properties.

These four topics on (1) the basic concepts regarding the creation of the universe; (2) composition of the human body; (3) drug composition and (4) the mechanism of drug action, described above are very important to the understanding and appreciation of the materia medica of ayurveda. At times, research workers, in their enthusiasm to develop the new drug from the plant sources, chemically and pharmacologically screen the drugs prescribed in the ayurvedic materia medica without paying any attention to these basic concepts and peculiar features of the system. They try to isolate alkaloids, glycosides and other similar active principles from these drugs. These so called active principles are often not found in some of these ayurvedic drugs and when they are found they do not necessarily produce the results which are attributed to the whole drug in the ayurvedic materia medica. No wonder, therefore, that the scientists are disappointed at the end of their hard labour and after considerable expenditure from the State exchequer. Sometimes they come to an erroneous conclusion that all ayurvedic drugs or at least most of them are therapeutically useless. This disappointment and wrong conclusion could be avoided if the research on ayurvedic drugs is planned and designed in the beginning, keeping in view these fundamental principles of ayurveda on drug composition and drug action.

In the present text on ayurvedic materia medica, only the single drugs—their synonyms and properties are described along with a few compound recipes, food articles and drinks. In actual ayurvedic practice, along with the single drugs, a number of compound preparations are used. These single drugs and compound preparations which are in use in ayurvedic therapeutics are not free from shortcomings.

## Classification of Ayurvedic Drugs

In Ayurveda, more than 8000 medicines—single drugs and compound preparations—have been described. In general, these ayurvedic drugs can be classified into five categories as follows :

(a) *Scientifically Studied Drugs* : Some single drugs and compound preparations, for example, *sarpa gandhā* and *yoga-rāja guggulu* have been studied scientifically and their therapeutic claims verified. *Sarpa gandhā* is useful for high blood pressure and *yoga rāja guggulu* for rheumatism. The gum resin of a plant called *guggulu* is the important ingredient of the latter medicine.

(b) *Popular Non-toxic Drugs* : Some ayurvedic medicines are popular for their therapeutic utility and of non-toxic character. One such medicine is *Cyavana prāśa*. *Āmalakī* is the important ingredient of this medicine which is useful in treating chronic diseases of the lungs like chronic bronchitis.

(c) *Effective but Toxic Drugs* : There are some drugs for example, *bhallātaka avaleha*, which have known therapeutic value but which also produce severe toxicity, if used injudiciously. *Bhallātaka* is the important ingredient of this medicine which is used in the treatment of chronic and obstinate skin diseases, among others.

(d) *Drugs of Rare Use* : Some drugs, for example, *Śrī viṣṇu taila*, though mentioned in ayurvedic classics, are not in extensive use. Only physicians of certain regions of India use them and claim their efficacy.

(e) *Hereditary and Patent Drugs* : Some physicians have specialised in curing certain diseases. The formulae and methods of preparation of the drugs they administer are known only to them or to the trusted members of their family. While some of the drugs are not as effective as the claims made for them, some others are found to be very effective. In most cases, physicians are not at all willing to disclose the formulae; and even if they give consent, it is associated with a demand for heavy financial compensation.

**Need For Standardization**

In olden days, the physician was rarely required to be consulted for minor ailments because the senior members of every family were well acquainted with the use of herbs available in their vicinity for treating such ailments. The physician's role in such cases was only to guide the family members to obtain the correct herb, to process it properly and to instruct the patient about the dietetic and other regimen to be followed. Only serious cases were brought to the physician for direct supervision, and in such cases, he had to prepare his own medicines. Things have changed now. At present, the physician is approached even for a minor ailment. People generally are not interested in knowing common household remedies or they do not believe in their efficacy. Thus, ayurvedic physicians, like modern doctors, have become busy practitioners who are also hard pressed for time to prepare their own medicines. Even for dispensing, these physicians are dependant entirely upon their compounders. As a result, many big commercial firms supplying medicines to ayurvedic physicians have come into existence. This, in turn, has led to a number of problems as follows :

(a) *Collection of Premature Herbs* : For therapeutic purposes different parts of medicinal plants are required to be used which are to be collected during specified periods. For example, *āmalakī* should be collected only when the fruits are fully ripe. Annual plants should be collected before the ripening of seeds, biennials during spring and perennials during autumn. Twigs must be of the first year's growth and roots, leaves and bark should be collected in the cold, hot and rainy seasons respectively. These instructions are seldom followed during the actual collection of herbs by large manufacturers of ayurvedic medicines.

(b) *Improper Processing and Preservation*: Usually, raw drugs are stored for some time before they are processed. Proper care in processing and preservation is required so that the active principles of the drugs may not get deteriorated. Dumping them in bundles or in gunny bags, and keeping them exposed to sun, rain and dust, adversely affect their therapeutic effectiveness.

(c) *Methods of Preparation* : Various methods are indicated in ayurvedic texts for the preparation of the same medicine. While some of the methods involve much time and labour, some others are less expensive. For reasons of economy, quite a few pharmacies follow the less expensive methods or develop some methods which make their products less expensive with no guarantee that the drugs so prepared are equally effective. According to ayurvedic texts, raw oil has to be processed before it is used for the preparation of medicated oil. This processing is known as *mūrchanā*. Pharmacies very rarely resort to this processing and in the absence of standard methods for testing these discrepancies in their drug preparation, the physicians cannot be sure about the effectiveness of the drugs they prescribe.

(d) *Use of Adulterated and Sub-standard Drugs* : Therapeutically important drugs like *vatsa nābha* and *yaṣṭi madhu* are often adulterated and sold in the market at a comparatively cheaper price. In the absence of any effective control over the sale of adulterated and spurious drugs, the dealers take full advantage and sell to their customers anything that resembles, or is made to resemble the genuine drug. The art of adulteration and prepration of spurious drugs has advanced to such an extent that even the most experienced among the *vaidyas* finds it difficult to distinguish between genuine and spurious samples. Ayurvedic physicians as well as commercial firms are often cheated and supplied with adulterated stuff. This obviously results in the circulation of sub-standard drugs in the market.

(e) *Substitution of Costly Drugs* : In some ayurvedic texts, of late, *pratinidhi dravyas* or official substitutes of many costly drugs have been prescribed; for example, *kuṣṭha* can be used in place of *puṣkara mūla* and *gaja pippalī* in the place of *cavya*. Instead of treating these usages as exceptional cases, the substitutes are often unscrupulously used as a rule (under the shelter of textual prescriptions) to make the medicinal preparations cheaper.

(f) *Omission of Ingredients*: Generally speaking, compound preparations are used in ayurvedic medicines. It is often the total effect of all the ingredients in the formula rather than the action of individual drugs that plays a vital role in therapeutics. Drug combinations are envisaged to serve the following important purposes :

(i) *Synergistic action* : *Tṛṇa-pañca-mūla-kvātha* presents a case of synergistic action. Even though all the ingredients of this group are known to be diuretics, still when given together, they produce marked diuresis which effect is not observed in individual drugs.

(ii) *Combined action* : The case of *Rāsnā-saptaka-kvātha* used for the treatment of rheumatic afflictions is illustrative of the combined action of an ayurvedic medicine. For curing rheumatism, which is known in ayurveda as *āma vāta*, the medicine should have sedative, digestive, laxative and anti-inflammatory action. Of all the ingredients of this drug, *rāsnā* is anti-inflammatory and sedative, ginger promotes digestion, and the root of *eraṇḍa* is a laxative.

(iii) *Neutralizing toxicity* : An example of this is the case of *Agni tuṇḍi vaṭi*. *Kupīlu* is an irritant to the nerves. It cannot be taken alone in a heavy dose as is required to make it therapeutically effective. But it is well tolerated when taken in combination with other drugs, specially after undergoing *śodhana*.

(iv) *Specific Action* : An example of this is the case of *Cyavana prāśa*. *Pippalī* added to this preparation has heating effect in addition to anti-tubercular property. The heating effect of the preparation is neutralized by the addition of other cooling drugs like *āmalakī*. Thus, the medicine is left with a marked anti-tubercular effect.

Keeping the above points in view, various formulae have been described for medicinal preparations in ayurvedic classics. Due to non-availability of drug ingredients or the expense involved, if any ingredient is accidentally or intentionally omitted from the preparation then not only is the efficacy reduced but adverse effects may also be produced at times.

(g) *Improper Storage* : Different categories of ayurvedic preparations which remain effective for a certain limited period are described in the classics. If these drugs are kept for a longer period, they lose their potency. Large manufacturing concerns, however, cannot help neglect this rule; for, the drugs prepared cannot be consumed immediately but will have to be sent to their various branches. Hence, there is considerable lapse of time before the medicine is actually used by the patient.

**Identification of Raw Drugs**

It is difficult to correctly identify certain drugs described in ayurvedic classics due to the following reasons :

(a) *Non-availability* : Some drugs like *Soma* and *Jīvaka* are not available now a days. It is probable that they have become extinct.

(b) *Multiplicity of Names* : In ayurvedic classics, drugs are often described with synonyms. Synonyms apart, the same drug is known by different names in different parts of the country. For example, *Clitoria ternatea* Linn. which is known in North India as *aparā jitā*, is called *śaṁkha puṣpī* in South India. But these two have distinct and different therapeutic attributes or characteristics.

(c) *Many Drugs with Same Name* : Under the name of *rāsnā*, thirteen different drugs are being made use of in different parts of the country for medicinal preparations.

(d) *Non-availability of Specific Varieties* : The drug *harītakī* is said to be of seven varieties. But presently, not more than four varieties are available. So is the case with other drugs like *bhṛṅgarāja* and *dūrvā*.

(e) *Exotic Plants* : Some plants, though introduced in India very recently, have grown profusely. Due to lack of proper knowledge, some of these plants have been given ayurvedic names which have led to their wrong identification.

For example, *Argemone mexicana* Linn. is often mistaken for *svarṇa-kṣirī*.

(f) *Adulteration* : Because of short supply, drugs, such as *yaṣṭi-madhu*, are often adulterated.

(g) *Synthetic Preparations* : Taking advantage of the heavy demand from consumers of certain drugs, such as *vaṁśa locana* or bamboo salt, some firms have started manufacturing imitations and synthetic preparations the therapeutic efficacy of which is in no way comparable to that of the genuine drug.

**Difficulties for Identification**

Most of the ayurvedic drugs can be identified conveniently. But there are some, which elude proper identification because of the following reasons :

(a) *Passage of Time* : Ayurvedic classics were written about 3000 years ago. Some of the drugs described at that time may have undergone modifications due to physical and genetic factors and some others may have become extinct. Thus, identification of a drug from the physical characteristics mentioned in the ayurvedic texts or commentaries thereon is not an easy task. The plant *soma*, which is mentioned even in the Vedas, is described by Suśruta as having 15 leaves in total. On new moon day, the plant, becomes leafless and every day thereafter, one leaf is added to it till it has 15 leaves on full moon day. Its root is said to contain a large quantity of an exhilarating sweet juice. Plants of this description are not, however, to be seen now.

(b) *Inadequate Description* : An important plant by name *svarṇa-kṣirī* is described as having golden latex and leaves like those of *sārivā*. This is said to grow in the Himalayas. This information is, however, very inadequate for identifying the plant correctly. Whether the contributors to the ayurvedic classics had a knowledge of systematic botany or not is a debatable point; but when these texts were compiled, there was no printing facility, so much so that brevity was always the rule in describing ayurvedic drugs.

(c) *Loss of Contact* : In olden days, learning had to be done through *guru-śiṣya paraṁparā*, which meant that the disciple had to seek and obtain first-hand knowledge from teachers. But with the advent of foreign influence, this traditional way of learning has been given up. Due to the inadequacy of written texts and the absence of direct links to gain deeper knowledge of the ayurvedic classics, it became difficult for later authors to appreciate what has been originally stated in the classics; and this has resulted in incoherent views. Personal knowledge of drugs available in various surroundings has become so meagre that ayurvedic physicians are often required to seek guidance from cow-herds and forest dwellers for the identification of such drugs.

(d) *Lack of Facility* : Even the available knowledge is not properly codified. Descriptions of plants and animals are also available in texts allied to ayurveda, such as *Smṛti śāstras* and *Dharma śāstras*. They are required to be critically screened.

(e) *Observance of Secrecy* : In the medieval period, in order to prevent the acquisition of ayurvedic knowledge by foreign invaders and unscrupulous natives, names having more than one meaning and also with allegorical meanings have been used in the texts. Due to the rigidity observed in the selection of disciples, some authors died without training even a single disciple and the knowledge acquired by them had thus been lost.

(f) *Short Supply* : Some important raw drugs, such as musk and bamboo salt, are in short supply. Hence, their prices are not only very high but spurious substitutes for them are also largely sold in the market.

**Procedure for Naming Formulae**

The names of the drug formulations are usually based on the following six factors :

(a) *Important Ingredient* : Some preparations are named after the important ingredient, for example, *Āmalakī rasāyana.*

(b) *Authorship* : The name of the sage or *ṛṣi* who first discovered or patronized the formula is used in naming the drug, for example, *Agastya harītakī*.

(c) *Therapeutic Property* : The disease for which the formula was indicated is at times used in naming the preparation, for example, *Kuṣṭhaghna lepa*.

(d) *First Ingredient of the Formula* : The drug that heads the list in the formula is sometimes used in naming the preparation, for example, *Pippalyāsava*.

(e) *Quantity of Drug* : At times, the preparation is named after the quantity of drug used, for example, *Ṣaṭpala ghṛta*.

(f) *Part of the Plant* : The drug is at times named after the part of the plant used, for example, *Daśa mūla kaṣāya*.

**Multiplicity of Formulae**

There are medicines having the same name but a number of different formulae, so much so that each differs from the other in composition, ratio of ingredients, method of preparation, mode of administration, mode of action, dosage and *anupāna*. Take, for example, *khadirādi vaṭi*. It has as many as eight formulae. In this preparation, the number of ingredients varies from 5 to 37, and the percentage of the main ingredient, namely, *khadira* (catechu) varies from 15 to 92. In four out of the eight formulae, costly drugs like *kasturī* or musk are added, the percentage of musk varying from formula to formula. In one formula, poisonous drugs like *bhallātaka* and *bākuci* are added as they are considered to be effective in obstinate skin diseases including leprosy. Thus, standardization of such medicines, which must also take into account of these variations, poses a very difficult problem.

**Pharmaceutical Processes**

In ayurveda, different pharmaceutical processes are followed in the preparation of drugs. Besides helping isolation of the active fraction of the drugs, these processes help make the medicines:

(a) easily administrable,
(b) tasteful,
(c) digestible and assimilable,
(d) therapeutically more effective,
(e) less toxic and more tolerable, and
(f) more preservable.

### *Śodhana* or Purification

Some raw drugs are required to be used after *Śodhana*. The literal meaning of the word *śodhana* is purification. But this is often misinterpreted to mean that the substance is rendered physically and chemically pure. *Śodhana*, no doubt, brings about physical and chemical purity to some extent but at times more physical and chemical impurities are added to the substance during certain stages of this processing. By such additions, the drug becomes less toxic and therapeutically more effective. Pure aconite, for example, cannot be administered so freely as *śodhita* aconite. Aconite, which is a cardiac depressant, becomes a cardiac stimulant after *śodhana* with cow's urine. Thus, the actual implications of *śodhana* processes require detailed study.

Some gum resins, such as *guggulu* and some drugs containing volatile oils, such as *kuṣṭha* are also described to undergo *śodhana* by boiling them with milk, *go-mūtra*, etc. Boiling of, these drugs however, definitely reduces the volatile oil content which is supposed to be therapeutically very active. The utility of such purificatory processes should, therefore, be studied before proceeding with the standardization of ayurvedic drugs.

Ayurveda should not be viewed from the point of history of medicine alone. It is both history and medicine. No doubt, there is a history of thousands of years behind it, but it is even now a living medical system catering to the health needs of millions of people living in India, Śrī laṅkā and Nepal including some of the Central Asian and South East Asian countries. There are several hundreds of trained and registered practitioners of ayurveda in these countries and people have implicit faith in the therapeutic efficacy of the drugs and therapies of this system. Like other medical systems it has, of course, its limitations. Advanced civilization and modernisation have not left ayurveda untouched. Accidental human errors and intentional profit motives coupled with the vicissitudes of time have created several problems for this system of medicine. Therefore, the Ayurvedic drug that is found in the market may not carry the same therapeutic effect as is claimed for it in the ayurvedic texts. The reasons for this are elaborated in the last eight topics of this 'Introduction' for the guidance of research workers, practitioners and well wishers of this system. The ayurvedic materia medica provides a rich storehouse of therapeutically effective drugs and these gems are to be selected with due care for mitigating the miseries of the suffering humanity."

> अमन्त्रमक्षरं नास्ति नास्ति मूलमनौषधम् ।
> अयोग्यः पुरुषो नास्ति योजकस्तत्र दुर्लभः ।

"There is no letter which is not a *mantra* (incantation); there is no root which is not a medicine and there is no human being who is not useful. Only their *yojaka* (co-ordinator) is a rare commodity."

# CHAPTER 1

भैषज्याहारचेष्टानां यो न वेन्ति गुणागुणं ।

न स वेन्ति भिषक् सम्यक् स्वस्थास्वस्थहिताहितम् ॥१॥

अतः समस्तवस्तूनां गुणदोषविनिश्चयः ।

ज्ञातव्यो यत्नतः सद्भिर्वैद्यैः[1] परहितार्थिभिः ॥ २ ॥

A physician who is not acquainted with the good and bad effects of drugs, diet and regimens, does not correctly know the things which are useful and harmful for healthy persons and patients. Therefore, a good physician who desires the welfare of others, should carefully ascertain the good and bad qualities of all these things.

संक्षिप्तं ग्रंथमिच्छंति भिषजो विस्तरद्विषः ।

संक्षिप्तोऽयमतः सूक्तः संप्रयुक्तो निगद्यते ॥ ३ ॥

Physicians generally do not like to go through details. They like books in condensed form. Therefore, this work is being composed in a condensed form by collecting useful material (from different sources).

वृद्धिं तुल्यगुणैर्भावैर्विपरितगुणैः क्षयं ।
2, 3
युक्तैर्यान्ति हि संक्षेपाद्दोषाद्याः सर्वधातवः ॥ ४ ॥

In brief, all *dhātus*, *doṣas* etc., get increased in quantity by the utilization of homologous material (having similar properties). They get decreased by the utilization of material having opposite properties.

**द्रव्यगुणरत्नमालायाम्**

द्रव्ये रसो गुणो वीर्यं विपाकः शक्तिरेव च ।
संवेदनक्रमादेताः पञ्चावस्था प्रकीर्तिताः ॥ ५ ॥

**According to *Dravyaguṇa Ratnamālā***

*Rasa* (taste), *guṇa* (property), *vīrya* (potency), *vipāka* (taste that emerges after digestion) and *śakti* (specific action)—these are the five consecutively manifested states of matter.

क्वचिद्रसो गुणः क्वापि वीर्यं विपाक एव च ।
क्वचित्प्रभावः स्वं कर्म द्रव्यस्थो विदधाति हि ॥ ६ ॥

While being lodged inside the matter, sometimes the *rasa*, sometimes the *guṇa*, sometimes the *vīrya*, sometimes the *vipāka* and sometimes the *prabhāva* manifest their effects on the individual's body.

मधुरोऽम्लः पटुश्चैव कटुतिक्तकषायकाः ।
इत्येते षड्रसाः ख्याताः नानाद्रव्यसमाश्रिताः ॥ ७ ॥

**Six Tastes**

*Madhura* (sweet), *amla* (sour), *paṭu* or *lavaṇa* (saline), *kaṭu* (pungent), *tikta* (bitter) and *kaṣāya* (astringent)—these are the six *rasas* (tastes) which are lodged in matter.

**मधुर रसगुण:**

4

रसो मधुरकः शीतो धातुस्तन्यबलप्रदः ।

चक्षुष्यो वातपित्तघ्न कुर्यात्स्थौल्यमलकृमीन् ॥ ८ ॥

[भावप्रकाशः पूर्वखण्डः वर्गप्रकरण ६:१७५]

बालबृद्धक्षतक्षीणवर्णकेशेन्द्रियौजसाम् ।

प्रशस्तो बृंहणः कण्ठ्यः गुरुः सन्धानकृन्मतः ॥ ९ ॥

[अष्टाङ्गहृदयः सूत्र १० : ७-८]

विषघ्नो पिच्छिलश्चापि स्निग्धः प्रीत्यायुषोहितः ।

**Attributes of Sweet taste**

Sweet taste is cooling, promoter of the growth of tissue elements *(dhātus)*, lactation *(stanya)* and strength. It promotes eyesight *(cakṣuṣya)*, alleviates *vāyu* and *pitta*, and causes obesity, excessive production of waste products *(mala)* and *kṛmi* (parasites). It is useful for children, old men and persons suffering from consumption and emaciation. It is also useful for complexion, hair, sense organ and *ojas*. It is nourishing and promoter of voice. It is heavy *(guru)* and it helps in uniting the broken or torn tissues *(sandhānakṛt)*. It is anti-toxic, slimy *(picchila)* and unctuous *(snigdha)*. It is conducive to pleasant feeling and longevity.

सोऽतियुक्तो ज्वरश्वासगलगण्डार्बुदकृमीन् ।

स्थौल्याग्निमान्द्यमेहांश्च कुर्यान्मेदःकफामयान् ॥ १० ॥

When used in excess, it causes *jvara* (fever) *śvāsa* (asthma), *galagaṇḍa* (goitre), *arbuda* (tumour), *kṛmi* (parasitic infestation), *sthaulya* (obesity), *agnimāndya* (suppression of digestive power), *meha* (obstinate urinary disorders including diabetes), and diseases caused by the vitiation of *medas* (adipose tissue) as well as *kapha*.

**अथाम्लः**

रसोऽम्लः पाचनो रुच्यः पित्तश्लेष्मप्रदो लघुः ।
[5] लेखनोष्णो वहिः शीतः क्लेदनः पवनापहः ॥ ११ ॥
[भावप्रकाशः पूर्वखण्डः वर्गप्रकरण ६ः१७६-१८०]

स्निग्धस्तीक्ष्णः सरः शुक्रविबन्धानाहदृष्टिहा ।
हर्षणो रोमदन्तानामक्षिभ्रूविनिकोचकः ॥ १२ ॥

**Attributes of Sour Taste**

Sour taste is carminative (*pācana*) and appetiser (*rucya*). It produces *pitta* and *śleṣman.* It is light, *lekhana* (which causes scraping), hot, *vahiḥ śīta* (cooling from outside) and *kledana* (promoter of stickiness). It alleviates *vāyu.* It is unctuous, sharp and *sara* (mobile). It reduces *śukra* (semen), *vibandha* (constipation), *ānāha* (tymphanitis) and eye sight. It causes horripilation and tingling sensation in teeth. It also causes twitchings in eyes and eyebrows.

सोऽतियुक्तो भ्रमं कुर्यात्तृड्दाहतिमिरज्वरान् ।
कण्डूपाण्डुत्वविस्फोटशोथवीसर्पकुष्ठकृत् ॥ १३ ॥

When used in excess, it causes *bhrama* (giddiness), *tṛṭ* (morbid thirst), *dāha* (burning sensation), *timira* (cataract), *jvara* (fever), *kaṇḍū* (itches), *pāṇḍutva* (anemia), *visphoṭa* (postules), *śotha* (oedema), *visarpa* (erysipelas) and *kuṣṭha* (obstinate skin diseases including leprosy).

**अथ लवण :**

लवणः शोधनो रुच्यः पाचनः कफपित्तदः ।
पुंस्त्ववातहरः कायशैथिल्यमृदुताकरः ॥ १४ ॥
बलघ्न आस्यजलदः कपोलगलदाहकृत् ।

**Attributes of Saline taste**

Saline taste is *śodhana* (cleansing), *rucya* (appetiser) and *pācana* (carminative). It produces *kapha* and *pitta*. It reduces virility (*puṁstva*) and *vāyu*. It causes slothfulness (*śaithilya*) and softness (*mṛdutā*) of the body. It reduces strength. It causes salivation and burning sensation in the cheek and throat.

सोऽतियुक्तोऽक्षिपाकास्रपित्त[6]कोपक्षतादिकृत् ।
वलीपलितखालित्यकुष्ठवीसर्पतृट्प्रदः ॥ १५ ॥
[भावप्रकाशः पूर्वखण्डः वर्गप्रकरण ६ : १८०-१८३]

When used in excess, it causes *akṣipāka* (conjunctivitis), *asrapitta* (bleeding from different parts of the body), *kṣata* (consumption), *valī* (premature wrinkling), *palita* (premature graying of hair), *khālitya* (baldness), *kuṣṭha* (obstinate skin diseases including leprosy), *visarpa* (erysipelas) and *tṛṭ* (morbid thirst).

**अथ कटु :**

'कटुकः पित्तलः श्लेष्मकृमिकण्डूविषापहः ।
आग्नेयो वातलः स्तन्यमेदःस्थौल्यहरो[7] लघुः' ॥ १६ ॥
'अश्रुदो नासिकाक्ष्यास्यजिह्वाग्रोद्वेजको मतः ।
दीपनः पाचनो रुच्यो नासिकाशोषणः परम् ॥ १७ ॥
क्लेदमेदोवसामज्जशकृन्मूत्रोपशोषणः ।
स्रोतःप्रकाशको रूक्षो मेध्यो वर्चोविबन्धकृत्' ॥ १८ ॥
[भावप्रकाशः पूर्वखण्डः वर्गप्रकरण ६ : १८५-१८६]

**Attributes of Pungent taste**

Pungent taste aggravates *pitta* and reduces *kapha*, *kṛmi* (parasitic infection), *kaṇḍū* (itching) and toxicity. It has properties of fire (*agni*) and it aggravates *vāyu*. It reduces *stanya* (lactation), *medas* (fat) and *sthaulya* (adiposity). It is light. It causes lacrimation and irritates nose, eyes, mouth and tip of the tongue. It is *dīpana* (stimulant of digestion), *pācana* (carminative) and *rucya* (appetiser). It causes dryness (*śoṣaṇa*) of the nose. It depletes (*śoṣaṇa*) *kleda* (sticky substance in the body), *medas* (fat), *vasā* (muscle fat), *majjā* (bone marrow), *śakṛt* (feces) and *mūtra* (urine). It opens up the channels of circulation. It is ununctuous (*rukṣa)*. It promotes intellect (*medhya*). It produces more of feces and constipation.

सोऽतियुक्तो भ्रमास्यौष्ठतालुशोषातिसारद:[8] ।
कण्ठादिपीड़ामूर्च्छातृट्कंपदो बलशुक्र [हृत्][9] ॥१९॥

When used in excess, it causes giddiness, dryness of mouth, lips and palate and diarrhoea. It also causes pain in throat etc., *mūrchā* (fainting), *tṛṭ* (morbid thirst) and *kampa* (shivering). It reduces strength and semen.

**अथ तिक्त** :

तिक्त: शीतस्तृषामूर्छाज्वरपित्तकफान् जयेत् ।
कृमिकुष्ठविषोत्क्लेशदाहरक्त [गदा][10] पहः ॥ २० ॥
रुच्य: स्वयमरोचिष्णु: कण्ठस्तन्यास्यशोधन: ।
वातलोऽग्निकरो नासाशोषणो रूक्षणो लघु: ॥ २१ ॥

**Attributes of Bitter taste**

Bitter taste is cooling and it cures morbid thirst, fainting and fever. It alleviates *pitta* and *kapha*. It cures *kṛmi* (parasitic infection), *kuṣṭha* (obstinate skin diseases including leprosy), *viṣa* (poisoning), *utkleśa* (nausea), *dāha* (burning sensation) and diseases caused by the vitiation of blood. Even though bitter taste itself is not relishing it is an appetiser. It cleanses the throat, lactation and mouth. It aggravates *vāyu* and stimulates *agni* (enzymes responsible for digestion and metabolism). It dries up the nose. It is ununctuous and light.

सोऽतियुक्त: शिर:शूलमन्यास्तम्भश्रमार्त्तिकृत् ।
कम्पमूर्च्छातृषाकारी बलशुक्रक्षयप्रद: ॥ २२ ॥

[भावप्रकाश: पूर्वखण्ड: वर्गप्रकरण ६ : १८८-१९१]

When used in excess, it causes *śiraḥ śūla* (headache), *manyāstambha* (torticolis), *śrama* (exhaustion), *arti* (pain), *kampa* (tremor), *mūrchā* (fainting) and *tṛṣā* (morbid thirst). It reduces strength and semen.

**अथ कषाय :**

कषायो रोपणो ग्राही शोषणो वातकोपनः ।

जिह्वाजाड्यकरः कण्ठस्रोतसां च विबन्धकृत् ।

**Attributes of Astringent taste**

Astringent taste is healing (*ropaṇa*), constipative (*grāhī*) and drying (*śoṣaṇa*). It aggravates *vāyu*. It causes sluggishness in the movement of the tongue and it obstructs the throat as well as the channels of circulation. It causes constipation.

'सोऽतियुक्तो ग्रहाध्मानहृत्पीडाक्षेपणादिकृत्' ॥ २३ ॥

[भावप्रकाशः पूर्वखण्डः वर्गप्रकरण ६ : १६४]

When used in excess it causes *graha* (obstruction), *ādhmāna* (tymphanitis), *hṛtpiḍā* (pain in cardiac region), *ākṣepaṇa* (convulsions) etc.

**अथ तत्रैवविशेषा**

मधुरं श्लेष्मलं सर्वमृते शालेः पुरातनात् ।

'मुद्गगोधूमतःक्षौद्रात्सिताया जाङ्गलामिषात् ॥ २४ ॥

[भावप्रकाशः पूर्वखण्डः वर्गप्रकरण ६ : १६५]

**Exceptions**

All sweet things aggravate *kapha* except old *śāli* rice, *mudga* (*Phaseolus mungo* Linn.), wheat, honey, sugar and meat of animals of *jāṅgala* type.

अम्लं पित्तकरं प्रायो विना धात्री च दाडिमात् ।

लवणं प्रायशो द्वेषी नेत्रयोः सैन्धवं विना ॥ २५ ॥

प्रायः कटु तथा तिक्तमवृष्यं वातकोपनम् ।

शुण्ठीकृष्णारसोनानि पटोलममृतां विना ।

प्रायशस्तम्भनं प्रोक्तं कषायमभयां विना ।। २६ ।।

All sour things aggravate *pitta* except *dhātrī* and *dāḍima*. Generally saline things afflict eyesight; but rock salt (*saindhava)* is an exception to it. Generally pungent and bitter things are not aphrodisiac and they aggravate *vāyu*. *Śunṭhī*, *kṛṣṇā*, *rasona*, *paṭola* and *amṛtā* are, however, exceptions. All astringent things are generally *stambhana* (constipative); but *abhayā* is an exception to this rule.

सामान्येनात्र निर्दिष्टा गुणाः षड्रससंभवाः ।

रसानां योगजेऽपि स्यादन्य एव गुणोदयः ।। २७ ।।

In the above, properties of drugs having six tastes are described in general. Combination of various tastes, however, produces new properties which were non-existent in the original tastes.

संयोगाद्विषतां याति सममाज्येन माक्षिकम् ।

अमृतत्वं विषं याति सर्पदष्टस्य वै यथा ।। २८ ।।

[भावप्रकाशः पूर्वखण्डः वर्गप्रकरण ६ : १९६—२०० ]

At times the combination of certain drugs produces poisonous effects; for example, ghee and honey in equal quantities. Even a poison at times works like ambrosia; for example, administration of poisonous drugs to a person afflicted by snake bite.

**अथ गुणानां गुणाः**

लघुपथ्यं परं प्रोक्तं कफघ्नं शीघ्रपाकि च ।

गुरुवातहरं पुष्टिः श्लेष्मकृत् चिरपाकि च ।। २९ ।।

**Actions of various *guṇas* (attributes)**

Things which are *laghu* (light) are wholesome. They

alleviate *kapha* and get digested immediately. Things that are *guru* (heavy) alleviate *vāta*. They cause nourishment and aggravate *kapha*. They take a long time for digestion.

स्निग्धं कफकरं वातहरं वृष्यं बलप्रदम् ।
रूक्षं परं कफहरं समीरणकरं मतम् ।
तीक्ष्णं पित्तकरं प्रायो लेखनं कफवातहृत् ।। ३० ।।
[भावप्रकाशः पूर्वखण्डः वर्गप्रकरण ६ : २०२—२०४]

*Snigdha* (unctuous) things aggravate *kapha* and alleviate *vāta*. They are aphrodisiac and they promote strength. *Rukṣa* (ununctuous) things alleviate *kapha* and aggravate *vāyu*. Things that are *tīkṣṇa* (sharp) aggravate *pitta* and they are generally *lekhana* (having scraping property). They alleviate *kapha* and *vāta*.

**अथ वीर्यम् :**

वीर्यमुष्णं तथा शीतं प्रायशो द्रव्यसंमतम् ।
यत्सर्वमग्निषोमीयं दृश्यते भुवनत्रये ।। ३१ ।।

***Vīrya* (Potency)**

*Vīrya* (potency) is of two categories viz., *uṣṇa* (hot) and *śīta* (cold). They are inherent in matter. They represent the *agni* and *soma* principles of the three worlds.

**अथ-तद्गुण :**

उष्णं वातकफौ हन्यात्पित्तं तु तनुते तराम् ।
शीतं वातकफातङ्कान्कुरुते पित्तहृत्परम् ।। ३२ ।।
[भावप्रकाशः पूर्वखण्डः वर्गप्रकरण ६ : २३८—२३९]

**Their attributes**

Those having *uṣṇa* (hot) potency alleviate *vāta* and *kapha* and they aggravate *pitta*.

Those having *śīta* (cooling) potency cause diseases of *vāyu* and *kapha*; but they alleviate *pitta*.

**अथ विपाक** :

12
स्वादुः पटुश्च मधुरमम्लोम्लं पच्यते रसः ।
[भावप्रकाशः पूर्वखण्डः वर्गप्रकरण ६ : २४२]

कटुतिक्तकषायाणां पाकः स्यात्प्रायशः कटुः ॥ ३३ ॥
[चरक : सूत्र २६ : ५८]

*Vipāka* **(Taste that emerges after digestion)**

The *vipāka* of sweet and saline things is *madhura* (sweet) and sour things have *amla* (sour) *vipāka*. The *vipāka* of pungent, bitter and astringent things is generally *kaṭu* (pungent).

**अथ विपाकानां गुणाः**

श्लेष्मकृन्मधुरः पाको वातपित्तहरो मतः ।
अम्लस्तु कुरुते पित्तं वातश्लेष्मगदापहः ।
कटुः करोति पवनं कफं पित्तं च नाशयेत् ॥ ३४ ॥
[भावप्रकाशः पूर्वखण्डः वर्गप्रकरण ६ : २४३—२४४]

**Attributes of** ***Vipākas***

Things having *madhura* (sweet) *vipāka* aggravate *kapha* and alleviate *vāta* and *pitta*. Those having *amla* (sour) *vipāka* aggravate *pitta* and alleviate diseases of *vāyu* and *kapha*. *Kaṭu* (pungent) *vipāka* aggravates *vāyu* but alleviates *kapha* and *pitta* (?).

**अथ प्रभाव** :

प्रभावस्तु यथा धात्री लकुचस्य रसादिभिः ।
समोऽपि कुरुते दोषत्रितयस्य विनाशनम् ॥ ३५ ॥
[भावप्रकाशः पूर्वखण्डः वर्गप्रकरण ६ : २४६—२४७]

***Prabhāva*** **or specific action**

The examples of *prabhāva* are *dhātrī* and *lakuca*. They have similar *rasa* (taste) etc. But the former alleviates all the three *doṣas* whereas the latter does not.

क्वचित्तु केवलं द्रव्यं कर्म कुर्यात्[13] प्रभावतः ।

ज्वरं हन्ति शिरोबद्धा सहदेवीजटा यथा ।। ३६ ।।

[भावप्रकाशः पूर्वखण्डः वर्गप्रकरण ६ : २४८]

At times the *dravya* (matter) itself produces action by its *prabhāva.* For example, the root of *sahadevī* cures fever when tied into the head (hair).

## NOTES AND REFERENCES

This is the eighth chapter of *Ayurveda Saukhyaṁ* in Toḍarānanda and the invocation reads as follows :

गोपांगनाप्रांगणभूमिभागे शनैरगच्छत्सुनिगृह्यधात्रीं ।
पायान्नृपं टंडणवंशजातं पदद्वयं यः कृतवान् स्वसृष्टेः ।

1. परिहिताय वै इति षष्ठ पुस्तके पाठ :
2. द्रष्टव्यम् चरकः सूत्र ४४-८५ ।
3. "औषधीषु सकल द्रववर्ग-धान्य-मांस-फल-शाक-रसाश्च ।
   कृत्यमन्नमनुपानकं युक्तं भाव-भावरचनाक्रमएषः" ।।
   पाठोऽयं आदर्शपुस्तकेषु अधिकंमुपलभ्यते ।
4. मधुरो हि रसः इति आकरे पाठः ।
5. लेखितोष्णो इति आकरे पाठः ।
6. पित्तकोठक्षतादिकृत् इति आकरे पाठः ।
7. द्रष्टव्यम् भावप्रकाशः पूर्वखण्डः वर्गप्रकरण ६ : १८४ ।
8. भ्रान्तिदाहमुखताल्वोष्ठशोधकृत् इति आकरे पाठः ।
9. बलशुक्रकृत् इति द्वितीयपुस्तके पाठ :
10. विषापहः इति द्वितीयपुस्तके पाठः ।
11. योगतस्तु इति आकरे पाठः ।
12. मिष्टः इति आकरे पाठः
13. कुर्यात्प्रधानतः इति षष्ठपुस्तके पाठः ।

# CHAPTER 2

हरस्य भवने जाता हरिता[1] च स्वभावतः ।
हरते सर्वरोगांश्च तेन प्रोक्ता **हरीतकी** ।।

*Harītakī* **(Terminalia chebula Retz.)**

It is called *harītakī* because of the following :

(1) it grows in the abode of Hara (Lord Siva) i.e. in the Himalayas ;

(2) it is green (*harita*) by nature ;

(3) it cures (*harate*) all diseases ;

जीवन्ती जीवनो योगान्[2] पावनात्पूतना मता ।
सुधावदमृता ज्ञेया विजया विजयप्रदा ।। २ ।।
नृणामभयदा यस्मादभया तत्प्रकीर्तिता ।
रोहिणी तु गुणरोहाच्चेतनाच्चेतकी मता ।। ३ ।।

The names of different varieties of *harītakī* have the following significance :

(a) *Jivantī* because it promotes life (*jīvana*) ;

(b) *Pūtanā* because it purifies (*pāvana*) ;

(c) *Amṛtā* because it is like ambrosia (*amṛta*) ;

(d) *Vijayā* because it endows the user with victory (*vijaya*) ;

(e) *Abhayā* because it takes away fear (*bhaya*) ;

(f) *Rohiṇī* because it promotes (*rohāt*) the attributes (*guṇas*) ;

(g) *Cetakī* because it promotes consciousness (*cetanā*).

जीवन्ती स्वर्णवर्णाभा पूतनास्थिमती मता ।
अमृता त्रिदला प्रोक्ता विजया तुंबरूपिणी ॥ ४ ॥
पंचागी त्वभया ज्ञया मता वृत्ता तु रोहिणी ।
[3] त्र्यंगी तु चेतकी ज्ञेया कर्म तासामिहोच्यते ॥ ५ ॥

Different varieties of *harītakī* have the following characteristics :

(a) *Jīvantī* is golden in colour ;

(b) *Pūtanā* has a bigger stone ;

(c) *Amṛtā* has three *dalas* (pieces or fruits in a bunch)

(d) *Vijayā* is like a *tumbī* ;

(e) *Abhayā* has five *aṅgas* (pieces) ;

(f) *Rohiṇī* is round in shape ;

(g) *Cetakī* has three *aṅgas* (pieces).

सर्वरोगेषु जीवन्ती प्रलेपे [4] पूतना मता ।

शुद्ध्यर्थममृता ज्ञेया विजया सर्वरोगहृत् ॥ ६ ॥

अस्थिरोगेऽभया प्रोक्ता रोहिणी व्रणरोहिणी ।

चेतकी चूर्णयोगे स्यात्सप्तधाऽत्र प्रकीर्तिता ॥ ७ ॥

Properties of different varieties of *harītakī* are as below :

(a) *Jīvantī* is useful in all diseases ;

(b) *Pūtanā* is useful in external application ;

(c) *Amṛtā* is useful in cleansing the body ;

(d) *Vijayā* cures all diseases ;

(e) *Abhayā* is useful in the diseases of bones ;

(f) *Rohiṇī* helps in the healing of ulcers ;

(g) *Cetakī* is useful in potions used in the form of powder.

These are the seven varieties of *harītakī*.

'हरीतकी पञ्चरसाऽलवणा तुवरोत्कटा ।

रूक्षोष्णा दीपनी मेध्या स्वदुपाका रसायनी ॥ ८ ॥

[5] सरा बुद्धिप्रदाऽऽयुष्या चक्षुष्या बृंहणी लघुः ।

**Attributes**

*Harītakī* has five tastes. It does not possess saline taste. It is extremely astringent. It is ununctuous, hot, *dīpana* (digestive stimulant), *medhya* (promoter of memory), *svādu pāka* (sweet in *vipāka*), *rasāyana* (rejuvenating), *sara* (laxative), *buddhi prada* (promoter of intellect), *āyuṣya* (promoter of longevity), *cakṣuṣya* (promoter of eye sight), *bṛmhaṇa* (nourishing) and *laghu* (light).

श्वास-कास-प्रमेहार्शः कुष्ठ-शोथोदरक्रमीन् ॥ ९ ॥
6
वैस्वर्यग्रहणीदोषविबन्धविषमज्वरान् ।
7
गुल्माध्मानव्रणच्छर्दिहिक्काकण्डूहृदामयान् ।
8
कामलां शूलमानाहं प्लीहानञ्चापि कर्षति' ॥ १० ॥

[भावप्रकाशः पूर्वखण्डः वर्गप्रकरण २ : १९-२२]

It cures *śvāsa* (asthma), *kāsa* (coughing), *prameha* (obstinate urinary disorders including diabetes), *arśas* (piles), *kuṣṭha* (obstinate skin diseases including leprosy), *śotha* (oedema), *udara* (obstinate abdominal diseases including ascitis), *kṛmi* (parasitic infections), *vaisvarya* (hoarseness of voice), *grahaṇī doṣa* (sprue syndrome), *vibandha* (constipation), *viṣamajvara* (malarial fever), *gulma* (phantom tumour), *ādhmāna* (tymphanitis), *vraṇa* (ulcer), *chardi* (vomiting), *hikkā* (hiccup), *kaṇḍū* (itching), *hṛdāmaya* (heart disease), *kāmalā* (jaundice), *śula* (colic pain), *ānāha* (wind formation in stomach) and *plihā* (splenic disorder).

अम्लत्वाद्वातशमनी पित्तघ्ना स्वादुतिक्ततः ।
कटोः कषायात्कफहृत् त्रिदोषघ्नी हरीतकी ॥

Because of sour taste it alleviates *vāyu* ; because of sweet and bitter tastes it alleviates *pitta* and because of pungent and astringent tastes it alleviates *kapha*. Thus, *harītakī* alleviates all the three *doṣas*.

मज्जाश्रितं तु मधुरं अम्लं स्नाय्वास्थिसंश्रितम् ।
त्वगाश्रितं तु कटुकं तिक्तं वृन्ताश्रितं मतम् ॥ १२ ॥
अस्थ्याश्रितं कषायं तु रसमाहुर्मनीषिणः ।

Tastes predominant in different parts of *harītakī* are as follows :

(1) Sweet taste in *majjā* or pulp ;
(2) Sour taste in fibres and stone ;

(3) Pungent taste in skin ;

(4) Bitter taste in stalk ;

(5) Astringent taste in stone.

नवा स्निग्धा घना वृत्ता गुर्वी क्षिप्ता च याम्भसि ॥ १३ ॥

[भावप्रकाशः पूर्वखण्डः वर्गप्रकरण २ :२ - ]

निमज्जेत्सा प्रशस्ता [9] स्यात्कथितातिगुणप्रदा ।

**Characteristics of good quality**

*Harītakī* which is fresh, unctuous, compact, round and heavy is the best. When put in water it should sink. This type of *harītakī* is extremely useful and therapeutically very effective.

चर्विता वर्धयत्यग्निं पेषिता [10] मलशोधिनी ।

स्विन्ना संग्राहिणी प्रोक्ता भृष्टा पथ्या त्रिदोषनुत् ॥१४॥

[भावप्रकाशः पूर्वखण्डः वर्गप्रकरण २ : २८, ३०]

**Different ways of Using**

Used in different ways it produces the following effects :

(1) when taken by chewing it promotes digestive power ;

(2) when used in paste form it cleanses the bowels ;

(3) when used by steam boiling it is constipative ;

(4) when used after frying it alleviates all the three *doṣas*.

ग्रीष्मे तुल्यगुडां सुसैन्धवयुतां मेघावनद्धेऽम्बरे ।

तुल्या शर्करया शरद्यमलया शुण्ठ्या तुषारागमे ॥१५॥

पिप्पल्या शिशिरे वसन्तसमये क्षौद्रेण संयोजिताम् ।

राजन्प्राप्य हरीतकीमिवरुजो नश्यन्तु ते शत्रवः ॥१६॥

**Use in different seasons**

In different seasons *harītakī* should be used as follows :

(1) In summer it should be used with equal quantity of *guḍa* ;

(2) In rainy season it is to be used with adequate quantity of *saindhava ;*

(3) In autumn season it is to be used with equal quantity of purified sugar ;

(4) In the beginning of winter it is to be used with *śuṇṭhī*.

(5) In the later part of winter it is to be used with *pippalī*.

(6) In the spring season it should be mixed with honey and then used.

O ! King, let your enemies be destroyed as diseases get destroyed by the use of *harītakī* in the above mentioned manner.

लवणेन कफं हन्ति पित्तं हन्ति सशर्करा ।

घृतेन वातजान् रोगान्सर्वरोगान्गुडान्विता ॥ १७ ॥

**Usage for different** ***doṣas***

It alleviates *kapha* when taken with salt. *Pitta* is alleviated when it is taken with sugar. When taken with *ghee* it cures all diseases caused by *vāyu*. Taken with *guḍa*, *harītakī* cures all types of diseases.

अध्वातिखिन्नः परिहीनतेजा रूक्षः कृशो लंघनकर्षितश्च ।

पित्ताधिको गर्भवती च नारी विमुक्तसत्वस्त्वभयां न सेवेत् ॥१८॥

**Contra-indications**

*Harītakī* should not be used by persons who are extremely exhausted by travelling, who have lost the lustre of their body, who have ununctuous skin, who are emaciated, whose body is dried up by fasting, whose *pitta* is aggravated, ladies who are pregnant and those who have lost their will power.

बिभीतकं स्वादुपाकं कषायं कफपित्तनुत् ।

उष्णवीर्यं हिमस्पर्शं भेदनं कासनाशनम् ॥ १९ ॥

रूक्षं नेत्रहितं केश्यं जंतुवैस्वर्यनाशनम् [11] ।

*Bibhītakī* **(Terminalia belerica Roxb.)**

*Bibhītakī* is sweet in *vipāka*. It is astringent in taste. It alleviates *kapha* and *pitta*. It is hot in potency. It is cooling in touch. It is *bhedana* (purgative), *kāsa nāśana* (cures coughing), *rūkṣa* (ununctuous), *netrahita* (useful for eyesight) and *keśya* (useful for hair). It cures parasitic infections and impaired voice.

बिभीतमज्जातृट्छर्दिकफवातहरो लघुः ॥ २० ॥

[भावप्रकाशः पूर्वखण्डः वर्गप्रकरण २ : ३७-३८]

The seed pulp of *bibhītaka* cures *tṛṭ* (morbid thirst), *chardi* (vomiting) and diseases caused by *kapha* and *vāta*. It is light.

कषायो मदकृत्स्वादुर्धात्रीमज्जापि [12] तद्गुणः ।

*Āmalakī* **(Emblica officinalis Gaertn.)**

The seed pulp of *āmalakī* has the same property as that of *bibhītakī*. It is intoxicating and sweet.

हरीतकीसमं **धात्रीफलं** किन्तु विशेषतः ॥ २१ ॥

रक्तपित्तप्रमेहघ्नं परं वृष्यं रसायनम् ।

The fruit of *dhātrī* is similar to *harītakī* in its properties. It has, however, some specific properties. It cures *raktapitta* (a disease characterised by bleeding from different parts of the body) and *prameha* (obstinate urinary disorders including diabetes). It is exceedingly aphrodisiac and rejuvenating.

हन्ति वातं तदम्लत्वात्पित्तं माधुर्यशैत्यतः ।

कफं रूक्षकषायत्वात्फलं धात्र्यास्त्रिदोषजित् [13] ॥ २२ ॥

[भावप्रकाशः पूर्वखण्डः वर्गप्रकरण २ : २८, ४०-४१]

It alleviates *vāta* because of its sour taste. Because of its sweet taste and cooling effect it alleviates *pitta*. *Kapha* is alleviated by its ununctuousness and astringent taste. The fruit of *dhātrī* alleviate all the three *doṣas*.

कुर्यापित्तं तदम्लत्वात्कफं माधुर्यशैत्यतः ।
वातं रूक्षकषायत्वादेवं किं न विपर्ययः ॥ २३ ॥

It should aggravate *pitta* by its sour taste. By its sweet taste and cooling effect *kapha* should get aggravated. Its ununctuousness and astringent taste should aggravate *vāyu*. Why does it not happen ?

धात्र्यास्त्रिदोषहंतृत्वं शक्त्यैव मुनिभिः स्मृतम् ।
संभावनावशादुक्ता रसादेरपि हेतुता ॥ २४ ॥

According to sages this property of *dhātrī* to alleviate all the three *doṣas* is because of its *prabhāva* (specific action) This property has been explained on the basis of its *rasa* etc., because of the existence of such a possibility.

यस्य यस्य फलस्येह वीर्यं भवति यादृशम् ।
तस्य तस्यैव वीर्येण मज्जानमपि निर्दिशेत् ॥ २५ ॥
[सुश्रुतः सूत्र ४६ : २०८]

The potency (*vīrya*) of the pulp of the seed will be the same as that of its fruit. This rule is applicable to all plants.

अभयैका योजनीया द्वावेव तु बिभीतकौ ।
14
धात्रीफलानि चत्वारि त्रिफलेयं प्रकीतिता" ॥२६॥

*Triphalā*

One fruit of *abhayā*, two fruits of *bibhītakī* and four fruits of *āmalakī*—taken together these are called *triphalā*.

"शिवा पंचरसायुष्या चक्षुष्याऽलवणा सरा ।
मेध्योष्णा दीपनी दोष-शोथ-कुष्ठ-व्रणापहा ॥ २७ ॥

*Sivā* has five tastes. It is *āyuṣya* (promoter of longevity), *cakṣuṣya* (promoter of eyesight), *alavaṇa* (free from saline taste), *sara* (laxative), *medhya* (promoter of intellect), *uṣṇa* (hot) and *dīpana* (stimulant of digestion). It alleviates *doṣas*, *śotha* (oedema), *kuṣṭha* (obstinate skin diseases including leprosy) and *vraṇa* (ulcer).

तद्वद्धात्री विशेषेण वृष्या शीतैव वीर्यतः ।

*Dhātrī* has similar properties. It has, however, some specific properties inasmuch as it is aphrodisiac and it is *śīta* (cooling) in potency.

'भेदनं कटुरुक्षोष्णं वैस्वर्यक्रिमिनाशनम् ।
चक्षुष्यं स्वादुपाक्यक्षं कषायं कफपित्तनुत्[15]' ॥ २८ ॥
[सुश्रुत : सूत्र ४६ : २००]

*Akṣa* is purgative, purgent, ununctuous and hot. It cures hoarseness of voice and parasitic infection. It promotes eyesight. It is sweet in *vipāka* and astringent in taste. It alleviates *kapha* and *pitta*.

'त्रिफला कफपित्तघ्नी मेह-कुष्ठ-विनाशिनी[16] ।
चक्षुष्या दीपनी रुच्या[17] विषमज्वरनाशिनी' ॥ २६ ॥
[भावप्रकाशः पूर्वखण्डः वर्गप्रकरण २ : ४४]

*Triphalā* alleviates *kapha* and *pitta*. It cures *meha* (obstinate urinary disorders) and *kuṣṭha* (obstinate skin diseases including leprosy). It is *cakṣuṣya* (promoter of eyesight), *dīpana* (digestive stimulant) and *rucya* (appetiser). It cures *viṣama-jvara* (malarial fever).

कफपित्तहरा रूक्षा मधुरा मृदुरेचनी[18] ।
वातकृत्कटुका पाके कषाया **त्रिवृताऽसिता** ॥ ३० ॥

*Trivṛt* **(Operculina turpethum Silva Manso)**

The black variety of *trivṛt* alleviates *kapha* and *pitta*, *rukṣa* (ununctuous), *madhura* (sweet), *mṛdu recana* (laxative), *vātakṛt* (aggravator of *vāta*), *kaṭu pāka* (pungent in *vipāka*) and astringent in taste.

तस्मादल्पांतरगुणा विज्ञेया त्रिवृताऽरुणा ।

The reddish (*aruṇa)* variety of *trivṛt* is slightly inferior in quality.

ज्वरहृद्रोगवातासृगुदावर्त्तादि—रोगिषु ॥ ३१ ॥

राजवृक्षोऽधिकं पथ्यो मृदुर्मधुरशीतलः ।

*Rājavṛkṣa* **(Cassia fistula Linn.)**

For patients suffering from *jvara* (fever), *hṛdroga* (heart disease), *vātāsṛk* (gout) and *udāvarta* (upward movement of wind in abdomen), *rājavṛkṣa* is extremely wholesome. It is *mṛdu* (soft), sweet and cooling.

तत्फलं मधुरं बल्यं वातपित्तामहृत्सरं ॥ ३२ ॥

पीतं तोयेन निन्नर्शिद्‌गृध्रसीं प्रबलामपि ।

Its fruit is sweet and strength promoting. It reduces *vāta*, *pitta* and *āma*. It is laxative. When taken with water it cures even the severe type of *gṛdhrasī* (sciatica).

कटुकाह्वा सरा रूक्षा कफपित्तज्वरापहा ॥ ३३ ॥

*Kaṭukā* **(Picrorhiza kurroa Royle ex Benth.)**

*Kaṭukā* is laxative and ununctuous. It alleviates *kapha*, *pitta* and fever.

त्रायन्ती कफपित्तास्रगुल्मज्वरहरी सरा ।

*Trāyantī* **(Gentiana kurroo Royle)**

*Trāyantī* cures vitiated *kapha*, *pitta* and blood, *gulma* (phantom tumour) and fever. It is laxative.

कफपित्तास्ररुक[19]च्छर्दिविषघ्नी तिक्तवल्कली[20] ॥ ३४ ॥

*Tikta valkalī*

*Tikta valkalī* alleviates vitiated *kapha*, *pitta* and blood, pain, *chardi* (vomiting) and *viṣa* (poisoning).

**यासः** सरो ज्वर-छर्दि-श्लेष्म-पित्त-विसर्पनुत् ।

*Yāsa* **(Alhagi pseudalhagi Desv.)**

*Yāsa* is laxative. It cures fever, vomiting, aggravated *kapha* and *pitta* and *visarpa* (erysipelas).

**भूधात्री** वातकृत्तिक्ता कषाया मधुरा हिमा ॥ ३५ ॥

पिपासा कास-पित्तास्र-कफ-पाण्डु-क्षयापहा ।

*Bhūdhātrī* **(Phyllanthus niruri Linn.)**

*Bhūdhātrī* aggravates *vāyu*. It is bitter, astringent and sweet in taste. It is cooling. It cures *pipāsā* (morbid thirst), *kāsa* (coughing), *pittāsra* (a disease characterised by bleeding from different parts of the body), vitiated *kapha*, *pāṇḍu* (anemia) and *kṣaya* (consumption).

**खदिरः** कुष्ठवीसर्पमेहपित्तविषापह ॥ ३६ ॥

*Khadira* **(Acacia catechu Willd.)**

*Khadira* cures *kuṣṭha* (obstinate skin diseases including leprosy), *visarpa* (erysipelas), *meha* (obstinate urinary disorders including diabetes), aggravated *pitta* and *viṣa* (poisoning).

**भूनिंबो** वातलो **रूक्षः** कफपित्तज्वरापहः ।

*Bhūnimba* **(Swertia chirata Buch.—Ham.)**

*Bhūnimba* aggravates *vāyu*. It is ununctuous and it alleviates aggravated *kapha* and *pitta* as well as fever.

**निंबः** पित्तकफच्छर्दिव्रणहृल्लासकुष्ठनुत् ॥ ३७ ॥

21

"शीतो ग्राह्यग्निकृत्कासज्वरतृट्क्रिमिमेहजित् ।

*Nimba* **(Azadirachta indica A. Juss.)**

*Nimba* cures aggravated *pitta* and *kapha*, *chardi* (vomiting), *vraṇa* (ulcer), *hṛllāsa* (nausea) and *kuṣṭha* (obstinate skin diseases including leprosy). It is cooling, constipative and digestive stimulant. It cures *kāsa* (coughing), *jvara* (fever), *tṛṭ* (morbid thirst), *kṛmi* (parasitic infection) and *meha* (obstinate urinary disorders including diabetes).

22

निम्बपत्रं तु चक्षुष्यं कृमिपित्तविषप्रणुत्" ॥ ३८ ॥

Leaf of *nimba* promotes eye sight. It cures *kṛmi* (parasitic infection), aggravated *pitta* and *viṣa* (poisoning).

23

तत्फलं भेदनं स्निग्धमुष्णं कुष्ठहर लघु ।

Fruit of *nimba* is purgative, unctuous and hot. It cures *kuṣṭha* (obstinate skin diseases including leprosy). It is light.

**महानिंबः परं ग्राही कषायो रूक्षशीतलः ॥ ३९ ॥**

*Mahā nimba* **(Melia azedarach Linn.)**

*Mahā nimba* is exceedingly constipative, astringent, ununctuous and cooling.

**पर्पटः पित्ततृट्दाहज्वरहृत् श्लेष्मशोषणः ।**

*Parpaṭa* **(Fumaria parviflora Lam.)**

*Parpaṭa* cures aggravated *pitta*, *tṛṭ* (morbid thirst), *dāha* (burning syndrome) and *jvara* (fever). It dries up *kapha*.

24

**पाठातीसारशूलघ्नी कफपित्तज्वरापहा ॥ ४० ॥**

*Pāṭhā* **(Cissampelos pareira Linn.)**

*Pāṭhā* cures *atisāra* (diarrhoea), *śūla* (colic pain), aggravated *kapha* and *pitta* and *jvara* (fever).

25

"द्विविधः कुटजो ज्ञेयः पुंस्त्रीभेदेन तद्विदा ।

बृहत्फलः श्वेतपुष्पः स्निग्धो दीर्घच्छदः पुमान् ॥ ४१ ॥

**तथातिरक्तवहलत्वचः प्रोक्तो विशारदैः ।**

*Kuṭaja* **(Holarrhena antidysenterica Wall.)**

According to scholars, *kuṭaja* is of two types viz., male

and female. The male variety has bigger fruits, white flowers and unctuous as well as long leaves. Its bark is exceedingly red and thick.

अणुफला वृत्तपुष्पा पुष्पैः श्यावारुणैर्युता ॥ ४२ ॥

धवलत्वक् भवेद्यासौ विज्ञेया स्त्री न संशयः ।

If the fruits are small, flowers are round in shape and grayish red in colour and bark is white, then this is undoubtedly the female variety of *kuṭaja*.

कुटजः पुरुषो ग्राही रक्तपित्तातिसारनुत् ॥ ४३ ॥

वातघ्नो प्रदरे योज्यो ततो हीनगुणाऽपरा ।

The male variety of *kuṭaja* is constipative and it alleviates *raktapitta* (a disease characterised by bleeding from different parts of the body) and *atisāra* (diarrhoea). It alleviates *vāyu* and is useful in *pradara* (menorrhagia and other allied gynaecological disorders).

The female variety is inferior in quality.

फलाच्च पुष्पतो ज्ञेया इति पाराशरोऽब्रवीत् ॥ ४४ ॥

According to the sage *Parāśara*; these varieties of *kuṭaja* should be determined from the characteristics of their fruits and flowers.

26

'कुटजः कफपित्तासृक् त्वग्दोषार्शोऽतिसारजित् ।'

*Kuṭaja* alleviates vitiated *kapha*, *pitta* and *rakta*. It cures *tvagdoṣa* (skin diseases), *arśas* (piles) and *atisāra* (diarrhoea).

तद्बीजं रक्तपित्तातिसारज्वरहरं हिमम् ॥ ४५ ॥

Its seed cures *raktapitta* (a disease characterised by bleeding from different parts of the body), *atisāra* (diarrhoea) and *jvara* (fever). It is cooling.

**ह्रीवेरं** छर्दिहृल्लासतृष्णातीसारनाशनम् ।

*Hrīvera* **(Coleus vettiveroides K. C. Jacob.)**

*Hrīvera* cures *chardi* (vomiting), *hṛllāsa* (nausea), *ṛṣṇā* (morbid thirst) and *atisāra* (diarrhoea).

कफघ्नं कटुकं तिक्तं **मुस्तं** संग्राहिपाचनम् ।

*Mustā* **(Cyperus rotundus Linn.)**

*Mustā* alleviates *kapha*. It is pungent and bitter in taste, *saṁgrāhi* (constipative) and *pācana* (carminative).

दोषघ्नं पाचनं ग्राहि तिक्तं **चातिविषाह्वयम्**[27] ।। ४६ ।।

*Ativiṣā* **(Aconitum heterophyllum Wall.)**

*Ativiṣā* alleviates *doṣas*. It is carminative, constipative and bitter.

संग्राही कफवातघ्नं **बिल्वं** दीपनपाचनं ।

बालं, वृद्धं त्रिदोषाय दुर्जरं पूतिमारुतं ।। ४७ ।।

*Bilva* **(Aegle marmelos Corr.)**

Unripe and immature fruit of *bilva* is constipative. It alleviates *kapha* and *vāta*. It is a digestive stimulant and carminative.

Ripe and matured fruit of *bilva* aggravates all the three *doṣas*. It is difficult of digestion and produces foul smelling wind.

कफवातामशूलघ्नी ग्राहिणी बिल्वपेशिका ।

The *peśi* (pulp or flesh) of *bilva* cures vitiated *kapha* and *vāyu*, *āma* and *śūla* (colic pain). It is constipative.

'फलेषु परिपक्वं यद्गुणवत्तदुदाहृतम् ।

बिल्वादन्यत्र विज्ञेयमामं तद्धिगुणोत्तरम् ।। ४८ ।।

[सुश्रुत: सूत्र ४६ : २०६]

Generally, among fruits, matured ones are considered to be of good quality. *Bilva* is an exception to this rule inasmuch as its immature fruits are better in quality.

कफानिलाम --दुर्नामव्रध्नशोफोदरापहम् ।

सरं **पुनर्नवायुग्ममुष्णवीर्यं** रसायनम् ॥ ४९ ॥

*Punarnavā* **(Boerhaavia diffusa Linn.)**

Two varieties of *punarnavā* alleviate *kapha* and *vāyu,* reduce *āma* and cure *durnāman* (piles), *vradhna* (inguinal lymphadenitis), *śopha* (oedema) and *udara* (obstinate abdominal diseases including ascitis.) They are laxative and hot in potency. They are *rasāyana* (rejuvenating).

**चित्रकोऽग्निसमः** पाके शोफार्शःकृमिकुष्ठहाः ।

*Citraka* **(Plumbago zeylanica Linn.)**

*Citraka* acts like fire during digestion i.e. it is a strong digestive stimulant. It cures *śopha* (oedema), *arśas* (piles), *kṛmi* (parasitic infection) and *kuṣṭha* (obstinate skin diseases including leprosy).

लोहितः केशरागश्च कृमिकुष्ठज्वरापहः ॥ ५० ॥

The red variety of *citraka* imparts colour to the hair and it cures *kṛmi* (parasitic infection), *kuṣṭha* (obstinate skin diseases including leprosy) and *jvara* (fever).

**तद्वद्दन्ती** प्रभावात्तु विरेचयति सा नरम् ।

*Dantī* **(Baliospermum montanum Muell.—Arg.)**

*Dantī* has properties similar to those of *citraka.* However, because of *prabhāva* (specific action) it causes purgation.

कफकृमिहरी तीक्ष्णा **हस्तिदन्ती** विरेचनी ॥ ५१ ॥

*Hasti danti* **(Trichosanthes bracteata Voigt)**

***Hasti dantī*** **alleviates** ***kapha*** **and** ***kṛmi*** **(parasitic infection). It is sharp and purgative.**

**जयपालो** गुरुस्निग्धो रेची पित्तकफापहः ।

*Jayapāla* **(Croton tiglium Linn.)**

*Jayapāla* is heavy, unctuous and purgative. It alleviates ***pitta*** **and** ***kapha*.**

स्नुही साष्ठीलिकाध्मानगुल्मोदरहरी सरा ॥ ५२ ॥

*Snuhī* **(Euphorbia neriifolia Linn.)**

*Snuhī* cures *aṣṭhilikā* (stony tumour in abdomen), *ādhmāna* (tymphanitis), *gulma* (phantom tumour) and *udara* (obstinate abdominal diseases including ascitis). It is *sarā* (purgative).

दूषीविषोदरप्लीहागुल्मकुष्ठप्रमेहिषु ।
[28] बहुदोषे प्रयोक्तव्यमग्नितुल्यं सुधापयः ॥ ५३ ॥

The latex of *snuhī* which is like fire should be used when the *doṣas* in a patient are aggravated very much in excess and also for patients suffering from *dūṣī viṣa* (artificial poison), *udara* (obstinate abdominal diseases including ascitis), *plīhā roga* (splenic disorder), *gulma* (phantom tumour), *kuṣṭha* (obstinate skin diseases including leprosy) and *prameha* (obstinate urinary disorders including diabetes).

हेमाह्वा रेचनी तिक्ता मदनुत् क्लेदकारिणी ।
कृमि-कंडू-कफानाह-विष- कुष्ठ-विनाशिनी ॥ ५४ ॥

*Hemāhvā* **(Argemone mexicana Linn.)**

*Hemāhvā* is purgative, bitter and *madanut* (cures intoxication). It produces *kleda* (stickiness) in body. It cures *kṛmi* (parasitic infection), *kaṇḍū* (itching), vitiated *kapha*, *ānāha* (constipation), *viṣa* (poisoning), and *kuṣṭha* (obstinate skin diseases including leprosy).

अर्कः[29] कृमिहरस्तीक्ष्णः सरोर्शः[30] कुष्ठनाशनः ।

*Arka* **(Calotropis gigantea R. Br. ex Ait.)**

*Arka* cures *kṛmi* (parasitic infection). It is sharp and purgative. It also cures *arśas* (piles) and *kuṣṭha* (obstinate skin diseases including leprosy).

तत्पयः कृमिदोषघ्नं हितं कुष्ठोदरार्शसाम् ॥ ५५ ॥

The latex of *arka* cures *kṛmidoṣa* (parasitic infection) and it is useful for patients suffering from *kuṣṭha* (obstinate skin diseases including leprosy), *udara* (obstinate abdominal diseases including ascitis).

आरुष्करं[31] तौवरकं[32] कषायं कटुपाकि च ।

उष्णं कृम्युदरानाहशोफदुर्नामनाशनम् ॥ ५६ ॥

ग्रहणीकफवाताग्निमांद्यामज्वरगुल्मनुत्[33] ।

*Āruṣkara & Tuvaraka* **(Semecarpus anacardium Linn. f. & Hydnocarpus wightiana Blume)**

*Āruṣkara* and *tauvaraka*—both are astringent in taste and pungent in *vipāka*. They are hot and they cure *kṛmi* (parasitic infection), *udara* (obstinate abdominal diseases including ascitis), *ānāha* (constipation), *śopha* (oedema) *durnāman* (piles), *grahaṇī* (sprue syndrome), vitiated *kapha* and *vāta*, *agnimāndya* (suppression of the power of digestion), *āma*, *jvara* (fever) and *gulma* (phantom tumour).

तन्मज्जा मधुरः पाके वृष्यश्चार्शोहरः परः ॥५७॥

The pulp of these drugs is sweet in *vipāka* and aphrodisiac. It also cures *arśas* (piles).

गुग्गुलुः पिच्छिलः स्पर्शो विशदोभ्यवहारतः ।

सुस्वादुः सकटुस्तिक्तः सकषायो रसायनः ॥ ५८ ॥

वर्ण्यः स्वर्यः कटुः पाके रूक्षः श्लक्ष्णोग्निदीपनः ।

क्लेदमेदोनिलश्लेष्मगंडमेहापचीकृमीन् ॥ ५९ ॥

पिडकाग्रंथिशोथार्शोहन्त्युष्णस्रंसनो लघुः ।

*Guggulu* **(Commiphora mukul Engl.)**

*Guggulu* is slimy in touch. But it has a non-slimy (*viśada*) effect on the body when used. It is sweet, pungent, bitter and astringent in taste. It is *rasāyana* (rejuvenating), *varṇya* (promoter of complexion), *svarya* (promoter of good voice), *kaṭupāka* (pungent in vipāka), *rūkṣa* (ununctuous), *ślakṣṇa* (smooth) and *agnidīpana* (promoter of digestive power). It alleviates *kleda* (sticky material in the body), *medas* (fat), vitiated *vāyu* and *kapha*, *gaṇḍa* (goitre), *meha* (obstinate urinary disorders including diabetes), *apacī* (cervical adenitis), *kṛmi* (parasitic infection), *piḍakā* (pimples), *granthi* (adenitis), *śotha* (oedema) and *arśas* (piles). It is hot, *sraṁsana* (laxative) and light.

स नवो बृंहणो वृष्यः पुराणस्त्वतिकर्षणः ॥ ६० ॥

Fresh *guggulu* is *bṛṁhaṇa* (nourishing) and *vṛṣya* (aphrodisiac). Old *guggulu* is extremely depleting (*karṣaṇa*).

"[34]महिषाक्षो महानीलः कुमुदः पद्म [35]इत्यपि ।
हिरण्यः पञ्चमो ज्ञेयो गुग्गुलोः पञ्चजातयः ॥६१ ॥
भृङ्गांजनसवर्णस्तु [36]महिषाक्ष इति स्मृतः ।
महानीलस्तु विज्ञेयः स्वनामसमलक्षणः ॥ ६२ ॥
कुमुदः कुमुदाभस्तु [37]पद्मश्चामिषसन्निभः ।
हिरण्याक्षस्तु[38]हेमाभः पञ्चैते समुदाहृताः ॥ ६३ ॥

There are five varieties of *guggulu*. They are *mahiṣākṣa*, *mahānīla*, *kumuda*, *padma* and *hiraṇya*. *Mahiṣākṣa* variety has the colour of either *bhṛnga* or *añjana*. *Mahānīla* is extremely blue in colour. *Kumuda* variety has the colour of a *kumuda* flower i.e. white. *Padma* variety of *guggulu* looks red like flesh. *Hiraṇākṣa* looks like gold. Thus all the five varieties of *guggulu* are illustrated.

[39]महिषाक्षो महानीलो गजेन्द्राणां हितावुभौ ।
[भावप्रकाशः पूर्वखण्डः तृतीय कर्पूरादिवर्ग ३३-३६]
हयानां कुमुदः [40]पद्मः स्वस्त्यारोग्यकरौ परौ ॥ ६४ ॥
विशेषेण मनुष्याणां कनकः परिकीर्त्तितः ।

41
कदाचिन्महिषाक्षस्तु मतः कैश्चिन्नृणामपि ॥ ६५ ॥

*Mahiṣākṣa* and *mahānīla*—these two varieties of *guggulu* are useful in the treatment of elephants. *Kumuda* and *padma* varieties are useful in the treatment of horses. *Kanaka* variety is specifically indicated for human beings. According to some scholars *mahiṣākṣa* is also useful for the treatment of human beings.

गुग्गुलुर्विशदस्तिक्तो वीर्योष्णः पित्तलः सरः ।
42
कषायः कटुकः पाके कटुरूक्षो लघुः परम् ॥ ६६ ॥
भग्नसंधानकृद्वृष्यः सूक्ष्मः स्वर्यो रसायनः ।
दीपनः पिच्छिलो बल्यः कफवातव्रणापचीः ॥ ६७ ॥
मेदो मेहांश्च वातास्रक्लेदकुष्ठाममारुतान् ।
पिडिकाग्रन्थिशोफार्शोगण्डमालाकृमीञ्जयेत् ॥६८ ॥

*Guggulu* is *viśada* (non-slimy), *tikta* (bitter) and *uṣṇa vīrya* (hot in potency). It aggravates *pitta*. It is laxative and astringent in taste. It is pungent in *vipāka* as also in taste. It is ununctuous and extremely light. It heals fracture of bones. It is *vṛṣya* (aphrodisiac), *sūkṣma* (subtle), *svarya* (promoter of voice), *rasāyana* (rejuvenator), *dīpana* (digestive stimulant), *picchila* (slimy) and *balya* (promoter of strength). It alleviates aggravated *kapha* and *vāta*. It cures *vraṇa* (ulcer), *apacī* (cervical adenitis), *meda* (adiposity), *meha* (obstinate urinary disorders including diabetes), *vatāsra* (gout), *kleda* (appearance of sticky material in excess in the body), *kuṣṭha* (obstinate skin diseases including leprosy), *āma māruta* (rheumatism), *piḍikā* (pimples), *granthi* (adenitis), *śopha* (oedema), *arśas* (piles), *gaṇḍamālā* (enlarged cervical glands) and *kṛmi* (parasitic infection).

माधुर्याच्छमयेद्वातं कषायत्वाच्च पित्तहा ।
तिक्तत्वात्कफजित्तेन गुग्गुलुः सर्वदोषहा ॥६९ ॥
[भावप्रकाशः पूर्वखण्डः तृतीय कर्पूरादिवर्ग ३६—४१]

Because of its sweet taste it alleviates *vāta. Pitta* is alleviated by its astringent taste. It alleviates *kapha* because of its bitter taste. Thus, all the three *doṣas* are alleviated by *guggulu*.

स नवो बृंहणो वृष्यः पुराणस्त्वतिलेखनः ।

स्निग्धः काञ्चनसङ्काशः पक्वजम्बूफलोपमः ।। ७० ।।

नूतनो गुग्गुलुः प्रोक्तः सुगन्धि यस्तु पिच्छिलः ।

शुष्को दुर्गन्धकश्चैव त्यक्तप्रकृतिवर्णकः ।। ७१ ।।

पुराणः स तु विज्ञेयो गुग्गुलुर्वीर्यवर्जितः ।

Fresh *guggulu* is *bṛṁhaṇa* (nourishing) and *vṛṣya* (aphrodisiac). Old *guggulu* is extremely depleting (*lekhana*).

Fresh *guggulu* is unctuous. It is golden in colour and it looks like a ripe fruit of *jambu.* It has fragrance and it is slimy. Old *guggulu* on the other hand emits a foul smell and it is devoid of its natural colour. Old *guggulu* does not possess the required potency.

अम्लं तीक्ष्णमजीर्णं च व्यवायं श्रममातपम् ।। ७२ ।।

मद्यं रोषं त्यजेत्सम्यक् गुणार्थी पुरसेवकः ।

The patient who is using *guggulu* should refrain from sour things, sharp things, things that are indigestible, sexual act, exhaustion, exposure to sun, alcoholic drinks and anger if he desires to have the prescribed therapeutic effects of this drug.

**श्रीवासो** मधुरस्तिक्तः स्निग्धोष्णस्तुवरः[43] सरः ।।७३।।

पित्तलो[44] वातमूर्धाक्षिस्वररुक्कफपीनसान् ।

रक्षोऽश्रीस्वेददौर्गन्ध्ययूकाकण्डूव्रणप्रणुत् ।। ७४ ।।

[भावप्रकाशः पूर्वखण्डः तृतीय कर्पूरादिवर्ग ४२-४७]

**Śrīvāsa (Pinus roxburghii Sargent)**

*Śrīvāsa* is sweet and bitter in taste, unctuous, hot, saline and laxative. It aggravates *pitta*. It cures aggravated *vāta*, diseases of head, eyes and voice, aggravated *kapha*, *pīnasa* (chronic sinusitis), attacks by evil spirits (*rakṣas*), unauspiciousness, excessive sweating, foul smell of the body, lice (*yūkā*), itching and ulcer.

यदाऽमृतं वैनतेयो जहार सुरसत्तमात् ।

तदा ततोऽपतद् बिन्दुः स **रसोनो** ऽभवद्भुवि ।। ७५ ।।

पञ्चभिश्च रसैर्युक्तो रसेनाम्लेन वर्जितः ।

45

तस्माद्रसोन इत्युक्तो द्रव्यनिश्चयकारकैः ।। ७६ ।।

कटुकश्चापि मूलेषु तिक्तः पत्रेषु संस्थितः ।

नाले कषाय उद्दिष्टो नालाग्रे लवणः स्मृतः ।। ७७ ।।

बीजे तु मधुरः प्रोक्तो रसस्तद्गुणवेदिभिः ।

*Rasona* **(Allium sativum Linn.)**

When *Garuḍa* took *amṛta* from *Indra*, then a drop of it fell down on the earth and *rasona* came out of it. According to scholars who are experts in the determination of various aspects of drugs, it is called '*rasona*' because it has five *rasas* (tastes) and it is devoid (*una*) of one *rasa* (taste) i.e. *amla* (sour). Pungent taste resides in its root (*bulb*); bitter taste in the leaf, astringent taste in the stem, saline taste at the top of the stem and sweet taste in the seed.

रसोनो बृंहणो वृष्यः स्निग्धोष्णः पाचनः सरः ।। ७८ ।।

रसे पाके च कटुकस्तीक्ष्णो मधुरको मतः ।

भग्नसन्धानकृत्कंठ्यो गुरुः पित्तास्रवृद्धिदः ।। ७९ ।

बलवर्णकरो मेधाहितो नेत्र्यो रसायनः ।

हृद्रोगजीर्णज्वरकुक्षिशूलविबन्धगुल्मारुचिकासशोफान् ॥८०॥

[भावप्रकाशः पूर्वखण्डः द्वितीय हरीतक्यादिवर्ग २२०—२२५]

दुर्नामकुष्ठानलसादजन्तुसमीरणश्वासकफांश्च हन्ति ।

*Rasona* is *bṛṁhaṇa* (nourishing), *vṛṣya* (aphrodisiac), unctuous, hot, carminative and laxative. In taste and *vipāka* it is pungent. It is sharp in property and sweet. It helps in the healing of fracture. It is good for throat and heavy. It aggravates *pitta* and blood. It promotes strength, complexion, intellect and eyesight. It is rejuvenating. It cures *hṛdroga* (heart disease), *jīrṇa jvara* (chronic fever), *kukṣi śūla* (colic pain in the pelvic region), *vibandha* (constipation), *gulma* (phantom tumour), *aruci* (anorexia), *kāsa* (coughing), *śopha* (oedema), *durnāman* (piles), *kuṣṭha* (obstinate skin diseases including leprosy), *anala sāda* (suppression of the power of digestion), *jantu* (parasitic infection), *samīraṇa* (aggravated *vāyu*), *śvāsa* (asthma) and aggravated *kapha*.

मद्यं मांसं तथाम्लं च हितं [46] लशुनसेविनः ॥ ८१ ॥

**Diet**

Alcoholic drink, meat and sour things are useful for a person using *rasona*.

व्यायाममातपं रोषमतिनीरं पयो गुडम् ।

रसोनमश्नन् पुरुषस्त्यजेदेतान्निरन्तरम्"[47] ॥ ८२ ॥

[भावप्रकाशः पूर्वखण्डः द्वितीय हरीतक्यादिवर्ग २२५—२२६]

**Prohibitions**

A person using *rasona* should avoid exercise, exposure to sun, anger, water in excess, milk and *guḍa* (jaggery).

पत्रे सक्षारमधुरो मध्ये मधुरपिच्छिलः ।

तीक्ष्णोष्णो लसुनः कंदः कटुपाकरसः सरः ॥ ८३ ॥

हृद्यः केश्यो गुरुर्वृष्यः स्निग्धो दीपनरोचनः ।

भग्नसंधानकृद्बल्यो रक्तपित्तप्रदूषणः ॥ ८४ ॥

किलास-कुष्ठ-गुल्मार्शोमेह-कृमि-कफानिलान् ।

सहिध्मापीनसश्वासकासान् हन्ति रसायनः[48]" ॥८५॥

[माधवद्रव्यगुणः विविधौषधिवर्गः ३७—३९]

Its leaf is alkaline and sweet; its stem is sweet and slimy and its bulb is sharp, hot, pungent both in taste and *vipāka* and laxative. *Lasuna* is *hṛdya* (cardiac tonic), *keśya* (promoter of hair), heavy, *vṛṣya* (aphrodisiac), unctuous, *dīpana* (digestive stimulant), *rocana* (appetiser), *bhagna sandhāna kṛt* (healer of fracture) and *balya* (strength promoting). It vitiates blood and *pitta*. It cures *kilāsa* (leucoderma), *kuṣṭha* (obstinate skin diseases including leprosy), *gulma* (phantom tumour), *arśas* (piles), *meha* (obstinate urinary disorders including diabetes), *kṛmi* (parasitic infection), aggravated *kapha* and *vāyu*, *hidhmā* (hiccup), *pīnasa* (chronic sinusitis), *śvāsa* (asthma) and *kāsa* (coughing). It is *rasāyana* (rejuvenating).

'पलाण्डुस्तद्गुणैस्तुल्यः कफहृन्नातिपित्तलः ।

अनुष्णः केवलं [वा] तं[49] स्वादुपाकरसो जयेत्[50]' ॥८६॥

***Palāṇḍu* (Allium cepa Linn.)**

*Palāṇḍu* has properties similar to those of *rasona*. It alleviates *kapha* but does not aggravate *pitta* in excess. It is not very hot. It alleviates *vāta* (which is not combined with other aggravated *doṣas*). It is sweet in *vipāka* and taste.

'पलांडुर्मधुरो वृष्यः कटुः स्निग्धोऽनिलापहः ।

बल्यः पित्ताविरोधी च कफहृद्[51]रोचनो गुरुः[52]' ॥ ८७ ॥

[माधवद्रव्यगुणः विविधौषधिवर्गः ८०]

*Palāṇḍu* is sweet, aphrodisiac, pungent and unctuous. It alleviates *vāyu*. It promotes strength and does not aggravate *pitta*. It alleviates *kapha*. It is an appetiser and heavy.

तीक्ष्णो गृंजनको ग्राही ग्रहण्यर्शोविकारनुत् ।

53
पुष्पाणि कफवातघ्नान्येतान्येषां फलानि च ॥ ८८ ॥

*Gṛñjanaka* **(Daucus carota Linn.)**

*Gṛñjanaka* is sharp and constipative. It cures *grahaṇī* (sprue syndrome) and *arśas* (piles). Its flowers and fruits alleviate *kapha* and *vāta*.

'कफानिलहरं स्वर्यं विबन्धानाहशूलनुत् ।
कटूष्णं रोचनं वृष्यं हृद्यं चैवार्द्रकं स्मृतम्' ॥ ८९ ॥
[सुश्रुत: सूत्र ४६ : २२७]

*Ārdraka* **(Zingiber officinale Rosc.)**

*Ārdraka* alleviates *kāpha* and *vāyu*. It promotes good voice. It cures *vibandha* (constipation), *ānāha* (obstruction to the movement of wind in the stomach) and *śūla* (colic pain). It is pungent, hot, appetiser, aphrodisiac and cardiac tonic.

54
वातश्लेष्मविबन्धेषु रसस्तस्योपदिश्यते ।

The juice of *ārdraka* is indicated in constipation caused by *vāyu* and *kapha*.

आर्द्रिका तिक्तमधुरा मूत्रला रक्तपित्तहृत् ॥ ९० ॥

*Ardrikā* (small variety of *ārdraka*) is bitter and sweet in taste. It is *mūtrala* (diuretic) and it cures *raktapitta* (a disease characterised by bleeding from different parts of the body).

"गुडार्द्रकं वातहरं चक्षुष्यं पित्तनाशनम् ।
क्षतघ्नं चैव वृष्यं च वर्चोभेदि कफापहम् ॥ ९१ ॥

*Guḍa* (jaggery) and *ārdraka*, taken together, alleviate *vāyu*. It promotes eye sight and alleviates *pitta*. It is *kṣataghna* (cures consumption), *vṛṣya* (aphrodisiac), purgative and *kaphāpaha* (alleviator of *kapha*).

चक्षुष्यं रोचनं स्वर्यं विपाके मधुरं सरम् ।
स्तम्भाटोपानिलघ्नं च कर्षणं लवणार्द्रकम् ॥ ९२ ॥

'भोजनाग्रे सदा पथ्यं लवणार्द्रकभक्षणम् ।

*Lavaṇa* (rock salt) and *ārdraka*, taken together, promote eyesight. It is appetiser and promoter of voice. It is sweet in *vipāka* and laxative. It cures *stambha* (rigidity), *āṭopa* (gurgling sound in the stomach) and aggravated *vāyu.* It is depleting (*karṣaṇa*). It is always useful to take salt and *ārdraka* before food.

कुष्ठे पाण्ड्वामये कृच्छ्रे रक्तपित्ते ज्वरे व्रणे ।
दाहे[55] शरन्निदाघे च नैव पूजितमार्द्रकम् ॥' ६३ ॥

[भावप्रकाश : पूर्वखण्ड: द्वितीय हरीतक्यादिवर्ग: ५२—५३]

**Contra-indications**

*Ārdraka* should not be taken by a patient suffering from *kuṣṭha* (obstinate skin diseases including leprosy), *pāṇḍu* (anemia), *kṛcchra* (dysuria), *raktapitta* (a disease characterised by bleeding from different parts of the body), *jvara* (fever), *vraṇa* (ulcer) and *dāha* (burning syndrome). It is contra-indicated in autumn and summer.

आर्द्रकं कृष्णलवणं रामठेन समन्वितम्[56]" ।
"रोचनं कफवातघ्नं [57][शूलघ्नं] जवणं तथा" ॥६४॥

*Ārdraka* and *kṛṣṇa lavaṇa* mixed with rock salt are appetiser. It alleviates *kapha* and *vāta* and colic pain and promotes digestion.

'नागरं कफवातघ्नं विपाके मधुरं कटु ।
वृष्योष्णं रोचनं हृद्यं सस्नेहं लघु दीपनम् ॥ ६५ ॥

[सुश्रुत: सूत्र ८६ : २२६]

*Nāgara* **(Zingiber officinalis Rosc.)**

*Nāgara* alleviates *kapha* and *vāta*. In *vipāka* it is sweet and it is pungent in taste. It is aphrodisiac, hot, appetiser, cardiac tonic, unctuous, light and digestive stimulant,

'विबन्धभेदिनी या च सा कथं ग्राहिणी भवेत् ।

58

शक्तिर्विबन्धभेदे स्याद् यतो न मलपातने" ॥ ६६ ॥

[भावप्रकाशः प्रथमखण्डः द्वितीय हरीतक्यादिवर्ग : ४६]

How can a drug which cures constipation also becomes a cure for diarrhoea ? It is because of its *prabhāva* or specific action by which it relieves constipation but does not cause diarrhoea and thus works as a remedy even for the latter.

स्निग्धोष्णा मधुरा वृष्या कटुका दीपनी सरा ।

**पिप्पली** मारुतश्लेष्मकासश्वासांश्च नाशयेत् ॥ ६७ ॥

"विबन्धश्वासशूलामवातकासघ्नं पाचनम् ।

वमिश्लीपदशोफार्शो हन्ति ग्राही जलांशहृत् ।

'कुष्ठप्रमेहगुल्मार्शः प्लीहशूलाममारुतान् ॥ ६८ ॥

[भावप्रकाशः पूर्वखण्डः द्वितीय हरीतक्यादि वर्ग ५६]

59

हन्तिज्वरोदरहरी सरा लघु रसायनी" ।

*Pippalī* **(Piper longum Linn.)**

*Pippalī* is unctuous, hot, sweet, aphrodisiac, pungent, digestive stimulant and laxative. It cures aggravated *vāyu* and *kapha*, *kāsa* (coughing) *śvāsa* (asthma) *vibandha* (constipation), *śūla* (colic pain) and *āmavāta* (rheumatism). It is carminative. It also cures *vami* (vomiting), *ślīpada* (filaria), *śopha* (oeḍema) and *arśas* (piles). It works as a constipative by absorbing water from the colon. *Kuṣṭha* (obstinate skin diseases including leprosy), *prameha* (obstinate urinary disorders including diabetes), *gulma* (phantom tumour), *plīhā* (splenic disorder), *jvara* (fever) and *udara* (obstinate abdominal diseases including ascitis) are also cured by the use of this drug. It is light and rejuvenating.

श्लेष्मला स्वादु शीतार्द्रा गुर्वी स्निग्धा च पिप्पली ॥६६॥

Green *pippalī* aggravates *kapha*. It is sweet, cooling, heavy and unctuous.

भेदनं **पिप्पलीमूलं** दीपनं कृमिनाशनम् ।

The root of *pippalī* is purgative, and digestive stimulant. It cures *kṛmi* (parasitic infection).

पित्तप्रकोपी तीक्ष्णोष्णं रूक्षं [60]दीपनपाचनम् ॥ १०० ॥

रसे पाके कटु [61]श्लेष्मवातघ्नं **मरिचं** लघु ।

*Marica* **(Piper nigrum Linn.)**

*Marica* aggravates *pitta*. It is sharp, hot, unctuous, digestive stimulant and carminative. It is pungent both in taste and *vipāka*. It alleviates *kapha* and *vāyu* and is light.

स्वादु पाक्याद्रं मरिचं गुरु श्लेष्मप्रसेकि च ॥ १०१ ॥

Green *marica* is sweet in *vipāka* and heavy. It eliminates *kapha*.

'नात्युष्णं नातिशीतं च वीर्यतो **मरिचं** [62]**सितम्**' ।

White variety of *marica* is neither hot nor cold in potency.

[63]कटूष्णं लघु चक्षुष्यमवृष्यं कफवातजित् ॥ १०२ ॥

**त्र्यूषणं** कासमेदोघ्नं मेहकुष्ठत्वगामयान् ।

निहन्याद्दीपनं गुल्मपीनसाग्न्यल्पतामपि ॥ १०३ ॥

*Tryūṣaṇa*

*Śuṇṭhī*, *pippalī* and *marica* taken together are called *tryūṣaṇa*. It is pungent, hot and light. It promotes eye sight. It is not an aphrodisiac. It alleviates *kapha* and *vāta*. It cures *kāsa* (coughing), *medas* (adiposity), *meha* (obstinate urinary disorders including diabetes), *kuṣṭha* (obstinate skin diseases including leprosy) and *tvagāmaya* (skin diseases). It is digestive stimulant. It also cures *gulma* (phantom tumour), *pipāsā* (morbid thirst) and *agnyalpatā* (suppression of the power of digestion.

**चविकागजपिप्पलौ** पिप्पलीमूलवत्स्मृतौ ।
तयोर्निःस्यंदिनी ज्ञेया विशेषाद्**गजपिप्पली**॥ १०४ ॥

*Cavikā* & *Gajapippalī* **(Piper chaba Hunter & Scindapsus officinalis Schott.)**

*Cavikā* and *gaja pippalī* are like the root of *pippalī* in their properties. *Gaja pippalī* is more expectorant than *cavikā*.

**पञ्चकोलं** कफानाहगुल्मशूलारुचीर्जयेत् ।
मरिचेन युतं तत्तु षडूषणमुदीरितम् ॥ १०५ ॥

*Pañcakola* **and** *Ṣaḍūṣaṇa*

*Pippalī*, *pippalī mūla*, *cavikā*, *citraka* and *nāgara*—these five drugs taken together are called *pañcakola*. It cures aggravated *kapha*, *ānāha* (obstruction to the movement of wind in the stomach), *gulma* (phantom tumour), *śūla* (colic pain) and *arucī* (anorexia).

These above mentioned five drugs along with *marica* are called *ṣaḍūṣaṇa*.

64
'**जलपिप्पलिका** हृद्या चक्षुष्या शुक्रला लघुः ।
65
संग्राहिणी हिमारूक्षा रक्तपित्तज्वरापहा' ॥ १०६ ॥

*Jala pippalī* **(Lippia nodiflora Mich.)**

*Jala pippalī* is *hṛdya* (cardiac tonic), *cakṣuṣya* (promoter of eyesight), *śukrala* (spermatopoetic), *laghu* (light) *saṁgrāhiṇī* (constipative), *hima* (cooling) and *rukṣa* (ununctuous). It cures *raktapitta* (a disease characterised by bleeding from different parts of the body) and *jvara* (fever).

66
'लघुष्णं पाचनं हिंगु दीपनं कफवातनुत् ।
67
स्निग्धं तीक्ष्णं कटुरसं शूलाजीर्णविबन्धनुत्" ॥१०७॥

[सुश्रुतः सूत्र ८६ : २२८]

68
'**कृमिगुल्मोदरानाहशूलाजीर्णविबन्धनुत्**' ।

[69] [70]
'लघूष्णं कटुकं पाके रुच्यं पित्ताग्निदीपनम् ॥ १०८ ॥

*Hiṅgu* **(Ferula foetida Regel.)**

*Hiṅgu* is light, hot, carminative and digestive stimulant. It alleviates *kapha* and *vāta*. It is unctuous, sharp and pungent in taste. It cures colic pain, indigestion, constipation, *kṛmi* (parasitic infection), *gulma* (phantom tumour), *udara* (obstinate abdominal diseases including ascitis) and *ānāha* (obstruction to the movement of wind in abdomen). It is pungent in *vipāka* and appetiser. It aggravates *pitta*.

कटु श्लेष्मानिलहरं गन्धाढ्यं **जीरकद्वयम्** ॥ १०९ ॥

[सुश्रुतः सूत्र ४६ : २२९]

"ग्राहि रूक्षं मेध्यं वृष्यं चक्षुष्यं छर्दिगुल्मनुत् ।
[71]
आध्मानहृत्पाचनं च गर्भाशयविशुद्धिकृत्" ॥ ११० ॥

*Jīraka* **(Cuminuṃ cyminum Linn.)**

Both the types of *jīrā* are pungent. They alleviate *kapha* and *vāyu*. They are full of aroma. They are constipative, ununctuous, promoter of memory, aphrodisiac and promoter of eyesight. They cure *chardi* (vomiting), *gulma* (phantom tumour) and *ādhmāna* (tymphanitis). They are carminative and they help in the cleansing of the uterus.

**कारवी** श्लेष्मवातघ्नी तद्वज्ज्ञेयोप**कुंचिका** ।

*Kāravī* **and** *Upakuñcikā* **(Carum carvi Linn. and Nigella sativum Linn.)**

*Kāravī* alleviates *kapha* and *vāta*. *Upakuñcikā* has similar properties.

**वाष्पिका** कटुतीक्ष्णोष्णा क्रिमिश्लेष्महरि सरा ॥१११॥

*Vāṣpikā* **(Carum bulbocastanum Koch)**

*Vāṣpikā* is pungent, sharp and hot. It cures *kṛmi* parasitic infection) and aggravated *kapha*. It is laxative.

तद्वच्च **राजिका** रुच्या दीपनी कोष्ठशूलनुत् ।

***Rājikā* (Brassica nigra Koch).**

Similarly *rājikā* is appetiser and digestive stimulant. It cures colic pain in the abdomen.

[72]यवानी पित्तला कुष्ठ-कृमि-वातकफापहा ॥ ११२ ॥

***Yavānī* (Trachyspermum ammi Sprague)**

*Yavānī* aggravates *pitta*. It cures *kuṣṭha* (obstinate skin diseases including leprosy), *kṛmi* (parasitic infection) and aggravated *vāyu* as well as *kapha*.

“छिछिका शीतली कुष्ठ-कृमि-[73]वातकफापहा” ।

***Chichikā***

*Chichikā* is cooling. It cures *kuṣṭha* (obstinate skin diseases including leprosy), *kṛmi* (parasitic infection) and aggravated *vāta* as well as *kapha*.

पुंस्त्वघ्नः कटुतीक्ष्णोष्णो [74]भुस्तृणो वक्त्रशोधनः ॥११३॥

***Bhūstṛṇa* (Cymbopogon martini Wats.)**

*Bhūstṛṇa* causes impotency. It is pungent, sharp and hot. It cleanses the mouth.

खराह्वा कफवातघ्नी [75]वस्तिरोगरुजापहा ।”

***Kharāhvā* (Apium graveolens Linn.)**

*Kharāhvā* alleviates *kapha* and *vāyu*. It alleviates diseases of the bladder and pain.

कषायं तिक्तमधुरं हृद्यं दीपनरोचनम् ॥ ११४ ॥
धान्यकं कासतृट्छर्दिः शमनं चक्षुषोर्हितम् ।

***Dhānyaka* (Coriandrum sativum Linn.)**

*Dhānyaka* is astringent, bitter and sweet in taste, cardiac tonic, digestive stimulant and carminative. It cures *kāsa* (coughing), *tṛṭ* (morbid thirst) and *chardi* (vomiting). It is useful for eyes.

76

"भव्यभोजनभोज्येषु विविधेष्ववचारिता ॥ ११५ ॥

**आर्द्रा कुस्तुंबरी** कुर्यात्स्वादुसौगन्ध्यहृद्यताम् ।

Green *kustumbarī (dhānyaka)*, when used in different ways, imparts good taste, fragrance and cardiac tonic property to various excellent types of eatables.

सा शुष्का मधुरा पाके स्निग्धा तृट्दाहनाशिनी ॥११६॥

77

दोषघ्नी कटुका किञ्चित् तिक्ता स्रोतोविशोधनी ।"

The dried *kustumbarī* is sweet in *vipāka* and unctuous. It cures *tṛṭ* (morbid thirst), *dāha* (burning syndrome) and aggravated *doṣas*. It is slightly pungent and bitter. It cleanses the channels of circulation.

**जम्बीरः** पाचनस्तीक्ष्णः कृमिवातकफापहः ॥ ११७ ॥

[सुश्रुतः सूत्र ४६ : २३०-२३२]

*Jambīra* **(Citrus limon Burm. f.)**

*Jambīra* is carminative and sharp. It cures *kṛmi* (parasitic infection) and aggravated *vāta* and *kapha*.

78

'**भंगा** कफहरा तिक्ता ग्राहिणी दीपनी लघुः ।

79

तीक्ष्णोष्णा पित्तला मोहमदकृद्वाग्विवर्धिनी' ॥११८॥

[धन्वन्तरिनिघण्टुः गुडूच्यादि प्रथमवर्ग १३१]

*Bhaṅgā* **(Cannabis sativa Linn.)**

*Bhaṅgā* alleviates *kapha*. It is bitter, constipative, digestive stimulant, light, sharp and hot. It aggravates *pitta*. It causes unconsciousness, intoxication and talkativeness.

80

**सुरभिर्दीपनो** रुच्यो मुखवैशद्यकारकः ।

[सुश्रुतः सूत्र ४६ : २३३]

पार्श्वशूलारुचिश्वासकासहिक्कानिलापहः ॥ ११९ ॥

*Surabhi*

*Surabhi* is digestive stimulant and appetiser. It causes non-sliminess (freshness) in mouth. It cures *pārśva sūla* (pain in the sides of chest), *aruci* (anorexia), *śvāsa* (asthma), *kāsa* (coughing) and aggravated *vāyu*.

**तुम्बरुः** पित्तकृद्वातकृमिदौर्गन्ध्यनाशनः ।

*Tumburu* **(Zanthoxylum alatum Roxb.)**

*Tumburu* aggravates *pitta*. It alleviates aggravated *vāyu*. It cures *kṛmi* (parasitic infection) and *daurgandhya* (foul smell coming out of the body).

'**वर्वरी** त्रितयं रूक्षं सरं कटुविदाहि च ।। १२० ।।
81
पित्तलं कफवातास्रदद्रूकृमिविषापहम् ।'

*Varvarī*

Three varieties of *varvarī* are ununctuous, laxative, pungent, *vidāhi* (causing burning sensation). They aggravate *pitta* and alleviate *kapha*, *vāta* as well as vitiated blood. They cure *dadrū* (ring worm), *kṛmi* (parasitic infection) and *viṣa* (poisoning).

शोथविद्रधिगंडघ्नी **कृष्णगन्धा** कफापहा ।। १२१ ।।

*Kṛṣṇagandhā* **(a variety of** *Śigru***)**

*Kṛṣṇagandhā* cures *śotha*, (oedema), *vidradhi* (abscess) and *gaṇḍa* (goitre). It alleviates *kapha*.

82
'**शिग्रुस्तीक्ष्णा** लघुर्ग्राही वह्निकृत्कफवातजित् ।'

*Śigru* **(Moringa pterigosperma Gaertn.)**

*Śigru* is sharp, light, constipative and digestive stimulant. It alleviates *kapha* and *vāta*.

**मधुशिग्रुः** सरस्तिक्तः शोथघ्नो दीपनः कटुः ।। १२२ ।।

*Madhu śigru* **(a variety of** *Śigru***)**

*Madhu śigru* is laxative and bitter (?). It alleviates *śotha* (oedema) and stimulates digestion. It is pungent.

उष्णोश्मरिहरो भेदी **वरुणो**ऽनिलशूलहृत् ।

*Varuṇa* **(Crataeva nurvula Buch. Ham.)**

*Varuṇa* is hot. It cures *aśmari* (stone in urinary tract), It is purgative. It alleviates aggravated *vāyu* and *śūla* (colic pain).

**पारिभद्रो**ऽनिलश्लेष्मशोथमेहकृमीन् जयेत् ॥ १२३ ॥

*Pāribhadra* **(Erythrina variegata Linn.)**

*Pāribhadra* cures aggravated *vāyu* and *kapha*, *śotha* (oedema), *meha* (obstinate urinary diseases including diabetes) and *kṛmi* (parasitic infection).

**बिल्वमूलं** मरुत्श्लेष्मछर्दिघ्नं न च पित्तकृत् ।

*Bilva* **(Aegle marmelos Corr.)**

The root of *bilva* alleviates *vāyu* and *kapha*. It cures *chardi* (vomiting) and it does not aggravate *pitta*.

83

**पाटला** कफवातघ्नी कट्वंशा ग्राहि दीपनीम् ॥१२४॥

*Pāṭalā* **(Stereospermum suaveolens DC.)**

*Pāṭalā* alleviates *kapha* and *vāta*. It is slightly pungent. It is constipative and digestive stimulant.

कषाया मधुरा तिक्ता **काश्मरी** च कफापहा ।

*Kāśmarī* **(Gmelina arborea Linn.)**

*Kāśmarī* is astringent, sweet and bitter. It alleviates *kapha*.

**शोथनुद्वह्निमन्थाश्च** हितो वातविकारिणाम् ॥१२५॥

*Vahnimantha* **(Clerodendrum phlomidis Linn. f.)**

*Vahnimantha* alleviates *śotha* (oedema) and it is useful for patients suffering from diseases caused by *vāyu*.

**एरण्डमूलं** शूलघ्नं वृष्यं वातहरं परम् ।

*Eraṇḍa* **(Ricinus communis Linn.)**

The root of *eraṇḍa* cures *śūla* (colic pain). It is aphrodisiac and is an excellent alleviator of *vāyu.*

**वृष्यस्त्रिकण्टको** बल्यो वातघ्नो मूत्रकृच्छ्रजित् ॥१२६॥

*Trikaṇṭaka* **(Tribulus terrestris Linn.)**

*Trikaṇṭaka* is aphrodisiac, strength promoter and alleviator of *vāyu.* It cures *mūtrakṛcchra* (dysuria).

उष्णा वातकफश्वासकासघ्नी **कंटकारिका** ।

*Kaṇṭakārikā* **(Solanum xanthocarpum Schrad & Wendle.)**

*Kaṇṭakārikā* is hot. It alleviates *vāyu* and *kapha.* It cures *śvāsa* (asthma) and *kāsa* (bronchitis).

पाचिनी ग्राहिणी सोष्णा वातघ्नी **बृहती** तथा ॥१२७॥

*Bṛhatī* **(Solanum indicum Linn.)**

*Bṛhatī* is carminative, constipative, hot, and alleviator of *vāyu.*

**पृश्निपर्णी स्थिरा** चैव पित्तश्लेष्मातिसारिणाम् ।

पानभोजनसंस्कारे शस्यते वातभूयसाम् ॥ १२८ ॥

*Pṛśniparṇī and Sthirā* **(Uraria picta Desv. & Desmodium gangeticum DC.)**

*Pṛśniparṇī* and *sthirā* are very useful for patients suffering from diarrhoea caused by *pitta* and *kapha* and for patients dominated by vitiated *vāta.* Their food and drinks should be boiled along with these two drugs.

84

**जिंगिनी** व्रणहृद्रोगवातातीसारजित्कटुः ।

*Jiṅginī* **(Lannea grandis Engl.)**

*Jiṅginī* cures *vraṇa* (ulcer), *hṛdroga* (heart disease), aggravated *vāyu* and *atisāra* (diarrhoea). It is pungent.

उष्णस्तस्यास्तु निर्यासो नस्याद्वाहुव्यथापहः ॥१२९॥

The gum resin extracted from this plant is hot. If this is

given for inhalation (*nasya*), then it cures pain in the arm.

वातपित्तापहं ग्राहि वृष्यं बल्यं **बलात्रयम्** ।

*Balā* **(Sida cordifolia Linn.)**

There are three varieties of *balā*. They alleviate *vāyu* and *pitta*. They are constipative and aphrodisiac.

85

स्निग्धं मधुरमायुष्यं **महती** मूत्रकृच्छ्रनुत् ॥ १३० ॥

*Mahābalā* **(Sida rhombifolia Linn.)**

*Mahābalā* is unctuous, sweet and promoter of longevity. It cures *mūtrakṛcchra* (dysuria).

क्षतक्षीणहितायुष्या वृष्या **नागबला**धिकम् ।

*Nāgabalā* **(Grewia populifolia Vahl.)**

*Nāgabalā* is specially useful for patients suffering from *kṣata kṣīṇa* (consumption). It promotes longevity and is aphrodisiac.

**बल्याश्वगन्धा** वातघ्नी कासश्वासक्षये हिता ॥१३१॥

*Aśvagandhā* **(Withania somnifera Dunal.)**

*Aśvagandhā* promotes strength, and alleviates *vāyu*. It is useful in *kāsa* (bronchitis), *śvāsa* (asthma) and *kṣaya* (phthisis).

**माषपर्णी** महावृष्या चक्षुष्या **मुद्गपर्णिका** ।

*Māṣaparṇī* & *Mudga parṇī* **(Teramnus labialis Spreng. & Phaseolus trilobus Ait.)**

*Māṣa parṇī* is exceedingly aphrodisiac. *Mudga parṇī* promotes eye sight.

**ऋद्धिर्बल्या** त्रिदोषघ्नी शुक्रला मधुरा गुरुः ॥ १३२ ॥

*Ṛddhi*

*Ṛddhi* promotes strength. It alleviates all the three *doṣas*. It is spermatopoetic (*śukrala*), sweet and heavy.

**वृद्धिर्गर्भप्रदा** शीता वृष्या कासक्षयापहा ।

*Vṛddhi*

*Vṛddhi* helps in conception (*garbhaprada*). It is cooling and aphrodisiac. It cures *kāsa* (bronchitis), and *kṣaya* (consumption).

**काकोलीयुगलं** शीतं शुक्रलं मधुरं गुरु ॥ १३३ ॥

86

जयेत्समीरदाहास्रपित्त-शोष-विष-ज्वरान् ।

*Kākolī*

*Kākolī* has two varieties. Both of them are cooling, spermatopoetic (*śukrala*), sweet and heavy. They cure aggravated *vāyu*, *dāha* (burning syndrome), *asrapitta* (a disease characterised by bleeding from different parts of the body), *śoṣa* (consumption), *viṣa* (poisoning) and *jvara* (fever).

**मेदायुग्मं** गुरुस्वादुवृष्यं स्तन्यं कफापहम् ॥ १३४ ॥

बृंहणं शीतलं पित्तरक्तक्षयसमीरजित् ।

*Medā*

There are two varieties of *medā*. They are heavy, sweet, aphrodisiac and *stanya* (galactogogue). They alleviate *kapha*. They are *bṛṁhaṇa* (nourishing) and cooling. They alleviate *pitta*, blood, *kṣaya* (consumption) and *vāyu*.

**जीवकर्षभकौ** बल्यौ शीतौ शुक्रकफप्रदौ ॥१३५॥

हरतः पित्तदाहास्रकार्श्यशोषक्षयापहौ ।

*Jīvaka & Ṛṣabhaka*

*Jīvaka* and *ṛṣabhaka* are strength promoting, cooling and spermatopoetic. They aggravate *kapha*. They cure aggravated *pitta*, *dāha* (burning syndrome), vitiated blood, *kārśya* (emaciation), *śoṣa* (consumption) and *kṣaya* (phthisis).

87

**अष्टवर्गो**ऽष्टभिर्द्रव्यैरेतैः शीतोऽतिशुक्रलः ॥ १३६ ॥

बृंहणः पित्तदाहास्र—शोषघ्नः स्तन्यगर्भकृत् ।

*Aṣṭavarga*

*Ṛddhi*, *bṛddhi*, *kākolī*, *kṣīra kākolī*, *medā*, *mahāmedā*, *jīvaka* and *ṛṣabhaka*—these eight drugs, taken together, are known as *aṣṭavarga*. It is cooling, exceedingly spermatopoetic and nourishing. It alleviates aggravated *pitta*, *dāha* (burning syndrome), *asra* (vitiated blood) and *śoṣa* (consumption). It promotes lactation and conception.

विशाला कफवातघ्नी मेहकुष्ठहरी सरा ॥ १३७ ॥

*Viśālā* **(Trichosanthes bracteata Voigt)**

*Viśālā* alleviates *kapha* and *vāta*. It cures *meha* (obstinate urinary disorders including diabetes) and *kuṣṭha* (obstinate skin diseases including leprosy). It is laxative.

सारिवा वातपित्तास्रविषमज्वरनाशिनी ।

*Sārivā* **(Hemidesmus indicus R. Br.)**

*Sārivā* alleviates *vāta*, *pitta* and blood. It cures *viṣama jvara* (malarial fever).

88

गवादनी त्वक्शोषघ्नी शोफ-कुष्ठव्रणापहा ॥१३८॥

*Gavādanī*

*Gavādanī* cures *tvak śoṣa* (emaciation or dryness of skin), *śopha* (oedema), *kuṣṭha* (obstinate skin diseases including leprosy) and *vraṇa* (ulcer).

अनंता ग्राहिणी रक्तपित्तप्रशमनी हिमा ।

*Anantā* **(Cryptolepis buchanani Roem. and Schult.)**

*Anantā* is constipative. It cures *raktapitta* (a disease characterised by bleeding from different parts of the body). It is cooling.

चक्षुष्या मूत्रकृच्छ्रघ्नी गुन्द्रा पित्तास्रदाहनुत् ॥१३९॥

*Gundrā* **(Typha elephantina Roxb.)**

*Gundrā* promotes eyesight. It cures *mūtrakṛcchra* (dysuria), aggravated *pitta* and blood and *dāha* (burning syndrome).

लोध्रोऽसृक्कफपित्तघ्नश्चक्षुष्यः शोथजित्सरः ।

*Lodhra* **(Symplocos crataegoides Buch.—Ham.)**

*Lodhra* alleviates vitiated blood, *kapha* and *pitta*. It promotes eyesight and cures *śotha* (oedema). It is laxative.

तद्वत्सावररोध्रोऽपि चक्षुष्यो मृदुरेचनः ।। १४० ।।

*Sāvara Lodhra* **(Symplocos racemosa Roxb.)**

*Sāvara lodhra* shares the properties of *lodhra*. Besides, it promotes eyesight and is a mild purgative.

89

**मधुकं** रक्तपित्तघ्नं व्रणशोधनरोपणम् ।

गुरुः स्वादुहिमं वृष्यं चक्षुष्यं स्वरवर्णकृत् ।।१४१।।

*Madhuka* **(Glycyrrhiza glabra Linn.)**

*Madhuka* cures *rakta pitta* (a disease characterised by bleeding from different parts of the body). It cleanses and heals the ulcer (*vraṇa*). It is heavy, sweet, cooling, aphrodisiac and promoter of eyesight, voice and complexion.

**प्रपौण्डरीकं** चक्षुष्यं शिशिरं व्रणरोपणम् ।

*Prapauṇḍarīka*

*Prapauṇḍṛīka* promotes eye sight. It is cooling and it heals ulcer.

**मंजिष्ठा** कुष्ठवीसर्पशोथघ्नी वर्णदा परम् ।।१४२।।

*Mañjiṣṭhā* **(Rubia cordifolia Linn.)**

*Mañjiṣṭhā* cures *kuṣṭha* (obstinate skin diseases including leprosy), *visarpa* (erysipelas) and *śotha* (oedema). It is an excellent drug for the promotion of complexion.

**लाक्षा** भग्नविसर्पघ्नी वर्ण्या त्वगदोषनाशिनी ।

*Lākṣā* **(Lac)**

*Lākṣā* helps in the healing of fracture. It cures *visarpa* (erysipelas). It promotes complexion and cures skin diseases.

90

**मुशली** मधुरा वृष्या वीर्योष्णा बृंहणी गुरुः ।।१४३।।

तिक्ता रसायनी हन्ति गुदजान्यनिलं तथा ।

*Muśalī* **(Chlorophytum tuberosum Baker)**

*Muśalī* is sweet, aphrodisiac, hot in potency, *bṛṁhaṇī* (nourishing), heavy, bitter and rejuvenating. It cures *gudaja* (piles) and aggravated *vāyu.*

द्विधा **शतावरी** ज्ञेया कण्टकैरधरोत्तरैः ॥१४४॥

91

द्विविधा तु भवेद् ग्राह्या गुणैस्त्वेषां न संशयः ।

शीता कषाया मधुरा पथ्या वृष्या रसायनी ॥१४५॥

वातपित्तविबन्धघ्नी वर्णौजोबलवर्द्धिनी ।

*Śatāvarī* **(Asparagus racemosus Willd.)**

*Śatāvarī* is of two varieties. One variety has thorns below and the other has thorns above. Both of them are therapeutically useful and there should be no doubt about it. It is cooling, astringent, sweet, wholesome (*pathya*), aphrodisiac and rejuvenating. It cures aggravated *vāyu* and *pitta* as well as constipation. It promotes complexion, *ojas* (vital fluid?) and strength.

92

**पार्थः** पथ्यः क्षते भग्ने रक्तस्तम्भनवद्गुणैः ॥ १४६ ॥

*Pārtha* **(Terminalia arjuna W. & A.)**

*Pārtha* is useful in *kṣata* (phthisis), *bhagna* (fracture) and *raktastambhana* (coagulation of blood).

अस्थिभग्नेऽ**स्थिसंहारो** हितो बल्योऽनिलापहः ।

*Asthi saṁhāra* **(Cissus quadrangularis Linn.)**

*Asthi saṁhāra* is useful in *asthi bhagna* (fracture of bone). It promotes strength and alleviates *vāyu.*

चक्षुष्यो **मार्कवः** केश्यः कफपाण्ड्वामयापहः ॥१४७॥

*Mṅrkava* **(Eclipta alba Hassk.)**

*Mārkava* promotes eye sight and hair growth. It cures vitiation of *kapha* and *pāṇḍu* (anemia).

कफामकामलाशोथकृमिघ्नी **द्रोणपुष्पिका** ।

*Droṇapuṣpīkā* **(Leucas cephalotes Spreng.)**

*Droṇapuṣpīkā* cures aggravated *kapha*, *āma*, *kāmalā* (jaundice), *śotha* (oedema) and *kṛmi* (parasitic infection).

शोषघ्नी विशदा कण्ठ्या विषघ्नी **गिरिकर्णिका** ॥१४८॥

*Girikarṇikā* **(Clitoria ternatea Linn.)**

*Girikarṇikā* cures *śoṣa* (consumption). It is *viśada* (non-slimy). It is useful for throat and it cures *viṣa* (poisoning).

कासजिद्वातशमनी **वृश्चिकाली** विषापहा ।

*Vṛścikālī* **(Pergularia extensa N. E. Br.)**

*Vṛścikālī* cures *kāsa* (bronchitis), aggravated *vāyu and viṣa* (poisoning).

**दुग्धिकोष्णा** गुरुर्वृष्या वातला गर्भकारिणी ॥१४९॥

93

स्वादुर्विष्टंभिनी चैव कफकुष्ठकृमीन् जयेत् ।

*Dugdhikā* **(Euphorbia thymifolia Linn.)**

*Dugdhikā* is hot, heavy and aphrodisiac. It aggravates *vāyu* and promotes conception. It is sweet and constipative. It cures aggravated *kapha*, *kuṣṭha* (obstinate skin diseases including leprosy) and *kṛmi* (parasitic infection).

**अहिंस्रा** विषशोथघ्नी तद्गुणैव **सुदर्शना** ॥१५०॥

*Ahiṁsrā & Sudarśanā* **(Copparis sepiarin Linn. & Crinum) asiaticum Linn.)**

*Ahiṁsrā* cures *viṣa* (poisoning) and *śotha* (oedema). *Sudarśanā* has similar properties.

94

कासश्वासहरी **भार्गी गुंजा** कुष्ठव्रणापहा ।

*Bhārgī & Gujñā* **(Clerodendrum serratum Moon & Abrus precatorius Linn.)**

*Bhargī* cures *kāsa* (bronchitis) and *śvāsa* (asthma).

*Guñjā* cures *kuṣṭha* (obstinate skin diseases including

leprosy) and *vraṇa* (ulcer).

**जयन्ती** विषदोषघ्नी **सैरीयः** कफवातजित् ॥१५१॥

*Jayantī* & *Sairīya* (**Sesbania sesban Merr. & Barleria cristata Linn.**)

*Jayantī* cures *viṣadoṣa* (poisoning). *Sairīya* alleviates *kapha* and *vāta*.

वातरक्तहरी सोष्णा वृष्या बल्या **प्रसारिणी** ।

*Prasāriṇī* (**Paederia foetida Linn.**)

*Prasāriṇī* cures *vāta rakta* (gout). It is hot, aphrodisiac and strength promoting.

आमवातानिलास्रघ्नौ **कोकिलाक्ष-कुलाहलौ** ॥१५२॥

*Kokilākṣa* & *Kulāhala* (**Astercantha longifolia Nees & Blumea balsamifera DC.**)

*Kokilākṣa* and *Kulāhala* cure *āmavāta* (rheumatism) and *anilāsra* (gout).

**धुत्तू**रोमदवर्णाग्निवान्तिकृज्ज्वरकुष्ठनुत् ।
[95]
उष्णो गुरुर्व्रणश्लेष्मकंडूकृमिविषापहः ॥१५३॥

*Dhuttūra* (**Datura stramonium Linn.**)

*Dhuttūra* produces *mada* (intoxication), *varṇa* (complexion), *agni* (digestive power) and *vānti* (vomiting). It cures *jvara* (fever) and *kuṣṭha* (obstinate skin diseases including leprosy). It is hot and heavy, It also cures *vraṇa* (ulcer), aggravated *kapha*, *kaṇḍū* (itching), *kṛmi* (parasitic infection) and *viṣa* (poisoning).

[96]
**हलिनी-करवीरौ** च कुष्ठदुष्टव्रणापहौ ।

*Halinī and Karaivīra* (**Gloriosa superba Linn. & Nerium indicum Linn.**)

*Halinī* and *karavīra* cure *kuṣṭha* (obstinate skin diseases including leprosy) and *duṣṭa vraṇa* (obstinate type of ulcer).

ऊर्ध्वाधःकफपित्तघ्नी कुष्ठ**मावर्त्तकी** हरेत् ॥१५४॥

*Āvartakī* **(Helicteres isora Linn.)**

*Āvartakī* cures aggrevated *kapha* and *pitta* both from upper and lower parts of the body. It also cures *kuṣṭha* (obstinate skin diseases including leprosy).

**कोशातकी** कफार्शोघ्नी पक्वामाशयशोधिनी ।

*Kośātakī* **(Luffa acutangula Roxb.)**

*Kośātakī* cures aggravated *kapha* and *arśas* (piles). It cleanses both the *pakvāśaya* (colon) and *āmāśaya* (stomach including small intestine).

मेध्या **ज्योतिष्मती** तीक्ष्णा व्रणविस्फोटनाशिनी ॥१५५॥

*Jyotiṣmatī* **(Celastrus paniculatus Willd.)**

*Jyotiṣmatī* promotes intellect. It is sharp and it cures *vraṇa* (ulcer) and *visphoṭa* (pustular eruptions).

वयसः स्थापिनी **ब्राह्मी** मेधायुःस्मृतिवर्धिनी ।

*Brāhmī* **(Bacopa monnieri Pennell)**

*Brāhmī* prevents aging. It promotes intellect, longevity and memory.

[97]कफवातास्रभूतघ्नी [98]**वचा**युःस्मृतिबुद्धिदा ॥१५६॥

*Vacā* **(Acorus calamus Linn.)**

*Vacā* cures aggravated *kapha*, *vāta* as well as blood and attacks by evil spirits (*bhūta*). It promotes longevity, memory and intellect.

[99]**कुक्कुरुंदः** कटुस्तिक्तो ज्वररक्तकफापहः ।

*Kukkurunda*

*Kukkurunda* is pungent and bitter. It cures fever and vitiated blood and *kapha*.

**शंखपुष्पी** सरा तिक्ता मेध्या कृमिविषापहा ॥१५७॥

*Śaṅkhapuṣpī* **(Convolvulus pluricaulis Chois)**

*Śaṅkha puṣpī* is laxative and bitter. It promotes *medhā*

(intellect) and cures *kṛmi* (parasitic infection) and *viṣa* (poisoning).

‘**हंसपादी** गुरुः शीता हन्ति रक्तगुरु( ? )व्रणान् ।

*Haṁsa pādī* (**Adiantum lunulatum Burm.**)

*Haṁsa pādī* is heavy and cooling. It alleviates vitiated blood and cures serious type (*guru*) of *vraṇa*.

**मुंडी** तिक्ता कटुपाके वीर्योष्णा मधुरा लघु ॥१५८॥

100

मेध्या गण्डापचीकृच्छ्रक्रिमियोन्यर्तिपाण्डुनुत् ।’

*Muṇḍī* (**Sphaeranthus indicus Linn.**)

*Muṇḍī* is bitter in taste and pungent in *vipāka*. It is hot in potency, sweet and *laghu*. It promotes intellect (*medhā*) and cures *gaṇḍa* (goitre), *apacī* (cervical adenitis), *kṛcchra* (dysuria), *kṛmi* (parasitic infection), *yonyarti* (pain in female genital tract) as well as *pāṇḍu* (anemia).

**मालती** कफपित्तास्ररुग्व्रणक्रिमिकुष्ठनुत् ॥१५९॥

*Mālatī* (**Aganosma dichotoma K. Schum.**)

*Mālatī* cures aggravated *kapha*, *pitta* and blood, *ruk* (pain), *vraṇa* (ulcer), *kṛmi* (parasitic infection) and *kuṣṭha* (obstinate skin diseases including leprosy).

चक्षुष्या मुकुलं तस्यास्तत्पुष्पं कफपित्तनुत् ।

Its bud (*mukula*) promotes eyesight. Its flowers alleviate *kapha* and *pitta*.

**स्यान्नागदमनी** वर्ण्या लूतासर्पविषापहा ॥१६०॥

*Nāgadamanī* (**Artemisia vulgaris Linn.**)

*Nāgadamanī* promotes complexion and cures poisoning by *lutā* (venomous spider) and *sarpa* (snake).

**शिरीषो** विषवीसर्पस्वेदत्वग्दोषशोथजित् ।

*Śirīṣa* (**Albizzia lebbeck Benth.**)

*Śirīṣa* cures *viṣa* (poisoning), *vīsarpa* (erysipelas), *sveda* (profuse sweating), *daurgandhya* (foul smell of body), *tvagdoṣa* (skin diseases) and *śotha* (oedema).

**सिक्थकं** व्रणवीसर्पकुष्ठवातास्रजित् परम् ॥१६१॥

*Sikthaka*

*Sikthaka* is an excellent cure for *vraṇa* (ulcer), *vīsarpa* (erysipelas), *kuṣṭha* (obstinate skin diseases including leprosy) and *vātāsra* (gout).

**आफूकं** शोषणं ग्राही श्लेष्मघ्नं वातपित्तलम् ।

*Āphūka* **(Papaver somniferum Linn.)**

*Āphūka* (opium) is *soṣaṇa* (drying) and *grāhī* (constipative). It alleviates *kapha* and aggravates *vāta* as well as *pitta.*

वृष्यो बल्यः **खसतिलः** श्लेष्मलो वातजिद्गुरुः ॥१६२॥

*Khasa tila* (seeds inside the poppy pod) is aphrodisiac and strength promoting. It aggravates *kapha* and alleviates *vāyu.* It is heavy.

वल्कलस्तत्फलोद्भूतो रुक्षो ग्राही विशोषणः ।

The *valkala* (outer layer) of the poppy pod is ununctuous, *grāhī* (constipative) and *viśoṣaṇa* (excessively drying).

रक्तपित्तहरी **दूर्वा** कंडूत्वग्दोषनाशिनी ॥ १६३ ॥

*Dūrvā* **(Cynodon dactylon Pers.)**

*Dūrvā* cures *rakta pitta* (a disease characterised by bleeding from different parts of the body), *kaṇḍū* (itching) and *tvagdoṣa* (skin disease).

101

पांडुमेहापचीपिल्लत्वग्दोषक्रिमिजि**न्निशा** ।

कफपित्तहरी शोथकंडूकुष्ठव्रणापहा ॥१६४॥

*Niśā* **(Curcuma longa Linn.)**

*Niśā* cures *pāṇḍu* (anemia), *meha* (obstinate urinary disorders including diabetes), *apacī* (cervical adenitis), *pilla* type of eye disease), *tvagdoṣa* (skin disease) and *kṛmi* (parasitic infection). It alleviates *kapha* and *pitta* and cures *śotha* (oedema), *kaṇḍū* (itching), *kuṣṭha* (obstinate skin diseases including leprosy) and *vraṇa* (ulcer).

तद्वद्दार्वी विशेषेण कफाभिष्यन्दनाशिनी ।

*Dārvī* **(Berberis aristata DC.)**

*Dārvī* shares the properties of *niśā*. It is specially useful for curing *abhiṣyanda* (conjunctivitis) caused by *kapha*.

त्वग्दोषमारुतश्लेष्मविषप्रशमनं स्मृतम् ॥१६५॥

अवल्गुजं फलं, तद्वत्प्रपुन्नाटस्य चोच्यते ।

'कुष्ठगुल्मोदरार्शोघ्नं कटुपाके तथैव च ॥ १६६ ॥

*Avalguja* **(Psoralea corylifolia Linn.)**

The fruit of *avalguja* cures *tvagdoṣa* (skin disease), aggravated *vāyu* and *kapha* and *viṣa* (poisoning).

*Prapunnāḍa* **(Cassia tora Linn.)**

*Prapunnāḍa* shares the properties of *avalguja*. Moreover, it cures *kuṣṭha* (obstinate skin diseases including leprosy), *gulma* (phantom tumour), *udara* (obstinate abdominal diseases including ascitis) and *arśas* (piles). It is pungent in *vipāka*.

102

करंजकिंशुकारिष्टफलं जंतु प्रमेहजित् ।'

रूक्षोष्णं कटुकं पाके लघुर्वातकफापहम् ॥ १६७ ॥

*Karañja*, *kiṁśuka* & *Ariṣṭa* **(Pongamia pinnata Merr., Butea monosperma Kuntze and Sapindus trifoliatus Linn.)**

The fruits of *karañja*, *kiṁśuka* and *ariṣṭa* cure *jantu* (parasitic infection) and *prameha* (obstinate urinary disorders including diabetes). They are ununctuous, hot, pungent in *vipāka* and light. They alleviate *vāta* and *kapha*.

तिक्तमीषद्विषहितं विडङ्गं क्रिमिनाशनम् ।

*Viḍaṅga* **(Embelia ribes Burm. f.)**

*Viḍaṅga* is slightly bitter. It is useful in the treatment

of poisoning and it cures *kṛmi* (parasitic infection).

**आस्फोता**[103] विषकुष्ठघ्नी **तिनिशा**[104] दाहपित्तनुत् ।।१६८।।

*Āsphotā* & *Tiniśā* **(Vallaris solanacea O. Ktze. & Ougeinia dalbergioides Benth.)**

*Āsphotā* cures *viṣa* (poisoning) and *kuṣṭha* (obstinate skin diseases including leprosy).

*Tiniśā* cures *dāha* (burning syndrome) and aggravated *pitta*.

**असनः**[105] कफपित्तघ्न **शिंशपा**दाहशोथनुत् ।

*Asana and Śiṁśapā* **(Pterocarpus marsupium Roxb. & Dalbergia sissoo Roxb.)**

*Asana* alleviates *kapha* and *pitta*. *Śiṁśapā* cures *dāha* (burning syndrome) and *śotha* (oedema).

**धातकी** रक्तपित्तघ्नी **कदरो** दन्तदार्ढ्यकृत् ।। १६९।।

*Dhātakī* & *Kadara* **(Woodfordia fruticosa Kurz. & Acacia suma Buch.—Ham.)**

*Dhātakī* cures *raktapitta* (a disease characterised by bleeding from different parts of the body).

*Kadara* makes teeth strongly embedded in the gums (*danta dārḍhya kṛt*).

**अपामार्गो**ऽग्निकृत्तीक्ष्णः **सिन्दुवारो**ऽनिलापहः ।

*Apāmārga and Sinduvāra* **(Achyranthes aspera Linn. & Vitex trifolia Linn.)**

*Apāmārga* stimulates digestion and it is sharp.

*Sinduvāra* alleviates *vāyu*.

**लज्जालुः** शीतला तिक्ता कषाया श्लेष्मपित्तहृत्[106] ।।१७०।।

रक्तपित्तमतीसारं योनिदोषं[107] विनाशयेत ।

*Lajjālu* **(Mimosa pudica Linn.)**

*Lajjālu* is cooling, bitter and astringent. It alleviates *kapha* and *pitta*. It cures *raktapitta* (a disease characterised by bleeding from different parts of the body), *atisāra* (diarrhoea) and *yonidoṣa* (diseases of the female genital tract).

**वंशो**[108] व्रणास्रसंहारो[109] भेदनः शोथनाशनः ॥ १७१ ॥

*Vaṁśa* **(Bambusa bambos Druce)**

*Vaṁśa* cures *vraṇa* (ulcer) and vitiated blood. It is purgative and it cures *śotha* (oedema).

**रोहीतको** यकृत्प्लीहगुल्मोदरहरः सरः ।

*Rohitaka* **(Tecomella undulata Seem.)**

*Rohitaka* cures diseases of *yakṛt* and *plīhan*, *gulma* (phantom tumour) and *udara* (obstinate diseases of the abdomen including ascitis). It is laxative.

शोथामकफवातघ्नो[110] **वृहद्दारो** रसायनः ॥ १७२ ॥

*Vṛhaddāra* **(Argyreia speciosa Sweet)**

*Vṛhaddāra* cures *śotha* (oedema), *āma* and aggravated *kapha* as well as *vāta*. It is rejuvenating.

भूयो व्रणकफास्रघ्नः[111] **तगरः** कुष्ठवद्गुणैः ।

*Tagara* **(Valeriana wallichii DC.)**

*Tagara* shares the properties of *kuṣṭha*. It is specifically useful in curing *vraṇa* (ulcer) and vitiated *kapha* as well as blood.

कफवातहरी **कौन्ती** दीपनी न च पित्तकृत् ॥१७३॥

*Kauntī* **(Vitex agnus-costus Linn.)**

*Kauntī* alleviates *kapha* and *vāta*. It stimulates digestive power. It does not aggravate *pitta*.

**श्रीवासः सरलं बोलः कुन्दरुर्ग्रन्थिपर्णकम्** ।
**तुरुष्कं सिह्लकं**[112] **स्पृक्का गुन्द्रा**[113] **सर्जोमुरा नखम्** ॥१७४॥

सर्वेऽमी पावनालक्ष्मीरक्षोघ्ना ज्वरनाशनाः ।

स्वादुतिक्तरसायुष्याः स्वेददौर्गन्ध्यनाशनाः ॥ १७५ ॥

*Śrīvāsa* **(Pinus roxburghii Sargent) etc.**

*Śrīvāsa, sarala, bola, kunduru, granthiparṇa, turuṣka, silhaka, spṛkkā, gundrā, sarja, murā* and *nakha*—all these drugs cure aggravated *vāyu, alakṣmī* (inauspiciousness), *rakṣa* (afflictions by *rakṣas*) and *jvara* (fever). They are sweet and bitter in taste. They promote longevity. They cure *svedadaurgandhya* (foul smell because of excessive sweating).

'**राला** हिमा गुरुस्तिक्ता कषाया ग्रहणीं जयेत् ।
114
ग्रहसंस्वेदवीसर्पज्वरव्रणविपादिकाः' ॥ १७६ ॥

*Rālā*

*Rālā* is cooling, heavy, bitter, and astringent. It cures *grahaṇī* (sprue syndrome), *graha* (affliction by unfavourably situated planets), *saṁsveda* (excessive sweating), *vīsarpa* (erysipelas), *jvara* (fever), *vraṇa* (ulcer) and *vipādikā* (cracking of the sole of the feet).

पित्तास्रविषतृट्दाहकृमिघ्नं गुरु रुक्षणम् ।
115
सर्वं सतिक्तमधुरं **चन्दनं** शिशिरं परम् ॥ १७७ ॥

*Candana (Śveta and Rakta)* **(Santalum album Linn. & Pterocarpus santalinus Linn. f.)**

Both the varieties of *candana* cure vitiated *pitta* and blood, *viṣa* (poisoning), *tṛṭ* (morbid thirst), *dāha* (burning syndrome) and *kṛmi* (parasitic infection). They are heavy, ununctuous, bitter, sweet and exceedingly cooling.

मनोज्ञं **चंदनं श्वेतं** रक्तपित्तविषापहम् ।

हृद्यं प्रह्लादनीयं च सतिक्तमतिशीतलम् ॥१७८॥

*Śveta candana* is *manojña* (pleasing to the mind) and it cures *rakta pitta* (a disease characterised by bleeding from different parts of the body) and *viṣa* (poisoning). It is *hṛdya* (cardiac tonic), *prahlādanīya* (which gives comfort), bitter and exceedingly cooling.

चक्षुष्यं रक्तपित्तघ्नं व्रण्यं **लोहितचंदनम्** ।

*Lohita candana* promotes eyesight. It cures *rakta pitta* (a disease characterised by bleeding from different parts of the body). It is useful in the treatment of ulcers (*vraṇya*).

**पतंगं**[116] तिक्तमधुरं व्रण्यं[117] पित्तकफास्रजित्[118] ॥ १७९ ॥

*Pataṅga* **(Caesalpinia sappan Linn.)**

*Pataṅga* is bitter and sweet. It is *vraṇya* (useful in the treatment of ulcer). It alleviates *pitta*, *kapha* and blood.

**पद्मकं** कुष्ठविस्फोटज्वरदाहव्रणापहम्[119] ।

*Padmaka* **(Prunus cerasoides D. Don.)**

*Padmaka* cures *kuṣṭha* (obstinate skin diseases including leprosy), *visphoṭa* (pustular eruption), *jvara* (fever), *dāha* (burning syndrome) and *vraṇa* (ulcer).

**सेव्यं** पित्तास्रजित्स्वेददाहदौर्गन्ध्यनाशनम् ॥१८०॥

*Sevya* **(Vetiveria zizanioides Nash)**

*Sevya* alleviates *pitta* and blood. It cures *sveda* (excessive sweating), *dāha* (burning syndrome) and *daurgandhya* (foul smell of body).

**वातघ्नं कुंकुमं** सोष्णं बल्यं[120] त्वग्दोषनाशनम् ।

*Kuṁkuma* **(Crocus sativus Linn.)**

*Kuṁkuma* alleviates *vāyu*. It is hot. It promotes strength and cures *tvagdoṣa* (skin disease).

**कस्तूरी** छर्दिदौर्गन्ध्यवातालक्ष्मीमलापहा ॥१८१॥

*Kastūrī* **(musk)**

*Kastūrī* cures *chardi* (vomiting), *daurgandhya* (foul smell of the body), aggravated *vāyu*, *alakṣmī* (inauspiciousness) and *mala* (excessive excretion of waste products).

कटुतिक्तोष्णमगुरु स्निग्धं वातकफापहम् ।

*Aguru* **(Aquilaria agallocha Roxb.)**

*Aguru* is pungent, bitter, hot and unctuous. It alleviates *vāyu* and *kapha.*

स्निग्धोष्णं कटुकं पाके **सुरदार्वं**निलापहम् ॥१८२॥

*Suradāru* **(Cedrus deodara Loud.)**

*Suradāru* is unctuous, hot and pungent in *vipāka.* It alleviates *vāyu.*

**कत्तृणं** तिक्तमधुरं वातश्लेष्मविषापहम् ।

*Kattṛṇa* **(Cymbopogon citratus Stapf.)**

*Kattṛṇa* is bitter and sweet. It alleviates *vāyu* and *kapha,* and cures *viṣa* (poisoning).

**कुष्ठं** सतिक्तमधुरं वातश्लेष्मविषापहम् ॥ १८३ ॥

*Kuṣṭha* **(Saussurea lappa C.B. Clarke.)**

*Kuṣṭha* is bitter and sweet. It alleviates *vāyu* and *kapha,* and cures *viṣa* (poisoning).

121

'**शटी** वातकफश्वासकासज्वरहरा मता' ।

*Śaṭī* **(Hedychium spicatum Ham. ex. Smith.)**

*Śaṭī* alleviates *vāyu* and *kapha.* It cures *śvāsa* (asthma), *kāsa* (bronchitis) and *jvara* (fever).

सुगन्धिः कटुको हृद्यः **कंकोलः** कफवातजित् ॥१८४॥

*Kaṅkola* **(Piper cubeba Linn. f.)**

*Kaṅkola* is fragrant, pungent and cardiac tonic. It alleviates *kapha* and *vāta.*

122

तद्वज्**जातीफलं** प्रोक्तं भ्रमपित्तकरं परं ।

*Jātīphala* **(Myrstica fragrans Houtt.)**

*Jātīphala* shares the properties of *kaṅkola.* In addition it causes *bhrama* (giddiness) and aggravates *pitta.*

जातीकोशो[123] लघुस्तिक्तः क्लेददौर्गन्ध्यजिन्मतः ।१८५।

*Jātikośa*

*Jātikośa* is light and bitter. It cures *kleda* and *daurgandhya* (foul smell of the body).

सतिक्तः कटुकश्चैव बलासस्य विनाशनः ।

कर्पूरः शीतलः पाके चक्षुष्यः कफनाशनः ॥१८६॥

*Karpūra* **(Cinnamomum camphora Nees. & Eberm)**

*Karpūra* is bitter and pungent. It alleviates *kapha*. It is cooling in *vipāka* (?). It promotes eyesight and is an expectorant.

'पक्वात्कर्पूरतः प्राहुरपक्वं गुणवत्तरम् ।

तत्रापि स्याद्यदक्षुद्रं स्फटिकाभं तदुत्तमम् ॥१८७॥

*Apakva karpūra* is better than *pakva karpūra*. There, also, *karpūra* which is not in small pieces and which is like crystal is the best.

पक्वं च सदलं स्निग्धं हरितद्युति चोत्तमम् ।

भङ्गे मनागपि न चेन्निपतन्ति कणास्ततः ॥१८८॥

*Pakva karpūra* which is in pieces (*sadala*), which is unctuous and which has greenish tinge is the best provided granules (even in small quantity) do not fall out of it when broken into pieces.

तिक्तदाहास्यवैरस्य मेद-शोथ-विषापहः[124] ।'

It cures *dāha* (burning syndrome), *āsya vairasyā* (distaste in mouth), *medas* (adiposity), *śotha* (oedema) and *viṣa* (poisoning).

'रास्ना हिमा गुरुस्तिक्ता कषाया ग्राहि[णी][125] जयेत् ॥१८९॥

ग्रहास्रस्वेदवीसर्प[126]ज्वरव्रणविपादिकाः ।

*Rāsnā* **(Pluchea lanceolata Oliver & Hiern.)**

*Rāsnā* is cooling, heavy, bitter, astringent and constipative. It cures *graha* (afflictions by evil spirits), vitiated blood, *sveda* (excessive sweating), *vīsarpa* (erysipelas), *jvara* (fever), *vraṇa* (ulcer) and *vipādikā* (cracking of the soul of the feet.)

127

**एला** तृट्छर्दिहृल्लासकंडूप्रित्तकफापहा ॥१९०॥

*Elā* **(Amomum subulatum Roxb.)**

*Elā* cures *tṛṭ* (morbid thirst), *chardi* (vomiting), *hṛllāsa* (nausea), *kaṇḍū* (itches) and aggravated *pitta* as well as *kapha*.

**सूक्ष्मैला** मूत्रकृच्छ्रार्शःश्वासकासकफे हिता ।

*Sūkṣmailā* (**Elettaria cardamomum Maton.**)

*Sūkṣmailā* is useful in *mūtrakṛcchra* (dysuria), *arśas* (piles), *śvāsa* (asthma), *kāsa* (bronchitis) and aggravation of *kapha*.

विबन्धानाहशूलघ्नं **लवङ्गं** भुक्तपाचनम् ॥ १९१ ॥

*Lavaṅga* **(Syzygium aromaticum Merr. & L.M.)**

*Lavaṅga* cures *vibandha* (constipation), *ānāha* (flatulence) and *śūla* (colic pain). It helps in the digestion of food.

चक्षुष्या मुखरोगघ्नी **लताकस्तूरिका** हिमा ।

*Latā kastūrikā* **(Hibiscus abelmoschus Linn.)**

*Latā kastūrikā* promotes eye sight and cures diseases of mouth. It is cooling.

128

**कट्फलं** मुखरोगघ्नं कासश्वासक्षयापहम् ॥१९२॥

*Kaṭphala* (**Myrica nagi Thunb.**)

*Kaṭphala* cures diseases of mouth, *kāsa* (bronchitis), *śvāsa* (asthma) and *kṣaya* (consumption).

**मदनो** वामनः तिक्तः वीर्योष्णो लेखनो लघुः ।

रूक्षः कुष्ठकफानाहशोफगुल्मव्रणापहः ॥ १९३ ॥

*Madana* **(Randia dumetorum Lam.)**

*Madana* is emetic, bitter, hot in potency, *lekhana* (scraping), light and ununctuous. It cures *kuṣṭha* (obstinate skin diseases including leprosy,) aggravated *kapha*, *ānāha* (flatulence), *śopha* (oedema), *gulma* (phantom tumour) and *vraṇa* (ulcer).

**शताह्वा**निलदाहास्रशूलतृट्छर्दिनाशिनी ।
मधुरा रोचनी वृष्या दाहासृक्पित्तनाशिनी ॥१९४॥

*Śatāhvā* **(Foeniculum vulgare Mill.)**

*Satāhvā* cures aggravated *vāyu*, *dāha* (burning syndrome), vitiated blood, *śūla* (colic pain), *tṛṭ* (morbid thirst) and *chardi* (vomiting). It is sweet, *rocana* (appetiser) and aphrodisiac. It alleviates *pitta*.

**फलिनी** गात्रदौर्गन्ध्यरक्तपित्तज्वरापहा ।

*Phalinī* **(Prunus mahaleb Linn.)**

*Phalinī* removes *gātra daurgandhya* (foul smell of the body) and cures *rakta pitta* (a disease characterised by bleeding from different parts of the body) and *jvara* (fever).

शस्ता शोणितपित्तातियोगे **गन्धप्रियंगुका**[129] ॥ १९५ ॥

*Gandha priyaṅgu* **(Callicarpa macrophylla Vahl)**

*Gandha priyaṅgu* is useful in the acute form of *śoṇita pitta* (a disease characterised by bleeding from different parts of the body).

**हपुषा** दीपनी तिक्ता कटूष्णा[130] तुवरा गुरुः ।
पित्तोदरसमीरार्शो-ग्रहणी-गुल्म-शूलहृत् ॥१९६॥

*Hapuṣā* **(Juniper communis Linn.)**

*Hapuṣā* is digestive stimulant, bitter, pungent, hot, saline and heavy. It cures aggravated *pitta*, *udara* (obstinate abdominal diseases including ascitis), aggravated *vāyu*, *arśas* (piles), *grahaṇī* (sprue syndrome), *gulma* (phantom tumour) and *śūla* (colic pain).

[131] 'राष्णोष्णा वातशोथामवातवातामयान् [132] जयेत् ।

*Rāṣṇā* **(Alpinia gulanga Willd.)**

*Rāṣṇā* is hot. It cures aggravated *vāyu, śotha* (oedema), *āmavāta* (rheumatism) and *vātāmaya* (diseases caused by the vitiation of *vāyu*).

**पौष्करं** पार्श्वरुक्श्वासकासहिक्काज्वरापहा ॥१६७॥

*Pauṣkara* **(Inula racemosa Hook. f.)**

*Pauṣkara* cures *pārśvaruk* (pain in the sides of chest), *śvāsa* (asthma), *kāsa* (bronchitis), *hikkā* (hiccup) and *jvara* (fever).

[133] शृंङ्गी कफानिलश्वासकासहिक्काज्वरापहा ।

*Śṛṅgī* **(Pistacia integerrmia Stew. ex Brandis)**

*Śṛṅgī* cures aggravated *kapha* as well as *vāyu, śvāsa* (asthma), *kāsa* (bronchitis), *hikkā* (hiccup) and fever (*jvara*).

[134] **वरांगं** कफशुक्रामवातघ्नं मधुरं कटु ॥ १६८ ॥

विषतृट्छर्दिहृल्लासकफपित्तविसर्पनुत् ।

*Varāṅga* **(Cinnamomum zeylanicum Blume.)**

*Varāṅga* alleviates *kapha* and reduces semen. It cures *āmavāta* (rheumatism). It is sweet and pungent. It cures *viṣa* (poisoning), *tṛṭ* (morbid thirst), *chardi* (vomiting), *hṛllāsa* (nausea), aggravated *kapha* as well as *pitta* and *visarpa* (erysipelas).

त्वग्दोषस्वेददौर्गन्ध्यनाशनो [135] **नागकेसरः** ॥ १६९ ॥

*Nāgakesara* **(Mesua ferrea Linn.)**

*Nāgakesara* cures *tvagdoṣa* (skin diseases), *sveda* (excessive sweating) and *daurgandhya* (foul smell of the body).

[136] **पत्रकं** कफवातार्शोहृल्लासारोचकापहम् ।

*Patraka* **(Cinnamomum tamala Nees and Eberm.)**

*Patraka* alleviates *kapha* and *vāta* and cures *arśas* (piles), *hṛllāsa* (nausea) and *arocaka* (anoxeria).

**तालीसपत्रं** तीक्ष्णोष्णं[137] कफवातक्षयापहम् ॥ २०० ॥
पित्तकृत्स्रंसनं स्वर्यं वह्निकृद्वक्त्रशोधनम् ।

*Tāḷisa patra* **(Abies webbiana Lindl.)**

*Tālisa patra* is sharp and hot. It alleviates *kapha* and *vāta*. It cures *kṣaya* (consumption). It aggravates *pitta*. It is laxative (*sraṁsana*). It promotes good voice and digestive power. It also cleanses mouth.

कषाया मधुरा रूक्षा कासघ्नी[138] **वंशरोचना** ॥ २०१ ॥

*Vaṁśa rocaṇā* **(Bamboo manna.)**

*Vaṁśa rocanā* is astringent, sweet and ununctuous. It cures *kāsa* (bronchitis).

**तुगाक्षीरी** क्षयश्वासकासघ्नी मधुरा हिमा ।

*Tugākṣīrī*

*Tugākṣīrī* cures *kṣaya* (consumption), *śvāsa* (asthma) and *kāsa* (bronchitis). It is sweet and cooling.

**बासकः** कासवैस्वर्यं रक्तपित्तकफापहः ॥ २०२ ॥
'तृषाश्वासज्वर[139]च्छर्दिमेह[140]कुष्ठक्षयापहः ।

*Vāsaka* **(Adhatoda vasica Nees)**

*Vāsaka* cures *kāsa* (bronchitis), *vaisvarya* (impairment of voice), *raktapitta* (a disease characterised by bleeding from different parts of the body), aggravated *kapha*, *tṛṣā* (morbid thirst), *śvāsa* (asthma), *jvara* (fever), *chardi* (vomiting), *meha* (obstinate urinary disorders including diabetes), *kuṣṭha* (obstinate skin diseases including leprosy) and *kṣaya* (consumption).

**कुमारी भेदनी** शीता यकृत्प्लीहकफज्वरान् ॥२०३॥
निहन्ति वह्निविस्फोटपित्तरक्तत्वगामयान् ।

*Kumārī* **(Aloe barbadensis Mill.)**

*Kumārī* is *bhedana* (purgative) and cooling. It cures *yakṛt* (diseases of liver), *plihan* (diseases of spleen), aggravated *kapha, jvara* (fever), *vahni visphoṭa* (carbuncle), aggravated *pitta* as well as *rakta* and *tvagāmaya* (diseases of skin).

बल्याऽ**मृता** त्रिदोषघ्नी ग्राहिण्युष्णारसायनी ।।२०४।।
[141]
दीपनी तृट्ज्वरछर्दीकामलावातरक्तजित् ।
कटुतिक्ता स्वादुपाका लघ्वी दाहामकुष्ठनुत् ।।२०५।।

*Amṛtā* **(Tinospora cordifolia Miers)**

*Amṛtā* promotes strength. It alleviates all the three *doṣas*. It is *grāhī* (constipative), hot, rejuvenating and digestive stimulant. It cures *tṛt* (morbid thirst), *jvara* (fever), *chardi* (vomiting), *kāmalā* (jaundice) and *vāta rakta* (gout). It is pungent, bitter, sweet in *vipāka* and light. It also cures *dāha* (burning syndrome), *āma* and *kuṣṭha* (obstinate skin diseases including leprosy).

**शालिपर्णीपृश्निपर्णीबृहतीद्वयगोक्षुरम्** ।
वातपित्तहरं वृष्यं **कनीयः पञ्चमूलकम्** ।।२०६।।

*Daśamūla*

*Śāliparṇī, pṛśni parṇī, bṛhatī, kaṇṭakārī* and *gokṣura*—these five drugs taken together, are called *kanīyas pañcamūla.* It alleviates *vāyu* and *pitta* and it is aphrodisiac.

[**श्रीफलः सर्वतोभद्रा पाटला गणिकारिका** ।
[142]
**श्योनाकः** पञ्चभिश्चैतैः **पञ्चमूलं मह**न्मतम् ।।२०७।।]

*Śrīphala, sarvato bhadrā, pāṭalā, gaṇikārikā* and *śyonāka*—these five drugs taken together are called *mahat pañcamūla.*

एताभ्यां पञ्चमूलाभ्यां **दशमूलमु**दाहृतम् ।
दोषत्रय-श्वासकासशिरःपीडापतन्त्रकान् ।
तन्द्रीशोथज्वरानाहारुचिपार्श्वरुजो जयेत् ।।२०८।।

All these ten drugs included both in *kanīyas pañcamūla* and *mahat pañcamūla* taken together are called *daśamūla*. It cures *doṣa traya* (aggravated *vāyu*, *pitta* and *kapha*), *śvāsa* (asthma), *kāsa* (bronchitis), *śiraḥ pīḍā* (headache), *apatantraka* (convulsion), *tandrī* (drowsiness), *śotha* (oedema), *jvara* (fever). *ānāha* (tymphanitis), *aruci* (anorexia) and *pārśva ruk* (pain in the sides of the chest).

मन्याहनुश्रवणलोचननासिकास्यभ्रूशंखदन्तगलतालुशिरोविकारान् ।

कुष्ठानि हन्ति दशमूलकषायपीतं क्वाथेन वा सहफलत्रितयोद्भवेन ॥२०९॥

Decoction of these ten drugs belonging to the group of *daśamūla* or the decoction of *harītakī*, *bibhītaka* and *āmalakī* (*triphalā*) along with these ten drugs belonging to *daśamūla* group cures diseases of *manyā* (sternomastoid region), *hanu* (mandibles), *śravaṇa* (ears), *locana* (eyes), *nāsikā* (nose), *āsya* (mouth), *bhrū* (eye brows), *śaṅkha* (temporal region), *danta* (teeth), *gala* (throat), *tālu* (palate) and *śiras* (head). It also cures *kuṣṭha* (obstinate skin diseases including leprosy).

143

**न्यग्रोधोदुम्बराश्वत्थपारिषप्लक्ष**पादपाः ।

पञ्चैते **क्षीरिणो वृक्षा**स्तेषां त्वक् **पञ्चवल्कलम्** ॥२१०॥

*Pañca kṣiri vṛkṣa* **and** *Pañca valkala*

*Nyagrodha*, *udumbara*, *aśvattha*, *pāriṣa* and *plakṣa*—these five are called *kṣiri vṛkṣas* (trees having milky latex). Barks of all these five trees taken together are called *pañca valkala*.

144

केचित्तु पारिषस्थाने **शिरीषं वेतसं** परम् ।

Some physicians use *śirīṣa* and some others use *vetasa* in the place of *pāriṣa* included in this group of drugs.

**क्षीरिवृक्षाः** हिमाः वर्ण्याः योनिदोषव्रणापहाः ॥२११॥

रूक्षाः कषायाः मेदोघ्नाः वीसर्पामयनाशनाः ।

शोथपित्तकफास्रघ्नाः स्तन्यभग्नास्थियोगदाः ।

*Kṣīri vṛkṣas* are cooling. They promote complexion (*varṇya*) and cure *yoni doṣa* (ailments of the female genital tract) and *vraṇa* (ulcer). They are ununctuous, and astringent. They cure *medas* (adiposity), *visarpa* (erysipelas), *śotha* (oedema) and vitiated *pitta, kapha* as well as blood. They promote lactation and help in the union of fractured bones.

त्वक्पञ्चकं हिमं ग्राहि व्रणशोथविसर्पजित् ॥२१२॥

*Pañca valkala* is cooling and constipative. It cures *vraṇa* (ulcer), *śotha* (oedema) and *visarpa* (erysipelas).

**अथ धातूपधातु-रसोपरस-रत्नोपरत्न-विषोपविषगुणाः**

**तत्रधातुलक्षणम्**

'स्वर्णं तारं च ताम्रं च वंगं नागस्तु पञ्चमः । [145]

रीतिका च तथा कांस्यं लोहं चेत्यष्टधातवः ॥२१३॥

**Properties of *Dhātu, Upadhātu, Rasa, Uparasa, Ratna, Uparatna, Viṣa* and *Upaviṣa*.**

**Description of *Dhātus***

*Svarṇa* (gold), *tāra* (silver), *tāmra* (copper) *vaṅga* (tin), *nāga* (lead), *rītikā* (bell metal), *kāṁsya* (brass), *loha* (iron) —these eight are called *dhātus*.

'वलीपलितखालित्यकार्श्याबल्यजरामयान् । [146]

निवार्यंनृणां दधति देहं तद्धातवो मताः ॥२१४॥

[भाव प्रकाशः पूर्वखण्डः धात्वादिवर्ग ८:२]

They are called *dhātus* because they sustain (*dadhati*) the body of human beings by curing *valī* (premature wrinkles), *palita* (premature graying of hair), *khālitya* (baldness), *kārśya* (emaciation), *abalya* (weakness), *jarā* (old age) and *āmaya* (diseases).

**सुवर्णोत्पत्तिलक्षणगुणाः** —

'पुरा निजाश्रमस्थानां सप्तर्षीणां जितात्मनाम् ।

पत्नीं विलोक्य लावण्यलक्ष्मीःसम्पन्नयौवनाः ॥२१५॥
कन्दर्पदर्पविध्वस्तचेतसो जातवेदसः ।
पतितं यद्धरापृष्ठे रेतस्तद्धेमताम[147]गात् । २१६ ॥
कृत्रिमञ्चापि भवति तद्रसेन्द्रस्य वेधतः ।

## Origin and description of Gold

**Mythology**

In the days of yore, *Jātavedas* (Agni or Fire god) became passionately excited when he saw the extremely beautiful, auspicious and youthful wives of the self controlled seven sages (*Saptarṣis*) in their hermitages. The semen he, thus, ejaculated fell upon the earth which became gold. Gold is also prepared artificially by the *vedhana* (a specific method of processing) of mercury.

दाहे रक्तं सितं छेदे निकषे[148] कुङ्कुमप्रभम् ॥ २१७ ॥
तारं शुल्वो[149]त्थितं स्निग्धं मृदु तद्गुरु[150] शस्यते ।

**Good quality**

The gold which becomes red when burnt, white when cut and like saffron when rubbed over *nikaṣa* (a specific type of stone used for testing the genuineness of gold), which is prepared out of silver or copper and which is unctuous, soft and heavy is the best.

[151]श्वेतांगं कठिनं रूक्षं विवर्णं समलं दलम्[152] ॥ २१८ ॥
दाहे छेदेऽसितं श्वेतं घर्षे[153]ऽस्फुटं लघु त्यजेत् ।

**Bad quality**

The gold which is partially white, hard, ununctuous and discoloured, which is associated with impurities, which has pieces like leaves, which becomes black in burning or cutting, which does not produce clear colour when rubbed over *nikaṣa* and which is light should not be used in medicine.

सुवर्णं शीतलं वृष्यं बल्यं गुरु रसायनम्' ॥ २१९ ॥

[भावप्रकाशः पूर्वखण्डः धातूपधातुवर्ग ८ : ३-५ ८-१०]

स्वादुपाकरसं तिक्तं हृद्यं तु वरलेखनम् ।

'पवित्रं बृंहणं नेत्र्यं मेधा[154]स्मृतिविशुद्धिदम् ॥ २२० ॥

[155]हृद्यमायुष्करं कान्तिवाग्विशुद्धिस्थिरत्वकृत् ।

विषद्वयक्षयोन्मादत्रिदोषज्वरशोषजित ॥ २२१ ॥

**Property**

Gold is cooling, aphrodisiac, strength promoting, heavy, rejuvenating, sweet in *vipāka* and taste, bitter, cardiac tonic exceedingly depleting (*vara lekhana*), *pavitra* (remover of sins), nourishing and promoter of eye sight. It purifies intellect and memory, and promotes longevity. It also purifies complexion and voice. It causes steadiness. It cures both the types of *viṣa* (poisoning), *kṣaya* (consumption), *unmāda* (insanity), vitiation of all the three *doṣas*, *jvara* (fever) and *śoṣa* (phthisis).

बलं सवीर्यं हरते नराणां [156]रोगव्रजं पोषयतीह काये ।

असौख्यकार्यं च सदैव हेमापक्वं सदोषं मरणं करोति ॥ २२२ ॥

**Adverse effects**

When gold is used without proper processing, it takes away strength and energy, helps manifestation of several diseases, causes discomfort and because of its toxicity even causes death.

त्रिपुरस्य वधार्थाय निर्निमेषैर्विलोचनैः ।

निरीक्षयामास शिवः क्रोधेन परिपूरितः ॥ २२३ ॥

ततस्तूलका [157]समापतत्तस्यैकस्माद्विलोचनात् ।

[158]तस्माद्रुद्रः समभवद्वैश्वानर इव ज्वलन् ॥ २२४ ॥

द्वितीयादपतन्नेत्रादश्रु बिन्दुस्ते वामकात् ।

159
तस्माद्रजतमुद्भूतमुक्तकर्मसु संस्थितम् ॥ २२५ ॥
[भावप्रकाशः पूर्वखण्डः धातूपधातुवर्ग ८ : ११-१२, १४-१६]

## Silver

**Mythology**

When lord *Śiva*, full of anger, looked without twinkling of eyes for killing the demon *Tripura*, then from one of his eyes a meteor (*ulkā*) fell down which gave birth to *Rudra* who was dazzling like fire. From the left eye drops of tears fell down which gave birth to silver and this is used for all different purposes.

160
कृत्रिमं चापि तत्प्रोक्तं वंगादेः रसयोगतः ।

It is also prepared artificially by adding *vaṅga* (tin) etc., to processed mercury.

गुरुः स्निग्धं मृदुः श्वेतं दाहच्छेदघनक्षमम् ॥२२६॥
161
वर्णाढ्यं चन्द्रवत्स्वच्छं तारे नवगुणाः स्मृताः ।

**Good quality**

Heaviness, unctuousness, softness, white colour, power to stand burning, cutting and pressure (*ghana*), good colour, pure appearance like moon—these are the nine qualities of good silver.

कठिनं कृत्रिम रूक्षं रक्तं पीतदलं लघुः ॥२२७॥

दाहच्छेदघनैर्नष्टं रूप्ये दोषा दशस्मृताः ।

**Bad quality**

Hardness, artificial preparation, unctuousness, redness, yellowness, fragility (*dala*), lightness and getting destroyed by burning, cutting or pressure (*ghana*)—these are the ten defects in silver.

162
रूप्यं शीतं कषायाम्लं स्वादुपाकरसं सरम् ॥२२८॥

वयसः स्थापनं स्निग्धं लेखनं वातपित्तजित् ।

प्रमेहादिकरोगांश्च [163] नाशयत्यचिरं ध्रुवम् ॥२२९॥

**Properties**

Silver is cooling, astringent and sour in taste, sweet both in *vipāka* and taste, and laxative. It prevents aging. It is unctuous and *lekhana* (depleting). It alleviates *vāta* and *pitta*. It certainly cures diseases like *prameha* (obstinate urinary disorders including diabetes).

तारं शरीरस्य करोति तापं [164] विध्वंसनं यच्छति शुक्रनाशम् ।

[165] सपाटवं वीर्यबलं निहन्ति महागदान्पोषयतीत्यशुद्धम् ॥२३०॥

**Adverse effects**

*Aśuddha* (not properly processed) silver produces excessive heat (*tāpa*) in the body and causes its destruction. It destroys semen, efficiency, energy and strength. It gives rise to many serious diseases (*mahāgada*).

[166] शुक्रं यत्कार्तिकेयस्य पतितं धरणीतले ।

तस्मादेतत्समुद्भूतं **ताम्र**माहुः पुराविदः ॥२३१॥

[भावप्रकाशः पूर्वखण्डः धातूपधातुवर्गः ८:१७,१९-२२]

## *Tāmra* (Copper)

**Mythology**

According to scholars well versed in the *purāṇas*, the semen of *Kārtikeya* which fell on the earth gave rise to *tāmra* (copper).

[167] कृष्णं रूक्षमतिस्तब्धं श्वेतं चापि घनासहम् ।

लौहनागयुतं चेति [168] शुल्वं स्याद्दोषसप्तकम् ।

**Bad quality**

Black colour, ununctuousness, excessive compactness, white colour, inability to tolerate pressure (*ghana*), mixture of iron and lead—these are the seven defects in copper of bad quality.

ताम्रं कषायं मधुरं सतिक्तं स्याद्रोपणं बृंहणमल्पमेव ।।२३२।।

[भावप्रकाशः पूर्वखण्डः धातूपधातुवर्ग ८:२५-२६]

पित्तोदरार्शःकृमिकुष्ठपीनसश्लेष्मक्षयघ्नं ज्वरशूलनुद्धिमम् ।

**Properties**

Copper is astringent, sweet and bitter. It is *ropaṇa* (healer of ulcers) and slightly *bṛṁhaṇa* (nourishing). It cures aggravated *pitta*, *udara* (obstinate abdominal diseases including ascitis), *arśas* (piles), *kṛmi* (parasitic infection), *kuṣṭha* (obstinate skin diseases including leprosy), *pīnasa* (chronic rhinitis), aggravated *kapha*, *kṣaya* (consumption), *jvara* (fever) and *śūla* (colic pain). It is cooling.

न विषं विषमित्याहुस्ताम्रं तु विषमुच्यते ।। २३३ ।।

एको दोषो विषे सम्यक् ताम्रे त्वष्टौ प्रकीर्तिताः ।

भ्रमो मूर्च्छा विदाहश्च स्वेदोत्क्लेदनवान्तयः ।। २३४ ।।

अरुचिश्चित्तसंताप एते दोषा विषोपमाः ।

**Adverse effects**

Poison is not the real poison. It is copper (not processed properly) which is the real poison. Poisons have only one adverse effect whereas copper (which is not processed properly) has eight types of adverse effects. These are *bhrama* (giddiness), *mūrcchā* (fainting), *vidāha* (burning sensation), *sveda* (excessive sweating), *utkledana* (production of stickiness in the body), *vānti* (vomiting), *aruci* (anorexia), *citta santāpa* (excessive discomfort in mind)—these are the eight types of adverse effects which are like poisoning effects.

खुरकं मिश्रकञ्चेति द्विविधं वङ्गमुच्यते ।। २३५ ।।

[आयुर्वेदप्रकाश ३ : १४८]



खुरकञ्च गुणैश्रेष्ठं मिश्रकं त्वहितं मतम् ।

## *Vaṅga* (Tin)

**Variety**

*Vaṅga* is of two types. They are called *khuraka* and *miśraka*. Of these two, *khuraka* type of *vaṅga* is very useful in therapeutics whereas the *miśraka* type is harmful.

[170] बंगं लघु सर रूक्षमुष्णं मेहकफकृमीन् ।
निहन्ति पाण्डुं सश्वासं [171] दृश्यमीषत्तु पित्तलम् ॥२३६॥

[आयुर्वेद प्रकाश ३:१५०]

**Property**

*Vaṅga* is light, laxative, ununctuous and hot. It cures *meha* (obstinate urinary diseases including diabetes), *kapha*, *kṛmi* (parasitic infection), *pāṇḍu* (anemia) and *śvāsa* (asthma). It is good for eye sight and it slightly aggravates *pitta*.

[172] सिंहो यथा हस्तिगणं निहन्ति तथैव बङ्गेऽखिलमेहवर्गम् ।
देहस्य सौख्यं प्रबलेन्द्रियत्वं [173] कृशस्य पुष्टिं कुरुते नरस्य ॥२३७॥

[आयुर्वेदप्रकाश ३:१५१]

As a lion kills a horde of elephants, similarly, *vaṅga* cures all types of *meha* (obstinate urinary disorders including diabetes). It causes happiness of the body and promotes the strength of sense organs. It nourishes an emaciated person.

दृष्ट्वा भोगिसुतां रम्यां वासुकिस्तु मुमोच यत् ।
वीर्यं जातस्ततो नागः सर्वरोगापहो नृणाम् ।

[आयुर्वेदप्रकाश ३:१८४]

## *Nāga* (Lead)

**Mythology**

The semen ejaculated by *Vāsuki* after seeing the beautiful daughter of Bhogi gave rise to *nāga* (lead). It cures all diseases of human beings.

सीसं वंगगुणं ज्ञेयं विशेषान्मेहनाशनम् ॥ २३८ ॥

[आयुर्वेदप्रकाश ३:१८५]

**Property**

*Nāga* shares all the properties of *vaṅga*. However, the former specifically cures *meha* (obstinate urinary disorders including diabetes).

न.गस्तु नागशततुल्यबलं ददाति
व्याधिं च नाशयति जीवनमातनोति ।

वह्निं प्रदीपयति कामबलं करोति
मृत्यु च नाशयति सततं सेवितः सः ।

[आयुर्वेदप्रकाश ३:१८७]

*Nāga* (Lead) endows a person with the strength of one hundred *nāgas* (cobras), cures diseases, promotes longevity, stimulates digestion, increases the strength for sexual act and prevents death if used constantly.

पाकेन हीनौ खलु वंगनागौ
कुष्ठानि गुल्मांश्च तथाऽतिकुष्ठान् ॥२३९॥

[आयुर्वेदप्रकाश ३ : १८९]

पाण्डुप्रमेहानपि वातशोफभगन्दरश्वित्रकिलासशूलान् ।

विषोपमं रक्तविकारवृन्दं क्षयं च कृच्छ्राणि कफं ज्वरं च ।

मेहाश्मरी विद्रधि मुखरोगान्नर्तींश्च नित्यं कुरुतेऽबलत्वम् ।

**Adverse effects**

Use of *nāga* (lead) and *vaṅga* (tin) without proper processing causes *kuṣṭha* (obstinate skin diseases including leprosy), *gulma* (phantom tumour), *atikuṣṭha* (?), *pāṇḍu* (anemia), *prameha* (obstinate urinary disorders including diabetes), *śopha* (oedema) caused by *vāyu*, *bhagandara* (fistula-in-ano), *śvitra* (leucoderma), *kilāsa* (a type of leucoderma) and *śūla* (colic pain). They are like poisons and cause *rakta vikāra* (diseases caused by the vitiation of blood), *kṣaya* (consumption), *kṛcchra* (dysuria), aggravation of *kapha*, *jvara* (fever), *aśmarī* (stone in urinary tract), *vidradhi* (abscess), *mukharoga* (diseases of mouth), *arti* (pain) and *nitya abalatva* (progressive weakness).

रीतिका काकतुण्डी च द्विविधा सा प्रकीर्तिता ।

संतप्ता कांजिके क्षिप्ता ताम्राभा रीतिका मता ॥२४१॥

एवं च जायते कृष्णा काकतुण्डीति सा मता ।

### *Rītikā* (Bell metal)

**Variety**

This is of two types viz., *rītikā* and *kākatuṇḍī*. If the metal is heated and dipped into *kāñji* (vinegar) and it becomes copper-coloured then it should be known as *rītikā*. If it becomes black in colour, then it is *kākatuṇḍī*.

गुर्वी मृद्वी च पीताभा स्फारांगी त्रोटनाक्षमा ॥२४२॥

सुस्निग्धा मसृणांगी च रीतिरेतादृशी शुभा ।

**Good quality**

*Rītikā* which is heavy, soft, yellowish in colour, dazzling (*sphārāṅgī*), *troṭanākṣama* (difficult to break), unctuous and smooth is of good quality.

स्तब्धा रूक्षा खरा श्वेता रक्तातीव घनासहा ॥२४३॥

174

पुटगा च मलैर्युक्ता रीतिका न शुभा मता ।

**Bad quality**

*Rītikā* which is *stabdha* (compact), ununctuous, rough, white, excessively red, *ghanāsaha* (intolerant of pressure), *puṭaga* (having layers) and associated with impurity (*mala*) is not useful.

'रीतिकायुगलं सूक्ष्मं सतिक्तं लवणं रसे ।

175

शोधनं पाण्डुरोगघ्नं कृमिघ्नं नातिलेखनं' ॥२४४॥

[भावप्रकाशः पूर्वखण्डः धातूपधातुवर्ग ८ : ७५]

**Property**

Both the types of *rītikā* are *sūkṣma* (subtle), bitter and saline in taste and cleansing. They cure *pāṇḍu* (anemia) and *kṛmi* (parasitic infection). It is not a depletive (*lekhana*) in excess.

कांस्यं कषायं तिक्तोष्णं लेखनं विशदं सरं ।

रूक्षं गुरु च चक्षुष्यं कफपित्तहरं परम् ।।२४५।।

### *Kāṁsya* (Brass)

*Kāṁsya* is astringent, bitter, hot, *lekhana* (depletive), *viśada* (non-slimy), laxative, ununctuous and heavy. It promotes eye sight and alleviates *kapha* and *pitta*.

पुरा लोमिलदैत्यानां[176] निहतानां सुरैर्युधि ।

उत्पन्नानि शरीरेभ्यो लोहानि विविधानि[177] च ।।२४६।।

[आयुर्वेदप्रकाश ३ : २०४]

### *Loha* (Iron)

**Mythology**

In the days of yore, different types of *lohas* came out from the bodies of the *lomila daityas* (a group of demons) when they were killed during their war with the gods.

'लोहं तिक्तं सरं शीतं कषायं मधुरं गुरु ।

रूक्षं वयस्यं चक्षुष्यं लेखनं वातलं जयेत् ।।२४७।।

कफं पित्तं गरं शूलं शोफार्शः प्लीहपाण्डुताम् ।

मेदोमेहक्रमीन्कुष्ठं तत्किट्टं तद्वदेव हि ।। २४८ ।।

**Property**

*Loha* is bitter, laxative, cooling, astringent. sweet, heavy, ununctuous, *vayasya* (promoter of longevity) and *cakṣuṣya* (promoter of eye sight). It aggravates *vāyu* and alleviates *kapha* and *pitta*. It cures *gara* (poisoning), . *śūla* (colic pain), *śopha* (oedema), *arśas* (piles), *plīhan* (splenic disorder), *pāṇḍutā* (anemia), *medas* (adiposity), *meha* (obstinate urinary disorders including diabetes), *kṛmi* (parasitic infection) and *kuṣṭha* (obstinate skin diseases including leprosy).

Its *kitta* which is called *maṇḍūra* (rust of iron) shares all the properties of iron.

गुरुता दृढतोत्क्लेद कश्मलं दाहकारिता ।

अश्मदोषः सुदुर्गन्धो दोषाः सप्तायसस्य च ॥२४६॥'

**Bad quality**

*Gurutā* (heaviness), *dṛḍhatā* (sturdiness), *utkleda* (stickiness), *kaśmala* (impurity), *dāhakāritā* (producing burning sensation), *aśmadoṣa* (adulteration with stone ?) *sudurgandha* (foul smell)—these are the seven defects of iron.

षंढत्वकुष्ठामयमृत्युदंतद्हृद्रोगशूलौ कुरुतेऽश्मरीं च ।

नानारुजानां च तथा प्रकोपं
करोति हृल्लासमशुद्धलोहम् ॥२५०॥

**Adverse effects**

*Loha,* which is not properly processed, causes *ṣaṇḍatva* (impotency), *kuṣṭha* (obstinate skin diseases including leprosy), *mṛtyu* (death), *hṛdroga* (heart disease), *śūla* (colic pain), *aṣmarī* (stone in urinary tract), aggravation of different types of pain and *hṛllāsa* (nausea).

जीवहारि मदकारि चायसं चेदशुद्धिमदसंस्कृतं[178] ध्रुवम् ।

पाटवं[179] न कुरुते शरीरके दारुणं हृदि रुजं च यच्छति ॥२५१॥

[आयुर्वेदप्रकाश ३:२१८-२२५]

If *loha* which is not properly processed is taken then it takes away the life, produces intoxication, does not produce energy in the body and causes acute pain in the heart.

कूष्माण्डं तिलतैलं च माषान्नं राजिकां तथा ।
मद्य[180]मम्लरसं चैव त्यजेल्लोहस्य सेवकः ॥ २५२ ॥

[आयुर्वेदप्रकाश ३ : २२६]

**Prohibition**

Persons using *loha* should give up *kuṣmāṇḍa*, *til* oil, *māṣa*, *rājikā*, *madya* (alcoholic drinks) and *amla rasa* (things having sour taste).

लोहं साराह्वयं श्रेष्ठं तस्य लक्षणमुच्यते ।
क्षमाभृच्छिखराकारन्यंगान्ये [न्यम्ले[181]नमर्दिते] ॥२५३॥
दृश्यन्ते यत्र सूक्ष्माणि सारं लोहेषु तद्वदेत् ।

*Sāra loha*

*Sāra loha* is the best among irons. It is *kṣamābhṛt* (stands to pressure) and *śikharākāra* (tapering in shape). When triturated with sour juice it leaves small dust-like particles.

लौहं साराह्वयं हन्याद्ग्रहणीमतिसारकम् ॥ २५४ ॥
अर्धंसर्वांगजं वातं शूलं च परिणामजम् ।
छर्दिपीनसपित्तं च श्वासं चाशु नियच्छति ॥२५५॥

**Property**

*Sārā lauha* immediately cures *grahaṇī* (sprue syndrome), *atisāra* (diarrhoea), aggravation of *vāyu* in half of the body or all over the body, *pariṇāmaja śūla* (colic pain which appears during the process of digestion of food), *chardi* (vomiting), *pīnasa* (chronic rhinitis), aggravated *pitta* and *śvāsa* (asthma).

यत्पात्रे न प्रसरति जले तैलबिन्दुः प्रतप्ते ।
हिंगु[182]र्गन्धं त्यजति च निजं तिक्त[183]तां निंबकल्कः ॥ २५६ ॥
तप्तं दुग्धं भवति शिखराकारकं नैति भूमिम् ।
कृष्णांगः स्यात्सजलचणकः कान्तलोहं तदुक्तम् ॥ २५७ ॥

*Kānta loha*

In a pot of *kānta loha* containing hot water if a drop of oil is put then the oil does not spread. *Hiṅgu* (asafoetida) loses its foul smell and the paste of *nimba* loses its bitterness when put in such a pot. If milk is boiled in this pot, then it goes up in the form of a *śikhara* (pyramid) but does not fall down. It becomes black when *caṇakāmla* (*sajala caṇaka*) is kept in this pot.

गुल्मोदरार्शः शूलममामवातं भगन्दरम् ।
कान्तं तत्कामलाशोफकुष्ठक्षयरुजोहरेत् ॥ २५८ ॥
देहपुष्टिवलस्थैर्यं दत्तं जनयते सुतान् ।
रक्तप्लीह[184]प्रशमनमम्लपित्तं शिरोरुजम् ॥ २५९ ॥
सर्वान् रोगान्विजयते कान्तलोहं न संशयः ।

**Property**

*Kānta loha* cures *gulma* (phantom tumour), *udara* (obstinate abdominal diseases including ascitis), *arśas* (piles), *śūla*, (colic pain), *āma*, *āmavāta* (rheumatism), *bhagandara* (fistula-in-ano), *kāmalā* (jaundice), *śopha* (oedema), *kuṣṭha* (obstinate skin diseases including leprosy), *kṣaya* (consumption) and *ruk* (pain). It gives nourishment to the body and promotes strength and stability. It helps in the procreation of children. It alleviates vitiation of blood, *plīhan* (diseases of spleen), *amla pitta* (hyper acidity of stomach) and *śiroruk* (headache). *Kānta loha* cures all these diseases undoubtedly.

शताब्द[185]मुत्तमं किट्टं मध्यं चाशीतिवार्षिकम् ।
अधमं पष्ठि[186]वार्षीयं ततो हीनं विषोपमम् ॥ २६० ॥

[आयुर्वेदप्रकाश ३ : २९०-२९१]

*Loha kiṭṭa* **(Rust of Iron)**

*Loha kiṭṭa* which is one hundred years old is the best, eighty years old is mediocre and sixty years old is inferior. Rust of iron which is less than sixty years old is like poison.

योजयेल्लोहवत्सर्वं लोहस्थाने च तन्मलम् ।
तत्किट्टं तद्गुणं ज्ञेयं विशेषात्पांडुनाशनम् ॥ २६१ ॥

In the place of *loha*, its *mala* (rust) can be used in all diseases because the latter shares all the properties of the former. Moreover, its *mala* (rust) is specifically indicated in the treatment of *pāṇḍu* (anemia).

किट्टाद्दशगुणं मुण्डं मुण्डातीक्ष्णं शताधिकम् ।
तीक्ष्णाल्लक्षगुणं कान्तं भक्षणात्कुरुते बलम् ॥ २६२ ॥

[आयुर्वेदप्रकाश ३ : २६४]

From *kiṭṭa* (*maṇḍūra* or rust of iron) *muṇḍa loha* is ten times effective, from *muṇḍa loha*, *tīkṣṇa loha* is hundred times effective and from *tīkṣṇa loha*, *kānta* is one lakh times effective in producing strength.

**अभ्रकं माक्षिकं तालं शिला नीलांजनं** तथा ।
**तुत्थकं रसकं** चैते प्रोक्ताः सप्तोपधातवः ॥ २६३ ॥

### *Upadhātus*

*Abhraka*, *mākṣika*, *tāla*, *śilā*, *nīlāñjana*, *tutthaka* and *rasaka*—these seven are known as *upadhātus*.

'पुरा वधाय वृत्रस्य वज्रिणा वज्रसुद्धृतम् ।
विस्फुलिंगास्ततस्तस्य गगनं परिसर्पिताः ॥ २६४ ॥
ते निपेतुर्घनध्वाना[187]च्छिखरेषु महीभृताम् ।
तेभ्य एव समुत्पन्नं तत्तद्गिरिषु **चाभ्रकम्**[188] ॥२६५॥

[आयुर्वेदप्रकाश ३ : ८६-८७]

### *Abhraka* (Mica)

**Mythology**

In the days of yore, when *Vajri* (*Indra*) took out the *vajra* to kill the demon *Vṛtra*, then *visphuliṅgas* (fire particles) from that *vajra* spread over the sky and because of the thundering sound of the clouds fell on the tops of mountains. Thus, *abhraka* took birth in those mountains.

कदाचिद्गिरिजा देवी हरं दृष्ट्वा मनोहरम् ।

मुमोचयत्तदावीर्यं तज्जातं शुभमभ्रकम् ॥ २६६ ॥

Once upon a time, the goddess *Girijā* saw the extremely handsome *Hara*. The genital fluid (ovum) she then ejaculated gave rise to pure *abhraka*.

तत्र दक्षिणशैलेऽर्कशोषादल्पगुणं हि तत् ।

अल्पसत्त्वं तदाधत्ते तस्य सत्त्वं गुणप्रदम् ॥ २६७ ॥

**Quality**

*Abhraka* which is available in the southern mountains is inferior in quality because it gets dried by the strong heat of the sun. It produces less of *sattva*. However, this *sattva* is therapeutically useful.

अतस्तूत्तरशैलोत्थं वहुसत्त्वं गुणाधिकम् ।

*Abhraka* which is available in northern mountains contains more of *sattva* and is therefore superior in quality.

तद्वज्रं वज्रजातत्वादभ्रमभ्ररवोद्भवात् ॥२६८॥

189 190

गगनात्पतितं यस्माद्गगनं च ततो मतम् ।

**Derivation**

It is called *vajra* because of its origin from thunder (*vajra*). It is called *abhra* because it is produced with the help of the cloud (*abhra*). Since it has fallen from the sky (*gagana*), it is called *gagana*.

विप्रक्षत्रियविट्शूद्रभेदात्तस्याच्चतुर्विधम् ॥२६९॥

क्रमेणैव सितं रक्तं पीतं कृष्णं च वर्णतः ।

प्रशस्यते सितं तारे रक्तं चैव रसायने ॥ २७० ॥

[191]
पीतं हेमनि कृष्णं तु गदेषु द्रुतयेऽपि च ।

**Variety**

It is of four types viz., *vipra, kṣatriya, viṭ* and *śūdra* and they are white, red, yellow and black respectively. The white variety is useful in the preparation of silver, red variety for rejuvenation therapy, yellow variety in the preparation of gold and the black variety for the treatment of diseases as well as for *druti kriyā.*

पिनाकं दर्दुरं नागं वज्रं चेति चतुर्विधम् ।।२७१।।

मुञ्चत्यग्नौ विनिक्षिप्तं पिनाकं दलसंचयम् ।

अज्ञानाद् भक्षणं तस्य महाकुष्ठप्रदायकम् ।।२७२।।

दर्दुरं त्वग्निगं चातिकुरुते दर्दुरध्वनिम् ।

गोलकान्बहुशः कृत्वा स स्यान्मृत्युप्रदायकः ।।२७३।।

[भावप्रकाशः धातूपधातुवर्ग ८:११५-१२०]

'नागं तु नागवद्वह्नौ फूत्कारं परिमुञ्चति ।

तद्भक्षितमवश्यं तु विदधाति भगन्दरम् ।।२७४।।

वज्रं तु वज्रवत्तिष्ठेत्तन्नाग्नौ विकृतिं व्रजेत् ।

[192]
सर्वाभ्रेषु वरं वज्रं व्याधिवार्धक्यमृत्युजित्' ।।२७५।।

It is also classified in four different ways viz., *pināka, dardura, nāga* and *vajra*. When placed on fire, the *pināka* variety of *abhraka* gives up leaves, and if because of ignorance, it is used, then it causes serious types of *kuṣṭha* (obstinate skin diseases including leprosy). The *dardura* variety of *abhraka* when placed on fire produces sound like a frog. It produces many *golakas* (abscesses?) and thus leads to death. The *nāga* variety of *abhraka* produces hissing (*phutkāra*) sound like that of a cobra, when placed on fire. This, when used, certainly produces *bhagandara* (fistula-in-ano). The *vajra* variety of *abhraka* stands on the fire like a *vajra* (thunder) without undergoing any change. Amongst all these varieties, the *vajra* type of *abhraka* is the best and it overcomes diseases, old age and even death.

अभ्रं कषायं मधुरं सुशीतमायुष्करं धातुविवर्धनं च ।

हन्यात्त्रिदोषं व्रणमेहकुष्ठं प्लीहोदरं ग्रन्थिविषं कृमींश्च ।।२७६।।

**Property**

*Abhraka* is astringent, sweet, exceedingly cooling and promoter of longevity and *dhātus* (tissue elements of the body). It alleviates all the three *doṣas* and cures *vraṇa* (ulcer), *meha* (obstinate urinary disorders including diabetes), *kuṣṭha* obstinate skin diseases including leprosy), *plīhan* (splenic disorders), *udara* (obstinate abdominal diseases including ascitis), *granthi* (adenitis), *viṣa* (poisoning) and *kṛmi* (parasitic infection).

रोगान्हन्ति दृढयति वपुर्वीर्यवृद्धिं विधत्ते ।

तारुण्याढ्यं रमयति शतं योषितां नित्यमेव ।।२७७।।

[193]

दीर्घायुष्याञ्जनयति सुतान् सिंहतुल्यप्रभावान् ।

मृत्योर्भीतिं हरति नितरां सेव्यमानं मृताभ्रम् ।

*Abhraka*, when used in *bhasma* form, cures diseases, produces sturdiness of the body and increases semen. It produces youthfulness because of which a person can enjoy sex with one hundred ladies daily. It helps in the procreation of children endowed with longevity and strength like a lion. It takes away the fear of untimely death for ever.

[194]

पीडां विधत्ते विविधां नराणां कुष्ठं क्षयं पाण्डुगदं च शोथम् ।

[भावप्रकाश: धातूपधातुवर्ग ८:१२०-१२२, १२४-१२६]

[195]

हृत्पार्श्वपीडां च करोत्यशुद्धमभ्रं त्वशुद्धं गुरुतापदं स्यात् ।

**Adverse effect**

*Abhraka*, which is not properly processed, produces

different types of pain, *kuṣṭha* (obstinate skin diseases including leprosy), *kṣaya* (consumption), *pāṇḍu* (anemia), *śopha* (oedema), *hṛṭ pīḍā* (pain in cardiac region), *pārśva pīḍā* (pain in the sides of the chest) and serious type of burning sensation in the body of human beings.

माक्षिकं द्विविधं प्रोक्तं पीतं शुक्लं च सर्वतः ॥२७९॥

तयो सुवर्णवर्णं तु विज्ञेयं प्रवरं जनैः ।

### *Mākṣika* (Copper pyrite)

**Variety**

*Mākṣika* is of two types viz., yellow and white. The golden colour (yellow) *mākṣika* is considered to be the better.

[196]'माक्षिकं मधुरं तिक्तं स्वर्यं वृष्यं रसायनम् ॥२८०॥

चक्षुष्यं वस्तिरुक्कुष्ठपांडुमेहविषोदरम्[197] ।

[198]अर्शः शोफं क्षयं कण्डूं त्रिदोषं[199] च नियच्छति ॥२८१॥

[आयुर्वेदप्रकाश ८:९-१०]

**Property**

*Mākṣika* is sweet, bitter, promoter of good voice, aphrodisiac and rejuvenating. It promotes eye sight and cures *vastiruk* (pain in bladder), *kuṣṭha* (obstinate skin diseases including leprosy), *pāṇḍu* (anemia), *meha* (obstinate urinary disorders including diabetes), *viṣa* (poisoning), *udara* (obstinate abdominal diseases including ascitis), *arśas* (piles), *śopha* (oedema), *kṣaya* (consumption), *kaṇḍū* (itching) and all the three aggravated *doṣas*.

'मंदानलत्वं बलहानिमुग्रां विष्टंभतां नेत्रगदान्सकुष्ठान् ।

[200]करोति मालां व्रणपूर्वकं च शुध्यादिहीनं खलु माक्षिकं च ॥२८२॥

[आयुर्वेदप्रकाश ४:११]

**Adverse effect**

If *mākṣika* is used without proper processing then it

causes indigestion, extreme loss of strength, constipation, diseases of the eye, *kuṣṭha* (obstinate skin diseases including leprosy), *mālā* (cervical adenitis) and *vraṇa* (ulcer).

> **हरितालं** कटु स्निग्धं कषायोष्णं हेरद्विषम् ।
> कंडूकुष्ठास्यरोगास्रकफपित्तकचव्रणान्[201] ॥ २८३ ॥
>
> [आयुर्वेदप्रकाश २ : १७४]

### *Haritāla* (Yellow arsenic)

**Property**

*Haritāla* is pungent, unctuous, astringent, and hot. It cures *viṣa* (poisoning), *kaṇḍū* (itching) *kuṣṭha* (obstinate skin diseases including leprosy), *āsyaroga* (diseases of the mouth), vitiated blood, *kapha* and *pitta*, *kaca* (diseases of hair) and *vraṇa* (ulcer).

> हरति च हरितालं सौष्ठवं[202] देहजातम् ।
> सृजति च बहुतापं मेहकृच्छ्राश्मपीडाम्[203] ॥ २८४ ॥
> वितरति कफवातान् स्नायुशोषं करोति ।
> ह्यमृतमिहसमन्तात्कुष्ठरोगांश्च वेगात् ॥ २८५ ॥

**Adverse effect**

*Haritāla* (which normally works as a nectar), when used without proper processing, takes away the beauty of the body and produces excessive heat, *meha* (obstinate urinary diseases including diabetes), *kṛcchra* (dysuria), *aśma* (stone in the urinary tract) and *pīḍā* (pain). It aggravates *kapha* and *vāta*, dries up *snāyu* (tendons and ligaments), and produces *kuṣṭharoga* (obstinate skin diseases including leprosy).

> **मनःशिला** मन्दबलं करोति जन्तुं ध्रुवं शोधनमन्तरेण ।
> मलस्य बन्धं किल मूत्ररोधं[204] सशर्करं कृच्छ्रगदं च कुर्यात् ॥२८६॥
>
> [आयुर्वेदप्रकाश २ : २१७]

### *Manaḥśilā* (Realgar)

**Adverse effect**

*Manaḥśilā* used without *śodhana* (processing) certainly causes weakness, constipation, obstruction to micturation, *śarkarā* (gravels in the urinary tract) and *kṛcchra* (dysuria).

अतिदुर्धरमाध्माघ्नं विषमज्वरनाशनम् ।
रसायनं सुवर्णघ्नं लोहमार्दवकारकम् ॥ २८७ ॥

**Property**

It cures serious types of *ādhmāna* (flatulence) and *viṣama jvara* (malarial fever). It is rejuvenating. It is *suvarṇaghna* (which reduces gold into *bhasma* form) and *lohamārdava kāraka* (which causes softness in iron).

नेत्रामयहरं हृद्यं सोष्णं **नीलाञ्जनं** मतम् ।

### *Nīlāñjana* (Lead sulphide)

*Nīlāñjana* cures eye diseases. It is cardiac tonic and hot.

**तुत्थकं**[205] कटुकं क्षारं कषायं[206] वामकं लघु ॥ २८८ ॥
लेखनं भेदनं शीतं चक्षुष्यं कफपित्तजित् ।
विषामकुष्ठकंडूघ्नं तद्गुणं **खर्परं** स्मृतम् ॥२८९॥
[आयुर्वेदप्रकाश ८:३८-३९]

### *Tutthaka* and *Kharpara* (Copper sulphate and Zinc ore)

*Tutthaka* is pungent, alkaline, astringent, emetic, *laghu*, *lekhana* (depleting), purgative and cooling. It promotes eye sight and cures *kapha* as well as *pitta*. Is cures *viṣa* (poisoning), *āma*, *kuṣṭha* (obstinate skin diseases including leprosy) and *kaṇḍū* (itching).

*Kharpara* shares the properties of *tuttha*.

ये गुणास्तुत्थके प्रोक्तास्ते गुणाः **रसके** मताः ।

### *Rasaka*

*Rasaka* has the same properties as those of *tuttha*.

रसायनार्थिभिर्लोकैः पारदोरस्यते यतः ॥२९०॥

ततो **रस** इति प्रोक्तः स च धातुरिति स्मृतः ।

### *Pārada* (Mercury)

**Derivation**

It is called *rasa* because persons desirous of rejuvenation commonly use (*rasyate*) it. It is also called *'dhātu'*.

[207] शिवाङ्गान्निर्गतं तेजः पतितं धरणी तले ॥२९१॥

[208] तद्देहसारजातत्वाच्छुक्लवर्णमभूच्च तत् ।

**Mythology**

It was produced from the *tejas* (semen) of Lord *Śiva* which fell on the earth because of which it is white in colour.

क्षेत्रभेदेन विज्ञेयं शिववीर्यं चतुर्विधम् ॥२९२॥

श्वेतं रक्तं तथा पीतं कृष्णं [209] च भवति क्रमात् ।

ब्राह्मणः क्षत्रियो वैश्यः शूद्रश्च खलु जातितः ॥२९३॥

**Variety**

Depending upon the nature of the earth on which it was produced it is of four types viz., white, red, yellow and black. They are called *brāhmaṇa*, *kṣatriya*, *vaiśya* and *śūdra* respectively.

शस्तं श्वेतं रुजां नाशे रक्तं किल रसायने ।

धातुवादे तु तत्पीतं खे गतौ कृष्णमेव च ॥२९४॥

[भावप्रकाशः धातूपधातुवर्ग ८:८७-८९]

The white variety is useful in curing diseases. Red variety is used in rejuvenation. For *dhātuvāda* (preparing gold out of ordinary metals) yellow variety is used. Black variety is used for *khe gati* (moving in the sky).

[210] स्वयं रसो भवेद्ब्रह्मा बद्धश्चैव जनार्दनः ।

रञ्जित [211] क्रामितः सूतः साक्षाद्देवो महेश्वरः ॥२९५॥

**Property**

*Pārada* itself is *Brahmā* and after *baddha* (a special process by which mercury is made to stand strong heat without vaporisation), it is *Janārdana*. After *rañjana* and *krāmaṇa samskāras* (processes), the mercury becomes *Maheśvara* himself.

मूर्छित्वा हरति रुजं बन्धनमनुभूय खे गतिं कुरुते ।

[212] अजरीकरोति हि मृतः कोऽन्यः करुणाकरः सूतात् ॥२९६॥

[भावप्रकाशः धातूपधातुवर्ग ८ : २३-२४]

After *mūrchanā saṁskāra*, *pārada* cures diseases. After *bandhana saṁskāra* it enables a person to move in sky. After *māraṇa* (lit. death) *saṁskāra* it prevents death. In view of the above, who else (other than *pārada*) is more blissful ?

पारदः षड्रसः स्निग्धस्त्रिदोषघ्नो रसायनः ।

योगवाही महावृष्यः सदा [213] दृष्टिबलावहः ।

सर्वामयहरः प्रोक्तो विशेषात्सर्वकुष्ठनुत् ॥२९७॥

*Pārada* has six *rasas* (tastes). It is unctuous. It alleviates all the three *doṣas*. It is rejuvenating, *yogavāhin* (which enhances the efficacy of other drugs when mixed) and exceedingly aphrodisiac. It always promotes eye sight and strength. It cures all diseases. It has special curative property for all types of *kuṣṭha* (obstinate skin diseases including leprosy).

मलं विषं [214] वह्निगिरीवचापलं

[215] नैसर्गिकं दोषमुशन्ति पारदे ।

उपाधिजौ द्वौ [216] त्रपुनागसंज्ञकौ

दोषौ च [217] सूते कथितौ [218] चिकित्सकैः ॥२९८॥

*Doṣas* **and adverse effects**

*Mala*, *viṣa*, *vahni*, *giri* and *capala*--these are the *naisargika* (natural) *doṣas* (defects) in *pārada*. It has two other *doṣas* called *trapu* and *nāga* which are artificial (*upādhija*).

मलेन मूर्च्छा मरणं [219] विषेन
दाहोऽग्निना कष्टतरः शरीरे ।
देहस्य जाड्यं गिरिणा सदा स्या— [220]
[221] च्चापल्यतो वीर्यहृतिं च पुंसः ।
वङ्गेन [222] कुष्ठं भुजगेन गण्डो
[223] भवेदतोऽसौ खलुशोधनीयः ॥२९९॥

*Mala doṣa* causes *mūrcchā* (fainting), *viṣa doṣa* causes death, *vahni doṣa* causes burning sensation of serious type. Numbness and rigidity *(jāḍya)* appear in the body because of *giridoṣa*. *Chapala doṣa* destroys semen in the man. *Vaṅga doṣa* produces *kuṣṭha* (obstinate skin diseases including leprosy) and *nāga doṣa* produces *gaṇḍa* (goitre). Therefore, it is necessary to make *pārada* free from all these *doṣas* through the process of *śodhana* before use.

संस्कारहीनं खलु सूतराजं यः सेवते तस्य करोति बाधाम् ।
देहस्य नाशं विदधाति [224] नूनं कुष्ठांश्च रोगाञ्जनयेन्नराणाम ॥३००॥
[भावप्रकाशः धातूपधातुवर्ग. ८:९१-९२, ९६-९७, १००]

If *pārada* is used without *śodhana*, than the person suffers from many serious maladies like *kuṣṭha* resulting in death.

अथोपरसाः

'गन्धको वज्रवैक्रान्तो वज्राभ्रं तालकं शिला ।
खर्परं शिखि तुत्थं च विमलं हेममाक्षिकम् ॥३०१॥
कासीसं कान्तपाषाणो [225] वराटांजनहिंगुलम् ।

**कंकुष्ठं शंखभूनागं टंकणं** च **शिलाजतु** ॥३०२॥

226

उक्ता **उपसरसा** जातेर्द्रव्यनिर्णयकारिभिः ।

*Uparasa*

*Gandhaka*, *vajra*, *vaikrānta*, *vajrābhra*, *tālaka*, *śilā*, *kharpara*, *śikhituttha*, *vimalā*. *hema mākṣika*, *kāsīsa*, *kānta pāṣāṇa*, *varāta*, *añjana*, *hingula*, *kaṁkuṣṭa*, *śaṁkha*, *bhūnāga*, *tankaṇa* and *śilājatu*—these are known as *uparasas* by persons well versed in the identification of drugs.

**दरद**स्त्रिविधः प्रोक्तश्चर्मारः शुकतुण्डकः ॥३०३॥

हंसपादस्तृतीयः स्याद्गुणवानुत्तरोत्तरम् ।

***Hiṅgula* (Cinnabar)**

**Variety**

*Darada* or *hiṅgula* is of three types viz., *carmāra*, *śuka tuṇḍaka* and *haṁsa·pāda*. The latter ones are therapeutically better than the former ones.

चर्मारः शुक्लवर्णः स्यात्सपीतः शुकतुण्डकः ।

जपाकुसुमसङ्काशो हंसपादो महोत्तमः ॥३०४॥

[भावप्रकाशः धातूपधातुवर्ग ८:१०२-१०४]

*Carmāra* is white, *śukatuṇḍaka* is yellow and *haṁsa pāda* is red like a flower of *japā*. The last one is the best.

तिक्त कषायं कटुहिंगुलं स्यान्नेत्रामयघ्नं कफपित्तहारि ।

हृल्लासकुष्ठज्वरकामलाश्च प्लीहामवातौ च गरं निहन्ति ॥३०५॥

[भावप्रकाशः धातूपधातुवर्ग ८ : १०५]

**Property**

*Hiṅgula* is bitter, astringent and pungent. It cures eye diseases, aggravated *kapha* as well as *pitta*, *hṛllāsa* (nausea), *kuṣṭha* (obstinate skin diseases including leprosy), *jvara* (fever), *kāmalā* (jaundice) *plīhan* (splenic disorders), *āmavāta* (rheumatism) and *gara* (poisoning).

'श्वेतद्वीपे पुरा देव्याः[227]
क्रीडन्त्या रजसा [ऽऽ] प्लुतम् ।
दुकूलं तेन वस्त्रेण स्नातायाः क्षीरे[228] नीरधौ ।
प्रसूतं यद्रजस्तस्माद्गन्धकः समजायत[229] ॥३०७॥

### *Gandhaka* (Sulphur)

**Mythology**

In the days of yore, in the *Śveta dvīpa*, goddess *Pārvati* was playing aquatic games in the *kṣīra sāgara* during her menstrual period. From her garments, the menstrual fluid got into the water from which *gandhaka* took its origin.

चतुर्धा गन्धकः प्रोक्तो रक्तः पीतः सितोऽसितः[230] ।
रक्तो हेमक्रियासूक्तः पीतश्चैव रसायजे ॥३०८॥
व्रणादिलेपने श्वेतः श्रेष्ठः कृष्णः सुदुर्लभः ।

**Variety**

*Gandhaka* is of four types viz., red, yellow, white and black. The red variety is used in processing (preparing) gold (*hema kriyā*). The yellow variety is used in rejuvenation therapy. The white variety is useful in ointments for ulcers. The black variety which is the best is extremely rare.

गन्धकः कटुकस्तिक्तो वीर्योष्णस्तुवरः सरः ॥३०९॥
पित्तलः कटुकः पाके कंडूविसर्पजन्तुजित् ।
हन्ति कुष्ठक्षयप्लीहकफवातान् रसायनम्[231] ॥३१०॥

[भावप्रकाशः धातूपधातुवर्ग ८:१०७-१११]

**Property**

*Gaudhaka* is pungent, bitter, hot in potency, saline,

laxative, aggravator of *pitta* and pungent in *vipāka*. It cures *kuṣṭha* (obstinate skin diseases including leprosy), *kṣaya* (consumption) and *plīhan* (splenic disorders). It alleviates *kapha* and *vāta*, and is rejuvenating.

'अशुद्धो गन्धकः कुष्ठं तापं देहे करोति हि ।
सौख्यं च रूपं च बलं
232
शुक्रमोजो हन्ति न संशयः ॥३११॥'

**Adverse effect**

Use of *gandhaka* which is not properly processed (*aśuddha*) causes *kuṣṭha* (obstinate skin diseases including leprosy) and *tāpa* (burning sensation). It undoubtedly takes away happiness, complexion, strength, semen and *ojas*.

233
'निदाघे धर्मसंतप्ता धातुसारं धराधराः ।
निर्यासवत्प्रमुञ्चन्ति तच्छिलाजतु कीर्तितम् ॥३१२॥

[आयुर्वेदप्रकाश ४:६६]

*Śilājatu* **(Mineral pitch)**

The essence of stones which exudates from the mountains by the heat of the sun in summer is called *śilājatu*.

मधुरं च सतिक्तं च जपापुष्पनिभं च यत् ।
विपाके कटुशीतं च तत्सुवर्णस्य निःसृतम् ॥३१३॥

**Variety**

The *śilājatu* which comes out of stones of gold is sweet and bitter in taste, like the flower of *japā* in colour, pungent in *vipāka* and cooling.

'राजतं पाण्डुरं शीतं कटुकं स्वादुपाकि च ।
ताम्रान्मयूरकण्ठाभं तीक्ष्णमुष्णं च जायते ॥ ३१४ ॥
234
'लौहं जटायुपक्षाभं सतिक्तं लवणं भवेत्' ।

विपाके कटुकं शीतं सर्वश्रेष्ठमुदाहृतम्' ॥३१५॥

[आयुर्वेदप्रकाश: ४ : ९९-१००]

The silver type of *śilājatu* is gray in colour, cooling, pungent in taste and sweet in *vipāka*. The *śilājatu* derived from *tāmra* is like the peacock throat in colour, sharp and hot. The *śilajatu* derived from iron stone is like the feather of *jatāyu* in colour and bitter and saline in taste. It pungent in *vipāka* and cooling. This is the best of all varieties.

यथाक्रमं वातपित्ते श्लेष्मापन्ने कफे त्रिषु ।

विशेषतः प्रशस्यन्ते भेदा अश्मजतूद्भवाः ॥३१६॥

The first variety is useful in alleviating *vāyu* and *pitta*, the second and third varieties alleviate *kapha* and the fourth one alleviates all the three *doṣas*.

शिलाजं कटुतिक्तोष्णं कटुपाकं रसायनम् ।

235

छेदि योगवहं हन्ति कफमेहाश्मशर्कराः ॥३१७॥

मूत्रकृच्छ्रं क्षयं श्वासं वातार्शांसि च पाण्डुताम् ।

236

अपस्मारं तथोन्मादं शोफकुष्ठोदरकृमीन् ॥३१८॥

[भावप्रकाशः धातूपधातुवर्ग ८:८०-८२]

**Property**

It is pungent and bitter in taste, hot, pungent in *vipāka* and rejuvenating. It is *chedi* (depleting) and *yogavaha* (which enhances the properties of other drugs). It cures aggravated *kapha*, *meha* (obstinate urinary diseases including diabetes), *aśma śarkarā* (stones and gravel in the urinary tract) *mūtra kṛcchra* (dysuria), *kṣaya* (consumption), *śvāsa* (asthma), aggravated *vāyu*, *arśas* (piles), *pāṇḍu* (anemia), *apasmāra* (epilepsy), *unmāda* (insanity), *śopha* (oedema), *kuṣṭha* (obstinate skin diseases including leprosy), *udara* (obstinate abdominal diseases including ascitis) and *kṛmi* (parasitic infection).

**अथरत्नोपरत्नलक्षणगुणा—**

गरुत्मतेन्द्रनीलाद्याः प्रस्तरा **रत्नसंज्ञकाः** ।

मौक्तिकाद्युपरत्नं स्यादुत्पत्तिस्तस्य कथ्यते ॥३१९॥

*Ratna* **and** *Uparatna* **(Jewels & costly stones)**

**Derivation**

Stones like *garutman* and *indranīla* are called *ratnas. Muktā* etc., are called *uparatnas*. Now the derivation of this term is being described.

धनार्थिनो जनाः सर्वे रमन्तेऽस्मिन्नतीव यत् ।

ततो रत्नमिति प्रोक्तं शब्दशास्त्रविशारदैः ॥३२०॥

[भावप्रकाशः धातूपधातुरत्नोपरत्नवर्ग ८:१६८]

[आयुर्वेदप्रकाश ५:२]

Since people desirous of wealth indulge (*ramante*) in excess in these stones, therefore scholars of linguistics call them *ratna*.

**इन्द्रपक्षीन्द्रसूर्येन्दुमणयः पुष्परागकः** ।

**वज्रवैडूर्यगोमेदपद्मरागा** अमीनव ॥३२१॥

**Type**

*Indra*, *paksīndra*, *sūryendu*, *maṇi*, *puṣpa rāga*, *vajra*, *vaiḍūrya*, *gomeda* and *padma rāga*—these are the nine *ratnas*.

मुक्ताविद्रुमशंखाद्या रत्नोपमणयतस्तथा ।

*Mukta*, *vidruma*, *śaṅkha* etc., are called *uparatnas*.

चक्षुष्याः लेखनाः शीताः कषाया मधुरा सराः ॥३२२॥

मंगल्या धारणादश्री ग्रहदुष्टिविषापहाः ।

**Property**

These *ratnas* and *uparatnas* are *cakṣuṣya* (promoter of eye sight), *lekhana* (depleting), cooling, astringent, sweet and laxative. Wearing them bestows auspiciousness and destroys the evil effects of *graha* (planets), *duṣṭi* (evil sight) and *viṣa* (poisoning).

पूजार्थमात्मयोनेश्च ब्रह्मणा सृजतः किल ।।३२३।।

237

अकरोद्विघ्नमसुरः कैटभाख्यः प्रतापवान् ।

तदाक्रुद्धस्य वदनाद्ब्रह्मणस्तेजसोनिधेः ।।३२४।।

क्रोधो विग्रहवान्भूत्वा निवपातातिदारुणः ।

स तं ददाहगर्जन्तमन्तकामं महाबलम् ।।३२५।।

ततोऽसुरं घातयित्वा तत्तेजोऽवर्धताद्भुतम् ।

ततो विषादो देवानामभवत्तं निरीक्ष्य च ।।३२६।।

विषादजननत्वाच्च **विषमित्यभिधीयते** ।

ततः स्पष्टा प्रजा शेषा तदा तं क्रोधमीश्वरः ।।३२७।।

न्यस्तवान्सर्वभूतेषु स्थावरेषु चरेषु च ।

## *Viṣa* (Poisons)

### Mythology

A powerful demon, who was created by *Brahmā*, created disturbance in the performance of rituals by the latter. Then *Brahmā*, the abode of all the powers (*tejas*) became very angry and from his mouth the terrifying anger came out in a corporeal form (*vigrahavān*) and fell on the roaring powerful demon and burnt him. After his death, that flame surprisingly expanded. Looking at this, the gods became exceedingly sad. Because of its property to cause sorrow (*viṣāda*), it is called *viṣa*. Then being requested by the remaining subjects, *Iśvara* withdrew that flame of anger and placed it in *sthāvaras* (those who do not move like vegetable kingdom, stone etc.,) and *cara* (those who move like animal kingdom).

यथाऽव्यक्तरसं तोयं आन्तरिक्षं महीगतम् ।।३२८।।

तेषु तेषु प्रदेशेषु रसं तं तं नियच्छति ।

एवमेव विषं यच्च द्रव्ये व्याप्यावतिष्ठते ॥३२९॥

स्वभावादेवतत्तस्य रसं समनुवर्तते ।

As the rain water which has no manifested taste while in the sky, carries different types of tastes when it falls on the earth and comes in contact with different types of soil, similarly the *viṣa* acquires the taste of the substance in which it resides.

विषे यस्माद्गुणाः सर्वे तीक्ष्णाः प्रायेण सन्ति हि ॥३३०॥

विषं सर्वमतो ज्ञेयं सर्वदोषप्रकोपनम् ।

**Property**

All the properties of *viṣa* are super imposed by sharpness (*tīkṣṇa*). Therefore, all types of poisons aggravate all the three *doṣas*.

238

**कालकूटोवत्सनाभः शृङ्गकश्च प्रदीपनः ॥ ३३१ ॥**

**हालाहलो ब्रह्मपुत्रो हारिद्रः सक्तुकस्तथा ।**

**सौराष्ट्रक** इति प्रोक्ता विषभेदा अमीनव ।

**Variety**

*Kālakūṭa*, *vatsanābha*, *śṛṅgaka*, *pradīpana*, *hālāhala*, *brahmaputra*, *hāridra*, *saktuka* and *saurāṣṭraka*—these are the nine varieties of *viṣa*.

239

**कालकूटः** कृष्णवर्णैरनन्तैर्विन्दुभिस्ततः ॥ ३३२ ॥

अयं तु देवासुरसमरे मालिनाम्नोऽसुरस्य शोणितात्समुत्पन्नस्य पिप्पल-सदृशस्य तरोः निर्यासः अहिछत्रमलयकोङ्कणश्रृङ्गवेरपर्वतादिषूत्पद्यते ।

*Kālakūṭa* is studded with innumerable black spots. It was originally produced from the blood of a demon called *Māli* during the war between the gods and the demons. It is the exudate of a tree having leaves like those of *pippala*. It is available in the mountains like *Ahichhatra, Malaya, Koṅkaṇa* and *Sṛṅgavera*.

वत्सनाभः सिन्दुवारसदृशपत्रो वत्सनाभ्याकृतिः एतत्समीपे वृक्षा न वर्धन्ते ॥ ३३३ ॥

*Vatsanābha* has leaves like those of *sinduvāra* and in shape it is like the umbilicus of a calf. No other tree grows near this plant.

240
'ब्राह्मणः पाण्डुरास्तेषु क्षत्रियो रक्तवर्णकः ।'

[भावप्रकाशः विषोपविषवर्ग ८ : २००]

वैश्यः पीतप्रभः शूद्रः कृष्णाभः स तु निन्दितः ।

'रसायने विषं विप्रं क्षत्रियं देहपुष्टये' ॥ ३३४ ॥

[भावप्रकाशः विषोपविषवर्ग ८ : २०१]

कुष्ठनाशे प्रयुञ्जीत वैश्यं शूद्रं च धातुषु ।

Among them, the *brāhmaṇa* variety is gray (*pāṇḍura*) in colour, *kṣatriya* is red, *vaiśya* is yellow and *śūdra* is black. The last variety is not useful therapeutically. The *brāhmaṇa* (*vipra*) type of *viṣa* is useful in rejuvenation therapy ; *kṣatriya* type is for nourishment of the body ; *vaiṣya* type is for curing *kuṣṭha* (obstinate skin diseases including leprosy) and *śūdra* is for processing *dhātus*.

विषं प्राणहरं युक्त्या प्राणकृच्च रसायनम् ॥ ३३५ ॥

योगवाहि परं श्लेष्मवातहृत्सन्निपातजित् ।

**Property**

*Viṣa* kills a person ; but when used judiciously it gives life and works as a rejuvenating agent. It is an excellent *yoga-vāhin* (which enhances the properties of other drugs). It alleviates *kapha* and *vāyu*, and cures *sannipāta* (a condition created by the aggravation of all the three *doṣas*).

**अर्कक्षीरं** **स्नुहीक्षीरं** **लांगली** **करवीरकः** ।

**गुंजाऽहिफेनो** **धुत्तूरः** **सप्तोपविषजातयः** ॥ ३३६ ॥

[भावप्रकाशः धातूपधातुरत्नोपरत्नविषोपविषवर्ग ८ : २०५]

*Upaviṣa* **(Subsidiary poisons)**

**Variety**

*Arka kṣīra*, *snuhīkṣīra*, *lāṅgalī*, *karavīraka*, *guñjā*, *ahiphena* and *dhuttūra*—these are the seven *upaviṣas* (subsidiary poisons).

विशदो **गैरिकः** स्निग्धः कषायो मधुरोहिमः ।

*Gairika* **(Red Ochre)**

*Gairika* is *viśada* (non slimy), unctuous, astringent, sweet and cooling.

**स्वर्णगैरिकस्तु** तद्वच्चक्षुष्यं तद्विशेषतः ॥ ३३७ ॥

A variety of it is known as *svarna gairika*. It shares all the properties of *gairika*. It is specially useful as a promoter of eyesight.

**स्रोतोञ्जनं** वरं तत्र ततः सौवीरकाञ्जनम् ।

*Srotoñjana* & *Sauvīrakañjana*

As a promoter of eyesight, *srotoñjana* is better than *svarna gairika* and *sauvīrakāñjana* is better than *srotoñjana.*

कफघ्नं कटुकं तिक्तं छेदि सोष्णं रसायनम् ॥३३८॥

'चक्षुष्यं **श्वेतमरिचं** चक्षुष्या पीतरोहिणी ।

*Śveta marica* & *Pītarohiṇī*

*Śveta marica* alleviates *kapha*. It is pungent, bitter, depleting, hot and rejuvenating. *Śveta marica* and *pītarohiṇī*—both are also promoters of eyesight (*cakṣuṣya*).

**वंदाकः** कफवातास्रक्षोव्रणविषापहः ॥ ३३९ ॥

*Vandāka*

*Vandāka* alleviates *kapha*, *vāta* and blood. It cures *rakṣas* (afflictions by evil spirits), *vraṇa* (ulcer) and *viṣa* (poison).

241

सक्षारं उष्णवीर्यश्च **काचो** दृष्टिकरोऽञ्जनात् ।

*Kāca*

*Kāca* is alkaline and hot in potency. It promotes eye sight when used as a collyrium.

**कासीसद्वय**मम्लोष्णं तिक्तं केश्यं दृशोर्हितम् ॥ ३४० ॥

हन्तिकण्डूविषश्वित्रशूलाघातकफानिलान् ।

*Kāsīsa* **(Iron sulphate)**

Both the types of *kāsīsa* are sour, hot, bitter and *keśya* (promoter of good hair). They also promote eyesight. They cure *kaṇḍū* (itching), *viṣa* (poison), *śvitra* (leucoderma), *śūla* (colic pain), *āghāta* (injury) and aggravated *kapha* as well as *vāyu*.

**शंखोदधिमलौ** शीतौ कषायावतिलेखनौ ।

*Śaṅkha* **and** *Udadhimala* **(Conch-shell and Cuttle fish bone)**

*Śaṅkha* and *samudraphena*—both are cooling, astringent and *atilekhana* (exceedingly depleting).

242

**लघुशंखादयः** शीतः नेत्ररुक्स्फोटनाशनाः ॥ ३४१ ॥

[माधवद्रव्यगुण : १५३-१५६]

*Laghu śaṅkha*

*Laghu śaṅkha* etc., are cooling. They cure *netraruk* (pain in eyes) and *sphoṭa* (pustular eruptions).

'कफपित्तविषार्तिघ्नी सौराष्ट्री व्रणशोधनी ।

### *Saurāṣṭrī* (Alum)

*Saurāṣṭrī* cures aggravated *kapha* as well as *pitta* and *viṣa* (poisoning). It is *vraṇaśodhana* (cleansing of ulcers).

**पंकः** पित्तास्रदाहघ्नो भग्नक्षयहितो हिमः ॥ ३४२ ॥

### *Paṅka* (Mud)

*Paṅka* alleviates *pitta*, vitiated blood and *dāha* (burning syndrome). It is useful in *bhagna* (fracture)and *kṣaya* (consumption). It is cooling.

243

केश्यो **हस्तिमद**श्वित्ररंजनो विषनाशनः ।

सर्वपित्तमपस्मारकुष्ठदुष्टव्रणापहः' ॥ ३४३ ॥

[माधवद्रव्यगुणः विविधौषधिवर्गः १६८-१६९]

'चक्षुष्यः कटुतीक्ष्णोष्णमुन्मादकृमिनाशनः ।

### *Hasti mada*

*Hastimada* is *keśya* (promoter of good hair). It gives colour to *śvitra* (leucoderma) and cures *viṣa* (poison), aggravated *pitta*, *apasmāra* (epilepsy), *kuṣṭha* (obstinate skin diseases including leprosy) and *duṣṭa vraṇa* (serious type of ulcer). It promotes eyesight. It is pungent, sharp and hot. It also cures *unmāda* (insanity) and *kṛmi* (parasitic infection).

**गोरोचना**तिमाङ्गल्या विषालक्ष्मीग्रहापहा' ॥ ३४४ ॥

[माधवद्रव्यगुण : विविधौषधिवर्ग : १७०]

### *Gorocana* (Ox bile)

Gorocana is exceedingly propitious and it cures *viṣa* (poison), *alakṣmī* (inauspiciousness) and *graha* (afflictions by evil planets).

244

'सिन्दूरमुष्णं वीसर्पकुष्ठकंडूविषापहम् ।

भग्नसंधानजननं व्रणशोधनरोपणम् ।। ३४५ ।।

[माधवद्रव्यगुणः विविधौषधिवर्ग : १६७]

### *Sindūra* (Red oxide of lead)

*Sindūra* is hot and it cures *visarpa* (erysipelas), *kuṣṭha* (obstinate skin diseases including leprosy) *kaṇḍū* (itching) and *viṣa* (poisoning). It helps in the healing of fracture. It cleanses and heals ulcers.

"**कमलं** शीतलं वर्ण्यं मधुरं कफपित्तजित् ।

245

"तृष्णादाहास्रविस्फोटविषविसर्पनाशनं" ।। ३४६ ।।

[भावप्रकाशः पुष्पवर्ग ५ : ३]

### *Kamala* (Nelumbo nucifera Gaertn.)

*Kamala* is cooling, *varṇya* (promoter of complexion) and sweet. It alleviates *kapha* and *pitta*. It cures *tṛṣṇā* (morbid thirst), *dāha* (burning syndrome), *asra* (vitiated blood), *visphoṭa* (pustular eruptions), *viṣa* (poisoning) and *visarpa* (erysipelas).

तस्मादल्पांतरगुणमन्य**द्रक्तोत्पला**दिकं ।

### *Raktotpala* (Nymphaea rubra Roxb.)

*Raktotpala* shares all the properties of *kamala* ; but it is slightly inferior.

**कुमुदं** पिच्छिलं स्निग्धं मधुरं ह्लादि शीतलं ।।३४७।।

[भावप्रकाशः पुष्पवर्ग ५ : १५]

### *Kumuda* (Nymphaea alba Linn.)

*Kumuda* is slimy, unctuous, sweet, *hlādi* (pleasing) and cooling.

जातीद्वयं लघूष्णं स्यात्तिक्तं दोषत्रयापहं ।

246

शिरोऽक्षिमुखदंतार्त्तिविषकुष्ठव्रणस्रजित् ॥ ३४८ ॥

*Jātī* **(Jasminum grandiflorum Linn.)**

Both the varieties of *jātī* are light, hot and bitter. They alleviate all the three *doṣas*. They cure diseases of head, eyes, mouth, teeth, *viṣa* (poisoning), *kuṣṭha* (obstinate skin diseases including leprosy), *vraṇa* (ulcer) and vitiated blood.

ईषदुष्णं मरुत्श्लेष्मनाशनं बहुगन्धकृत् ।

कामसंजननं चापि **करुणकुसुमं** मतम् ॥ ३४९ ॥

*Karuṇa*

The flower of *karuṇa* is slightly hot. It alleviates *vāyu* and *kapha*. It is very fragrant and it stimulates passion.

'मल्लिकोष्णालघुर्वृष्यातिक्ता च कटुका हरेत् ।

247

वातपित्तास्यहृद्रोगकुष्ठारुचिविषव्रणान् ॥ ३५० ॥

*Mallikā* **(Jasminum sambac Ait.)**

*Mallikā* is hot, light, aphrodisiac, bitter and pungent. It alleviates *vāyu* and *pitta* and cures diseases of mouth and heart, *kuṣṭha* (obstinate skin diseases including leprosy), *aruci* (anorexia), *viṣa* (poisoning) and *vraṇa* (ulcer).

248

माधवी मधुरा शीता लघुर्दोषत्रयापहा' ।

[भावप्रकाश: पुष्पवर्ग ५ : ३९-४०]

*Mādhavī* **(Hiptage benghalensis Kurz)**

*Mādhavī* is sweet, cooling and light. It alleviates all the three *doṣas*.

यूथिकायुगलं शीतं तिक्तं च कटुकं लघु ॥ ३५१ ॥

तुबरं मधुरं हृद्यं पित्तघ्नं कफवातलम् ।

व्रणास्रमुखदन्ताक्षिशिरोरोगविषापहम्'' ॥ ३५२ ॥

[भावप्रकाशः पुष्पवर्ग ५ : २९]

### *Yūthikā* (Jasminum auriculatum Vahl.)

Both the types of *yūthikā* are cooling, bitter, pungent, light, astringent, sweet and cardiac tonic. It alleviates *pitta* and aggravates *kapha* as well as *vāyu*. It cures *vraṇa* (ulcer), *asra* (vitiated blood), diseases of mouth, teeth, eyes and head, and *viṣa* (poisoning).

'कुब्जकः सुरभिः स्वादुः कषायानुरसः सरः ।

249

त्रिदोषशमनो वृष्यः शीत हर्त्ता च स स्मृतः ॥ ३५३ ॥

[भावप्रकाशः पुष्पवर्ग 4 : 37]

### *Kubjaka* (Rosa Moschata Herrm.)

*Kubjaka* is fragment, sweet, astringent (as subsidiary taste or *anurasa*) and laxative. It alleviates all the three *doṣas*. It is aphrodisiac and alleviator of cold.

'शतपत्री हिमा हृद्या ग्राहिणी शुक्रला लघुः ।

दोषत्रयास्रजिद्वर्ण्या कट्वी तिक्ता च पाचिनी' ॥ ३५४ ॥

[भावप्रकाशः पुष्पवर्ग ५ : २२]

### *Śatapatrī*

*Śatapatrī* is cooling, cardiac tonic, constipative, promoter of semen and light. It alleviates all the three *doṣas* and vitiated blood and promotes complexion. It is pungent, bitter and carminative.

शतपत्रीभवं वारिश्रमघ्नं वातपित्तजित् ।

मनोह्लादकरं नेत्र्यं दुर्गन्धाश्रीविषापहम् ॥ ३५५ ॥

The water (after distillation?) of *śatapatrī* alleviates exhaustion, *vāyu* and *pitta*. It is pleasing to the mind, promoter of eye sight and remover of foul smell of the body as well as inauspiciousness. It cures *viṣa* (poisoning).

**केतकी** युगलं तिक्तं कटुस्वादुविषापहम् ।

*Ketakī* **(Pandanus tectorius Soland ex Parkinson)**

Both the varieties of *ketakī* are bitter, pungent and sweet. It cures *viṣa* (poisoning).

250 **नैपाली** शीतला तिक्ता लघ्वी दोषत्रयापहा ॥ ३५६ ॥

कर्णाक्षि मुखरोगघ्नी तद्गुणा 251 **वार्षिकी** मता ।

*Naipālī* & *Vārṣikī*

*Naipālī* is cooling, bitter and light. It alleviates all the three *doṣas*. It cures the diseases of ear, eyes and mouth. *Vārṣikī* has similar properties.

'**चंपकः** कटुकस्तिक्तः कषायो मधुरो हिमः ।

विषक्रिमिहरः कृच्छ्रकफपित्तास्रवातजित्' ॥ ३५७ ॥

[भावप्रकाशः पुष्पवर्ग ५ : ३१]

*Campaka* **(Michelia champaca Linn.)**

*Campaka* is pungent bitter, astringent, sweet and cooling. It cures *viṣa* (poisoning), *kṛmi* (parasitic infection), *kṛcchra* (dysuria), aggravated *kapha*, *pitta*, blood and *vāyu*.

अक्षिरोगहरश्चापि विशेषाद्**राजचंपकः** ।

*Rāja campaka*

*Rāja campaka* is specifically useful for eye diseases.

252 **बकुलस्तुवरो**रूक्षः कटुपाकरसो गुरुः ।

कफपित्तविषश्वित्रक्रिमिदन्तगदापहः' ॥ ३५८ ॥

[भावप्रकाशः पुष्पवर्ग ५ : ३२]

### *Bakula* (**Mimusops elengi Linn.**)

*Bakula* is astringent and ununctuous. It is pungent both in *vipāka* and *rasa*. It is heavy. It cures aggravated *kapha* as well as *pitta*, *viṣa* (poisoning), *śvitra* (leucoderma), *kṛmi* (parasitic infection) and *danta gada* (diseases of teeth).

[253] '**वको** रूक्षः कटुस्तिक्तः कफपित्तविषापहः ।
योनिशूलतृषादाहकुष्ठशोफास्रनाशनः[254]' ॥ ३५९ ॥
[भावप्रकाशः पुष्पवर्ग ५ : ३४]

### *Vaka*

*Vaka* is ununctuous, pungent and bitter. It cures aggravated *kapha* as well as *pitta*, *viṣa* (poisoning), *yoni śūla* (pain in female genital tract), *tṛṣā* (morbid thirst), *dāha* (burning syndrome), *kuṣṭha* (obstinate skin diseases including leprosy), *śopha* (oedema) and *asra* (vitiated blood).

**पाटल**स्तु महाशीतः कफवातप्रकोपनः ।
मन्दाग्निपित्तरोगघ्नः कफव्याधिविनाशकृत् ॥३६०॥

### *Pāṭala* (**Stereospermum suaveolens Dc.**)

*Pāṭala* is exceedingly cooling. It aggravates *kapha* and *vāta*. It cures indigestion, diseases caused by *pitta* as well *kapha* (?).

वातपित्तप्रशमनो मनोज्ञो **देववल्लभः** ।

### *Deva vallabha*

*Deva vallabha* alleviates *vāta* and *pitta*. It is pleasing to the mind.

पवित्रं **नीपकुसुमं** तद्वदेव**कदंबजम** ॥३६१॥

### *Nīpa* & *Kadamba* (**Adina cordifolia Benth and Hook. f and Anthocephalus cadamba Miq.**)

The flowers of both *nīpa* and *kadamba* are sacred,

'**तुलसी** कटुका तिक्ता हृद्योष्णा दाहपित्तकृत् ।

दीपनी कुष्ठकृच्छ्रास्रपार्श्वरुक्कफवातजित्' ॥३६२॥

[भावप्रकाशः पुष्पवर्ग ५:६२]

विषकृमिवमिश्वासदुर्नामाक्षिरुजापहा ।

*Tulasī* (**Ocimum sanctum Linn.**)

*Tulasī* is pungent, bitter, cardiac tonic and hot. It causes *dāha* (burning syndrome) and aggravation of *pitta*. It stimulates digestion, and cures *kuṣṭha* (obstinate skin diseases including leprosy), *kṛcchra* (dysuria), *asra* (vitiation of blood) and *pārśvaruk* (pain in the sides of chest). It alleviates *kapha* and *vāta*. It also cures *viṣa* (poisoning), *kṛmi* (parasitic infection), *vami* (vomiting), *śvāsa* (asthma), *durnāma* (piles) and *akṣiruk* (pain in eyes).

[255] '**दमन**स्तुवरस्तिक्तः शीतो वृष्यः सुगन्धिकः ।

[256] ग्रहणीविषकुष्ठास्रक्लेदकण्डूत्रिदोषजित्' ॥ ३६३ ॥

[भावप्रकाशः पुष्पवर्ग ५:६७]

*Damana*

*Damana* is astringent, bitter, cooling, aphrodisiac and fragrant. It cures *grahaṇī* (sprue syndrome), *viṣa* (poisoning), *kuṣṭha* (obstinate skin diseases including leprosy), *asra* (vitiation of blood), *kleda* (stickiness), *kaṇḍū* (itching) and aggravation of all the three *doṣas*.

**फणिज्झको**ऽग्निदोहृद्यस्तिक्तोष्णः पित्तलो लघुः ।

'वृश्चिकादिविषश्लेष्मवातकुष्ठकृमिप्रणुत् ।

कटुपाकरसो रुच्यस्तिक्तो रूक्षः सुगन्धिकः[257] ॥ ३६४ ॥

[भावप्रकाशः पुष्पवर्ग ५:६५]

*Phaṇijjhaka* (**Ocimum basilicum Linn.**)

*Phaṇijjhaka* stimulates digestion. It is cardiac tonic,

bitter and hot. It aggravates *pitta*. It is light. It cures the poisoning by scorpion stings, aggravation of *kapha* and *vāyu*, *kuṣṭha* (obstinate skin diseases including leprosy) and *kṛmi* (parasitic infection.) In *vipāka* and taste it is pungent. It is appetiser, bitter, unusuctuous and fragrant.

**कुमुदोत्पलनालाश्च** सपुष्पाः सफलाः स्मृताः ।

शीतस्वादुकषायाश्च कफमारुतकोपनाः ॥ ३६५ ॥

*Kumuda* & *Utpala* **(Nymphaea alba Linn. & Nymphaea stellata Willd.)**

The stalk, flower and fruit of *kumuda* and *utpala* are cooling, sweet and astringent. They aggravate *kapha* and *vāyu*.

**शणस्य कोविदारस्य कर्बुदारस्य शाल्मलेः** ।

पुष्पं ग्राहिप्रशस्तं च रक्तपित्ते विषे क्षये ॥ ३६६ ॥

*Śaṇa*, *Kovidāra*, *Karbudāra* & *Śālmalī* **(Crotalaria juncea Linn., Bauhinia variegata Linn., Bauhinia purpurea Linn., & Salmalia malabarica Schott and Endl.)**

The flowers of *śaṇa*, *kovidāra*, *karbudāra* and *śālmalī* are constipative and they are useful in *rakta pitta* (a disease characterised by bleeding from different parts of the body), *viṣa* (poisoning) and *kṣaya* (consumption).

**मधूकं** श्लेष्मलं ग्राही तद्वदेव च **यूथिका** ।

*Madhūka* & *Yūthika* **(Madhuca indica J.F. Gmel. & Jasminum auriculatum Vahl.)**

*Madhūka* and *Yūthika* aggravate *kapha* and they are constipative.

रक्तपित्तातिसारघ्नं **धातकी** कुसुमं हिमम् ॥३६७॥

*Dhātakī* (**Woodfordia fruticosa Kurz.**)

*Dhātakī* flower cures *rakta pitta* (a disease characterised by bleeding from different parts of the body) and *atisāra* (diarrhoea). It is cooling.

**मुचुकुन्दं** शिरोर्तिघ्नं पित्तास्रघ्नं महद्गुणम् ।

*Mucukunda* (**Pterospermum acerifolium Wild.**)

*Mucukunda* is exceedingly useful in curing headache, aggravation of *pitta* and vitiation of blood.

वातघ्नी **मल्लिका** तिक्ता, रंजनी स्तंभिनी **जया** ।।३६८।।

*Mallikā & Jayā* (**Jasminum sambac Ait** & **Sesbania sesban Merr.**)

*Mallikā* alleviates *vāyu* and is bitter. *Jayā* imparts colour and is constipative.

**वृषागस्तिकयोः** पुष्पं तिक्तं पित्तकफापहम् ।

क्षयकासापहं पाके कटुकं वातकोपनम् ।। ३६९ ।।

*Vṛṣa & Agastya* (**Adhatoda vasica Nees & Sesbania grandiflora Pers**)

The flowers of *vṛṣa* and *agastya* are bitter and they alleviate *pitta* as well as *kapha*. They cure *kṣaya* (consumption) and *kāsa* (bronchitis). In *vipāka*, they are pungent and they aggravate *vāyu*.

**अगस्त्यं** नातितिक्तं स्यात् नक्तान्ध्यानां प्रशस्यते ।

*Agastya* is not exceedingly bitter and is useful for patients suffering from *naktāndhya* (night blindness).

**ब्रह्मवृक्षस्य निंबस्य मुष्ककस्यासनस्य च** ।। ३७० ।।

कफपित्तहरं पुष्पं कुष्ठघ्नं कुटजस्य च ।

*Brahma, Nimba, Muṣkaka Asana & Kuṭaja* **(Butea monosperma Kuntze, Azadirachta indica A. Juss., Schrebera swietenioides Roxb., Pterocarpus marsupium Roxb., & Holarrhena antidysenterica Wall.)**

The flowers of *brahma, nimba, muṣkaka asana* and *kuṭaja* alleviate *kapha* and *pitta*. They cure *kuṣṭha* (obstinate skin diseases including leprosy).

कफघ्नं केतकं[258] तिक्तं सैरेयं[259] विषहारि च ॥ ३७१ ॥

॥ इति नानौषधिवर्गः ॥

*Ketaka & Saireya* **(Pandanus tectorius Soland ex Parkinson & Barleria cristata Linn.)**

*Ketaka* alleviates *kapha* and is bitter. *Saireya* cures *viṣa* (poisoning).

***Thus ends the group of miscellaneous drugs.***

## NOTES AND REFERENCES

1. रेचका इति द्वितीयपुस्तके पाठः ।
2. पावनी पूतना इति षष्ठपुस्तके पाठः ।
3. त्र्यब्दी इति षष्ठपुस्तके पाठः ।
4. पूतनामृता इति द्वितीयपुस्तके पाठः ।
5. चक्षुष्या लघुरायुष्या बृंहणी चानुलोमिनी इति आकरे पाठः।
6. ०ग्रहणीरोग० इति आकरे पाठः ।
7. ०तृंषाच्छर्दि० इति आकरे पाठः ।
8. प्लीहानञ्च यकृत्तथा इति आकरे पाठः
9. च कथिताऽतिगुणप्रदा इति आकरे पाठः ।
10. भ्रष्टा इति द्वितीयपुस्तके पाठः ।

11. क्रमि इति आकरे पाठः ।
12. मदकृच्चाथ धात्रीमज्जाऽपि इति आकरे पाठः ।
13. धान्यास्त्रिदोषनुत् इति द्वितीयपुस्तके पाठः ।
14. द्रव्यगुणरत्नमालायाम्.........त्रिफलेयं प्रकीर्तिता पाठोऽयं द्वितीयपंचम-पुस्तकयोः नोपलभ्यते ।
15. शिवा..........कफपित्तनुत् पाठोऽयं द्वितीयषष्ठपुस्तकयोः नोपलभ्यते ।
16. कुष्ठहरासरा इति आकरे पाठः ।
17. चैव इति द्वितीयपुस्तके पाठः ।
18. मृदुरोचनी इति द्वितीयपुस्तके पाठः ।
19. कफपित्तस्यरुक् इति द्वितीयपुस्तके पाठः ।
20. वल्कल्ला इति द्वितीयपुस्तके पाठः ।
21. शीतो..........क्रमिपित्तविषप्रणुत् पाठोऽयं प्रथमपंचमपुस्तकयोः नोपलभ्यते ।
22. क्रमिपित्तविनाशनं इति षष्ठपुस्तके पाठः ।
23. हृद्यं इति प्रथमपुस्तके पाठः ।
24. कफपित्तहरं लघु इति षष्ठपुस्तके पाठः ।
25. द्विविधः........पाराशरोऽब्रवीत पाठोऽयं प्रथमपुस्तके नोपलभ्यते ।
26. कुटजः..........त्वग्दोषार्शोतिसारजित् पाठोऽयं द्वितीयषष्ठपुस्तकयोः नोपलभ्यते ।
27. चातिविषाद्वयम् इति प्रथमद्वितीयपुस्तकयोः पाठः ।
28. दोषं इति पंचमपुस्तके पाठः ।
29. अर्कः इति प्रथमपुस्तके पाठः ।
30. सुरोक्तं इति द्वितीयपुस्तके पाठः ।
31. तौवरक्तं इति द्वितीय पुस्तके पाठः ।
32. मधुरं इति द्वितीयपुस्तके पाठः ।
33. ग्रहणी..........गुल्मनुत् पाठोऽयं प्रथमपंचमपुस्तकयोः नोपलभ्यते ।
34. महिषाख्यो इति द्वितीयषष्ठपुस्तकयोः पाठः ।
35. एव च इति द्वितीयपुस्तके पाठः ।
36. महिषाख्य इति षष्ठपुस्तके पाठः ।
37. कुमुदः कुमुदाभः स्यात्पद्मौ माणिक्यसन्निभः इति आकरे पाठः ।

38. पञ्चानां लिंगमीरितम् इति आकरे पाठः ।
39. महिषाख्यो इति षष्ठपुस्तके पाठः ।
40. परम् इति द्वितीयपुस्तके पाठः ।
41. कदाचिन्महिषाक्षश्च इति आकरे पाठः ।
कदाचिन्महिषाख्यस्तु इति षष्ठपुस्तके पाठः ।
42. कटू रूक्षो लघुः परः इति आकरे पाठः ।
43. स्मृतः इति षष्ठपुस्तके पाठ ।
44. पत्तलो इति आकरे पाठः ।
45. द्रव्याणां गुणवेदिभिः इति आकरे पाठः ।
46. लशुनसेविनाम् इति आकरे पाठः ।
47. महिषाख्यो·······निरन्तरम् पाठोऽयं प्रथमपंचमपुस्तकयोः नोपलभ्यते ।
48. पत्रे············रसायनः पाठोऽयं द्वितीयषष्ठपुस्तकयोः नोपलभ्यते ।
49. नातं इति द्वितीयषष्ठपुस्तकयोः पाठः ।
50. पलाण्डु······· ····स्वादुपाकरसो जयेत् पाठोऽयं प्रथमपंचमपुस्तकयोः नोपलभ्यते ।
51. कफकृद्रोचणो इति पंचमपुस्तके पाठः ।
52. पलांडु.......गुरु पाठोऽयं द्वितीयषष्ठपुस्तकयोः नोपलभ्यते ।
53. शुष्काणि इति प्रथमपुस्तके पाठः ।
54. वातश्लेष्मविबंधघ्नो इति प्रथमपुस्तके पाठः ।
55. निदाघशरदोर्नैव पूजितमार्द्रकम् इति आकरे पाठः ।
56. गुडार्द्रकं·······समन्वितम् पाठोऽयं प्रथमपंचमषष्ठपुस्तकेषु नोपलभ्यते ।
57. शलघ्न इति षष्ठपुस्तके पाठः ।
58. विबन्ध भेदिनी···········मलपातने पाठोऽयं प्रथमद्वितीयपुस्तकयोः नोपलभ्यते ।
59. विबन्ध... ...रसायनी पाठोऽयं प्रथमपंचमपुस्तकयोः नोपलभ्यते ।
60. दीपनरोचनम् इति द्वितीयपुस्तके पाठः ।
रोचनदीपनम् इति प्रथमपुस्तके पाठः ।
61. च कटुकं कफघ्नं इति प्रथमपुस्तके पाठः ।
62. नात्युष्णं.... ...सितम् पाठोऽयं प्रथमपंचमपुस्तकयोः नोपलभ्यते ।
63. कटुकं इति षष्ठपुस्तके पाठः ।

64. वृष्या इति षष्ठपुस्तके पाठः ।
65. जलपिप्पलिका..........रक्तपित्तज्वरापहा पाठोऽयं प्रथमपंचमपुस्तकयोः नोपलभ्यते ।
66. कफवातजित् इति आकरे पाठः ।
67. रुच्यं पित्तविमर्दनम् इति द्वितीयपुस्तके पाठः ।
68. कृमि........विबन्धनुत् पाठोऽयं द्वितीयपुस्तके अधिकमुपलभ्यते ।
69. तीक्ष्णोष्णं इति प्रथमपंचमपुस्तकयोः आकरे च पाठः ।
70. पित्ताग्निवर्धनम् इति आकरे पाठः ।
71. ग्राहि........गर्भाशयविशुद्धिकृत् पाठोऽयं प्रथमपंचमपुस्तकयोः नोपलभ्यते ।
72. जवानी इति प्रथमपुस्तके पाठः ।
73. छिछिका.......वातकफापहा पाठोऽयं प्रथमपंचमपुस्तकयोः नोपलभ्यते ।
74. भूतृणो इति द्वितीयपुस्तके पाठः ।
75. पुंस्त्वघ्न........वस्तिरोगरुजापहा पाठोऽयं षष्ठपुस्तके नोपलभ्यते ।
76. भक्ष्यव्यञ्जनभोज्येषु इति आकरे पाठः ।
77. भव्य........स्रोतोविशोधनी पाठोऽयं प्रथमपंचमपुस्तकयोः नोपलभ्यते।
78. भङ्गी कफहरी तिक्ता ग्राहिणी पाचनी लघुः इति आकरे पाठः ।
79. मोहमन्दवाग्वह्निवर्धिनी इति आकरे पाठः ।
80. हृद्यो इति द्वितीयपुस्तके पाठः ।
81. वर्वरी........विषापहम् पाठोऽयं प्रथमपंचमपुस्तकयोः नोपलभ्यते।
82. शिग्रुः.......वातजित् पाठोऽयं प्रथमपंचमपुस्तकयोः नोपलभ्यते ।
83. कट्वंगो इति षष्ठपुस्तके पाठः ।
84. जिंगणी इति षष्ठपुस्तके पाठः ।
85. मूत्रकृच्छ्रजित् इति प्रथमपुस्तके पाठः ।
86. तृषा इति प्रथमपुस्तके पाठः ।
87. भवति इति प्रथमपुस्तके पाठः ।
88. गवादिनी इति षष्ठपुस्तके पाठः ।
89. मधूकं इति द्वितीयपुस्तके पाठः ।
90. मुसली इति द्वितीयपुस्तके पाठः ।
91. द्विगुणा इति षष्ठपुस्तके पाठः ।
92. रक्तस्तम्भनहृद्गुणैः इति द्वितीयपुस्तके पाठः ।

93. वृष्या इति प्रथमपुस्तके पाठः ।

94. फंजी इति प्रथमपुस्तके पाठः ।

95. गुरुर्व्रणश्लेष्मकटुकृमिविषापहः इति द्वितीयपुस्तके पाठः ।

96. फलिनी इति षष्ठपुस्तके पाठः ।

97. कफवातामभूतघ्नी इति द्वितीयपुस्तके पाठः ।

98. बलायुः इति द्वितीयपुस्तके पाठः ।

99. कुक्कुतुंदुः इति प्रथमपुस्तके पाठः ।

100. हंसपादी ·······पाण्डुनुत् पाठोऽयं प्रथमपंचमपुस्तकयोः नोपलभ्यते ।

101. पित्त इति प्रथमपंचमपुस्तकयोः पाठः ।

102. कुष्ठं........प्रमेहजित् पाठोऽयं द्वितीयषष्ठपुस्तकयोः नोपलभ्यते ।

103. ग्रास्फोटा इति द्वितीयपुस्तके पाठः ।

104. तिनीशा इति प्रथमपुस्तके पाठः ।

105. अशणः इति प्रथमपुस्तके पाठः ।

106. श्लेष्मपित्तजित् इति प्रथमपुस्तके पाठः ।

107. योनिदोषान् इति प्रथमपुस्तके पाठः ।

108. व्रणे इति द्वितीयपुस्तके पाठः ।

109. व्रणास्रसंभारभेदनः इति द्वितीयपुस्तके पाठः ।

110. शोथामवातवातघ्नो इति द्वितीयपुस्तके पाठः ।

111. व्रण्यकफास्रघ्नस्तगरः इति द्वितीयपुस्तके पाठः ।

112. शिह्लकं इति प्रथमपुस्तके पाठः ।

113. गुञ्जासर्ज्जोमुरानखम् इति प्रथमपुस्तके पाठः।

114. राला ·······विपादिकाः पाठोऽयं प्रथमपंचमपुस्तकयोः नोपलभ्यते ।

115. शिशिरप्रदम् इति षष्ठपुस्तके पाठः ।

116. पत्रांगं इति षष्ठपुस्तके पाठः ।

117. बर्ण्यं इति प्रथमपुस्तके पाठः ।

118. पित्तविषकफापहं इति प्रथमपुस्तके पाठः ।

119. पित्तविस्फोटज्वरदाहविषापहं इति प्रथमपुस्तके पाठः ।

120. व्रण्यं इति प्रथमपुस्तके पाठः ।

121. शटी·······हरामता पाठोऽयं प्रथमपंचमपुस्तकयोः नोपलभ्यते ।

122. कफपित्तहरं इति षष्ठपुस्तके पाठः ।

123. लघुस्तष्णा इति प्रथमपुस्तके पाठः ।

124. पक्वात्कर्पूरतः······शोथ-विषापहः पाठोऽयं प्रथमपंचमपुस्तकयोः नोपलभ्यते ।

125. ग्राहिनी इति प्रथमपुस्तके पाठः ।

126. राष्णा······व्रणविपादिका पाठोऽयं द्वितीयषष्ठपुस्तकयोः नोपलभ्यते ।

127. तृट्छर्दिहृल्लासकटुपित्तकफापहा इति द्वितीयपुस्तके पाठः ।
तृट्छर्दिहृल्लासकटुपित्तविषापहा इति षष्ठपुस्तके पाठः ।

128. कासश्वासव्रणापहम् इति प्रथमपुस्तके पाठः ।

129. गन्धप्रजागुका इति प्रथमपुस्तके पाठः ।

130. शूलजित् इति प्रथमपुस्तके पाठः ।
शूलनुत् इति षष्ठपुस्तके पाठः ।

131. राष्ट्रोष्णा इति द्वितीयपुस्तके पाठः ।

132. राष्णावातशोथाना[म]वातवातामयान् जयेत् इति प्रथमपुस्तके पाठः ।

133. शटीवातकफश्वासकासहिक्काज्वरापहा इति प्रथमपुस्तके पाठः ।

134. तजगं इति प्रथमपुस्तके पाठः ।

135. नागकेशरः इति षष्ठपुस्तके पाठः ।

136. कटुवातार्शो इति षष्ठपुस्तके पाठः ।

137. कफकाशक्षयापहम् इति प्रथमपुस्तके पाठः ।

138. वंशलोचना इति षष्ठपुस्तके पाठः ।

139. कुष्ठज्वरापहः इति षष्ठपुस्तके पाठः ।

140. तृषा——क्षयापहः पाठोऽयं प्रथमपंचमपुस्तकयोः नोपलभ्यते ।

141. पाण्डुरक्तजित् इति द्वितीयपुस्तके पाठः ।

142. श्रीफलः——महन्मतम् पाठोऽयं आदर्शपुस्तिकासु नोपलभ्यते द्वितीय-षष्ठपुस्तकयोः——"पञ्चमूलमिदं महत्" इतिमात्रं पाठः प्राप्तः । तस्मात् भावप्रकाशात् उद्धृत्य पाठपूरणं कृतम् (भावप्रकाशः गुडूच्यादि चतुर्थवर्ग २९:३०) ।

143. न्यग्रोधोदुम्बराश्वत्थपारिसप्लक्षपादयाः इति द्वितीयपुस्तके पाठः ।

144. पारिसस्थाने इति द्वितीयपुस्तके पाठः ।

145. द्रष्टव्यम्—आयुर्वेदप्रकाशः ३:१
भावप्रकाशः पूर्वखण्डः धात्वादिवर्गं ८:१ ।

146. दधते देहं नृणां हति आयुर्वेदप्रकाशे पाठः ।
देहं दधति नृणां इति भावप्रकाशे पाठः ।
147. मियात् इति षष्ठपुस्तके पाठः ।
148. निषेके इति आकरे पाठः ।
149. शुल्बोज्झितं इति आकरे पाठः ।
150. हेमगुरुक्षमम् इति द्वितीयपुस्तके पाठः ।
151. तच्छेवतं इति आकरे पाठः ।
152. दलिम् इति द्वितीयपुस्तके पाठः ।
153. कषेत्याज्यं लघु स्फुटम् इति आकरे पाठः ।
154. बुद्धिदम् इति द्वितीयपुस्तके पाठः ।
मेधास्मृतिप्रदम् इति आकरे पाठः ।
155. स्वर्णमायुःकरं इति द्वितीयपुस्तके पाठः ।
156. रोगव्रजान् पोषुयतीह काये इति आकरे पाठः ।
157. समापतत्तत्स्थैकस्माद्विलोचनात् इति द्वितीयपुस्तके पाठः ।
158. तस्माद्भद्र इति आदर्शपुस्तिकासु पाठः ।
159. तस्माद्रजतमुत्पन्नमुक्तकर्मसु योजयेत् इति आकरे पाठः ।
160. च भवेत्तद्धि वङ्गादिरसयोगतः इति आकरे पाठः ।
161. स्वर्णाभं इति आदर्शपुस्तिकासु पाठः ।
162. रूक्षं इति आदर्शपुस्तिकासु पाठः ।
163. नाशयत्यचिराद् इति आकरे पाठः ।
164. करोति विड्बन्धनं इति द्वितीयपुस्तके पाठः ।
165. वीर्यं बलं हन्ति तनोश्चापुष्टिं महागदान्पोषयति ह्यशुद्धम् इति आकरे पाठः ।
166. शुल्वं इति षष्ठपुस्तके पाठः ।
167. कुष्णं इति भावप्रकाशे पाठः ।
168. शुल्यं दुष्टं प्रकीर्त्तितम् इति आकरे पाठः ।
169. नरसेहितम् इति द्वितीयपुस्तके पाठः ।
170. रङ्गं इति आकरे पाठः ।
171. चक्षुष्यं पित्तलं मनाक् इति आकरे पाठः ।
172. "सिंहौ गजौघं तु यथा" इति आदर्शपुस्तिकासु पाठः ।
173. पुष्टिं विदधाति नूनम् इति आकरे पाठः ।

174. च इति षष्ठपुस्तके पाठः ।

175. रीतिकायुगलं——लेखनं पाठोऽयं द्वितीयपुस्तके नोपलभ्यते ।

176. लोमिलदंत्यस्य निहतस्य इति आकरे पाठः ।

177. व इति आकरे पाठः ।

178. देहशूलकृदसंस्कृतं ध्रुवम् इति आकरे पाठः ।

179. तनुते इति आकरे पाठः ।

180. मद्यमम्लं मसूरांश्च इति आकरे पाठः ।

181. न्यंगान्येवाम्लिते सति इति द्वितीयपुस्तके पाठः ।

182. विसृजति इति द्वितीयपुस्तके पाठः ।
सृजति इति षष्ठपुस्तके पाठः ।

183. तत्कृतां इति द्वितीयपुस्तके पाठः ।

184. रक्तपित्तप्रशमनमम्लपित्तं इति षष्ठपुस्तके पाठः ।

185. शतोत्थमुत्तमं इति आकरे पाठः ।

186. षष्ठिवर्षीयं इति आकरे पाठः ।

187. निपेतुर्घनध्वानाच्छिखरेषु इति आकरे पाठः ।

188. पुरा——चाभ्रकम् पाठोऽयं प्रथमपञ्चमपुस्तकयोः नोपलभ्यते ।

189. गगनात्स्खलित इति आकरे पाठः ।

190. गगनच्युति जातत्वाद् गगनं च जगुः सुराः इति द्वितीयषष्ठपुस्तकयोः पाठः ।

191. गदे शुद्धतयाऽपि च इति द्वितीयपुस्तके पाठः ।

192. 'नागं वह्निस्थितं शब्दं फूत्कारं परिमुञ्चति ।
तच्छरीरं गतं नित्यं व्याधिं कुर्याद्भगन्दरम् ।
वज्रं तु वज्रवत्तिष्ठेत्तन्नाग्नौ विकृतिं व्रजेत् ।
यत्नतो वर्जयेद्धीमानभ्रकत्रितयं भिषक् ।
चतुर्थं पीवरं वज्रं व्याधिवार्द्धक्यनुत् ।'
पाठोऽयं द्वितीयषष्ठपुस्तकयोः उपलभ्यते ।

193. सुतान् विक्रमैः सिंहतुल्यान् इति आकरे पाठः ।

194. दुष्टम् इति द्वितीयपुस्तके पाठः ।
कुष्टम् इति षष्ठपुस्तके पाठः ।

195. करोत्यसह्यामसिद्धमभ्रं इति द्वितीयषष्ठपुस्तकयोः पाठः ।

196. सुवर्णमाक्षिकं स्वादु इति आकरे पाठः ।

197. बस्तिहृत्कण्ठपाण्डुमेहविषोदरम् इति आकरे पाठः ।

198. विषं इति आकरे पाठः।

199. अपि नाशयेत् इति आकरे पाठः।

200. मालां विधत्तेऽपि च गण्डपूर्वां शुद्धयादिहीनं खल माक्षिकं तु इति आकरे पाठः।

201. कण्डूकुष्ठादि इति आकरे पाठः।
कण्डूकुष्ठार्शरोगासृक्कफपित्तमरुद्व्रणान् इति द्वितीयपुस्तके पाठः।

202. चारुतां इति आकरे पाठः।

203. बहुतापानङ्गसङ्कोचपीडाः इति आकरे पाठः।

204. मलानुबन्धं खलुमूत्ररोधं इति द्वितीयपुस्तके पाठः।

205. तु कटुकं इति आकरे पाठः।

206. विशदं इति द्वितीयपुस्तके पाठः।

207. शिवाङ्गात्प्रच्युतं रेतः इति आकरे पाठः।

208. छुक्लमच्छामभूच्च इति आकरे पाठः।

209. तत्तु भवेत् इति आकरे पाठः।

210. स्वस्थो इति आकरे पाठः।

211. कामितश्चापि इति आकरे पाठः।
क्रामिता इति षष्ठपुस्तके पाठः।

212. अजरीकृतो इति षष्ठपुस्तके पाठः।

213. दृष्टिबलप्रदः इति आकरे पाठः।

214. वह्निगिरीत्वचापलं इति आकरे पाठः।

215. पारदो इति द्वितीयपुस्तके पाठः।

216. त्रपुनागयोगजौ इति आकरे पाठः।

217. रसेन्द्र इति आकरे पाठः।

218. भिषक्रमैः इति षष्ठपुस्तके पाठः। मुनीश्वरैः इति आकरे पाठः।

219. विषेण इति आकरे पाठः।

220. स्याच्चाञ्चलयतो इति आकरे पाठः।

221. पुंसाम् इति आकरे पाठः।

222. षण्ढो इति आकरे पाठः।

223. परिशोधनीयः इति आकरे पाठः।

224. कष्टांश्च इति षष्ठपुस्तके आकरे च पाठः।

225. वरारांजनहिंगुलम् इति द्वितीयपुस्तके पाठः ।

226. गन्धो हिंगुलमभ्रतालकशिलाः स्रोतोऽञ्जनं टकणं,
राजावर्तकचुम्बकौ स्फटिकयाशङ्खखटीगैरिकम् ।
कासीसं रसकं कपर्दसिकताबोलाश्च कङ्कुष्टकं ।
सौराष्ट्री च मता अमी उपरसाः सूतस्य किञ्चिद् गुणैः । इति भावप्रकाशे पाठः ।

227. देव्या इति आकरे पाठः ।

228. क्षीरनीरधौ इति आकरे पाठः ।

229. समभूत्ततः इति आकरे पाठः ।

230. सितोसितः इति आकरे पाठः ।

231. रसायनः इति आकरे पाठः ।

232. द्रष्टव्यम्-भावप्रकाशः धातूपधातुवर्ग ८:११२ ।

233. धातुसंतप्ता इति आकरे पाठः ।

234. यज्जटायु प्रतीकाशं सतिक्तं लवणान्वितम् इति द्वितीयपुस्तके पाठः ।

235. कफमेदोश्मशर्कराः इति द्वितीयपुस्तके पाठः ।

236. शोथकुष्ठोदरक्रिमीन् इति आकरे पाठः ।

237. सुदुर्म्मदः इति षष्ठपुस्तके पाठ ।

238. प्रदीपनं इति षष्ठपुस्तके पाठः ।

239. कृष्णवर्णैरनन्तैर्विन्दुभिर्युतः इति षष्ठपुस्तके पाठः ।

240. लोहितप्रभः इति आकरे पाठः ।

241. दृष्टिकृदजनात् इति आकरे पाठ:: ।

242. नेत्रदोषापहाः स्मृताः इति आकरे पाठः ।

243. हस्तिमदश्चित्तरंजनो इति आकरे पाठः ।

244. च कुष्ठपाण्डुविषापहम् इति आकरे पाठः ।

245. तृष्णादाहास्रविस्फोटविषवीसर्पनाशनम् इति आकरे पाठः ।

246. तृष्णा··········व्रणास्रजित् पाठोऽयं प्रथमद्वितीयपंचमपुस्तिकासु नोपलभ्यते ।

247. वातपित्तास्यदृग्व्याधि इति आकरे पाठः ।

248. लघ्वी दोषत्रयापहा इति आकरे पाठः ।

249. शीतघ्न इतरः मतम् इति आदर्शपुस्तिकासु पाठः ।

250. वासन्ती इति भावप्रकाशे पाठः। (भावप्रकाशः पुष्पवर्ग ५ : २३)।
251. तत्तैलं तद्गुणं स्मृतम् इति भावप्रकाशे पाठः (भावप्रकाशः पुष्पवर्ग ५:२५)।
252. बकुलस्तुवरोऽनुष्णः इति आकरे पाठः।
253. बकोऽनुष्णः इति आकरे पाठः।
254. ०शोथास्रनाशनः इति आकरे पाठः।
255. दमनस्तुवरस्तिक्तो हृद्यो इति आकरे पाठः।
256. ग्रहणाद् इति आकरे पाठः।
257. सुगन्धिके इति आदर्शपुस्तिकासु पाठः।
258. द्रष्टव्यम्-भावप्रकाशः पुष्पवर्ग ५ : ४२।
259. भावप्रकाशः पुष्पवर्ग ५ : ५३।

# CHAPTER 3

'भिष्यन्दि **लवणं** सर्वं सूक्ष्मं सृष्टमलं विदुः ।
वातघ्नं पाकि तीक्ष्णोष्णं रोचनं कफपित्तकृत् ॥१॥
[माधवद्रव्यगुणः लवणवर्ग २:१]

### *Lavaṇa* (Salt)

All types of *lavaṇa* are *abhiṣyandi* (which obstruct channels of circulation), *sūkṣma* (subtle), *sṛṣṭamala* (which eliminates waste products) and alleviator of *vāta*. They cause suppuration. They are sharp, hot and appetisers. They aggravate *kapha* and *pitta*.

**सैन्धवं** मधुरं हृद्यं दीपनं शीतलं लघु ।
चक्षुष्यं पाचनं स्निग्धं वृष्यं दोषत्रयापहम् ॥२॥

### *Saindhava* (Rock salt)

*Saindhava* is sweet, cardiac tonic, digestive stimulant, cooling, light, promoter of eye sight, carminative, unctuous, and aphrodisiac. It alleviates all the three *doṣas*.

**गजाह्वयं** लघुवातघ्नमत्युष्णं भेदि पित्तलम् ।

तीक्ष्णं व्यवायि सूक्ष्मं चाभिष्यन्दि कटुपाकि च ॥३॥

*Gaja*

The *gaja* type of salt is *laghu*, alleviator of *vāta*, extremely hot, purgative, aggravator of *pitta*, sharp, *vyavāyi* (a substance whose digestion and metabolism take place after it has pervaded all over the body), *sūkṣma* (subtle), *abhiṣyandi* (which obstructs the channels of circulation) and pungent in *vipāka*.

सामुद्रं मधुरं पाके स्निग्धं नातिसरं गुरु ।
नात्युष्णं दीपनं भेदि सक्षारमविदाहि च ॥ ४ ॥
श्लेष्मलं वातनु[1]त्तिक्तमरूक्षं नातिपित्तलम् ।

***Sāmudra* (Sea salt)**

*Sāmudra* is sweet in *vipāka* and unctuous. It does not possess strong laxative effect. It is heavy. It is not very hot. It is digestive stimulant, purgative (?), alkaline, *avidāhi* (which does not cause burning sensation). It aggravates *kapha* and alleviates *vāyu*. It is bitter and *arukṣa* (not un-unctuous).

विडं [सक्षार][2]मूर्ध्वाधो कफवातानुलोमनम् ॥ ५ ॥

*Viḍa*

*Viḍa* is alkaline. It helps in the elimination of *kapha* as well as *vāyu* both through upward and downward tracts.

दीपनं लघु तीक्ष्णोष्णं रुच्यं पाक्यं व्यवायि च ।
विबन्धानाहविष्टम्भहृद्रुग्गौरवशूलनुत् ॥६॥

*Pākya*

*Pākya* is digestive stimulant, light, sharp, hot, appetiser and *vyavāyi* (which gets digested and metabolised after it has pervaded all over the body). It cures *vibandha* (constipation), *ānāha* (flatulence), *viṣṭambha* (impairment of the peristaltic movement of the colon), *hṛdruk* (heart disease), *gaurava* (heaviness) and *śūla* (colic pain).

अग्निदीप्तिकरस्तीक्ष्णष्टंकणक्षार उच्यते ।

*Taṅkaṇa kṣāra* (**Borax**)

*Taṅkaṇa kṣāra* is a digestive stimulant and it is sharp.

'सुधाक्षारोऽग्निना तुल्यः क्लेदी पक्ता विदारणः ॥७॥

*Sudhākṣāra*

*Sudhākṣāra* is like fire. It is *kledi* (produces stickiness), *paktā* (stimulant of digestion and metabolism) and *vidāraṇa* (which causes perforation).

श्वादंष्ट्रो[3] मधुरः शीतो लघुः स्रोतोविशोधनः ।

*Śvadaṁṣṭrā kṣāra*

The *kṣāra* of *śvadaṁṣṭrā* is sweet, cooling and light. It cleanses the channels of circulation.

अनपत्यकरः श्रेष्ठः पालाशः सर्वकर्मसु ॥८॥

*Palāśa kṣāra*

The *kṣāra* of *palāśa* prevents conception and is the most useful.

पूतीकनक्तमालार्कधवमुष्ककपाटलाः ।
सर्षपत्रपुसैर्वा[4]रुकदलीतिलशिग्रुजाः ॥९॥
कोशातकीन्द्रतर्कारी शिखरी[5] वरुणाग्निजाः ।
क्षाराश्चान्येऽपि गुल्मार्शोग्रहणीरुक्छिदः सराः ॥१०॥
पाचनाः कृमिपुंस्त्वघ्नाः शर्कराश्मरिनाशनाः ।
चक्षुःकेशौजसां नेष्टा रक्तपित्तकराः परम् ॥ ११ ॥'

[माधवद्रव्यगुणः लवणवर्ग २:६-१३]

॥ इति क्षाराः ॥

### *Other kṣāras*

*Kṣāras* prepared of *pūtīka*, *naktamāla*, *arka*, *dhava*, *muṣkaka*, *pāṭalā*, *sarṣapa*, *trapusa*, *ervāru*, *kadalī*, *tila*, *śigru*, *kośātaki*, *indra*, *tarkārī*, *śikhari*, *varuṇa*, *agni* and such other drugs cure *gulma* (phantom tumour), *arśas* (piles) and *grahaṇī* (sprue syndrome). They are laxative and carminative. They cure *kṛmi* (parasitic infection). They cause impotency. They cure *śarkarā* (gravel) and *aśmari* (stone in the urinary tract). They are harmful for the eyesight, hair and *ojas*. They cause *rakta pitta* (a disease characterised by bleeding from different parts of the body).

[6]

**रुचकं** रोचनं हृद्यं दीपनं पाचनं परम् ।
सस्नेहं वातनुन्नातिपित्तलं विशदं लघु ॥ १२ ॥
उद्गारशुद्धिदं सूक्ष्मं विबन्धानाहशूलनुत् ।

### *Rucaka*

***Rucaka*** is an excellent appetiser, cardiac tonic, digestive stimulant and carminative. It is unctuous. It alleviates *vāyu* but does not aggravate *pitta* in excess. It is *viśada* (non-slimy) and light. It cleanses *udgāra* (eructation). It is subtle. It cures *vibandha* (constipation), *ānāha* (flatulence) and *śūla* (colic pain).

सौवर्चलगुणाः **कृष्णे लवणे** गन्धवर्जिताः ॥ १३ ॥

### *Kṛṣna lavaṇa*

*Kṛṣna lavaṇa* shares all the properties of *sauvarcala* except the smell.

रोचनं दीपनं स्वादु **रोमकं** मारुतापहम् ।

### *Romaka*

*Romaka* is an appetiser, digestive stimulant, sweet and alleviator of *vāyu*.

सतिक्तं कटुकं क्षारं तीक्ष्णमुत्क्लेदि चोद्भिदम् ॥१४॥

*Udbhida*

*Udbhida* is bitter, pungent, alkaline and sharp. It produces *kleda* (sticky material) in the body.

'पांशुजं तिक्तमुष्णं च शोफपित्तकफापहम् ।

*Pāṁśuja*

*Pāṁśuja* is bitter and hot. It cures *śopha* (oedema) and aggravation of *pitta* and *kapha*.

गुल्महृद्ग्रहणीपाण्डुप्लीहानाहगलामयम् ॥ १५ ॥

श्वासार्शः कफवातांश्च शमयेद्यावशूकजः ।

*Yavaśūkaja kṣāra*

The *kṣāra* of *yavaśūka* cures *gulma* (phantom tumour), *hṛdroga* (heart disease), *grahaṇī* (sprue syndrome), *pāṇḍu* (anemia), *plīhan* (splenic disorder), *ānāha* (flatulence), *galāmaya* (diseases of throat), *śvāsa* (asthma), *arśas* (piles) and aggravation of *kapha* as well as *vāyu*.

तस्मादल्पान्तरगुणः सर्जिकाक्षार उच्यते ॥ १६ ॥'

[माधवद्रव्यगुणः लवणवर्ग २:७-९]

*Sarjikā kṣāra*

*Sarjikā kṣāra* is slightly inferior in property in comparison with *yavaśūkaja kṣāra*.

उष्णोऽनिलघ्नः प्रक्लेदी उषःक्षारोऽग्निनाशनः ।

*Uṣaḥ kṣāra*

*Uṣaḥ kṣāra* is hot, alleviator of *vāyu* and *prakledī* (which produces sticky matter). It destroys the power of digestion.

मेदोघ्नः पाचितः क्षारः मुखबस्तिविशोधनः ।

विरूक्षणोऽनिलकरः श्लेष्मघ्नः पित्तदूषणः ॥ १७ ॥

### *Pācita kṣāra*

*Pācita kṣāra* cures *medas* (adiposity). It cleanses the mouth and *vasti* (urinary bladder). It is un-unctuous. It aggravates *vāyu*, alleviates *kapha* and vitiates *pitta*.

## NOTES AND REFERENCES

1. वातनत्तिक्तमरूक्षं इति षष्ठपुस्तके पाठः ।
2. साक्षरं इति आदर्शपुस्तिकासु पाठः ।
3. स्वाद्वम्लो इति आकरे पाठः ।
4. सर्षपत्रपुषैर्वारुकदलीतिलशिग्रुजाः इति आकरे पाठः ।
5. शिरीषवरुणाग्निजाः इति आकरे पाठः ।
6. रुचिकं इति षष्ठपुस्तके पाठः ।

# CHAPTER 4

वातासृक्पित्तजित् स्वादुः स्निग्धः प्रीणनबृंहणः ।

जीवनस्तर्पणो वृष्यः शीतश्चेक्षुरसः सरः ॥ १ ॥

[माधवद्रव्यगुणः इक्षुवर्ग ३:१०]

*Ikṣurasa* (**Sugarcane juice**)

The juice of *ikṣu* alleviates *vāyu*, blood and *pitta*. It is sweet, unctuous, pleasing, nourishing, life giver, refreshing, aphrodisiac, cooling and laxative.

**इक्षवो** मधुरा बल्या विपाके मधुरा सराः ।

स्निग्धाः कृमिकराश्चेति ते चानेकविधाः मताः ॥२॥

*Ikṣu* (**Sugarcane**)

Different types of *ikṣu* are sweet, strength promoting, sweet in *vipāka*, laxative, and unctuous. They cause *kṛmi* (parasitic infection).

**'पौण्ड्रको भीरुकश्चेति वंशकः शतपोरकः ।**

**कान्तारेक्षुस्तापसेक्षुः काष्ठेक्षुः सूचिपत्रकः ।**

1
'नैपालो दीर्घपत्रश्च नीलपोरो[ऽ] थ कोशकृत् ॥३॥'

[भावप्रकाशः इक्षुवर्ग २३:३-४]

2
इत्येता जातयः स्थौल्यात् गुणान्वक्ष्याम्यतः परम् ।

*Ikṣu* is of different types viz., *pauṇḍraka*, *bhīruka*, *vaṁśaka*, *śataporaka*, *kāntārekṣu*, *tāpasekṣu*, *kāṣṭhekṣu*, *sūci patraka*, *naipāla*, *dīrgha patra*, *nīlapora*, and *kośakṛt*. These are the varieties in general and now their properties will be described.

3
सुशीतो मधुरः स्निग्धो बृंहणः श्लेष्मलः सरः ॥ ४ ॥"

[माधवद्रव्यगुणः इक्षुवर्ग ३:३-४]

4
दीर्घपोरः सुकठिनः सक्षारो वंशको मतः ।

[भावप्रकाशः इक्षुवर्ग २३:८]

*Dīrghapora & Vaṁśaka*

*Dīrghapora* is exceedingly cooling, sweet, unctuous, nourishing, aggravator of *kapha* and laxative.

*Vaṁśaka* is hard and alkaline.

5
'वंशवच्छतपोरस्तु किञ्चिदुष्णः स वातहा ॥ ५ ॥

*Śatapora*

*Śatapora* is like *vaṁśa*. It is slightly hot and it alleviates *vāyu*.

कांतारतापसाविक्षू वंशकानुगतौ मतौ ।

*Kāntāra & Tāpasa*

*Kāntāra* and *tāpasa* types are like *vaṁśaka*.

6
एवंगुणस्तु काण्डेक्षुर्वातपित्तप्रकोपनः ॥' ६ ॥

[माधवद्रव्यगुणः इक्षुवर्ग ३:६-७]

*Kāṇḍekṣu*

*Kāṇḍekṣu* has similar properties but it aggravates *vāyu* and *pitta*.

7

सूचीपत्रो नीलपोरो नेपालो दीर्घपत्रकः ।

वातलाः कफपित्तघ्नाः सकषाया विदाहिनः ॥ ७ ॥

*Sūcīpatra* **etc.**

*Sūcīpatra*, *nīlapora*, *nepāla* and *dīrgha patraka* aggravate *vāyu*. They alleviate *kapha* and *pitta*. They are astringent and they cause burning sensation.

कोशकारो गुरुः शीतो रक्तपित्तक्षयापहः ।

*Kośakāra*

*Kośakāra* is heavy and cooling. It cures *raktapitta* (a disease characterised by bleeding from different parts of the body) and *kṣaya* (consumption).

अतीव मधुरो मूले मध्ये मधुर एव च ।

8

अग्रेत्विक्षुश्च विज्ञेय इक्षूणां लवणो रसः ॥ ८ ॥

[माधवद्रव्यगुणः इक्षुवर्ग ३ : ७-९]

**Taste of the different parts of *Ikṣu***

The root (lower part of the stem) of *ikṣu* is extremely sweet. The middle portion of the stem of this plant is (moderately) sweet. The upper part of the stem bears saline taste.

अविदाही कफकरो वातपित्तनिवर्हणः ।

चक्षुःप्रह्लादनो वृष्यो दन्तनिष्पीडितो रसः ॥ ९ ॥

**Juice extracted by chewing**

The juice of *ikṣu* that comes out by chewing does not cause any burning sensation. It aggravates *kapha* but alleviates *vāyu* and *pitta*. It is nourishing to the eyes and aphrodisiac.

'गुर्विदाही विष्टम्भी यान्त्रिकस्तु प्रकीर्तितः ।

**Juice extracted by a machine**

The juice of *ikṣu* that is extracted by a machine is heavy and it causes burning sensation. It is constipative.

9 पक्वो गुरुः सरः स्निग्धः सतीक्ष्णः कफवातनुत् ।

**Boiled juice**

The boiled juice of *ikṣu* is heavy, laxative, unctuous and sharp. It alleviates *kapha* and *vāta*.

10 "फाणितं गुर्वभिष्यन्दि बृंहणं कफशुक्रलम्' ॥ १० ॥

[माधवद्रव्यगुणः इक्षुवर्ग ३ : १२-१३]

वातपित्तश्रमं हन्ति मूत्रवस्तिविशोधनम् ।

*Phāṇita* **(Penidium)**

*Phāṇita* is heavy, *abhiṣyandi* (which obstructs the channels of circulation) and *bṛṁhaṇa* (nourishing). It produces more of *kapha* and semen. It alleviates *vāta* and *pitta*. It relieves exhaustion and cleanses urine and urinary bladder.

रूक्षं मधूकपुष्पोत्थं फाणितं वातपित्तजित्" ॥ ११ ॥

*Phāṇita* prepared of the flower of *madhūka* is un-unctuous. It alleviates *vāta* and *pitta*.

'गुड़ो वृष्यो गुरुः स्निग्धो वातघ्नो मूत्रशोधनः ।

नातिपित्तहरो मेदःकफकृमिबलप्रदः' ॥ १२ ॥

[भावप्रकाशः इक्षुवर्ग २३ : २५]

*Guḍa* **(Molasses)**

*Guḍa* is aphrodisiac, heavy and unctuous. It alleviates *vāyu* and cleanses urine. It does not alleviate *pitta* in excess. It produces *medas* (adiposity), *kapha*, *kṛmi* (parasitic infection) and strength.

'पित्तघ्नो मधुरः स्निग्धो वातहासृक्प्रसादनः ।

सः पुराणोऽधिकंगुणो गुड़पथ्यतमः स्मृतः' ॥ १३ ॥

[माधवद्रव्यगुणः इक्षुवर्ग ३ : १५]

हृद्यः पुराणो तर्पण्यो नवः श्लेष्मग्निसादकृत् ।

*Guḍa* which is preserved for a long time (*purāṇa*) alleviates *pitta*. It is sweet and unctuous. It alleviates *vāyu* and promotes blood. It is superior in therapeutic property and is wholesome par excellence. It is a cardiac tonic.

Freshly collected (*nava*) *guḍa* reduces *kapha* and the power of digestion.

**'गुडमत्स्यण्डिका खण्डशर्कराविमलाः परा:**[11] ॥ १४ ॥

यथा यथैषां वैमल्यं भवेच्छैत्यं तथा तथा ।

"स्नेहगौरवमाधुर्य्यं[12] रसत्वं च तथा तथा[13]" ॥ १५ ॥

*Guḍa, matsyaṇḍikā, khaṇḍa, śarkarā* and *vimalā*—they are progressively free from impurity, cooling, unctuous, heavy, sweet and delicious.

वातपित्तहरं शीतं स्निग्धं हृद्यं[14] मुखप्रियम् ।

चक्षुष्यं बृंहणं बल्यं खंडं वृष्यतमं मतम् ।

*Khaṇḍa* **(Candied sugar)**

*Khaṇḍa* alleviates *vāyu* and *pitta*. It is cooling, unctuous, cardiac tonic, delicious, promoter of eyesight, nourishing and strength promoting. It is an aphrodisiac par excellence.

क्षीणक्षतहिता वृष्या स्निग्धा **पौण्ड्रकशर्करा**[15]' ॥ १६ ॥

[माधवद्रव्यगुण इक्षुवर्ग ३ : १५-१७, १८]

*Pauṇḍraka śarkarā*

*Pauṇḍraka śarkarā* is useful in *kṣīṇa* (emaciation) and

*kṣata* (phthisis). It is aphrodisiac and unctuous.

'छर्द्यतीसारतृष्णाघ्नी विरूक्षा **मधुशर्करा**' ।

[माधवद्रव्य इक्षुवर्ग ३ : २१]

*Madhu śarkarā*

The *śarkarā* prepared of *madhu* (honey) cures *chardī* (vomiting), *atisāra* (diarrhoea) and *tṛṣṇā* (morbid thirst). It is exceedingly un-unctuous.

'मूत्रकृच्छ्राश्मरी[16]प्लीह्नि हिता सामुद्रिकोद्भवा ॥१७॥

ज्वरासृक्पित्ततृट्छर्दिमोहमूर्च्छाविषार्तिषु ।

*Sāmudrikodbhavā śarkarā*

The *sāmudrikodbhavā śarkarā* is useful in the treatment of *mūtrakṛcchra* (dysuria), *aśmari* (stone in the urinary tract), *plīhan* (splenic disorder), *jvara* (fever), *asṛkpitta* (a disease characterised by bleeding from different parts of the body), *tṛṭ* (morbid thirst), *chardi* (vomiting), *moha* (unconsciousness), *mūrchā* (fainting) and *vīṣa* (poisoning).

सर्वा एवामृतप्रख्याः शर्कराः समुदाहृताः ॥ १८ ॥

*Śarkarā* **in general**

All types of *śarkarā* are like ambrosia.

सारे[17] स्थिता निर्मलाश्च त्यक्त[18]क्षारा यथा यथा ।

तथा तथा वीर्यवत्यः शीतवीर्यास्तथा तथा' ॥ १९ ॥

[माधवद्रव्यगुणः इक्षुवर्ग ३ : १९-२१]

॥ इत्यिक्षुवर्गः ॥

Depending upon these three factors viz., (1) extraction from the most useful part, (2) freedom from impurity and (3) freedom from alkalinity, the *śarkarā* becomes progressively more potent and more cooling in potency.

Thus ends the group dealing with sugarcane and its derivatives.

## NOTES AND REFERENCES

1. नेपालो इति आकरे पाठः ।
2. इत्येते ज्ञातयः स्थौल्याद् गुणत्वक्सारतो मताः इति आकरे पाठः ।
3. सुशीतो——सरः पाठोऽयं द्वितीयपुस्तके नोपलभ्यते ।
4. वंशकः स्मृतः इति आकरे पाठः ।
5. वंशवत् शतपोनस्तु इति आकरे पाठः ।
6. कान्तेक्षुः स च वातप्रकोपणः इति आकरे पाठः ।
7. नैपालो इति भावप्रकाशे पाठः ।
8. अग्रे ग्रन्थित्वचोर्ज्ञेयो लवणो रस एव च इति आकरे पाठः ।
9. कफवातजित् इति आकरे पाठः ।
10. फाणितं——वातपित्तजित् पाठोऽयं षष्ठपुस्तके नोपलभ्यते ।
11. परम् इति आकरे पाठः ।
12. सञ्चरेच्च इति आकरे पाठः ।
13. स्नेह——तथा तथा पाठोऽयं द्वितीयपुस्तके नोपलभ्यते ।
14. स्निग्धं शीतं बल्यं इति आकरे पाठः ।
15. स्निग्धा खण्डस्य शर्करा इति आकरे पाठः ।
16. प्लीहहिता इति आकरे पाठः ।
17. सारोत्थिता इति आकरे पाठः ।
18. त्यक्तक्षीरा इति द्वितीयपुस्तके पाठः ।

# CHAPTER 5

"पौतिकं [1]भ्रामरं क्षौद्रं माक्षिकं छात्रमेव च ।
आर्घ्यमौद्दालकं दालमित्यष्टौ मधुजातयः ॥ १ ॥'

[भावप्रकाशः मधुवर्ग २२:६]

## *Madhu* (Honey)

**Variety**

*Paittika*, *bhrāmara*, *kṣaudra*, *mākṣika*, *chātra*, *ārghya*, *auddālaka* and *dāla*—these are the eight varieties of *madhu*.

कषायानुरसं रूक्षं शीतलं मधुरं **मधु** ।
दीपनं लेखनं बल्यं व्रणशोधनरोपणम् ॥ २ ॥
संधानं लघु चक्षुष्यं स्वर्यं हृद्य [2]त्रिदोषनुत् ।

**Property**

*Madhu* is astringent in *anurasa* (after-taste), un-unctuous, cooling, sweet, a digestive stimulant, *lekhana* (depleting) and strength promoting. It cleans and heals ulcers and helps in the joining of fractured bones. It is light, promoter of eyesight and good voice, cardiac tonic and alleviator of all the three *doṣas*.

छर्दिहिक्काविषश्वास[3]कासशोथातिसारजित् ॥ ३ ॥[4]

रक्तपित्तहरं ग्राही कृमिघ्नं मोहहृत्परम् ।

It cures *chardi* (vomiting), *hikkā* (hiccup), *viṣa* (poisoning), *śvāsa* (asthma), *kāsa* (bronchitis), *śotha* (oedema), *atisāra* (diarrhoea) and *raktapitta* (a disease characterised by bleeding from different parts of the body). It is constipative. It cures *kṛmi* (parasitic infection). It is an excellent drug for curing *moha* (unconsciousness).

पैच्छिल्यात्स्वादुभूयस्त्वात्पैत्तिकं गुरु संस्मृतम् ॥ ४ ॥

*Paittika*

*Paittika* type of *madhu* is slimy and sweet in excess. Therefore it is known to be heavy.

भ्रामरं कुरुते जाड्यं भूयिष्ठं मधुरं च तत्[5] ।

*Bhrāmara*

*Bhrāmara* type of *madhu* produces *jāḍya* (numbness and rigidity). It is excessively sweet.

क्षौद्रं विशेषतो ज्ञेयं शीतलं लघु लेखनम् ॥ ५ ॥

*Kṣaudra*

*Kṣaudra* type of *madhu* is specifically cooling, light and *lekhana* (depleting).

तस्माल्लघुतरं रूक्षं माक्षिकं प्रवरं स्मृतम् ।

श्वासादिषु च रोगेषु प्रशस्तं तद्विशेषतः ॥ ६ ॥"

[माधवद्रव्यगुणः मधुवर्ग ४ : १-७]

*Mākṣika*

*Mākṣika* type of *madhu* is lighter than the former. It is

exceedingly un-unctuous. It is specifically, useful in diseases like *śvāsa* (asthma).

बृहणीयं मधु नवं नातिश्लेष्महरं परम्[6] ।

[माधवद्रव्यगुण: मधुवर्ग ४ : १२]

**Freshly Collected *Madhu***

Freshly collected (*nava*) *madhu* is nourishing. It does not alleviate *kapha* in excess. It is very useful.

"स्वादुपाकं गुरु हिमं पिच्छिलं रक्तपित्तजित् ॥७॥

श्वित्रमेहक्रमिघ्नं च विद्याच्छात्रं[7] गुणोत्तरम् ।

*Chātra*

*Chātra* type of *madhu* is sweet in *vipāka*, heavy, cooling and slimy. It cures *raktapitta* (a diseases characterised by bleeding from different parts of the body), *śvitra* (leucoderma), *meha* (obstinate urinary disorders including diabetes) and *kṛmi* (parasitic infection). It is of superior quality.

'आर्घ्यमध्वतिचक्षुष्यं कफपित्तहरं परम् ।

कषायं कटुकं पाके[8] तिक्तं[9] बल्यमवातकृत् ॥ ८ ॥'

[भावप्रकाश: मधुवर्ग २२ : १९]

*Ārghya*

*Ārghya* type of *madhu* is an excellent promoter of eyesight. It is also an excellent alleviator of *kapha* and *pitta*. It is astringent in taste and pungent in *vipāka*. It is bitter and does not aggravate *vāyu*.

औद्दालिकं रुचिकरं स्वर्यं कुष्ठविषापहम् ।

कषायमुष्णमम्लं च पित्तकृत्कटुपाकि च ॥ ९ ॥

[भावप्रकाश: मधुवर्ग २२ : २१] [माधवद्रव्यगुण: मधुवर्ग ४: ९]

*Auddālika*

*Auddālika* type of *madhu* is appetiser and promoter of good voice. It cures *kuṣṭha* (obstinate skin diseases including leprosy) and *viṣa* (poisoning). It is astringent, hot and sour. It aggravates *pitta*. It is pungent in *vipāka*.

छर्दिमेहप्रशमनं मधुरूक्षं दलोद्भवम् ।

*Dalodbhava*

*Dalodbhava* type of *madhu* cures *chardi* (vomiting) and *meha* (obstinate urinary disorders including diabetes). It is un-unctuous.

विशेषात्पौत्तिकं तेषु रक्षोघ्नं सर्पिषान्वयात् ।

**Special attribute of *Paittika***

*Paittika* type of *madhu* is specially *rakṣoghna* (which cures afflictions by evil spirits including germs) when used mixed with ghee.

मेदःस्थौल्यापहं ग्राहि पुराणमतिलेखनम् ॥ १० ॥

[माधवद्रव्यगुणः इक्षुवर्ग ४:८-१२]

10

तद्युक्तं विविधैर्द्रव्यैः निहन्यादामयान्बहून् ।

नाना द्रव्यात्मकत्वाच्च योगवाहि मधु स्मृतम् ॥ ११ ॥

[माधवद्रव्यगुणः मधुवर्ग ४ : १५]

दोषत्रयहरं पक्वं मध्वामं तत्त्रिदोषकृत् ।

***Madhu* in general**

*Madhu* in general cures *medas* (fat) and *sthaulya* (obesity). It is constipative and when preserved for a long time (*purāṇa*), it is exceedingly depleting. It is a mixture of many drugs; therefore, it cures many diseases. In view of its association with many drugs it is known to be *yogavāhin* (which enhances the property of other drugs). It alleviates all the three *doṣas* when properly digested. If *āma* is produced by its improper digestion it vitiates all the three *doṣas*.

[11]उष्णार्त्तस्योष्णकाले च ज्ञेयं विषसमं मधु ॥ १२ ॥

**Adverse effect**

In a person who is afflicted with heat and during the summer season, *madhu* works like a poison.

तत्सौकुमार्याच्च तथैव शैत्यान्नानौषधीनां रससंभवाच्च ।

उष्णैर्विरुद्धेन विशेषतस्तु
तथान्तरिक्षेण जलेन वापि ॥ १३ ॥

*Madhu* is tender (*sukumāra*) and cooling. It is produced by the mixture of the juices (*rasa*) of many drugs. Therefore, it is specifically opposed to heat. It also produces adverse effects when used by mixing with rain water (?).

उष्णेन मधु संयुक्तं वमनेष्ववचारितम् ।
अपाकादनवस्थानात् विरुद्धेत्त[न्न][12] पूर्ववत् ॥ १४ ॥

In emetic therapy, *madhu* is mixed with hot water and administered. It does not produce any adverse effect because it does not stay in the stomach (comes out along with vomiting), and therefore, does not get digested to produce such an effect.

लवणं मधुना नैव तच्च क्षीरेण संयुतम् ।
कदाचिन्नैव दातव्ये तुल्ये च मधु सर्पिषी ॥ १५ ॥

**Combination**

Salt should not be used in combination with either honey or milk. Honey and ghee should never be used together in equal quantities.

अन्यद्रव्ययुतं पूर्वं सर्पिर्वाप्यथवा मधु ।
समं न कुरुते दोषमाहु भेषजवेदिनः ॥ १६ ॥

॥ इति मधुवर्गः ॥

When honey and ghee are used in equal quantities but mixed with other drugs, then such a combination, according to scholars, does not produce any adverse effect.

Thus ends the group of different types of *madhu.*

## NOTES AND REFERENCES

1. भ्रामरी इति षष्ठपुस्तके पाठः ।
2. त्रिदोषजित् इति आकरे पाठः ।
3. छर्दिहिक्काविषश्वासकासशोषातिसारनुत् इति आकरे पाठः ॥
4. क्रिमितृण्मोहहृत्परम् इति आकरे पाठः ॥
5. यत् इति आकरे पाठः ।
6. वातश्लेष्महरं इति द्वितीयपुस्तके पाठः ॥
7. तृष्णावान्त्यतिसारनुत् इति आदर्श पुस्तिकासु पाठः ॥
8. बल्यं पित्तामवातकृत् इति माधवद्रव्यगुणे पाठः ।
   तिक्तञ्च बलपुष्टिकृत् इति भावप्रकाशे पाठः ।
9. बल्यामवातकृत् इति षष्ठपुस्तके पाठः ।
10. लघूष्णं इति आदर्शपुस्तकेषु पाठः ॥
11. उष्णार्त्तमुष्णैरुष्णैर्वातं निहन्ति यथा विषम् इति द्वितीयपुस्तके पाठः ॥
12. विरुद्धेत्तच्च पूर्ववत् इति द्वितीयपुस्तके पाठः ।

# CHAPTER 6

“गव्यमाजं तथौरभ्रं माहिषं चौष्ट्रकं[1] च यत् ।
अश्वायाश्चैव[2] नाग्याश्च मानुषांणां च यत्पय: ॥ १ ॥
तत्त्वनेकौषधिरसं[3] प्राणिनां प्राणदं गुरु ।
मधुरं पिच्छिलं स्निग्धं शीतं सूक्ष्मं सरं स्मृतम् ॥ २ ॥

*Payas* **(Milk)**

**Variety**

The milk of *go* (the cow), *ajā* (the goat), *urabhra* (the sheep), *mahiṣa* (buffalo), *uṣṭra* (the camel), *aśva* (the horse), *nāga* (the elephant) and *manuṣya* (woman) is used in medicine. The milk of these animals contains the essence (*rasa*) of many drugs, and therefore, it is life giver, heavy, sweet, slimy, unctuous, cooling, subtle and laxative.

पथ्यं रसायनं बल्यं हृद्यं मेध्यं गवां पय: ।
आयुष्यं पुंस्त्वकृद्वातरक्तपित्तविकारनुत् ॥ ३ ॥

*Go payas* **(Cow's milk)**

Cow's milk is wholesome, rejuvenating, strength promoting and cardiac tonic. It promotes intellect, longevity and virility. It cures aggravation of *vāyu* and *raktapitta* (a disease characterised by bleeding from different parts of the body).

'छागं कषायं मधुरं शीतं ग्राहि पयो लघु ।
रक्तपित्तातिसारघ्नं क्षयकासज्वरापहम् ॥ ४ ॥

### *Chāga payas* (Goat's milk)

Goat's milk is astringent, sweet, cooling, constipative and light. It cures *raktapitta* (a disease characterised by bleeding from different parts of the body), *atisāra* (diarrhoea), *kṣaya* (consumption), *kāsa* (bronchitis) and *jvara* (fever).

अजानामल्पकायत्वात्कटुतिक्तनिषेवणात् ।
[4] स्तोकाम्बुपानाद् व्यायामात्सर्वव्याधिहरं पयः ॥ ५ ॥"
[भावप्रकाशः दुग्धवर्ग १४:१६-१७]

Goats have a small physique. They eat mostly pungent and bitter things and drink very little water. They perform a lot of physical exercise. (They are agile). Therefore, goat's milk cures all diseases.

'औरभ्रं मधुरं [5] स्निग्धं गुरुपित्तकफापहम् ।
[6] उष्णं शुद्धेऽनिले पथ्यं कासे चानिलशोणिते ॥ ६ ॥'
[माधवद्रव्यगुणः क्षीरवर्ग ५:१-६]

### *Urabhra payas* (Sheep's milk)

The milk of the sheep is sweet, unctuous and heavy. It alleviates *pitta* and *kapha*. It is hot and is wholesome for patients having an aggravation of *vāyu* alone. It cures *kāsa* (bronchitis) and *anilaśoṇita* (gout).

[7] महाभिष्यन्दि मधुरं माहिषं पक्तिनाशनम् ।

निद्राकरं शीतकरं गव्यात्स्निग्धतरं गुरु ॥ ७ ॥

*Mahiṣa payas* **(Buffalo milk)**

The milk of the buffalo is exceedingly *abhiṣyandi* (which obstructs channels of circulation) and sweet. It suppresses the power of digestion. It induces sleep and produces a cooling effect. It is more unctuous and heavy than cow's milk.

रूक्षोष्णं लवणं **क्षीरमौष्ट्रं**[8] स्वादुरसं लघु ।

शस्तं वातकफानाहकृमिशोफोदरार्शसाम्[9] ॥ ८ ॥

*Uṣṭra payas* **(Camel milk)**

The milk of the camel is un-unctuous, hot, saline, sweet and light. It is useful in the aggravation of *vāta* and *kapha*, *ānāha* (flatulence), *kṛmi* (parasitic infection), *śopha* (oedema), *udara* (obstinate abdominal diseases including ascitis) and *arśas* (piles).

**उष्णमेकशफं**[10] बल्यं शाखावातहरं पयः ।

मधुराम्लरसं रूक्षं लवणानुरसं कटुः ।

स्निग्धं स्थैर्यंकरं शीतं चक्षुष्यं बलवर्धनम् ॥ ९ ॥

[माधवद्रव्यगुणः क्षीरवर्ग ५:७-१०]

*Ekaśapha payas* **(Mares milk)**

The milk of the mare is hot. It promotes strength. It cures affliction of the limbs by *vāyu*. It is sweet and sour in taste, un-unctuous, saline in *anurasa* (subsidiary taste) and pungent.

**हस्तिन्या** मधुरं वृष्यं कषायानुरसं गुरु ।

*Hasti payas* **(Elephant's milk)**

The milk of the elephant is unctuous, *sthairyakara* (producing steadiness) and cooling. It promotes eyesight and strength. It is sweet, aphrodisiac and astringent in *anurasa* (subsidiary taste) and heavey.

जीवनं बृंहणं सात्म्यं स्नेहनं **मानुषी** पयः[11] ।
नावनं रक्तपित्तेषु[12] तर्पणं चाक्षिशूलनुत्[13] ॥ 10 ॥

*Mānuṣi payas* **(Woman's milk)**

The woman's milk promotes longevity and nourishment. It is wholesome and unctuous. Its inhalation cures *raktapitta* (a disease characterised by bleeding from different parts of the body). When used in *akṣatarpaṇa* therapy (application of cotton swab soaked in the milk over the eyes) it cures pain in the eyes.

अथ वर्णभेदे गुणा :—

कृष्णायार्गोर्भवेद्दुग्धं वातहारि गुणाधिकम् ।

पीताया हरते पित्तं तथा वातहरं भवेत् ॥ 11 ॥

श्लेष्मलं गुरु शुक्लायाः रक्तायाः वातकृत्पयः ।

**Property of the milk of cows of different colours**

The milk of a black cow alleviates *vāyu* and it is superior in quality. The milk of a yellow cow alleviates *pitta* and *vāyu*. The milk of a white cow aggravates *kapha*. The milk of a red cow aggravates *vāyu*.

वालवत्सविवत्सानां गवां क्षीरं त्रिदोषकृत्[14] ॥ 12 ॥

वष्कयिण्यास्त्रिदोषघ्नं तर्पणं बलकृत्पयः ।

**Other Varieties**

The milk of the cow having a very young calf or without a calf aggravates all the three *doṣas*. The milk of a cow long after her delivery (*baṣkayiṇī*) alleviates all the three *doṣas*. It is refreshing and strength promoting.

जांगलानूपशैलेषु चरन्तीनां यथोत्तरम् ॥ १३ ॥

पयो गुरुतरं स्नेहो यथाचारं प्रवर्त्तते ।

The heaviness and unctuousness of the milk progressively increases depending upon the arid, marshy and hilly areas in which the cow grazes.

स्वल्पान्नभक्षणाज्जातं क्षीरं गुरु कफापहम् ॥ १४ ॥

तत्तु बल्यं परं वृष्यं स्वस्थानां गुणदायकम् ।

पलालतृणकार्पासवीजनं रोगिणे हितम् ॥ १५ ॥

The milk of the cow which takes less food is heavy and it alleviates *kapha*. For healthy persons it is very useful inasmuch as it promotes strength and virility. The milk of the cow which eats straw, grass and cotton seed is useful for patients.

धारोष्णं गोपयो बल्यं लघुशीतं[15] सुधासमम् ।

त्रिदोषनुद्दीपनं तद्धाराशीतं त्रिदोषकृत् ॥ १६ ॥

The warm milk of the cow immediately after milking (*dhāroṣṇa*) promotes strength. It is light and cooling. It is like ambrosia. It alleviates all the three *doṣas* and it stimulates the digestion. When it becomes cold after milking (*dhārā śīta*) it aggravates all the three *doṣas*.

वर्जयित्वा स्त्रियाः स्तन्यमामेव हि तद्धितम् ।

The Woman's milk is an exception to this rule inasmuch as it is useful only when it is cold.

आमवातकरं चाम धारोष्णममृतं पयः ॥ १७ ॥

Cold milk causes *āmavāta* (rheumatism) and *dhāroṣṇa* (when it is warm immediately after milking) milk is like ambrosia.

'धारोष्णं शस्यते गव्यं धाराशीतं तु माहिषम् ।
श्रृतोष्णमाविकं क्षीरं श्रृतशीतमजापयः ॥ १८ ॥

Cow's milk is useful when it is *dhāroṣṇa* and buffalo's milk is useful when it becomes cold after milking (*dhārā śīta*). Sheep's milk is useful when it is warm after boiling. Goat's milk should be used when it is cold after boiling.

श्रृतोष्णं कफवातघ्नं श्रृतशीतं तु पित्तनुत् ।

Boiled and hot milk alleviates *kapha* and *vāta*. The milk which is cooled after boiling alleviates *pitta*.

अर्द्धोदकं क्षीरशिष्टं मानाल्लघुतरं हितम् ॥ १९ ॥

The milk which is boiled with half of water till the original quantity of milk remains is lighter and useful.

जलेन रहितं दुग्धमतिपक्वं यथा यथा ।
तथा तथा गुरु स्निग्धं वृष्यं बलविवर्धनम् ॥ २० ॥

[भावप्रकाशः दुग्धवर्ग १४:२५-२८]

The milk which is excessively boiled by which it becomes free from its water content, depending upon the time of boiling, becomes progressively more and more heavy, unuctuous, aphrodisiac and promoter of strength.

क्षीरसंतानिका बल्या वृष्या पित्तानिलापहा ।

The *santānikā* (the layer of cream which is formed on the surface when the milk is boiled on low heat) of milk promotes strength and virility. It alleviates *pitta* and *vāyu*.

16
रात्रौ क्षीरं न सेवेत सेवेत यदि न स्वपेत् ॥ २१ ॥
यदि स्वपेद्धरत्यायुस्तस्मात्पथ्यं दिवा पयः ।

**Time of taking milk**

Milk should not be taken at night. If one happens to

to take milk at night, then he should not sleep. If he sleeps after taking milk, then it reduces longevity. Therefore, milk is wholesome if taken during day time.

रात्रौ चन्द्रगुणाधिक्याद्व्यायामपरिवर्जनात् ॥२२॥
प्रभातिकं पयः प्रायो विष्टम्भि गुरु दोषलम् ।
दिवाकरकराघाताद् व्यायामानिलसेवनात् ।
17
प्रादोषं श्रमनुद्बल्यं चक्षुष्यं वातपित्तहृत् ॥ २३ ॥

During night the attributes of the moon become predominant and there is no exercise. Therefore early morning (*prabhāta*) milk is generally constipative, heavy and aggravator of *doṣas*. On the other hand, there is exposure to sun shine, exercise and wind, for which the evening (*pradoṣa*) milk alleviates fatigue. It promotes strength and eye sight. It alleviates *vāyu* and *pitta*.

**सेवनसमयभेदे गुणभेदः —**

"वृष्यं बृंहणमग्निदीप्तिजननं पूर्वाह्णकाले पयो ।

**Time of intake**

Milk taken in the forenoon produces aphrodisiac and nourishing effects. It stimulates the power of digestion.

मध्याह्ने बलवर्धनं कफहरं पित्तापहं दीपनम् ॥ २४ ॥

Milk taken during noon-time promotes strength. It alleviates *kapha* and *pitta*. It is a digestive stimulant.

18 19
बाले वृद्धिकरं क्षये क्षय[ह]रं वृद्धेषु रेतोवहम् ।
20
रात्रौ पथ्यमनेकरोगशमनं क्षीरं सदा चाक्षुषम्" ॥२५॥

[भावप्रकाशः दुग्धवर्ग १४ : ३६]

Milk taken during the night promotes strength in children, cures consumption, increasingly produces semen in oldmen. It is wholesome and it cures many diseases. It invariably promotes eye sight.

'शर्करासहितं क्षीरं कफकृत्पवनापहम् ।

**Combination**

When used in combination with *śarkarā*, milk produces *kapha* and alleviates *vāyu.*

सितासितोपलायुक्तं शुक्रदं दोषनाशनम् ।

In combination with *sitā* and *sitopalā*, milk produces semen and alleviates *doṣas.*

सगुडं मूत्रकृच्छ्रघ्नं पित्तश्लेष्मकरं भवेत् ॥ २६ ॥

[भावप्रकाशः दुग्धवर्ग १४ : ३६]

If taken in combination with *guḍa*, milk cures *mūtra kṛcchra* (dysuria) and it aggravates *pitta* and *kapha.*

'वदन्ति पेयं निशि केवलं पयो
भोज्यं न तेनेह सहौदनादिकम् ।
भवेदजीर्णं[21] यदि न स्वपेन्निशि
क्षीरस्य पीतस्य न शेषमृत्सृजेत् ॥ २७ ॥

**Intake of milk at night**

Some scholars hold the view that milk alone can be taken at night. But along with milk no other food like rice should be taken. If there is indigestion, then one should not sleep at night. One should not leave a part of the milk after drinking.

विदाहीन्यन्नपानानि दिवा भुंक्ते हि मानवः[22] ।
तद्विदाहप्रशान्त्यर्थं[23] रात्रौ क्षीरं प्रशस्यते ॥ २८ ॥

[भावप्रकाशः दुग्धवर्ग १४:४०-४१]

Generally, human beings take food and drinks during, the day time which cause burning sensation (*vidāhin*). To alleviate this burning sensation, milk is useful at night.

'विवर्णं विरसं चाम्लं दुर्गन्धं ग्रथितं पयः ।
वर्जयेदम्ललवणं युक्तं[24] कुष्ठादिरोगकृत् ॥ २९ ॥'

[भावप्रकाशः दुग्धवर्ग १४ : ४६]

**Bad quality**

Milk whose colour and taste are changed, which has become sour, which produces a putrid smell and which is of knotted appearance should not be used. It should not be used when mixed with sour things and salt because this type of milk produces diseases like *kuṣṭha* (obstinate skin diseases including leprosy).

'दीप्तानले कृशे पुंसि बाले वृद्धे रतप्रिये[25] +
मतं हिततमं दुग्धं सद्यः शुक्रकरं पयः[26] ॥ ३० ॥

**Indication**

For persons whose digestive power is very strong, who are emaciated, for infants and old persons and for those who indulge in sex, milk is exceedingly useful. It produces semen instantaneously.

क्षीरं गव्यमथाजं वा कोष्णं दण्डाहतं भवेत्[27] ।
लघु वृष्य ज्वरहरं वातपित्तकफापहम् ॥ ३१ ॥

[भावप्रकाशः दुग्धवर्ग १४ : ४२-४३]

**Special Processing**

When the luke-warm (*koṣṇa*) milk of either a cow or a goat is stirred with a wooden rod (*daṇḍāhata*), it becomes light and aphrodisiac. It cures fever and alleviates *vāyu*, *pitta* and *kapha*.

[28]'क्षीरफेनं त्रिदोषघ्नं रोचनं बलवर्धनम् ।
वह्निवृद्धिकरं पथ्यं सद्यस्तृप्तिकरं लघु ।

अतीसारेऽग्निमान्द्ये च ज्वरे जीर्णे प्रशस्यते' ॥ ३२ ॥

[भावप्रकाश: दुग्धवर्ग १४:४४-४५]

शूलशोफामकासघ्नं विषमज्वरनाशनम् ।

उर: संधानजननं हिक्काश्वासनिषूदनम् ॥ ३३ ॥

*Kṣīra phena* **(foam of the milk)**

The foam that comes out of the milk (*kṣīra phena*) alleviates all the three *doṣas*. It is an appetiser and promoter of strength as well as the power of digestion. It is wholesome, instantaneously refreshing and light. It is beneficial in *atisāra* (diarrhoea), *agnimāndya* (suppression of the power of digestion) and *jīrṇajvara* (chronic fever). It cures *śūla* (colic pain), *śopha* (oedema), *āma, kāsa* (bronchitis) and *viṣama jvara* (irregular fever). It heals the wound in the chest (*uraḥ sandhāna*) and cures *hikkā* (hic cup), and *śvāsa* (asthma).

नान्नहीनं प्रदातव्यं क्षीरं तक्रं भिषग्वरै: ।

**Precaution**

Milk and butter milk (*takra*) should not be given without food (*anna*) by a physician.

ताम्रे वातहरं क्षीरं सौवर्णे पित्तनाशनम् ॥ ३४ ॥

रौप्ये कफहरं चैव कांस्ये रक्तप्रसादनम् ।

**Container**

Milk in a copper container alleviates *vāyu*. In a gold container it alleviates *pitta*, in silver it alleviates *kapha* and in a brass container it promotes blood.

29

क्षीरं तत्कालं सूताया: **घनं पीयूषमुच्यते** ॥ ३५ ॥

*Ghana & Pīyūṣa*

The milk of the cow immediately after delivery is called *ghana* and *pīyūṣa*.

सप्तरात्रात्परं क्षीरमप्रसन्नं तु **मोरटम्** ।
'नष्टदुग्धासवं मस्तु मोरटं [30] जय्यटोऽब्रवीत्' ॥ ३६ ॥

[भावप्रकाशः दुग्धवर्ग १४ : ३२]

*Moraṭa*

After seven days of the delivery, the milk is called *moraṭa*. According to *Jayyaṭa*, the *āsava* or *mastu* prepared of the curdled (*naṣṭa*) milk is called *moraṭa*.

पक्वं दध्नासमं क्षीरं विज्ञेया **दधिकूर्चिका** ।
तक्रेण **तक्रकूर्चीस्यात्**तयोः पिण्डः **किलाटकः** ॥ ३७ ॥
पाकं विना स एव स्यात् **क्षीरसीकः** सितान्वितः ।

*Dadhi kūrcikā, Takra kurcikā, Kilāṭa* **etc.**,

The preparation made out of boiling curd and milk (in equal quantity) is called *dadhi kūrcikā*. When this is done with buttermilk and milk it is called *takra kūrcikā*. If the preparation is made out in a solid form (*piṇḍa*) then it is called *kilāṭaka*. If the preparation is done without boiling but by adding sugar, then it is called *kṣīrasīka*.

तक्रनष्टं स तक्रं यद्दुग्धं [31] [वस्त्रावगालितम्] ॥ ३८ ॥
द्रवगुणपरित्यक्तं तत्र **पिण्डः** स उच्यते ।

*Piṇḍa*

When the curdled (*naṣṭa*) milk (?) or butter milk is filtered through a cloth and the residue is completely free from water, it is called *piṇḍa*.

पीयूषं मोरटश्चापि कूर्चिका दधितक्रयोः ॥ ३९ ॥
किलाटः क्षीरसीकश्च तक्रपिण्डश्च पुष्टिदः ।
गुरवः श्लेष्मला वृष्या हृद्या वाताग्निनाशनाः ॥ ४० ॥

दीप्ताग्नीनामनिद्राणां व्यवाये चातिपूजिताः ।

**Property of *Pīyūṣa* etc.**

*Pīyūṣa*, *moraṭa*, *dadhi kūrcikā*, *takra kūrcikā*, *kilāṭa*, *kṣīrasīka* and *takra piṇḍa* are nourishing and heavy. They aggravate *kapha*. They are aphrodisiacs and cardiac tonics. They alleviate *vāyu* and suppress the power of digestion. They are exceedingly useful for those having a strong power of digestion, those suffering from sleeplessness and those indulging in sex.

घर्मे तु माहिषं सेव्यं हेमन्ते चाप्यजाविकम् ।

गव्यं क्षीरं तु वर्षासु नराणाममृतोपमम् ॥ ४१ ॥

**Milk in different Seasons**

Buffalo's milk should be used in the summer season. The milk of goat and sheep is useful in *hemanta* (beginning of winter). Cow's milk is like ambrosia for human beings during the rainy season.

॥ इति क्षीरवर्गः ॥

Thus ends the group dealing with various types of milk.

## NOTES AND REFERENCES

1. कारंभं तथा इति आकरे पाठः ।
2. अश्वायाश्चापि नार्याश्च करेणूनां इति आकरे पाठः ।
3. तत्त्वेनैकोषधिरसं इति षष्ठपुस्तके पाठः ।
4. नात्यम्बुपानाद् इति आकरे पाठः ।
5. स्निग्धमुष्णं वातकफापहम् इति आकरे पाठः ।
6. गुरु इति आकरे पाठः ।

7. महाभिष्यन्दि इति आकरे पाठः ।
8. क्षीरमुष्ट्रीणामीषत्सलवणं लघु इति आकरे पाठः ।
9. शोथो इति आकरे पाठः ।
10. उष्णमैकशफं इति आकरे पाठः ।
11. मानुषं इति आकरे पाठः ।
12. रक्तपित्ते तु इति आकरे पाठः ।
13. चाक्षिशूलनाम् इति आकरे पाठः ।
14. क्षीरत्रिदोषहृत् इति षष्ठपुस्तके पाठः ।
15. सुधासमम् इति षष्ठपुस्तके पाठः ।
16. रात्रि इति द्वितीयपुस्तके पाठः ।
17. अदोषं इति षष्ठपुस्तके पाठः ।
18. वाते इति द्वितीयपुस्तके पाठः ।
19. क्षयकरं इति द्वितीयपुस्तके पाठः ।
20. वृष्यं बृंहणमग्निदीपनकरं पूर्वाह्णकाले पयो ।
    मध्याह्ने बलवर्धनं रतिकरं कामाग्निसंदीपनम् ।
    बालेष्वग्निकरं क्षये हितकरं वृद्धेषु वीर्यप्रदम् ।
    रात्रौ पथ्यमनेकदोषहरणं क्षीरं हितं चक्षुषाम् ।
    इति माधवद्रव्यगुणे पाठः ।
21. भवत्यजीर्णं न शयति शर्वरीं इति आकरे पाठः ।
22. यन्नरः इति आकरे पाठः ।
23. सदा पिबेत् इति आकरे पाठः ।
24. कुष्ठादिकृद् यतः इति आकरे पाठः ।
25. पयः प्रिये इति आकरे पाठः ।
26. यतः इति आकरे पाठः ।
27. पिबेत् इति आकरे पाठः ।
28. भवेत् फेनं इति आकरे पाठः ।
29. पीयूषसममुच्यते इति षष्ठपुस्तके पाठः ।
30. जैज्जटोऽब्रवीत् इति षष्ठपुस्तके पाठः ।
31. वाससा·······। इति द्वितीयपुस्तके पाठः ।
    वसा गालितां इति षष्ठपुस्तके पाठः ।

# CHAPTER 7

'दध्युष्णं दीपनं स्निग्धं कषायानुरसं गुरु ।
पाकेऽम्लं ग्राहि पित्तास्रशोथमेदःकफप्रदम् ॥ १ ॥
मूत्रकृच्छ्रे[1] प्रतीश्याये शीतगे विषमज्वरे ।
अतीसारेऽरुचौ कार्श्ये शस्यते बलशुक्रकृत् ॥ २ ॥

*Dadhi* (**curd**)

Dadhi is hot, a digestive stimulant, unctuous, astringent in *anurasa* (subsidiary taste), heavy, sour in *vipāka* and constipative. It vitiates *pitta* and blood and aggravates *śotha* (oedema), *medas* (adiposity) and *kapha*. It is useful in *mūtra kṛcchra* (dysuria), *pratiśyāya* (cold), *śītaga viṣamajvara* (irregular fever which is associated with a feeling of cold), *atisāra* (diarrhoea), *aruci* (anorexia) and *kārśya* (emaciation). It promotes strength and semen.

आदौ मन्दं ततः स्वादुः स्वाद्वम्लं च ततः परम् ।
अम्लं चतुर्थमत्यम्लं पञ्चमं दधि पञ्चधा ॥ ३ ॥

**Variety**

The first stage of *dadhi* is called *manda* (in which there is no manifested taste). The second stage of it is called ***svādu*** (sweet) and the third stage is *svādvamla* (both sweet and sour in taste). During the fourth stage it is called *amla* (sour) and the fifth stage is called *atyamla* (excessively sour). These are the five varieties of *dadhi.*

**मंदं** दुग्धवदव्यक्तरसं किञ्चिद् घृतं मतम् ।

*Manda*

Like milk, *manda* has no manifested taste and there is less of ghee in it.

मन्दं स्यात्सृष्टविण्मूत्रं दोषत्रयविदाहकृत् ॥ ४ ॥

It helps in the elimination of stool and urine. It vitiates all the three *doṣas* and causes burning sensation.

यत्सम्यग्घनतां यातं व्यक्तं स्वादुरसं भवेत् ।

2

अव्यक्ताम्लरसं तत्तु **स्वादु**स्तज्ज्ञैरुदीरितम् ॥ ५ ॥

*Svādu*

When it gets properly condensed and there is the manifestation of a sweet taste it is called *svādu.* The sour taste in it is not manifested.

स्वादुः स्यादल्पाभिष्यन्दि वृष्यं 'मेदःकफापहम् ।

वातघ्नं मधुरं पाके रक्तपित्तप्रसादनम्' ॥ ६ ॥

[भावप्रकाशः दधिवर्ग १५:१-६]

3

प्राभातिकं तु मधुरं वातपित्तनिवर्हणम् ।

*Svādu* is slightly *abhiṣyandi* (which obstructs the channels of circulation). It is aphrodisiac and it reduces *medas* (fat), *kapha* and *vāta.* It is sweet in *vipāka.* It produces more of blood and *pitta.* If this is taken during the early morning then it alleviates both *vāyu* and *pitta.*

'**स्वाद्वम्लं** साम्लमधुरं कषायानुरसं भवेत् ॥ ७ ॥

### *Svādvamla*

The *svādvamla* variety of *dadhi* is both sweet and sour in taste. It is astringent in *anurasa* (subsidiary taste).

[4] स्वाद्वम्लस्य गुणा ज्ञेया सामान्यदधिवज्जनैः ।

In properties, it is like *dadhi* in general.

[5] यत्तिरोहितमाधुर्यं [व्य]क्ताम्लं च तदम्लकम् ॥८॥

### *Amlaka*

When *dadhi* is deprived of its sweet taste, and its sour taste is well manifested, then it is called *amlaka*.

अम्लं तु दीपनं रक्तपित्तश्लेष्मविवर्धनम् ।

It stimulates digestion and aggravates blood, *pitta* and *kapha*.

[6] तदत्यम्लं दन्तरोमहर्षकण्ठादिदाहकृत् ।

### *Atyamla*

When *dadhi* becomes exceedingly sour it is called *atyamla*. It causes a tingling sensation (*harṣa*) in the teeth and horripilation (*roma harṣa*). It produces burning sensation in the throat etc.

[7] अत्यम्लं दीपनं रक्तपित्तदुष्टिकरं परम् ॥ ९ ॥'

(भावप्रकाशः दधिवर्ग १५:७-९)

It stimulates digestion and exceedingly vitiates blood and *pitta*.

[8] 'गव्यं दध्युत्तमं बल्यं पाके स्वादुरुचिप्रदम् ।

'पवित्रं दीपनं स्निग्धं पुष्टिकृत्पवनापहम् ॥ १० ॥

### *Gavya dadhi* (Curd of cow's milk)

***Dadhi*** prepared from Cow's milk is an excellent promoter of strength. In *vipāka*, it is sweet. It is an appetiser, sacred, a digestive stimulant, unctuous and nourishing. It alleviates *vāyu.*

[9]उक्तं दध्नामशेषाणां मध्ये गव्यं गुणाधिकम् ।

Among the several varieties of *dadhi*, the one prepared from cow's milk is known to be the best.

**माहिषं दधि** सुस्निग्धं श्लेष्मलं वातपित्तनुत् ।
स्वादुपाकमभिष्यन्दि वृष्यं गुर्वस्रदूषणम् ॥ ११ ॥

[भावप्रकाशः दधिवर्ग १०-११]

### *Māhiṣa dadhi* (Curd of buffalo's milk)

***Dadhi*** prepared from buffalo milk is exceedingly unctuous. It aggravates *kapha* and alleviates *vāyu* as well as *pitta*. It is sweet in *vipāka*, *abhiṣyandi* (which obstructs the channels of circulation), an aphrodisiac and heavy. It vitiates blood.

'**आजं** दध्युत्तमं ग्राहि लघु दोषत्रयापहम् ।
शस्यते श्वासकासार्शःक्षयकार्श्येषु दीपनम् ॥ १२ ॥

### *Āja dadhi* (Curd of goat's milk)

*Dadhi* prepared from goat's milk is very useful. It is constipative and light. It alleviates all the three *doṣas*. It is useful in *śvāsa* (asthma), *kāsa* (bronchitis), *arśas* (piles), *kṣaya* (consumption) and *kārśya* (emaciation). It stimulates the digestive power.

[10]पक्वदुग्धभवं रुच्यं **दधि स्निग्धं** गुणोत्तमम् ।
पित्तनिलापहं सर्वधात्वग्निबलवर्धनम् ॥ १३ ॥

### *Dadhi* of boiled milk

*Dadhi* prepared from boiled milk is an appetiser, unctuous and exceedingly useful. It alleviates *pitta* and *vāyu*, and promotes all the tissue elements (*dhātus*), digestive power and strength.

असारं दधि संग्राहि कषायं वातलं लघु ।
विष्टम्भि दीपनं रुच्यं ग्रहणीरोगनाशनम् ॥ १४ ॥

*Asāra dadhi*

*Dadhi* which is free from fat is constipative, astringent, aggravator of *vāyu* and light. It produces flatulence (*viṣṭambhi*). It is a digestive stimulant and appetiser. It cures *grahaṇī* (sprue syndrome).

गालितं दधि सुस्निग्धं वातघ्नं श्लेष्मलं गुरु ।
बलपुष्टिकरं रुच्यं मधुरं नातिपित्तलम् ॥ १५ ॥

*Gālita dadhi*

If the watery portion of *dadhi* is removed by filteration, then it becomes exceedingly unctuous. It alleviates *vāyu* and aggravates *kapha*. It is heavy. It promotes strength and nourishment. It is an appetiser and sweet. It does not aggravate *pitta* in excess.

सशर्करं दधि श्रेष्ठं तृष्णापित्तास्रदाहनुत् ।
सगुडं वातनुद्वृष्यं बृंहणं तर्पणं गुरु ॥ १६ ॥

**Combination**

Combined with sugar, *dadhi* in very useful in curing *tṛṣṇā* (morbid thirst), vitiated *pitta* as well as blood and *dāha* (burning syndrome).

Along with *guḍa*, *dadhi* alleviates *vāyu*. It is aphrodisiac, nourishing, refreshing and heavy.

न नक्तं दधि भुञ्जीत न चाप्यघृतशर्करम् ।

न मुद्गसूपं नाक्षौद्रं नोष्णं नामलकैर्विना ॥ १७ ॥'

[भावप्रकाशः दधिवर्ग १५ : १२-१७]

**Contra-indications**

*Dadhi* should not be taken at night, nor should it be taken without ghee, sugar, *mudga sūpa* or honey. It should not be taken when it is hot nor without *āmalaki.*

'शस्यते दधि नो रात्रौ शस्तं चाम्बुघृतान्वितम् ।
रक्तपित्तकफोत्थेषु विकारेषु [12] हितं न तत्' ॥ १८ ॥

[भावप्रकाशः दधिवर्ग १५ : प्रक्षिप्तपाठ]

At night, *dadhi* should not be taken. It is useful when mixed with water and ghee. It is not useful in diseases caused by blood, *pitta* and *kapha.*

'हेमन्ते शिशिरे [13] चैव वर्षासु दधि शस्यते ।
शरद्ग्रीष्मवसन्तेषु प्रायशस्तद्विगर्हितम् ॥ १९ ॥

In *hemanta* (first part of winter), *śiśira* (later part of winter) and in the rainy season intake of *dadhi* is beneficial. Generally, it is not useful in autumn, summer and spring season.

ज्वरासृक्पित्तवीसर्पकुष्ठपाण्ड्वामयभ्रमान् ।
प्राप्नुयात्कामलां चोग्रां विधिं हित्वा दधिप्रियः ॥२०॥

[भावप्रकाशः दधिवर्ग १५:१८-१९]

**Adverse effect**

A person who takes *dadhi* without following the prescribed procedure succumbs to acute form of *jvara* (fever), *asṛk pitta* (a disease characterised by bleeding from different parts of the body), *visarpa* (erysipelas), *kuṣṭha* (obstinate skin diseases including leprosy), *pāṇḍvāmaya* (anemia), *bhrama* (giddiness) and *kāmalā* (jaundice).

विपाके कटुसक्षारमम्लं **भेद्यौष्ट्रिकं** **दधि** ।

[14]'वातमर्शांसि कुष्ठानि क्रमीन्हन्त्युदराणि च ॥ २१ ॥

*Auṣṭrika dadhi* **(Curd of camel's milk)**

*Dadhi* prepared from camel's milk is pungent in *vipāka,* alkaline and sour. It cures aggravated *vāyu, arśas* (piles), *kuṣṭha* (obstinate skin diseases including leprosy), *kṛmi* (parasitic infection) and *udara* (obstinate abdominal diseases including ascitis).

कोपनं कफवातानां दुर्नाम्नां **चाविकं** **दधि** ।'

*Āvika dadhi* **(Curd of sheep milk)**

*Dadhi* prepared from the milk of the sheep aggravates *kapha, vāta* and *durnāman* (piles).

दीपनीयमचक्षुष्यं वातलं **दधि** **वाडवम्** ॥ २२ ॥

रूक्षमुष्णं कषायं च कफमू[त्रा][15]पहं च तत् ।

*Vāḍava dadhi* **(Curd of mare's milk)**

*Dadhi* prepared from mare's milk is a digestive stimulant and harmful for the eye. It aggravates *vāyu.* It is un-unctuous, hot and astringent. It reduces *kapha* and urine.

स्निग्धं विपाके मधुरं बल्यं संतर्पणं गुरु ॥ २३ ॥

चक्षुष्यमग्र्यं दोषघ्नं **दधि** **नार्या** गुणोत्तरम् ।

*Nārī dadhi* **(Curd of woman's milk)**

Dadhi prepared from woman's milk is unctuous, sweet in *vipāka,* promoter of strength, refreshing and heavy. It is an excellent promoter of eye sight. It alleviates *doṣas.* It is extremely useful.

लघुपाके बलासघ्नं वीर्योष्णं पक्तिनाशनम् ॥ २४ ॥

कषायानुरसं **नार्या** **दधि** वर्चोविवर्धनम् ।

### *Nāga dadhi* (Curd of elephant's milk)

*Dadhi* prepared from elephant's milk is light in *vipāka*. It alleviates *kapha*. It is hot in potency and it reduces the power of digestion. It is astringent in *anurasa* (subsidiary taste). It increases the quantity of stool.

दधीन्युक्तानि यान्येवं गव्यादीनि पृथक् पृथक् ॥ 25 ॥

विज्ञेयमेव सर्वेषु गव्यमेव गुणोत्तरम् ।

**General**

Properties of different types of *dadhi* are described above. Among them, the *dadhi* prepared from cow's milk is the best.

कपित्थमज्जकल्केन यद्वामलरसेन तु ॥ २६ ॥

16

'पिष्टैश्चित्रकमूलैर्वा पक्वाम्रस्य रसेन तु ।'

लिप्तभाण्डेऽथ कठिनं मधुरं दधि जायते ॥ २७ ॥

If the inside wall of the *bhāṇḍa* (jar in which curd is prepared) is smeared with the paste of the pulp of *kapittha*, juice of *āmalaka*, paste of the root of *citraka* or the juice of ripe mango, then the curd becomes hard (increased density) and sweet.

लवणं रूप्यं विडं वा दध्नो भवति जीवनम् ।

Salt, silver and *viḍa*—these are very essential (lit. life) for *dadhi*.

दध्नस्तूपरि यो भागो घनः स्नेहसमन्वितः ॥ २८ ॥

लोके **सर** इति ख्यातो दध्नो मंडस्तु **मस्त्विति** ।

### *Sara* & *Mastu*

The upper layer of the milk which is dense and unctuous is called *sara* (cream) and the watery portion of the curd is called *mastu*.

सरः स्वादुर्गुरुर्वृष्यो वातवह्निप्रणाशनः ।। २९ ।।

वस्तेर्विधमनश्चाम्लः पित्तश्लेष्मविवर्धनः ।

*Sara* is sweet, heavy and aphrodisiac. It reduces *vāyu* and the power of digestion. It stimulates (*vidhamana*) the bladder. When it becomes sour, it aggravates *pitta* and *kapha*.

मस्तु क्लमहरं बल्यं लघु भक्ताभिलाषदम् ।। ३० ।।

17

स्रोतोविशोधनं क्लेदि कफतृष्णानिलापहम् ।

अवृष्यं प्रीणनं शीघ्रं भिनत्ति मलसंग्रहम् ।। ३१ ।।

*Mastu* cures mental fatigue (*klama*). It is a strength promoter and light. It promotes appetite for food. It cleanses the channels of circulation and produces *kleda* (sticky material). It alleviates *kapha*, *tṛṣṇā* (morbid thirst) and *vāyu*. It is not aphrodisiac. It is refreshing and works as an instant laxative.

।। इति दधिवर्गः ।।

Thus ends the group dealing with various types of *dadhi*.

## NOTES AND REFERENCES

1. अतीसारे शुचौ इति आदर्शपुस्तिकासु पाठः ।
2. स्वादु विज्ञैरुदाहृतम् इति आकरे पाठः ।
3. वातपित्तकफाधिकं इति षष्ठपुस्तके पाठ ।
4. सामान्यस्य इति षष्ठपुस्तके पाठः ।
5. वात्ताम्लं इति द्वितीयपुस्तके पाठः ।
6. दध्यम्लं इति षष्ठपुस्तके पाठः ।
7. रक्तवातपित्तकरं इति आकरे पाठः ।

8. गव्यं दधि विशेषेण स्वाद्वम्लं च रुचिप्रदम् इति आकरे पाठः ।
9. "दध्यामशोषाणां" इति आदर्शपुस्तिकासु पाठः ।
10. शृतक्षीरमयं द्रव्यं इति आदर्शपुस्तिकासु पाठः ।
11. रुच्यं.........बलपुष्टिकरं पाठोऽयं षष्ठपुस्तके नोपलभ्यते ।
12. तु नैव तत् इति आकरे पाठः ।
13. चापि इति आकरे पाठः ।
14. वातमर्शांसि.........दधि पाठोऽयं षष्ठपुस्तके नोपलभ्यते ।
15. कफमूत्रपहं इति द्वितीयपुस्तके पाठः ।
16. पिष्टै..........तु पाठोऽयं द्वितीयपुस्तके नोपलभ्यते ।
17. लघुतृष्णानिलापहम् इति षष्ठपुस्तके पाठः ।

# CHAPTER 8

तक्रं[1] लघुकषायोष्णं दीपनं कफवातजित् ।

शोथोदरार्शो[2] — ग्रहणीदोषमूत्रग्रहारुचीन् ॥ १ ॥

गुल्मप्लीहघृतव्यापत्हरं पांड्वामयान् जयेत् ।

### *Takra* (Butter milk)

*Takra* is light, astringent, hot and digestive stimulant. It alleviates *kapha* and *vāta*. It cures *śotha* (oedema), *udara* (obstinate abdominal diseases including ascitis), *arśas* (piles), *grahaṇī* (sprue syndrome), *mūtra graha* (anuria), *aruci* (anorexia), *gulma* (phantom tumour), *plīhan* (splenic disorder), *ghṛta vyāpat* (complications because of wrong administration of ghee) and *pāṇḍvāmaya* (anemia).

समुद्धृतघृतं तक्रमर्द्धोद्धृतघृतं च यत्[3] ॥ २ ॥

अनुद्धृतघृतं चान्यदित्येतत्त्रिविधं स्मृतम्[4] ।

**Variety**

*Takra* is of three types depending upon the content of fat

which is either completely removed, half removed or not removed at all.

पूर्वं च लघु पथ्यं च [5]गुरुवृष्यतमं परम् ॥ ३ ॥

ततः परं वृष्यतमं यथाक्रममुदाहृतम् ।

The first variety from which fat is completely removed is light and wholesome. The second variety from which half of the fat is removed is exceedingly heavy and aphrodisiac. The third variety from which fat is not removed is exceedingly aphrodisiac.

यान्युक्तानि दधीन्यष्टौ तद्गुणं तक्रमादिशेत् ॥ ४ ॥

The properties of the different types of *dadhi* prepared from the milk of different animals are also shared by the *takra* prepared out of them.

तक्रं तु **घोलं** **मथितोदश्वित्तक्र**प्रभेदतः ।

सुश्रुताद्यैर्मुनिश्रेष्ठैश्चतुर्विधमुदीरितम् ॥ ५ ॥

ससरं [6]निर्जलं घोलं मथितं त्वसरोदकम् ।

तक्रं पादजलं प्रोक्तं उदश्विच्चार्द्धवारिकम् ।

[भावप्रकाशः तक्रवर्ग १६:१-२]

वातपित्तहरं **घोलं** [7]**मथितं** कफपित्तनुत् ॥ ६ ॥

[माधवद्रव्यगुणः तक्रवर्ग ७ : १०]

By the great sages like *Suśruta*, *takra* is described to be of four types viz., *ghola*, *mathita*, *udaśvit* and *takra*. The butter-milk which contains cream and to which water is not added is called *ghola*. When the cream is removed but no water is added then it is called *mathita*. When one fourth quantity of water is added then it is called *takra*. In *udaśvit* half the quantity of water is added.

**तक्रं** त्रिदोषशमनम**ुदश्वित्कफदं** भवेत् ।

उदश्वित्कफदं बल्यं श्रमघ्नं परमं मतम् ।। ७ ।।

*Takra* alleviates all the three *doṣas*. *Udaśvit* aggravates *kapha*, promotes strength and alleviates fatigue par excellence.

**अथ मन्दादितक्रगुणा :**

8
मंदजातं भवेत्तक्रं रूक्षाभिष्यन्दिदुर्जरम् ।

**Property of different types**

Butter milk prepared of the *manda* variety of *dadhi* is unctuous, *abhiṣyandi* (which obstructs the channels of circulation), and difficult of digestion.

9
तक्रं तु मधुरं स्निग्धं श्लेष्मलं वातपित्तनुत् ।। ८ ।।

Buttermilk prepared of the sweet variety of *dadhi* is unctuous. It aggravates *kapha* and alleviates *vāyu* and *pitta*.

अम्लं वातघ्नंमत्यम्लं रक्तपित्तप्रकोपनम् ।

Buttermilk prepared of the sour variety of *dadhi* alleviates *vāyu*. Buttermilk prepared of *dadhi* which is extremely sour, aggravates *rakta* (blood) and *pitta*.

तत्तु सान्द्रं सान्द्रतरं गुरुविद्याद्यथोत्तरम् ।। ९ ।।

The heaviness of *takra* progressively increases depending upon the increase in density.

वातेऽम्लं सैन्धवोपेतं पित्ते स्वादुसशर्करम् ।
पिवेत्तक्रं कफे रूक्षं क्षारव्योषसमन्वितम् ।
'मूत्रकृच्छ्रे तु सगुडं पांडुरोगे सचित्रकम् ।। १० ।।'

[भावप्रकाशः तक्रवर्ग १६ : १३]

**Combination**

When there is aggravation of *vāyu*, sour variety of *takra* should be taken by adding rock salt. In *pitta*, sweet variety of *takra* should be taken mixed with sugar. In *kapha* the unctuous variety of *takra* should be used by adding alkalies, *śuṇṭhi*, *pippalī* and *marica*. In *mūtrakṛcchra* (dysuria), *guḍa* should be added and in *pāṇḍu citraka* should be added to the *takra*.

'हिंगुजीरयुतं घोलं सैन्धवेनावचूर्णितम्[10] ।
[11]भवेत्तदतिवातघ्नमर्शोतीसारहृत्परम् ॥ ११ ॥'

[भावप्रकाश: तक्रवर्ग १६ : १२]

सरुच्यं पुष्टिदं बल्यं वस्तिशूलविनाशनम् ।

If *hiṅgu* and *jīrā* are added and the powder of rock salt is sprinkled over takra, then it becomes an excellent alleviator of *vāyu*. It also becomes an excellent curative for *arśas* (piles) and *atisāra* (diarrhoea). It is an appetiser, nourishing and strength promoting. It also cures colic pain in the region of *vasti* (urinary bladder).

"तक्रमामं कफं कोष्ठे हन्ति कण्ठे करोति च ॥ १२ ॥
पीनसश्वासकासादौ [12]पक्वमेव विशिष्यते ।

**Process of preparation**

Unboiled (*āma*) *takra* alleviates *kapha* in the *koṣṭha* (colon) but produces *kapha* in the throat. The boiled (*pakva*) *takra* is specifically useful in *pīnasa* (chronic cold), *śvāsa* (asthma) and *kāsa* (bronchitis).

शीतकालेऽग्निमान्द्ये च कफवातामयेषु च ॥ १३ ॥
अरुचौ स्रोतसां रोधे तक्रं स्यादमृतोपमम् ।
[13]तत्तु हन्ति कफच्छर्दिप्रसेकविषमज्वरान् ॥ १४ ॥
पाण्डुमेदो — ग्रहण्यर्शो — मूत्रग्रहभगन्दरान् ।
मेहगुल्ममतीसार शूलप्लीहोदरारुचीः ॥ १५ ॥

[14]
श्वित्रकोठघृतव्यापत्कुष्ठशोफतृषाक्रमीन् ।

**Properties in general**

*Takra* works like ambrosia in winter season, when there is suppression of the power of digestion, in the diseases caused by *kapha* and *vāyu*, in *aruci* (anorexia) and *srotorodha* (obstruction to the channels of circulation). It cures diseases caused by *kapha*, *chardi* (vomiting), *praseka* (salivation), *viṣama jvara* (irregular fever), *pāṇḍu* (anemia), *medas* (adiposity), *grahaṇī* (sprue syndrome), *arśas* (piles), *mūtragraha* (suppression of urination), *bhagandara* (fistula-in-ano), *meha* (obstinate urinary disorders including diabetes), *gulma* (phantom tumour), *atīsāra* (diarrhoea), *śūla* (colic pain), *plīhan* (splenic disorder), *udara* (obstinate abdominal disorders including ascitis), *arucī* (anorexia), *śvitra* (leucoderma), *koṭha* (urticaria), *ghṛta vyāpat* (complications arising out of improper use of ghee), *kuṣṭha* (obstinate skin diseases including leprosy), *śopha* (oedema), *tṛṣā* (morbid thirst) and *kṛmī* (parasitic infection),

नैव तक्रं क्षते दद्यान्नोष्णकाले न दुर्बले ।
[15] [16]
न मूर्च्छाभ्रमदाहेषु न रोगे रक्तपैत्तिके ॥ १६ ॥"

[भावप्रकाशः तक्रवर्ग १६:१४-१८]

**Contra-indication**

*Takra* should not be used in *kṣata* (phthisis), during hot season, when a person is weak and in *mūrchā* (fainting), *bhrama* (giddiness), *dāha* (burning syndrome) and *raktapitta* (a disease characterised by bleeding from different parts of the body).

न तक्रसेवी व्यथते कदाचिन्न तक्रदग्धाः प्रभवन्ति रोगाः ।

यथा सुराणाममृतं सुखाय तथा नराणां भुवि तक्रमाहुः ।

[भावप्रकाशः तक्रवर्ग १६ : ७]

**Excellence**

A person who habitually takes *takra* never suffers and being impregnated with *takra*, diseases do not attack him. As ambrosia gives happiness to the gods, so also *takra* produces happiness in human beings on this earth.

अम्लेन वातं मधुरेण पित्तं
कफं कषायेण निहन्ति तक्रम् ।

तस्मान्न तक्रं ज्वरितेषु देयं
न तक्रदग्धाः प्रभवन्ति रोगाः ॥ १८ ॥

It cures *vāyu* because of its sour taste, *pitta* because of its sweet taste and *kapha* because of its astringent taste. Therefore (?) *takra* should not be given to a patient suffering from fever and being impregnated with *takra*, diseases do not attack him.

॥ इति तक्रवर्गः ॥

Thus ends the group dealing with various types of *takra*.

## NOTES AND REFERENCES

1. लघु कषायाम्लं इति आकरे पाठः ।
2. शोफोदरार्शोग्रहणीदोषमूत्रग्रहारुचीः इति आकरे पाठः ।
3. तत् इति आकरे पाठः ।
4. मतम् इति आकरे पाठः ।
5. गुरु वृष्यमतः इति आकरे पाठः ।
6. सजलं इति षष्ठपुस्तके पाठः ।
7. घोलमुदश्विच्छ्लेष्मलं भवेत् इति आकरे पाठः ।
8. रूक्षाभिष्यन्दि तद्गुणं इति षष्ठपुस्तके पाठः ।
9. सर्वं इति द्वितीयपुस्तके पाठ :
10. सैन्धवे नावधूलितम् इति द्वितीयपुस्तके पाठः ।

11. तद्भवे इति द्वितीयपुस्तके पाठः ।
12. सिद्धमेव तदिष्यते इति प्रथमपुस्तके पाठः ।
13. तक्रं इति षष्ठपुस्तके पाठः ।
14. ०शोथ०……इति षष्ठपुस्तके पाठः ।
15. भ्रमतृष्णासु इति षष्ठपुस्तके पाठः ।
16. रक्तपित्तजे इति आकरे पाठः ।

# CHAPTER 9

नवनीतं हितं गव्यं वृष्यं वर्णबलाग्निकृत् ।
संग्राहि वातपित्तासृक्क्षयार्शो[ऽ]दितकासजित् ॥ १ ॥

*Navanīta* (**Butter**)

Butter (*navanīta*) prepared from cow's milk is very useful. It is aphrodisiac, promoter of complexion, strength and the power of digestion and constipative. It cures aggravated *vāyu*, *pitta* and blood, *kṣaya* (consumption), *arśas* (piles), *ardita* (facial paralysis) and *kāsa* (bronchitis).

तद्धितं बालके वृद्धे विशेषादमृतं शिशोः ।

It is useful both for young and old and it is like ambrosia for infants.

नवनीतं महिष्यास्तु वातश्लेष्मकरं गुरु ॥ २ ॥
दाहपित्तश्रमहरं मेदःशुक्रविवर्द्धनम् ।

*Māhiṣa Navanīta*

The butter collected from buffalo milk aggravates *vāyu*

and *kapha*. It is heavy. It cures *dāha* (burning syndrome), vitiated *pitta* and *śrama* (physical fatigue). It promotes *medas* (adiposity) and semen.

3 क्षीरोत्थं तदतिस्निग्धं चक्षुष्यं रक्तपित्तजित् ।। ३ ।।
4 वृष्यं बलकरं ग्राहि मधुरं शीतलं परम् ।

**Milk butter**

The butter collected from milk is extremely unctuous. It promotes eye sight and cures *rakta pitta* (a disease characterised by bleeding from different parts of the body). It is aphrodisiac, promoter of strength, constipative, sweet and extremely cooling.

नवनीतं तु सद्यस्कं स्वादु ग्राहि हिमं लघु ।। ४ ।।
मेध्यं किञ्चित्कषायाम्लमीषत्तक्रांशसंक्रमात् ।

**Freshly collected butter**

Freshly collected butter is sweet, constipative, cooling, light and promoter of intellect. It is slightly astringent and sour because of its association with a small quantity of butter milk.

5 सक्षारकटुकाम्लत्वाच्छर्द्यर्शःकुष्ठकोपनम् ।
श्लेष्मलं गुरु मेदस्यं नवनीतं चिरन्तनम् ।। ५ ।।

[भावप्रकाशः नवनीतवर्ग १७ १-६]

**Preserved butter**

Butter preserved for a long time is alkaline, pungent and sour because of which it aggravates *chardi* (vomiting), *arśas* (piles) and *kuṣṭha* (obstinate skin diseases including leprosy). It aggravates *kapha*. It is heavy and it produces more of fat.

।। इति नवनीतवर्गः ।।

Thus ends the group dealing with various types of butter.

स्मृति—वुद्धयग्निशुक्रौजः—कफमेदोविवर्धनम् ।
6
वातपित्तकफोन्मादशोषालक्ष्मीविषापहम् ॥ ६ ॥
[माधवद्रव्यगुणः घृतवर्ग ६ : १]
7
"चक्षुष्यं दीपनं बल्यं गव्यं सर्पिर्गुणोत्तरम् ।

**Ghee**
**Cow's milk ghee**

Ghee prepared from cow's milk increases memory, intellect, power of digestion, semen, *ojas*, *kapha* and *medas* (fat). It cures *unmāda* (insanity) caused by *vāyu*, *pitta* and *kapha*, *śoṣa* (consumption), *alakṣmī* (inauspiciousness) and *viṣa* (poisoning). It promotes eyesight, digestive power and strength. Cow's ghee is the best among the ghees.

आजं सर्पिर्दीपनीयं चक्षुष्यं बलवर्द्धनम् ॥ ७ ॥
कासे श्वासे क्षये चापि पथ्यं पाके च तल्लघु ।

**Goat's milk ghee**

Ghee prepared from goat's milk stimulates the digestive power and promotes eyesight and strength. It is useful in *kāsa* (bronchitis), *śvāsa* (asthma) and *kṣaya* (consumption). It is light for digestion.

मधुरं रक्तपित्तघ्नं गुरु पाके कफावहम् ॥ ८ ॥
8
वातपित्तप्रशमनं सुशीतं माहिषं घृतम् ।

**Buffalo milk ghee**

The ghee prepared from buffalo-milk is sweet. It cures *raktapitta* (a disease characterised by bleeding from different parts of the body). It is heavy for digestion. It aggravates *kapha* and alleviates *vāyu* and *pitta*. It is cooling.

'औष्ट्रं कटु घृतं पाके शोथकृमिविषापहम् ॥ ९ ॥
दीपनं कफवातघ्नं कुष्ठगुल्मोदरापहम् ।

### Camel's milk ghee

Ghee prepared from camel's milk is pungent in *vipāka*. It cures *śotha* (oedema), *kṛmi* (parasitic infection) and *viṣa* (poisoning). It stimulates digestion and alleviates *kapha* and *vāyu*. It cures *kuṣṭha* (obstinate skin diseases including leprosy), *gulma* (phantom tumour) and *viṣa* (poisoning).

पाके लघ्वाविकं सर्पिर्न च पित्तप्रकोपणम् ॥ १० ॥'

[भावप्रकाशः घृतवर्ग ६-१०]

9

कफेऽनिले योनिदोषे शोथे कंपे च तद्धितम् ।''

[माधवद्रव्यगुणः घृतवर्ग ६ : ३-७]

### Sheep's milk ghee

Ghee prepared from sheep's milk is light for digestion and it does not aggravate *pitta*. It is useful in aggravated *kapha* and *vāyu*, *yoni doṣa* (diseases of the female genital tract), *śotha* (oedema) and *kampa* (trembling).

10

'पाके लघूष्णवीर्यं च कषायं कफनाशनम् ॥ ११ ॥

11

दीपनं वद्धविण्मूत्रं विद्यादैकशफं घृतम् ।

### Mare's milk ghee

Ghee prepared from mare's milk is light for digestion, hot in potency, astringent, alleviator of *kapha* and stimulant of the digestive power. It obstructs proper elimination of stool and urine.

कषायं बद्धविण्मूत्रं तिक्तमग्निकरं लघु ॥ १२ ॥

हन्ति कारेणवं सर्पिः कफकुष्ठविषक्रमीन् ।

### Elephant's milk ghee

The ghee prepared from elephant's milk is astringent. It obstructs proper elimination of stool and urine. It is bitter, stimulant of digestion and light. It cures aggravated *kapha*, *kuṣṭha* (obstinate skin diseases including leprosy), *viṣa* (poisoning) and *kṛmi* (parasitic infection).

[12]चक्षुष्यमग्र्य **स्त्रीणां च सर्पिः** स्यादमृतोपमम् ॥१३॥

वृद्धिं करोति [13]देहाग्न्योर्लघुपाके विषापहम् ।

**Ghee of woman's milk**

The ghee prepared from woman's milk is an excellent promoter of eyesight. It is like ambrosia. It promotes the physique and the power of digestion. It is light for digestion and it cures *viṣa* (poisoning).

तर्पणं नेत्ररोगघ्नं दाहनुत्पयसो घृतम् ॥ १४ ॥

**Ghee prepared of milk**

The ghee prepared of milk is refreshing. It cures eye diseases and *dāha* (burning syndrome).

**सर्पिः पुराणं** तिमिरं [14]पीनसश्वासकासजित् ।

मूर्च्छाकुष्ठविषोन्माददाहापस्मारनाशनम् ॥ १५ ॥

**योनिकर्णाक्षिशिरसां** [15]शूलं **शोथगरज्वरान्** ।

**हन्ति दोषत्रयं भेदि व्रणशोधनरोपणम्** ॥ १६ ॥

[माधवद्रव्यगुणः घृतवर्ग ९ : ८-१३]

**Preserved ghee**

The ghee which is kept preserved for a long time (*purāṇa*) cures *timira* (cataract), *pīnasa* (chronic cold), *śvāsa* (asthma), *kāsa* (bronchitis), *mūrchā* (fainting), *kuṣṭha* (obstinate skin diseases including leprosy), *viṣa* (poisoning), *unmāda* (insanity), *dāha* (burning syndrome), *apasmāra* (epilepsy), colic pain in *yoni* (female genital tract), ear, eye and head, *śotha* (oedema), *gara* (a type of poisoning) and fever. It alleviates all the three *doṣas*. It is purgative. It cleanses and heals ulcers.

**घृतमण्डो** घृतस्योर्ध्वभागः स्यात्सुश्रुतस्य यः ।

'तद्वच्च घतमण्डोऽपि रूक्षस्तीक्ष्णस्तनुस्तु सः ॥ १७ ॥'

[माधवद्रव्यगुणः घृतवर्ग १८ : १३]

*Ghṛta maṇḍa*

The upper portion of the ghee is called *ghṛta maṇḍa* according to *Suśruta*. It is un-unctuous, sharp and thin.

16 यो गो दोहाद्भवं सर्पिर्भवेद्धैयङ्**गवीनकम्** ।

हैयङ्गवीनं चक्षुष्यं दीपनं रोचनं परम् ॥ १८ ॥'

[भावप्रकाशः घृतवर्ग १८ : १५]

*Hayaṁgavīna*

The ghee that is taken out from the cream produced at the time of milking the cow is called *hayaṁgavīna*. It promotes eyesight and the power of digestion. It is digestive stimulant and appetiser par excellence.

बल्यं वृष्यं निगदितं विशेषाज्ज्वरनाशनम् ।

सर्पिः पुराणं विज्ञेयं दशवर्षस्थितं तु यत् ॥ १९ ॥

**Preservation**

The ghee which is preserved for ten years is strength promoting and aphrodisiac. It specifically cures fever.

दशसम्वत्सराद्दूर्ध्व**माज्य**मुक्तं रसायनम् ।

The ghee which is preserved for more than ten years is called *ājya*. It is rejuvenating.

शतवर्षस्थितं यत्तु **कुंभसर्पि**स्तदुच्यते ॥ २० ॥

रक्षोघ्नं कुम्भसर्पिः स्यात्तत्परस्तु **महाघृतम्** ।

पेयं महाघृतं भूतैः सर्वतोऽपि गुणाधिकम् ॥ २१ ॥

The ghee which is preserved for one hundred years is

called *kumbha sarpi*. It cures the afflictions by *rakṣas* (evil spirits). The ghee which is preserved for more than one hundred years is called *mahāghṛta*. It is the best among all the ghees.

यथा यथा जरां याति गुणवत्स्यात्तथा तथा ।

Depending upon the duration of preservation, the ghee becomes progressively more and more useful.

राजयक्ष्मणि वाले च वृद्धे श्लेष्माश्रये गदे ।। २२ ।।

रोगे सामे विसूच्यां च विबन्धे च मदात्यये ।

ज्वरे च शमिते वह्नौ न सर्पिर्बहुमन्यते ।। २३ ।।

**Contra-indication**

Ghee is not very useful in *rāja yakṣmā* (tuberculosis), young age, old age, in diseases caused by *kapha*, in the *āma* stage of diseases, *visūcikā* (cholera), constipation, *madātyaya* (alcoholism), fever and in the suppression of the power of digestion.

।। इति घृतवर्गः ।।

Thus ends the group dealing with various type of ghee.

## NOTES AND REFERENCES

1. क्षयार्शोऽर्दिकासहृत् इति आकरे पाठः ।
   क्षयार्शोर्दितकासजित् इति आदर्शपुस्तकेषु पाठः ।
2. वातश्लेष्महरं इति षष्ठपुस्तके पाठः ।
3. दुग्धोत्थं नवनीतं तु चक्षुष्यं रक्तपित्तनुत् इति आकरे पाठः ।
4. वृष्यं बल्यमतिस्निग्धं मधुरं ग्राहि शीतलम् इति आकरे पाठः ।
5. सक्षारकटुलाम्लत्वाच्छर्द्यर्शःकुष्ठकारकम् इति आकरे पाठः ।

6. लक्ष्मीज्वरापहम् इति आकरे पाठः ।
7. बृंहणं इति आकरे पाठः ।
8. सुश्रुतं इति आदर्शपुस्तिकासु पाठः ।
9. शोफे इति आकरे पाठः ।
10. तु इति आकरे पाठः ।
11. लघु इति षष्ठपुस्तके पाठः ।
12. चक्षुष्यमग्र्यं इति आदर्शपुस्तिकासु पाठः ।
13. देहास्य लघु पाकि इति षष्ठपुस्तके पाठः ।
14. तिमिरप्रतिश्याश्वासकासनुत् इति आकरे पाठः ।
15. शूलघ्नं शोकजित् परम् इति आकरे पाठः ।
16. हयो इति षष्ठपुस्तके पाठः ।

# CHAPTER 10

'कषायानुरसं स्वादु सूक्ष्ममुष्णं व्यवायि च ।

पित्तलं बद्धविण्मूत्रं न च श्लेष्मविवर्धनम् ॥ १ ॥'

[माधवद्रव्यगुणः तैलवर्ग १० : १]

'तैलं संयोगसंस्कारात्सर्वरोगहर[1] सरम् ।

## Oil

Oil is astringent in *anurasa* (subsidiary taste), sweet, subtle; hot and *vyavāyi* (which pervades all over the body before digestion). It aggravates *pitta*. It obstructs the proper elimination of stool and urine. It does not aggravate *kapha*. By combination and processing it cures all diseases. It is laxative.

छिन्नभिन्नच्युतोत्पिष्टमथितक्षतपिच्चिते ॥ २ ॥

भग्नस्फुटितविद्धाग्निदग्ध[2]श्लिष्टविदारिते ।

[3]तथाभिहतनिर्भुग्नमृगव्यालादिभक्षिते ॥ ३ ॥

सेकाभ्यंगावगाहेषु तिलतैलं प्रशस्यते ।

तथा[4] वस्तिषु पानेषु नस्ये कर्णाक्षिपूरणे ।। ४ ।।

अन्नपानविधौ चापि प्रयोज्यं वातशान्तये ।

*Tila taila* **(Gingili oil)**

*Til* oil is useful in excised, incised, dislocated, macerated, lacerated, ulcerated, pressed, fractured, broken, perforated, burnt, separated and scraped wounds and injury and eating away by wild animals. It is used in the form of *seka* (sprinkling), *abhyaṅga* (massage), *avagāha* (bath), *vasti* (enema), *pāna* (drinking through mouth), *nasya* (inhalation), *karṇapūraṇa* (ear drop) and *akṣipūraṇa* (pouring over eyes). It is used in food and drinks for the alleviation of *vāyu*.

वातघ्नं मधुरं तेषु **क्षौमं तैलं** बलावहम् ।। ५ ।।

कटुपाकमचक्षुष्यं स्निग्धोष्णं कटुपित्तलम् ।

*Kṣauma taila* **(Linseed oil)**

The oil of *kṣauma* alleviates *vāyu*. It is sweet and a promoter of strength. It is pungent in *vipāka*. It is not useful for eyes. It is unctuous, hot and pungent. It aggravates *pitta*.

कृमिघ्नं **सार्षपं तैलं** कंडूकुष्ठापहं लघु ।। ६ ।।

कफमेदोऽनिलहरं लेखनं कटु दीपनम् ।

*Sārṣapa taila* **(Mustard oil)**

The oil of *sarṣapa* cures *kṛmi* (parasitic infection), *kaṇḍū* (itching) and *kuṣṭha* (obstinate skin diseases including leprosy). It is light and reduces *kapha*, *medas* (fat) and *vāyu*. It is *lekhana* (depleting), pungent and a digestive stimulant.

हृद्बस्तिपार्श्वजानूरुकटि[5]पृष्ठास्थिशूलिनाम् ।। ७ ।।

आनाहाष्ठील[6]वातासृक्प्लीहोदावर्त्त[7] शूलिनाम् ।

हितं वातामयश्वास[8]ग्रन्थिहिध्मविकारिणाम् ।। ८ ।।

तैलमेरण्डजं बल्यं गुरूष्णं मधुरं सरम् ।

### *Eraṇḍa taila* (Castor oil)

The oil of *eraṇḍa* is useful in the pain of the heart, bladder, sides of the chest, knee joint, thigh, waist, back and bone. It is also useful in *ānāha* (flatulence), *aṣṭhīlā* (hard tumour in the abdomen), *vātāsṛk* (gout), *plīhan* (splenic disorder) *udāvarta* (tymphanitis), *śūla* (colic pain), diseases caused by *vāyu*, *śvāsa* (asthma), *granthi* (adenitis) and *hidhmā* (hic cup). It is strength promoting, heavy, hot, sweet and laxative.

तीक्ष्णोष्णं पित्तलं[9] विस्रं रक्तैरण्डोद्भवं भृशम् ॥ ९ ॥

The oil of the red variety of *eraṇḍa* is exceedingly sharp and hot. It strongly aggravates *pitta* and is extremely putrid.

कुसुम्भतैलमुष्णं च विपाके कटुकं गुरु ।
विदाही तु[10] विशेषेण सर्वदोषप्रकोपणम्[11] ॥ १० ॥

### *Kusumbha taila*

The oil of *kusumbha* is hot, pungent in *vipāka*, heavy and *vidāhī* (producing burning sensation). It specifically aggravates all the *doṣas*.

सरं कोशाम्रजं तैलं क्रिमिकुष्ठव्रणापहम् ।

### *Kośāmra taila*

The oil of *kośāmra* is laxative. It cures *kṛmi* (parasitic infection), *kuṣṭha* (obstinate skin diseases including leprosy) and *vraṇa* (ulcer).

दन्तीमूलकरक्षोघ्नकरञ्जारिष्टशिग्रुजम् ॥ ११ ॥
सुवर्चले[12]ङ्गुदीपीलुशंखिनीनीपसंभवम् ।
सरलागुरुदेवाह्वशिंशपासारजन्म च ॥ १२ ॥
तुवरारुष्करोत्थं च नीक्ष्णं कट्वम्लपित्तजित्[13] ।

अर्शः कुष्ठकृमिश्लेष्मशुक्रमेदोऽनिलापहम् ॥ १३ ॥

*Taila* of *Danti* etc.,

The oils of *dantī*, *mūlaka*, *rakṣoghna*, *karañja*, *ariṣṭa*, *sigru*, *suvarcalā*, *iṅgudī*, *pīlu*, *śaṁkhinī*, *nīpa*, heart wood of *sarala*, *aguru*, *devāhva* and *śiṁśapā*, *tuvara* and *āruṣkara* are sharp, pungent and sour. They alleviate *pitta* and cure *arśas* (piles), *kuṣṭha* (obstinate skin diseases including leprosy) and *kṛmi* (parasitic infection). They reduce *kapha*, semen, fat and *vāyu*.

**करंजारिष्टजे**[14] तिक्ते नात्युष्णे तत्र निर्दिशेत् ।
कषायतिक्तकटुकं सरलं[15] व्रणशोधनम् ॥ १४ ॥

Of these, the oils of *karañja* and *ariṣṭa* are bitter and they are not very hot. The oil of *sarala* is astringent, bitter and pungent and it cleanses ulcer.

[16]भृशोष्णतीक्ष्णकटुके तुवरारुष्करोद्भवे ।
विशेषात्कृमिकुष्ठघ्ने तथोर्ध्वाधोविरेचने ॥ १५ ॥

[माधवद्रव्यगुणः तैलवर्ग १० : १-१६]

Oils of *tuvara* and *āruṣkara* are exceedingly hot, sharp and pungent. They specifically cure *kṛmi* (parasitic infection) and *kuṣṭha* (obstinate skin diseases including leprosy). They are emetic and purgative.

सर **ज्योतिष्मतीतैलं** वातश्लेष्मशिरोर्तिनुत् ।

*Jyotiṣmatī taila*

The oil of *jyotiṣmatī* is laxative. It alleviates *vāta*, *kapha* and headache.

**अक्षातिमुक्तकाक्षोटनालिकेलमधूकजम्**[17] ॥ १६ ॥

18

**त्रपुसैर्वारु — कुष्माण्डश्लेष्मातकपियालजं ।**

वातपित्तहरं केश्यं श्लेष्मलं गुरु शीतलम् ॥ १७ ॥

### *Taila* of *Akṣa* etc.

The oil of *akṣa*, *atimukta*, *akṣoṭa*, *nālikela*, *madhūka*, *trapusa*, *ervāru*, *kuṣmāṇḍa*, *śleṣmātaka* and *piyāla* alleviates *vāyu* and *pitta*. It promotes good hair and aggravates *kapha*. It is heavy and cooling.

19

पित्तश्लेष्मप्रशमनं **श्रीपर्णकिंशुकोद्भवम्** ।

दोषघ्नं दीपनं मेध्यं किञ्चित्तिक्तं रसायनम् ॥ १८ ॥

[माधवद्रव्यगुण : तैलवर्ग १० : १६-१८]

### *Taila* of *Śrīparṇa* & *Kiṁśuka*

The oil of *śrīparṇa* and *kiṁśuka* alleviates *pitta* and *kapha*. It is *doṣaghna* (correcting morbid factors) and digestive stimulant. It promotes intellect. It is slightly bitter and rejuvenating.

**श्लेष्मातकाक्षपिचुमंदककाकिनीनां,**

**काश्मर्यकस्य** यदि वापि **हरीतकीनाम्** ॥ १९ ॥

तैलं निहन्ति पलितान्युपयुज्य **नस्ये** ।

गोक्षीरभोज्यनिरतस्य सदैव पुंसः ॥ २० ॥

### *Taila* of *Śleśmātaka* etc.

The oil of *śleṣmātaka*, *akṣa*, *picumandaka*, *kākini*, *kāṣmaryaka* and *harītakī* cures premature graying of hair when used for inhalation. For this purpose, patients should constantly use cow's milk as their food.

20

**'यवतिक्ताभवं** तैलं स्वादुपाकं विलेखनम् ।

कफवातहरं रूक्षं कषायं नातिपित्तकृत् ॥ २१ ॥

### *Taila* of *Yavatiktā*

The oil of *yavatiktā* is sweet in *vipāka* and depleting. It alleviates *kapha* and *vāta*. It is un-unctuous and astringent. It does not aggravate *pitta* in excess.

[21] सहकारभवं तैलं तिक्तं सुरभिरोचनम् ।

### *Taila* of *Sahakāra*

The oil of *sahakāra* is bitter, fragrant and an appetiser.

फलोद्भवानि तैलानि [22] यान्युक्तानीह कानिचित् ।

गुणान्कर्म च विज्ञाय [23] फलानां च विनिर्दिशेत् ॥ २२ ॥

[माधवद्रव्यगुणः तैलवर्ग १०:१६-२१]

### *Taila* of other fruits

The oil extracted from other fruits which are described elsewhere in this text shares the properties of fruits from which it is extracted.

तैलं सर्जरसोद्भूतं विस्फोटव्रणनाशनम् ।

कुष्ठपामाकृमिहरं वातश्लेष्मामयापहम् ॥ २३ ॥

### *Taila* prepared of *Śarjarasa*

The oil prepared of *sarjaraṣa* cures *visphoṭa* (pustular eruptions), *vraṇa* (ulcer), *kuṣṭha* (obstinate skin diseases including leprosy), *pāmā* (itching), *kṛmi* (parasitic infection) and diseases caused by *vāyu* and *kapha*.

तैलं स्वयोनिवत्सर्वं कीर्तितं वाग्भटेन यत् ।

ततः शेषस्य बोद्धव्या योनेरेव गुणा जनैः ॥ २४ ॥

'यावन्तः स्थावराः स्नेहाः समासात्परिकीर्तिताः ।

24
सर्वे तैलगुणा ज्ञेया सर्वेष्यनिलनाशनाः ॥ २५ ॥
[माधवद्रव्यगुणः तैलवर्ग १०:२१-२२]

**Miscellaneous**

*Vāgbhaṭa* has stated that the oil shares the properties of the source plant from which it is extracted. Following this principle, the properties of the remaining types of oil should be determined.

वसा मज्जा च वातघ्नौ बलपित्तकफप्रदौ ।

मांसानुगस्वरूपौ च विद्यान्मेदोऽपि ताविव ॥ २६ ॥

**Muscle fat and Bone marrow**

*Vasā* (muscle fat) and *majjā* (bone marrow) alleviate *vāta* and increase strength, *pitta* as well as *kapha*. They share the properties of the meat of the respective animals. *Medas* (fat) has also similar properties.

औलूकी सौकरी वा च हंसजा कुक्कुटोद्भवा ।

वसा श्रेष्ठा स्ववर्गेषु कुंभीरमहिषोद्भवा ॥ २७ ॥

काकमृगवसा तद्वत्कारण्डोत्था च निन्दिता ।

The *vasā* (muscle fat) of *ulluka*, *sukara*, *haṁsa*, *kukkuṭa*, *kumbhīra*, *mahiṣa*, *kāka* and *mṛga* is the best among their respective groups. The *vasā* (muscle fat) of *kāraṇḍa* is not useful.

सुस्वादु मेदश्छागं तु हास्तिकं तु वराद्वरम् ॥ २८ ॥

The *medas* (fat) of goat is delicious and that of the elephant is exceedingly useful.

मधुरौ बृंहणौ वृष्यौ बल्यौ मज्जा तथा वसा ।

यथा सत्त्वं तु शैत्योष्णैर्वसामज्जा विनिर्दिशेत् ॥ २९ ॥

**Property**

Both *vasā* (muscle fat) and *majjā* (bone marrow) are

sweet, nourishing, aphrodisiac and strength promoting. The potency, viz., hot and cold of *vasā* and *majjā* should be determined on the basis of the nature of the animal from which they are collected.

'घृतमब्दात्परं[25] पक्वं हीनवीर्यं प्रजायते ।
तैलं पक्वमपक्वं वा चिरस्थायि गुणाधिकम् ॥ ३० ॥'

[माधवद्रव्यगुणः तैलवर्ग २३]

**Miscellaneous**

Boiled ghee loses its potency after one year. But oil whether boiled or not maintains its potency for ever and therefore it is better.

॥ इति तैलवर्गः ॥

Thus ends the group dealing with various types of oils etc.

## NOTES AND REFERENCES

1. संयोगसंस्कारात्सर्वरोगापहं मतम् इति आकरे पाठः ।
2. भग्नस्फुटितविद्धाग्निदग्धविश्लिष्टदारिते इति आकरे पाठः ।
3. तथाभिहतनिर्भुग्ने मृगव्यालादिभक्षिते इति आकरे पाठः ।
4. तद्बस्तिषु च इति आकरे पाठः ।
5. हृद्बस्तिपार्श्वजानूरुत्रिकपृष्ठास्थिशूलिनाम् इति आकरे पाठः ।
6. आनाप्तष्ठीलपित्तासृक् इति आकरे पाठः ।
7. प्लीहोदावर्त्तशूलिनाम् इति आकरे पाठः ।
8. वातामयश्वासग्रन्थिवर्त्मविकारिणाम् इति आकरे पाठः ।
9. पिच्छिलं इति आकरे पाठः ।
10. च इति आकरे पाठः ।

11. सर्वरोगप्रकोपणम् इति आकरे पाठः ।
    सर्वरोगहरं परं इति षष्ठपुस्तके पाठः ।
12. सौवर्चलेङ्गुदीपीलु इति आकरे पाठः ।
13. कंड्वस्रपित्तकृत् इति आकरे पाठः ।
14. तापोष्णे इति द्वितीयपुस्तके पाठः ।
15. सारलं इति आकरे पाठः ।
16. भृशोष्णं कटुतीक्ष्णे च इति पाठः ।
17. अक्षातिमुक्तकाक्षोडनालिकेरमधूकजम् इति आकरे पाठः ।
18. पियज्जलम् इति द्वितीयपुस्तके पाठः ।
19. श्रीपर्णीकिंशुकोद्भवम् इति आकरे पाठः ।
20. स्वादु पाके विरेचनम् इति आकरे पाठः ।
21. सतिक्तं सहकारस्य तैलं सुरभि रोचनम् इति आकरे पाठः ।
22. तानि च इति आकरे पाठः ।
23. फलानीव विनिर्दिशेत् इति आकरे पाठः ।
24. सर्वे चानिलनाशनाः इति आकरे पाठः ।
25. घृतमद्वाद्वात्परं इति द्वितीयषष्ठपुस्तकयोः पाठः ।

# CHAPTER 11

‘दीपनं रोचनं **मद्यं** तीक्ष्णोष्णं [1] तुष्टिपुष्टिदम् ।
सुस्वादुतिक्तकटुकमम्लपाकरसं सरम् ॥ १ ॥
सकषायं स्वरारोग्यप्रतिभावर्णकृल्लघु ।
नष्टनिद्रातिनिद्रेभ्यो हितं पित्तास्रदूषणम् ॥ २ ॥
कृशस्थूलहितं रूक्षं सूक्ष्मं स्रोतोविशोधनम् ।
वातश्लेष्महरं युक्त्या पीतं विषवदन्यथा ॥ ३ ॥

[माधवद्रव्यगुणः मद्यवर्ग १२:१-३]

### *Madya* (Alcoholic drinks)

Alcoholic drink (*madya*) is a digestive stimulant, appetiser, sharp, *uṣṇa*, refreshing, nourishing, sweet, *tikta*, pungent, sour in *vipāka* and taste, laxative and astringent. It promotes good voice, health, intuition (*pratibhā*) and complexion. It is light. It is useful for persons who do not get sleep and also for persons who get sleep in excess. It vitiates *pitta* and blood. It is useful for both emaciated and corpulent persons. It is un-unctuous and subtle. It cleanes the channels of circulation. It alleviates *vāyu* and *kapha*. All the above mentioned properties are manifested when alcohol is taken only in appropriate dose. Otherwise it works like a poison.

यदपक्वौषधाम्बुभ्यां सिद्धं मद्यं स आसवः ।

अरिष्टः क्वाथसाध्यः स्यात्तयोर्मानं पलोन्मितम् ॥४॥

*Āsava & Ariṣṭa*

The alcoholic drink prepared of unboiled drugs and water is called *āsava*. *Ariṣṭa* is prepared of decoctions and the dose of both the *āsava* and *ariṣṭa* is one *pala* (48 ml approx.).

आसवादधिकोऽरिष्टो गुणैः पाकेन लाघवात् ।

बीजद्रव्येण विज्ञेया आसवारिष्टयोर्गुणाः ॥ ५ ॥

*Ariṣṭa* is better than *āsava* because the former is light because of boiling. Their properties are determined on the basis of the property of drugs used in their preparation.

'शालिषष्टिकपिष्टादिकृतं मद्यं सुरा[2] मता ।

*Surā*

The alcoholic drink prepared of the paste of *śāli* and *ṣaṣṭika* types of rice is called *surā*.

सुरा[3] गुर्वी बलस्तम्भपुष्टिमेदःकफप्रदा ॥ 6 ॥'

ग्राहिणी शोफगुल्मार्शोग्रहणी[4]मूत्रकृच्छ्रनुत् ।

*Surā* in heavy. It promotes strength, power of retention (*stambha*), plumpness, *medas* (fat) and *kapha*. It is constipative. It cures *śopha* (oedema), *gulma* (phantom tumour), *arśas* (piles), *grahaṇī* (sprue syndrome) and *mūtrakṛcchra* (dysuria).

पुनर्नवा[5]शालिपिष्टैर्विहिता वारुणी मता ॥ ७ ॥

[6]यत्तालखर्जूररसैः सहिता सापि वारुणी ।

### *Vāruṇī*

The alcoholic drink prepared of the paste of *punarnavā* and *śāli* is called *vāruṇī*. It is also prepared of the juice of *tāla* and *kharjūra*.

सुरावद्वारुणी लघ्वी पीनसाध्मानशूलनुत् ॥ ८ ॥'

[भावप्रकाशः सन्धानवर्ग ११ : २३-२४]

*Vāruṇī* shares the properties of *surā*. However, it is light and it cures *pīnasa* (chronic cold), *ādhmāna* (flatulence) and *śūla* (colic pain).

**प्रसन्ना** स्यात्सुरामण्डस्ततः **कादम्बरी** घना ।

जगलस्तदधः प्रोक्तो **मेदको** जगलादधः ॥ ९ ॥

**Different parts**

The upper portion of *surā* (which is very thin) is called *prasannā*. The portion below that which is more dense is called *kādambarī*. The portion below that is called *jagala*. The *surā* which is at the bottom of the container is called *medaka*.

सद्यो गृहीत सारो यः कल्को ज्ञेयः स **वक्कसः** ।

**किण्वं** स्यान्मदिराबीजमसंजातं मधूलकम् ॥ १० ॥

The fermenting material from where alcohol has been taken out is called *vakkasa*. The material that is used for initiating fermentation of alcoholic drinks is called *kiṇva*. If *kiṇva* is not matured then it is called *madhūlaka*.

**प्रसन्ना**नाहगुल्मार्शः — छर्द्यरोचकवातनुत् ।

### *Prasannā*

*Prasannā* cures *ānāha* (flatulence), *gulma* (phantom tumour), *arśas* (piles), *chardi* (vomiting), *arocaka* (anorexia) and aggravated *vāyu*.

दीपन्याध्मानहृत्कुक्षितोदशूलप्रणाशिनी ॥ ११ ॥

कादंबरी गुरुर्वृष्या दीपनी वातहृत्सरा ।

*Kādambarī*

*Kādambarī* type of alcoholic drink is a digestive stimulant. It cures *ānāha* (flatulence), pain in the heart and pelvic region and colic pain. It is heavy, aphrodisiac, alleviator of *vāyu* and laxative.

जगलः कफनुद्ग्राही शोफार्शोग्रहणीहरः ॥ १२ ॥

रूक्षोष्णः पाचनो बल्यः क्षुत्तृष्णारुचिनाशनः ।

*Jagala*

*Jagala* alleviates *kapha*. It is constipative. It cures *śopha* (oedema), *arśas* (piles) and *grahaṇī* (sprue syndrome). It is ununctuous, hot, carminative and strength promoting. It cures *kṣut* (morbid hunger), *tṛṣṇā* (morbid thirst) and *aruci* (anorexia).

मेदको मधुरो बल्यः स्तम्भनः शीतलो गुरुः ॥ १३ ॥

*Medaka*

*Medaka* is sweet, strength promoting, *stambhana* (which increases the power of retention), cooling and heavy.

'[8]बक्कसो हृतसारत्वाद् विष्टंभी [9]वातकोपनः ।

[माधवद्रव्यगुणः मद्यवर्ग १२:६]

*Vakkasa*

*Vakkasa* from which alcohol is taken out is constipative and it aggravates *vāyu.*

किण्वकं वातशमनमहृद्यं दुर्जरं गुरुः ॥ १४ ॥

*Kiṇvaka*

*Kiṇvaka* alleviates *vāyu*. It is not good for heart. It is difficult of digestion and heavy.

10

मधूलकं कफकरं स्निग्धं विष्टम्भिदुर्जरम् ।

*Madhūlaka*

*Madhūlaka* aggravates *kapha.* It is unctuous, constipative and difficult of digestion.

मृद्वीकाभिः कृतं मद्यं **मार्द्वीकं कापिशं** च तत् ॥ १५ ॥

कापिशं मदिरा श्रेष्ठं स्निग्धं स्वादुसरं लघु ।

रोचनं पाचनं हृद्यं बृंहणं बलवीर्यदम् ॥ १६ ॥

अल्पपित्तानिलकरमविदाहि कफापहम् ।

पाण्डुताक्षयमेहार्शो विषमज्वरनाशनम् ॥ १७ ॥

*Mārdvīka*

The alcoholic drink prepared of grapes is called *mārdvīka* or *kāpiśa.* It is the best among the alcoholic drinks. It is unctuous, sweet, laxative, light, appetiser, carminative, cardiac tonic and nourishing. It promotes strength and semen. It causes *amlapitta* (acidity in stomach) and aggravation of *vāyu.* It does not cause burning sensation and it alleviates *kapha.* It cures *pāṇḍu* (anemia), *kṣaya* (consumption), *meha* (obstinate urinary disorders including diabetes), *arśas* (piles) and *viṣama jvara* (irregular fever).

"तस्मादल्पान्तरगुणं **खार्जूरं** वातलं गुरु ।

हृद्यं कषायमधुरं सुगन्धेन्द्रियबोधनम् ॥ १८ ॥"

[माधवद्रव्यगुणः मद्यवर्ग १२ : ११]

*Khārjūra madya*

The alcoholic drink prepared of *kharjūra* is slightly inferior in quality in comparison to the *mārdvīka* type of alcohic drink. It aggravates *vāyu* and is heavy. It is a cardiac tonic, astringent, sweet and fragrant. It activates the senses (*indriya bodhana*).

धातक्यम्बुगुडैर्गौडो[11] भिषग्भिः परिकीर्तितः ।
गौडोऽग्निवर्धनो[12] वर्णबलकृत्तर्पणः कटुः ॥ १६ ॥

तिक्तको बृंहणः स्वादुः सृष्टविण्मूत्रमारुतः ।

*Gauḍa madya*

The alcoholic drink prepared of *dhātakī*, water and *guḍa* is called by physicians "*gauḍa*". It promotes the power of digestion, complexion and strength. It is refreshing, pungent, bitter, nourishing and sweet. It promotes the elimination of stool, urine and flatus.

मधूककुसुमैर्मद्यं माधूकमिति कथ्यते ॥ २० ॥

वातपित्तकरं रूक्षं माधूकं परिकीर्तितम ।

*Mādhūka madya*

The alcoholic drink prepared of the flower of *madhūka* is called *mādhūka*. It aggravates *vāyu* and *pitta*. It is ununctuous.

'इक्षोः[13] पक्वैरसैः सिद्धः सीधुः[14] पक्वरसश्च सः ॥२१॥
आमैस्तैरेव[15] विहितः स च शीतरसो[16] भवेत् ।

*Sidhu*

The alcoholic drink prepared of boiled sugar cane juice is called *pakvarasa sidhu*. If unboiled sugar cane juice is used in the preparation, then it is called *śīta rasa*.

सीधुः पक्वरसः श्रेष्ठः स्वराग्निबलवर्णकृत् ॥ २२ ॥
वातपित्तकरो हृद्यः[17] स्नेहनो[18] रोचनो जयेत् ।
विबन्धमेदो[19] — शोफार्शः — श्वासोदरकफामयान्[20] ।

*Pakvarasa* type of *sidhu* is the better of the two. It promotes good voice, digestive power, strength and complexion. It aggravates *vāyu* and *pitta*. It is a cardiac tonic, unctuous and an appetiser. It cures *vibandha* (constipation), *medas* (adiposity), *śopha* (oedema), *arśas* (piles), *śvāsa* (asthma), *udara* (obstinate abdominal diseases including ascitis) and diseases caused by *kapha*.

तस्मादल्पगुणः शीतरसः संलेखनः स्मृतः ॥ २३ ॥

[भावप्रकाशः सन्धानवर्ग २१ : २५-२७]

*Śītarasa* type of *sidhu* is slightly inferior in quality. It is known for its depleting action.

'**शार्करो** मधुरो हृद्यो दीपनो बस्तिशोधनः ।

वातघ्नो मधुरः पाके रुच्य इन्द्रियबोधनः ॥ २४ ॥'

[माधवद्रव्यगणः मद्यवर्ग १२ : १३]

*Śārkara*

*Śārkara* type of alcoholic drink is sweet, cardiac tonic and digestive stimulant. It cleanses the urinary bladder and alleviates *vāyu*. It is sweet in *vipāka*, appetiser and stimulant of senses (*indriya bodhana*).

'छेदी **मध्वासवस्ती**क्ष्णो मेहपीनसकासजित् ।'

[माधवद्रव्यगुणः मद्यवर्ग १२ : १६]

*Madhvāsava*

*Madhvāsava* in *chedi* (which takes away tissues by cutting) and sharp. It cures *meha* (obstinate urinary disorders including diabetes), *pīnasa* (chronic rhinitis) and *kāsa* (bronchitis).

[21] **आक्षिकः** पाण्डुरोगघ्नो बल्यः संग्राहिको लघु ॥ २५ ॥

कषायो मधुरः शीतः पित्तघ्नो[22]ऽसृक्प्रसादनः ।

---

*Ākṣika*

*Ākṣika* type of alcoholic drink cures *pāṇḍu* (anemia). It

is a promoter of strength, constipative, light, astringent, sweet and cooling. It alleviates *pitta* and promotes blood formation.

**जाम्बवो**[23] बद्धनिष्यंदो तौवरो वातकोपनः ।
तीक्ष्णः कषायो मदकृत् दुर्नामकफगुल्मनुत् ॥ २६ ॥'

[माधवद्रव्यगुणः मद्यवर्ग १२ : १७-१८]

### *Jāmbava* & *Tauvara*

*Jāmbava* type of alcoholic drink helps in the prevention of excretion (*baddha niṣyanda*).

*Tauvara* aggravates *vāyu*. It is sharp, astringent and intoxicating. It cures *durnāma* (piles), aggravated *kapha* and *gulma* (phantom tumour).

'निर्दिशेद् द्रव्यतश्चान्यान् कंदमूलफलासवान् ।'

[माधवद्रव्यगुणः मद्यवर्ग १२ : २१]

'अरिष्टासवसीधूनां गुणान् कर्माणि चादिशेत् ।
बुद्ध्या[24] यथास्वसंस्कारमवेक्ष्य कुशलो भिषक् ॥ २७ ॥'

[माधवद्रव्यगुणः मद्यवर्ग १२ : २३-२४]

**Miscellaneous**

Many other types of alcoholic drinks viz., *āsavas*, *ariṣṭas* and *sīdhus* are prepared from rhizomes, roots and fruits of different plants. Their properties should be determined by an expert physician on the basis of the properties of their ingredients and the pharmaceutical processes followed in their preparation.

पिप्पल्यादि कृतो गुल्मकफरोगहरो भवेत् ।

The alcoholic drink prepared from *pippalī* etc., cures *gulma* (phantom tumour) and diseases caused by *kapha*.

चिकित्सितेषु वक्ष्यन्तेऽरिष्टा रोगहराः पृथक् ॥ २८ ॥

In a separate section on the "treatment of diseases"

*ariṣṭas* which cure different ailments will be described.

नवं मद्यमभिष्यन्दि त्रिदोषशमनं सरम् ।

25

अहृद्यं विरसं दाही दुर्गन्धं विशदं गुरु ॥ २९ ॥

**Fresh and Preserved wines**

Freshly prepared alcoholic drinks are *abhiṣyandi* (which obstructs channels of circulation). It alleviates all the three *doṣas* and is a laxative. It is not a cardiac tonic and is not tasteful (*virasa*). It causes burning sensation and produces putrid smell. It is *viśada* (non-slimy) and heavy.

'जीर्णं तदेव रोचिष्णुः क्रिमिश्लेष्मानिलापहम् ।

हृद्यं सुगन्धिगुणवल्लघु स्रोतोविशोधनम् ॥ ३० ॥'

[भावप्रकाशः सन्धानवर्ग २१ : ३१]

The same alcoholic drink, when preserved for a long time and used, is relishing. It cures *kṛmi* (parasitic infection) and aggravation of *kapha* as well as *vāyu*. It is cardiac tonic, fragrant, endowed with good qualities and light. It cleanses the channels of circulation.

व्यक्तं पञ्चरसं शुद्धं गंधयुक्तं गुणावहम् ।

**Good and bad quality**

The alcoholic drink in which five tastes are manifested, which is pure and which is endowed with good smell is of a good quality.

त्याज्यं विदाहि दुर्गन्धि विरसं क्रिमिलं घनम् ॥ ३१ ॥

The alcoholic drink which causes burning sensation, which is putrid in smell, which is of bad taste, which contains *kṛmis* (maggots) and which is thick should be rejected.

'सात्त्विके गीतहास्यादि राजसे साहसादिकम् ।

26

तामसे निन्द्यकर्माणि निद्रां च कुरुते मदः ॥ ३२ ॥

**Action on different types of individuals**

Alcoholic drink makes a person of *sāttvika* type to sing and laugh. In a *rājasika* type of person it promotes strength. In *tāmasika* type of persons it produces despisable acts and they get sleep after taking alcoholic drinks.

विधिना मात्रया काले हितैरन्नैर्यथाबलम् ।
27
प्रहृष्टो यः पिवेन्मद्य तस्य स्यादमृतोपमम् ॥ ३३ ॥

**Proper method of drinking**

An alcoholic drink, taken according to the prescribed procedure, in proper doses, at the proper time, along with wholesome food, according to the capacity of the individual and in an exhilerating mood produces effects like ambrosia.

किन्तु मद्यं स्वाभावेन यथैवान्नं तथा स्मृतम् ।
अयुक्तियुक्तं रोगाय युक्तियुक्तं यथाऽमृतम् ॥ ३४ ॥

[भावप्रकाशः सन्धानवर्ग २१ : ३२-३८]

By nature, an alcoholic drink is like a food. When used inappropriately, it causes diseases and in appropriate circumstances it works like ambrosia.

प्राणाः प्राणभृतामन्नं तदयुक्त्या निहन्त्यसून् ।
विषं प्राणहरं तच्च युक्तियुक्तं रसायनम् ॥ ३५ ॥

Food, when taken appropriately, gives life and it takes away life when used inappropriately. A poison normally kills a person but when taken appropriately it works as a rejuvenating drug.

॥ इति मद्यवर्गः ॥

Thus ends the group dealing with alcoholic drinks.

1. परम् इति आदर्शपुस्तिकासु पाठः ।
2. स्मृता इति आकरे पाठः ।
3. गुर्वी वलस्तन्यपुष्टिमेदः कफप्रदा इति आकरे पाठः ।
4. शोथगुल्मार्शोग्रहणीमूत्रकृच्छ्रनुत् इति आकरे पाठः ।
5. पुनर्नवाशालिषिष्टिविहिता वारुणी स्मृता इति आकरे पाठः ।
6. संहितैस्तालखर्जूररसैर्या साऽपि वारुणी इति आकरे पाठः ।
7. बीजं समं जातं इति आकरे पाठः ।
8. वक्वसो इति द्वितीयपुस्तके पाठः ।
9. वातवर्धनः इति द्वितीयपुस्तके पाठः ।
10. विष्टम्भिस्वादुदुर्जरम् इति षष्ठपुस्तके पाठः ।
11. धातक्यचन्नगुडैगौंडो इति षष्ठपुस्तके पाठः ।
12. गौडोनिषेवितो इति षष्ठपुस्तके पाठः ।
13. रसो इति षष्ठपुस्तके पाठः ।
14. पक्वः इति आदर्शपुस्तिकासु पाठः ।
15. यः सीधुः इति आकरे पाठः ।
16. शीतरसः स्मृतः इति आकरे पाठः ।
17. वातपित्तकरः सद्यः स्नेहनो रोचनो हरेत इति आकरे पाठः ।
18. स्नेहनो रेचने जयेत् इति षष्ठपुस्तके पाठः ।
19. विबन्दमेदः इति आकरे पाठः ।
20. शोफोदरकफामयान् इति आकरे पाठः ।
21. आक्षकः इति आकरे पाठः ।
22. पित्तघ्नोऽसृकप्रसादनः इति आकरे पाठः ।
23. बद्धनिस्यन्दस्तुवरो इति आकरे पाठः ।
24. यथास्वं संस्कारमवेक्ष्य इति आकरे पाठः ।
25. दाहि इति षष्ठपुस्तके पाठः ।
26. मदिराऽऽचरेत् इति आकरे पाठः ।
27. नस्य स्यादमृतं यथा इति आकरे पाठः ।

# CHAPTER 12

कदमूलफलादीनि सस्नेहलवणानि च ।
यत्र द्रवेऽभिधीयन्ते तच्छुक्तमभिधीयते ॥ १ ॥

## *Śukta* (Vinegar)

The potion prepared by adding rhizomes, roots and fruits along with fat and salt in water (lit. liquid) is called *śukta*.

'रक्तपित्तकरं शुक्तं छेदि भुक्तविपाचनम् ।
भेदनं लेखनं[1] पाण्डुरोगकृमिहरं[2] लघु ॥ २ ॥
तीक्ष्णोष्णं मूत्रलं हृद्यं कफघ्नं[3] कटुपाकि च ।

It produces *raktapitta* (a disease characterised by bleeding from different parts of the body). It causes *chedana* (which takes away tissues by cutting). It helps in the digestion of food. It is purgative and depleting. It cures *pāṇḍu* (anemia) and *kṛmi* (parasitic infection). It is light, sharp, hot, diuretic, cardiac tonic, alleviator of *kapha* and pungent in *vipāka*.

तद्वत्तदासुतं सर्वं राचनं च[4] विशेषतः ॥ ३ ॥'

[माधवद्रव्यगुणः काञ्जिकवर्ग १३ : १-२]

When prepared by the process of fermentation (*āsuta*), it also produces the same effect. It, however, becomes a good appetiser.

"संधितं धान्यमण्डादि प्रोच्यते **कांजिकं** जनैः[5] ।

*Kāñjika*

The potion prepared by fermenting *dhānya manda* etc., is called *kāñjika*.

काञ्जिकं भेदितीक्ष्णोष्णं रोचनं पाचनं लघु ॥ ४ ॥

'दाहज्वरहरं स्पर्शात् पानाद्वातकफापहम्' ।"

[माधवद्रव्यगुणः काञ्जिकवर्ग १३ : ७]

[भावप्रकाशः सन्धानवर्ग २१ : १-२]

It is purgative, sharp, hot, appetiser, carminative and light. When applied externally, it cures *dāha* (burning syndrome) and fever. When taken internally, it alleviates *vāyu* and *kapha*.

'**तुषोदकं** यवैरन्यैः[6] सतुषैः शकलीकृतैः ॥ ५ ॥'

[भावप्रकाशः सन्धानवर्ग २१ : ८६]

*Tuṣodaka*

*Tuṣodaka* is prepared by the coarse powder of *yava* along with its husk and some other drugs.

'तुषांबु दीपनं हृद्यं पाण्डुक्रिमिगदापहम्[7] ।'

[माधवद्रव्यगुणः काञ्जिकवर्ग १३ : ६]

तीक्ष्णोष्णं पाचनं पित्तरक्तकृद्वस्तिशूलजित् ॥ ८ ॥

It is a digestive stimulant and a cardiac tonic. It cures *pāṇḍu* (anemia) and *kṛmi* (parasitic infection). It is sharp, hot and carminative. It vitiates *pitta* and blood and cures pain in the urinary bladder.

सौवीरं तु यवैरामैः पक्वैर्वा निस्तुषैः कृतम् ।
गोधूमैरपि सौवीरमिति[8] क्वचन[9] कीर्तितम् ॥ ७ ॥

### *Sauvīra*

*Sauvīra* is prepared of dehusked *yava*—either unboiled or boiled. In some places *sauvīra* is also prepared of *godhūma.*

सौवीरकं[10] ग्रहण्यर्शःकफघ्नं भेदि दीपनम् ।
[उ]दावर्त्ताङ्गमर्दास्थिशूलानाहेषु शस्यते ॥ ८ ॥

*Sauvīraka* cures *grahaṇī* (sprue syndrome), *ārśas* (piles) and aggravation of *kapha*. It is purgative and digestive. It is useful in *udāvarta* (flatulence), *aṅga marda* (malaise), *asthi śūla* (pain in bones) and *ānāha* (tymphanitis).

आरनालं तु गोधूमैस्तत्सौवीरगुणं[11] मतम् ।

### *Āranāla*

*Āranāla* is prepared of *godhūma* and it shares all the properties of *sauvīraka.*

धान्याम्लं शालिचूर्णादि[12] कोद्रवादिकृतं मतम्[13] ।
अरुचौ वातरोगेषु सर्वेष्वास्थापने हितम् ॥ ९ ॥

[भावप्रकाशः सन्धानवर्ग २१ : ८-११]

समुद्रमाश्रितानां च जनानां सात्म्यमुच्यते ।

### *Dhānyāmla*

*Dhānyāmla* is prepared of the powder of *śāli*, *kodrava* etc. It is useful in anorexia and diseases caused by *vāyu*. It is useful in *āsthāpana* type of enema for all patients. It is *sātmya* (wholesome) for persons residing on the sea coast.

मूलकच्छदसंथानं[14] शाण्डाकी रोचनी मता ॥ १० ॥

मुद्गादिवटकैर्यातु क्रियते सा गुणोत्तमा ॥ ११ ॥

सा तु वातहरी लघ्वी रोचनी पाचनी परम् ।

शूलाजीर्णविबन्धामनाशिनी बस्तिशोधनी ॥ १२ ॥

*Śāṇḍākī*

The potion prepared by the fermentation of the leaves of *mūlaka* is called *śāṇḍākī*. It is purgative. The *śāṇḍākī* prepared of the *vaṭaka* of *mudga* etc., is superior in quality. It alleviates *vāyu*. It is light, appetiser and carminative par excellence. It cures *śūla* (colic pain), *ajīrṇa* (indigestion), *vibandha* (constipation) and *āma*. It cleanses the urinary bladder.

'का[ञ्जि]कार्द्रं[15] सलवणं पाचनं दीपनं लघु ।

वातश्लेष्महरं[16] रुच्यं विशेषादामवातनत् ॥ १३ ॥'

[माधवद्रव्यगुणः काञ्जिकवर्ग १३ : ११]

**Special preparation of *Kāñjika***

The potion prepared of *kāñjika* mixed with *ārdraka* and salt is carminative, digestive stimulant and light. It alleviates *vāyu* and *kapha*. It is an appetiser. It specifically alleviates *āmavātā* (rheumatism).

॥ इति शक्तवर्गः ॥

Thus ends the group dealing with various types of vinegar.

## NOTES AND REFERENCES

1. जरणं इति आकरे पाठः ।
2. श्लेष्मपाण्डुकृमिहरं इति आकरे पाठः ।

3. कफजं इति आकरे पाठः ।
4. सुविशेषतः इति द्वितीयपुस्तके पाठः ।
   तु विशेषतः इति आकरे पाठः ।
5. काञ्जिकं कथ्यते इति आकरे पाठः ।
6. यवैरामैः इति आकरे पाठः ।
7. हृत्पाण्डुक्रिमिरोगनुत् इति आकरे पाठः
8. सौवीरमाचार्य्याः इति आकरे पाठः ।
9. केचिदूचिरे इति आकरे पाठः ।
10. सौवीरं इति आकरे पाठः ।
11. गोधूमैरामैः स्यान्निस्तुषीकृतैः इति आकरे पाठः ।
12. च इति आकरे अधिकं पाठः ।
13. भवेत् इति आकरे पाठः ।
14. मूलकच्छंदसंधाने इति षष्ठपुस्तके पाठः ।
15. काञ्चिकाद्रैं इति द्वितीयपुस्तके पाठः ।
16. वातपित्तहरं इति षष्ठपुस्तके पाठः

# CHAPTER 13

'मूत्रं [1]गोऽजाविमहिषीगजाश्वोष्ट्रखरोद्भवम् ।

*Mūtra* (Urine)

**Variety**

The urine of cow, goat, sheep, buffalo, elephant, horse, camel and donkey is commonly used in medicine.

पित्तलं तीक्ष्णरूक्षोष्णं लवणानुरसं कटु ॥ १ ॥

कृमिशोफोदरानाहशूलपाण्डुकफानिलान् ।

गुल्मारुचिविषश्वित्रकुष्ठार्शांसि जयेल्लघु ॥ २ ॥

**General Property**

Urine aggravates *pitta*. It is sharp, un-unctuous, hot, saline in *anurasa* (subsidiary taste) and pungent. It cures *kṛmi* (parasitic infection), *śopha* (oedema), *udara* (obstinate abdominal diseases including ascitis), *ānāha* (flatulence), *śūla* (colic pain), aggravation of *kapha* as well as *vāyu*, *gulma* (phantom tumour), *aruci* (anorexia), *viṣa* (poisoning), *śvitra* (leucoderma) and *kuṣṭha* (obstinate skin diseases including leprosy). It is light.

गोमूत्रं लघु[2] तीक्ष्णोष्णं सक्षारत्वान्न वातलम् ।
लघ्वग्निदीपनं मेध्यं पित्तलं कफवातजित् ॥ ३ ॥

**Cow's urine**

Cow's urine is light, sharp, hot and alkaline. Therefore, it does not aggravate *vāyu*. It is light, digestive stimulant, promoter of intellect, aggravator of *pitta* and alleviator of *kapha* as well as *vāyu*.

शूलगुल्मोदरानाहविरेकास्थापनादिषु[3] ।
मूत्रप्रयोगसाध्येषु[4] गव्यं मूत्रं प्रयोजयेत् ॥ ४ ॥

In diseases which are amenable to urine like *śūla* (colic pain), *gulma* (phantom tumour), *udara* (obstinate abdominal diseases including ascitis) and *ānāha* (flatulence) and for the purpose of purgation therapy and *āsthāpana* therapy cow's urine should be used.

कासश्वासापहं शोफकामलापाण्डुरोगनुत्[5] ।
छागं रूक्षोष्णकटुकं नाडीव्रणविषापहम्[6] ॥ ५ ॥

**Goat's urine**

The urine of goat cures *kāsa* (bronchitis), *śvāsa* (asthma), *śopha* (oedema), *kāmalā* (jaundice) and *pāṇḍu* (anemia). It is ununctuous, hot and pungent. It also cures *nāḍīvraṇa* (sinus) and *viṣa* (poisoning).

प्लीहोदरश्वासकासशोफवर्चोग्रहे[7] हितम् ।
सक्षारं तिक्तकटुकमुष्णं वातघ्नमाविकम् ।

**Sheep's urine**

The urine of sheep cures *plīhan* (splenic disorder), *udara* (obstinate abdominal disorders including ascitis), *śvāsa* (asthma), *kāsa* (bronchitis), *śopha* (oedema) and *varcograha* (retention of stool). It is alkaline, bitter, pungent and hot. It alleviates *vāyu*.

दुर्नामोदरशूलेषु कुष्ठमेही[8] विशुद्धिषु ॥ ६ ॥
आनाहशोथगुल्मेषु पाण्डुरोगेषु[9] **माहिषम्** ।

**Buffalo's urine**

The urine of buffalo is useful in *durnāma* (piles), *udara* (obstinate abdominal diseases including ascitis), *śūla* (colic pain), *kuṣṭha* (obstinate skin diseases including leprosy), *meha* (obstinate urinary disorders including diabetes), *viśuddhi* (elimination therapy), *ānāha* (tymphanitis), *śotha* (oedema), *gulma* (phantom tumour) and *pāṇḍu* (anemia).

सतिक्तलवणं भेदि वातघ्नं पित्तकोपनम् ॥ ७ ॥
तीक्ष्णं क्षारं किलासे च **नागमूत्रं** प्रयोजयेत् ।

**Elephant's urine**

The urine of elephant is bitter, saline and purgative. It alleviates *vāyu* and aggravates *pitta*. It is sharp and alkaline. It is useful in *kilāsa* (a type of leucoderma).

दीपनं कटु तीक्ष्णोष्णं वातचेतोविकारनुत्[10] ॥ ८ ॥
**आश्वं** कफहरं[11] मूत्रं[12] क्रिमिदद्रुविनाशनम्[13] ।

**Urine of Horse**

The urine of horse is a digestive stimulant, pungent, sharp and hot. It cures diseases caused by aggravation of *vāyu* and of the mind. It alleviates *kapha* and cures *kṛmi* (parasitic infection) and *dadru* (ring worm).

**औष्ट्रं** कुष्ठोदरोन्मादशोफार्शःक्रिमिवातनुत् ॥ ९ ॥

**Camel's urine**

The urine of camel cures *kuṣṭha* obstinate skin

diseases including leprosy), *udara* (obstinate abdominal diseases including ascitis), *unmāda* (insanity), *arśas* (piles) and *kṛmi* (parasitic infection). It alleviates *vāyu.*

गरचेतोविकारघ्नं तीक्ष्णं जठररोगनुत् ।
दीपनं **गार्दभं** मूत्रं कृमिवातकफापहम्[14] ॥ १० ॥

**Urine of donkey**

The urine of donkey cures *gara* (poisoning) and *cetovikāra* (mental disease). It is sharp. It cures *jaṭhara* (obstinate abdominal diseases including ascitis). It is a digestive stimulant. It also cures *kṛmi* (parasitic infection). It alleviates *vāyu* and *kapha*.

कषायतिक्तमेतेषां हिक्काश्वासहरं[15] **शकृत्**[16] ।
पित्तरक्तकृमिहरं रोचनं कफवातजित् ॥ ११ ॥'

[माधवद्रव्यगुण: मूत्रवर्ग १४ : १-१२]

**Stool**

The stool of these animals is astringent and bitter. It alleviates *hikkā* (hiccup), *śvāsa* (asthma), vitiation of *pitta* and blood and *kṛmi* (parasitic infection). It is appetiser and it alleviates *kapha* and *vāyu.*

'**नरमूत्रं** गरं हन्ति सेवितं तद्रसायनम् ।
रक्तपामाहरं तीक्ष्णं सक्षारलवणं स्मृतम् ॥ १२ ॥

**Human urine**

The urine of human beings cures *gara* (poisoning). It is rejuvenating. It alleviates vitiation of blood and *pāmā* (itching). It is sharp, alkaline and saline.

गोजाविमहिषीणां[17] तु स्त्रीणां मूत्र प्रशस्यते ।
खरोष्ट्रेभनराश्वानां पुंसां मूत्रं[18] हितं मतम् ॥ १३ ॥'

[भावप्रकाश: मूत्रवर्ग १९ : ७-८]

**Male and Female urine**

The urine of females of cattle, goat, sheep and buffalo is more useful On the other hand, the urine of the males of donkey, camel, elephant, human being and horse is known to be useful.

स्त्रीपुंसयोरनियमश्चरकादौ यतो मतः ।
तस्मादन्यतमं शास्त्रं विशेषात्स्त्रीसमुद्भवम् ॥ १४ ॥

In classics like *Caraka*, this distinction between male and female urine has not been made. Therefore, in actual practice urine of either the male or female animal can be used. However, the urine of female animal is more useful.

Thus ends the group dealing with various types of urine.

## NOTES AND REFERENCES

1. गोजाविमहिषीगजाश्वोष्ट्रखरोद्भवम् इति आकरे पाठः ।
2. कटु इति आकरे पाठः ।
3. शूलगुल्मोदरानाहविलेपास्थापनादिषु इति आकरे पाठः ।
4. मूत्रप्रयोगे सर्वेषु इति आकरे पाठः ।
5. (क) शोथकामलापाण्डुरोगनुत् इति आकरे पाठः ।
   (ख) शोफकामलापाण्डुदाहनुत् इति षष्ठपुस्तके पाठः ।
6. नाडीविषगरापहम् इति आकरे पाठः ।
7. प्लीहोदरश्वासकासशोथवर्चोग्रहे इति आकरे पाठः ।
8. कुष्ठमेहविशुद्धिषु इति आकरे पाठः ।
9. पाण्डुरोगे च इति आकरे पाठः ।
10. वातरोगविकारनुत् इति आकरे पाठः ।
11. कासहरं इति आकरे पाठः ।

12. रुक्षं इति आकरे पाठः ।
13. कृमिकण्डुविनाशनम् इति षष्ठपुस्तके पाठः ।
14. कृमिवातविषापहम् इति आकरे पाठः ।
15. हिध्माश्वासहरं इति आकरे पाठः ।
16. सकृत् इति द्वितीयपुस्तके पाठः ।
17. गोऽजाऽविमहिषीणां इति आकरे पाठः ।
18. स्मृतम् इति आकरे पाठः ।

# CHAPTER 14

**सामान्यतो जलगुणा :**

'**पानीय**ं श्रमनाशनं क्लमहरं मूर्च्छापिपासाहरम् ।
तन्द्रास्वप्नविनाशनं बलकरं स्याज्जीवनं तर्पणम् ।।१।।
हृद्यं गुप्तरसं ह्यजीर्णशमनं चैकान्तपथ्यं परम् ।
शीतं लघ्वमृतोपमं रसगणानां कारणं छर्दिहृत्[1] ।। २ ।।

## Water

**General properties**

Water removes physical and mental fatigue, *mūrchā* (fainting), thirst, *tandrā* (drowsiness) and *svapna* (sleep). It promotes strength. It is life giving, refreshing and caradiac tonic. It has unmanifested tastes. It cures indigestion. It is wholesome par excellence. It is cooling, light and like ambrosia. It helps in the manifestation of all tastes. It cures *chardi* (vomiting).

**अथ तद्भेदा :**

पानीयं प्रथमं प्रोक्तं **दिव्यं भौम**मिति द्विधा ।

**Varieties**

Water is first classified into two categories viz., *divya* (which falls from the sky) and *bhauma* (which is available on the earth).

दिव्यं त्वनिर्देश्यरसं जीवनं तर्पणं लघु ॥ ३ ॥

रसायनं तृषामूर्च्छातन्द्रादाहक्लमापहम् ।

सौम्यं च पाचनं बल्यं मदनिद्रा त्रिदोषनुत् ॥ ४ ॥

आश्वासजननं ह्लादि श्रमघ्नमतिबुद्धिकृत् ।

The former type of water has no manifested taste. It is life-giving, refreshing, light and rejuvenating. It cures *tṛṣā* (morbid thirst), *mūrchā* (fainting), *tandrā* (drowsiness), *dāha* (burning syndrome) and *klama* (mental fatigue). It is *saumya* (cooling) and carminative. It promotes strength and cures *mada* (intoxication), *nidrā* (excessive sleep) and vitiation of all the three *doṣas*. It gives consolation and happiness. It removes physical fatigue and promotes intellect.

**धाराजं करकाजातं तौषारं हैममेव च ॥ ५ ॥**

चतुर्द्धा[2] सलिलं दिव्यं तेषु धारं गुणाधिकम् ।

**Classification of *divya* type of water**

*Divya* type of water is of four types viz., *dhārāja*, *karakājāta*, *tauṣāra* and *haima*. Of them, *dhārāja* is the best.

पतितं यत्तु गगनात्तद्धारमिति कीर्तितम् ॥ ६ ॥

तत्तु धौतशिलाहर्म्यपटादिभ्यो विनिःसृतम् ।

हेमाद्रिपात्रगं पेयं यावन्न विकृतं भवेत् ॥ ७ ॥

तत्तु तावद्भवेद्दिव्यं यावत्प[त][3]ति [न][4]भुवि ।

धारं नीरं मरुत्पित्त कफान्संहरते लघु ॥ ८ ॥

### *Dhārāja* water

The water that falls from the sky is called *dhārāja.* It should be collected on a clean roof made of stones or through a piece of cloth and collected in vessels of gold and stone. It should be used before it gets spoiled. The rain water which is collected before it falls on the earth is called *divya*. *Dhāra* type of *divya* water alleviates *vāyu, pitta* and *kapha* and it is light.

धारं वारि द्विधा ज्ञेयं गांगसामुद्रभेदतः ।

**Variety**

The *dhāra* type of water is of two type viz., *gāṅga* (which is derived from the river (?) Ganges and *sāmudra* (which is derived from the sea).

'आकाशगंगा संभूतं[5] जलमादाय दिग्गजाः ॥ ९ ॥
मेघैरन्तरिता वृष्टिं कुर्वन्तीति वचः सताम् ।

According to the saints, *diggajas* (elephant guiding different directions as described in the epic) collect water from *ākāśa gaṅgā* (the gaṅgā river in the sky as described in the epic) and release it on the earth in the form of rain through the cloud.

गंगामाश्वयुजे मासि यत्प्रवर्षति[6] तोयदः ॥ १० ॥
सर्वदा[7] तज्जलं पेयं तथा[8] च चरके वचः ।

The *gaṅgā* water which rains from the clouds in the month of *aśvina* (September-October) is always useful for drinking. This is described in *Caraka saṁhitā*.

[9]स्थापितं हेमजे पात्रे राजते मृण्मयेऽपि वा ॥ ११ ॥
शाल्यन्नं येन संसिक्तं भवेदक्लेदि वर्णवत् ।
तद्गांगं सर्वदोषघ्नं ज्ञेयं सामुद्रमन्यथा ॥ १२ ॥'

[भावप्रकाशः वारिवर्ग १३ : १०-१३]

If this *gāṅga* type of water is collected in a vessel of gold, silver or stone and *śāli* rice is kept in it soaked then this rice does not deteriorate (*akledi*) and it retains its colour for a long time. This is the characteristic feature of *gāṅga* type of water. In *sāmudra* type of water this *śāli* rice deteriorates.

‘आश्विने मासि सामुद्रं गुणैर्गांगवदादिशेत्[10] ।’

The *sāmudra* type of water which rains in the month of *aśvina* (September-October) shares all the properties of the *gāṅga* type of water.

‘फूत्कारविषवातेन नागानां व्योमचारिणाम् ।। १३ ।।
वर्षासु सविषं तोयं दिव्यमप्याश्विनादृते[11] ।
अनार्त्तवं प्रमुञ्चन्ति वारि वारिधरास्तु यत् ।। १४ ।।
तत्त्रिदोषाय सर्वेषां देहिनां परिकीर्तितम् ।

## Poisonous Water

The *nāgas* (snakes as described in the epic) moving in the sky emit (*phutkāra*) poisonous air which impregnates the rain water and such rain falls take place from clouds unseasonally i.e. during months other than *aśvina* (September and October). This type of water aggravates all the three *doṣas* in living creatures.

[12]दिव्यं वाय्वग्निसंयोगात्संहताः स्वात्पतन्ति याः ।।१५।।
शिला[13]शकलवच्चापस्ताः कारक्योऽमृतोपमाः ।

## *Karakājāta* (Water from hail stone)

The *divya* type of water gets condensed because of the impact of wind and heat (*agni*) and falls from the sky in the form of pieces of stone. This is called *karakājāta* water which is like ambrosia.

कारक्योत्थं[14] जलं रूक्षं विशदं गुरु च स्थिरम् ॥ १६ ॥
दारणं[15] शीतलं सान्द्रं पित्तहृत्कफवातकृत् ।

This type of water is un-unctuous, non slimy (*viśada*), heavy and *sthira* (stable). It is penetrating (*dāraṇa*), cooling and dense. It alleviates *pitta* and aggravates *kapha* as well as *vāta*.

अपितात्[16] याः समुद्रान्ते वह्ने[17] राप[18][श्च]तद्भवा ॥१७॥
धूमावयवनिर्मुक्तास्तुषाराख्यास्तु ता[19] मताः[20] ।
अपथ्याः प्राणिनां प्रायो भूरुहाणां तु ता हिताः ॥१८॥

### *Tauṣāra* (Water from dew & frost)

The water on the sea coast gets impregnated with heat (*vahni*). It is free from portions of smoke and is called *tuṣāra*. It is generally unwholesome for living creatures but it is useful for plants.

तौषारं[21] वातलं शीतं रूक्षं सान्द्रमपित्तलम् ।
कफोरुस्तम्भकुष्ठाग्नि[22]मेदोगण्डादिरोगनुत् ॥ १९ ॥

*Tauṣāra* types of water aggravates *vāyu*. It is cooling, un-unctuous and dense. It does not aggravate *pitta*. It cures ailments like aggravation of *kapha*, *urustambha* (a disease characterised by immobility of thigh), *kuṣṭha* (obstinate skin diseases including leprosy), *agni* (digestive power), *medas* (adiposity) and *gaṇḍa* (goitre).

हिमवच्छिखरादिभ्यो द्रवीभूयाभिवर्षति ।
यत्तदेव हिमं हैमं जलमाहुर्मनीषिणः ।

### *Haima* (Water from snow)

When the snow (*hima*) collected on the top of hills melts and this water comes through rain fall, it is called *haima* water.

[23] हैमं गुरुतरं शीतं पित्तनुद्वातवर्धनम् ॥ २० ॥

This water is heavier and cooling. It alleviates *pitta* and aggravates *vāyu.*

**अन्ये तु :**

[24] जलमनलधूमेरितमन्तःसमुद्रस्य यद्घनीभूतम् ।
पवनानीतमुदीच्यां [25] तद्धिममिति कीर्त्यते मुनिभिः ॥२१॥

[भावप्रकाशः वारिवर्ग १३ : १६-२३]

**Another view**

The sea water being impelled by heat (*anala*) and smoke gets condensed (solidified). It is carried by the wind to the north which is called *hima* (snow) by sages.

'हिमन्तु शीतलं रूक्षं दारणं सूक्ष्ममेव च ।
कफं न तद्दूषयति न पित्तं न च मारुतम्' [26] ॥ २२ ॥

This snow (*hima*) water is cooling, ununctuous, *dāraṇa* (which causes excission) and subtle. It does not vitiate either *kapha* or *pitta* or *vāyu.*

एतेन हिमस्य द्वैविध्यमा[ख्या]तम्' [27] ।

Thus, there are two types of *haiṁa* water.

अथ **भौमं** जलं वक्ष्ये [28] यथा देशगुणान्वितम् ॥ २३ ॥

भौममम्भः प्रथमतस्त्रिविधं मुनिभिर्मतम् ।
**आनपं जाङ्गलं** चैव तथा **साधारणं** क्रमात् ॥ २४ ॥

*Bhauma* **(Water on earth)**

Depending upon the attributes of the land, the *bhauma*

type of water is first classified into three types viz., *ānūpa*, *jāṅgala* and *sādhāraṇa*.

देशः प्रचुरपानीयो बहुवृक्षसमाकुलं ।
बहुवातकफव्याधिरानूप इति कीर्तितः ॥ २५ ॥
अल्पोदकः स्वल्पवृक्षः प्रायः पित्तासृगामयः ।
विज्ञेयो जाङ्गलो देशस्ताभ्यां साधारणः परः ॥ २६ ॥

The area which contains a lot of water, which is surrounded by many trees and where many diseases caused by *vāyu* and *kapha* are manifested is called *ānūpa* (marshy land). The land which has less of water and fewer trees and where diseases of *pitta* and blood occur is called *jāṅgala* (arid land). The land which is in between these two categories is called *sādhāraṇa* (moderate land).

आनूपोद्भवमानूपं जांगलं जङ्गलोद्भवम् ।
साधारणस्थलोत्थं च जल साधारण मतम् ॥ २७ ॥

The water found in marshy areas is called *ānūpa*, that of arid areas is called *jāṅgala* and that of the moderate type of land is called *sādhāraṇa*.

'आनूपं वार्यभिष्यन्दि स्वादुस्निग्धं [29] तथा गुरु ।
वह्निहृत्[30]कफकृन्नित्यं विकारान्कुरुते बहून् ॥ २८ ॥
[भावप्रकाशः वारिवर्ग १३ : ३०]

ज्ञेयं जांगलमानूपं विपरीतगुणान्वितम् ।
'साधारणं तु मधुरं दीपनं शीतलं लघु ।
तर्पणं [31] प्रीतिजनकं तृष्णाघ्नं दाहदोषनुत् ॥ २९ ॥'
[भावप्रकाशः वारिवर्ग १३ : ३१]

**Attributes**

The *ānūpa* type of water reduces the power of digestion

and aggravates *kapha.* It is despisable. It causes many diseases. The *jāṅgala* type of water has properties which are just opposite to *ānūpa* type. The *sādhāraṇa* type of water is sweet, digestive stimulant, cooling, light and refreshing. It producess the feeling of comfort and cures *tṛṣṇā* (morbid thirst) and *dāha* (burning syndrome).

भौमस्य पयसोऽन्येऽपि भेदाः सन्ति वदामि तान् ।
नादेय प्रभृतिस्तेषां लक्षणानि गुणानपि ॥ ३० ॥

**Another Classification**

The *bhauma* type of water is also classified in a different way like *nādeya* (which is derived from *nadī* or river) etc. Their characteristics and properties will now be described.

'नद्या नदस्य वा नीरं नादेयमिति कीर्तितम् ।

**River Water**

The water of a *nadī* (small river) or *nada* (big river) is called *nādeya.*

नादेयमुदकं रूक्षं वातलं लघु दीपनम् ।
32
अनभिष्यन्दि विशदं कटुकं कफपित्तजित् ॥ ३१ ॥

This is ununctuous, aggravator of *vāyu,* light, digestive stimulant, *anabhiṣyandi* (which does not obstruct the channels of circulation), *viśada* (non-slimy) and pungent. It alleviates *kapha* and *pitta.*

नद्यः शीघ्रप्रवाहाश्च सर्वा याश्चामलोदकाः ।
गुर्व्यः शैवालसंछन्ना मंदगाः कलुषाश्च याः' ॥ ३२ ॥

[भावप्रकाशः वारिवर्ग १३: ३३-३४]

All rivers which have a strong flow carry pure water. The water of the river which flows very slowly, is heavy. It is covered with moss etc. and its water is not pure.

'नदीसरस्तडागस्थे कूपप्रस्रवणादिजे ।

उदके देशभेदेन गुणान् दोषांश्च लक्षयेत् ।। ३३ ।।

**Other Varieties**

The good and bad qualities of the water of rivers, lakes, ponds, wells and springs should be determined on the basis of the attributes of the land in which they are situated.

विदार्यभूमिं निम्नां यन्महत्या धारया स्रवेत् ।
तत्रोयमौद्भिदं नाम भिषजः[33] प्राक्तना जगुः ।। ३४ ।।

*Audbhida* **(Water coming out from earth)**

The water which comes out in a strong current by penetrating the low lying land is called *audbhida* by ancient physicians.

**औद्भिदं** वारि पित्तघ्नमविदाह्यतिशीतलम् ।
प्रीणनं मधुरं बल्यं ईषद्वातकरं लघु ।। ३५ ।।

The *audbhida* type of water alleviates *pitta*. It does not produce burning sensation. It is exceedingly cold, refreshing, sweet and strength promoting. It is a mild aggravator of *vāyu* and is light.

शैलसानुस्रवद्वारिप्रवाहो **निर्झरो** मतः[34] ।
सानु[35] प्रस्रवणं चापि तज्जलं नैर्झरं भवेत् ।। ३६ ।।

*Nirjhara* **(Water from Spring)**

The water that flows from the peak of the mountain is called *nirjhara*. The water of the spring that is found in the peak is also called *nirjhara*.

नैर्झरं रुचिकृन्नीरं कफघ्नं दीपनं लघु ।
मधुरं कटुपाकं च वातलं चातिपित्तकृत्[36] ।। ३७ ।।

The water of *nirjhara* is appetiser, alleviator of *kapha*, digestive stimulant, light, sweet in taste and pungent in *vipāka*.

It aggravates *vāyu* and excessively aggravates *pitta.*

नद्याः शैलवराच्चापि स्रुतमेकत्र संस्थितम् ।
कुमुदांभोजसंछन्नं वारि सारसमुच्यते ।। ३८ ।।

### *Sārasa* (Water of pond)

The water that flows down from the big mountain and gets accumulated in the valley is called *sārasa.* It is covered with *kumuda* and *padma.*

**सारसं** सलिलं बल्यं तृष्णाघ्नं मधुरं लघु ।
तुवरं रोचनं रूक्षं बद्धमूत्रमलं[37] शुचिः ।। ३९ ।।

The *sārasa* type of water is strength promoting, alleviator of *tṛṣṇā* (morbid thirst), sweet, light, astringent, appetiser and un-unctuous. It causes retention of urine and stool. It is pure.

अल्पं सरः **पल्वलं** स्याद्यत्र दक्षिणगे[38] रवौ ।
न तिष्ठति जलं किञ्चित्तत्रत्यं वारि पाल्वलम् ।।४०।।

### *Pālvala* (Water of small pond)

A small pond is called *palvala.* During the southern solstice when the sun moves towards a southernly direction, these small ponds get dried. The water of these small ponds is called *pālvala.*

पाल्वलं वार्यभिष्यन्दि गुरु स्वादु त्रिदोषकृत् ।

This water is *abhiṣyandi* (which obstructs the channels of circulation), heavy and sweet. It aggravates all the three *doṣas.*

प्रशस्तभूमिभागस्थं नैकसंवत्सरोषितम् ।
मुनिभिः किल तत्तोयं **ताडाग**मिति कीर्तितम् ।। ४१ ।।

### *Tāḍāga* (Water from lake)

The water that gets accumulated for many years in a plain land is called *tāḍāga* by the sages.

39

ताडागमुदकं स्वादुः कषायं कटुपाकि च ।
वातलं बद्धविण्मूत्रमसृक्पित्तकफापहम् ॥ ४२ ॥

The water of *taḍāga* is sweet and astringent in taste and pungent in *vipāka*. It aggravates *vāyu*. It causes retention of stool and urine. It alleviates vitiation of blood, *pitta* and *kapha*.

शिलादिभिरबद्धो यः सतीर्था वापिकाकृति ।
सगर्तः कथितश्चुण्डस्तज्जलं चौण्डमुच्यते ॥ ४३ ॥

### *Cauṇḍa* water

The receptacle of water dug in the earth of the size of a *vāpi* (big well) which has no boundary wall of stone and which has a staircase to go down is called *cuṇḍa*. Its water is called *cauṇḍa*.

40

चौण्ड्यं नीरं वह्निकरं रूक्षं कफहरं लघु ।
मधुरं पित्तनुद्रुच्यं पाचनं विशदं मतम् ॥ ४४ ॥

This water stimulates digestion. It is ununctuous, alleviator of *kapha*, light, sweet, alleviator of *pitta*, appetiser, carminative and *viśada* (non slimy).

"पाषाणैरिष्टिकाभिर्बद्धास्याद्या तु कूपवत् ।
वापी सा खलु विज्ञेया कृतसोपानपङ्क्तिका ॥४५॥

### *Vāpī* water

The water reservoir which is like a well, which has a boundary wall of stone or brick and which has a staircase to go down, is called *vāpī*.

वाप्यं क्षारं जलं पित्तकरं वातकफापहम्

तदेव यदि मिष्टं स्यात्तदा पित्तानिलापहम् ।। ४६ ।।

The water of the *vāpī* is alkaline. It aggravates *pitta* and alleviates *vāyu* as well as *kapha*. If this water is sweet in taste then it alleviates *pitta* and *vāyu*.

भूमौ खातोऽल्पविस्तारो गाम्भीयणाधिकोभृशम् ।

41

इष्टिकादिनिबद्धश्च स कूप इति कीर्तितः ।। ४७ ।।"

### *Kūpa* water

The water reservoir prepared by digging earth which has no wide opening but which is very deep and which has a boundary wall of bricks is called *kūpa* (well).

'कौपं पयो यदि स्वादु त्रिदोषघ्नं हितं लघु ।

तत्क्षारं कफवातघ्नं दीपनं पित्तकृत्परम्' ।। ४८ ।।

[भावप्रकाशः वारिवर्ग १३ : ४६]

If the water of this well is sweet in taste, then it alleviates all the three *doṣas*. It is wholesome and light. If the taste of this water is alkaline, then it alleviates *kapha* and *vāyu*. It is a digestive stimulant and it aggravates *pitta*.

'नद्यादिनिकटे भूमिर्या भवेद्वालुकामयी ।

उद्भाव्यते ततो यत्तु तज्जलं विकिरं विदुः ।। ४९ ।।

### *Vikira* water

The water that is taken out by digging small hole in the sandy river bed is called *vikira*.

विकिरं शीतलं स्वच्छं निर्दोषं लघु च स्मृतम् ।

तुवरं स्वादु पित्तघ्नं क्षारं तत्पित्तलं मनाक् ।। ५० ।।

This water is cooling, pure, free from defects and light.

If it is either astringent or sweet then it alleviates *pitta*. If it is alkaline then it slightly aggravates *pitta*.

केदारं[42] क्षेत्रमुद्दिष्टं **कैदारं** तज्जलं भवेत्[43] ।

**_Kedāra_ water**

*Kedāra* means a field. The water of the field is called *kaidāra*.

कैदारं वार्यभिष्यन्दि मधुरं गुरु दोषकृत् ।। ५१ ।।

This water is *abhiṣyandi* (which obstructs the channels of circulation), sweet and heavy. It aggravates *doṣas*.

वार्षिकं तदहर्वृष्टं भूमिष्ठमहितं[44] जलम् ।

त्रिरात्रमुषितं तत्तु प्रसन्नममृतोपमम् ।। ५२ ।।

**Rain water**

The rain water which is collected from the ground on the same day is unwholesome. If it remains on the ground for three nights then it becomes clear and acts like ambrosia.

हेमन्ते सारसं नीरं[45] ताडागं वा गुणावहम्[46] ।

शिशिरे[47]ऽपि हितं तोयं सारसं वा तडागजम् ।। ५३ ।।

वसन्तग्रीष्मयोः कौप्यं[48] वाप्यं वा नैर्झरं जलम् ।

नादेयं वारि नादेयं वसन्तग्रीष्मयोर्बुधैः' ।। ५४ ।।

[भावप्रकाशः वारिवर्ग १३ : ५५-६०]

[49]'विषवत्पत्रपुष्पादिदुष्टनिर्झरयोगतः ।

[50]औद्भिदं वान्तरिक्षं वा वारि वर्षासु शस्यते ।। ५५ ।।

शस्तं शरदि नादेयं नीरमंशूदकं परम् ।

**Water in different seasons**

In the *hemanta* (early winter) and *śiśira* (later part of winter) seasons the water of *saras* (big pond) and *taḍāga* (small pond) is useful. In spring and summer the water of a well, *vāpī* (big well) and *nirjhara* (spring) is useful. In the spring and summer seasons, river water should not be used because it gets polluted by poisonous leaves, flowers etc., and also by the polluted springs. During the rainy season, *audbhida* type of water (that comes out by piercing the earth) and the water that is collected directly from the sky (*āntarikṣa*) is useful. During autumn, river water and *aṁśūdaka* (described below) are useful.

[51]
दिवा रविकरैर्पुष्टं निशि शीतकरांशुभिः ।
ज्ञेयमंशूदकं नाम स्निग्धं दोषत्रयापहम् ।। ५६ ।।
अनभिष्यंदिनिर्दोषमांतरिक्षजलोपमम् ।
बल्यं रसायनं मेध्यं शीतं लघु सुधासमम् ।। ५७ ।।

*Aṁśūdaka*

The water which is exposed to the sun's rays during the day time and the moon's rays during the night time is called *aṁśūdaka*.

It is unctuous. It alleviates all the *doṣas*. It is *anabhiṣyandi* (which does not obstruct the channels of circulation) and free from defects. It is like *āntarikṣa jala* (water collected directly from the sky). It is strength promoting, rejuvenating, intellect promoting, cold and light. It is like ambrosia.

**अन्यच्च :**

[52]
शरदि स्वच्छमुदक[म]गस्त्यस्याखिलं हितम् ।

**Another view**

The clean water of autumn which is impregnated with the rays of *agastya* (star canopus) is always useful.

**अथवृद्धसुश्रुतमतम् :**

पौषे वारि सरोजातं माघे तत्तु तडागजम् ।
फाल्गुने[53] कूपसंभूतं चैत्रे चौण्ड्यं[54] हितं मतम् ॥ ५८ ॥
वैशाखे नैर्झरं नीरं ज्येष्ठे शस्तं तदौद्भिदम्[55] ।
आषाढे शस्यते कौपं श्रावणे दिव्यमेव च ॥ ५९ ॥
भाद्रे कौपं पयः शस्तमाश्विने चौण्ड्यमेव[56] च ।
कार्त्तिके मार्गशीर्षे च पयोमात्रं[57] प्रशस्यते ॥ ६० ॥

**Water in different months according to *Vṛddha Suśruta***

In the month of *pauṣa* (December-January) the water of *saras* (big pond) is useful. In the month of *māgha* (January-February) the water of *taḍāga* (small pond) is useful. In *phālguna* (February—March) well water is useful. In *caitra* (March—April) the water of *cauṇḍya* (a big well without a boundary wall) is useful. In *vaiśākha* (April—May) spring water is useful. In *jyeṣṭha* (May—June) *audbhida* (the water that comes out penetrating the earth) is useful. Well-water is useful in *āṣāḍha* (June—July) and the water collected directly from the sky (*divya*) is useful in *śrāvaṇa* (July—August). In *bhādrapada* (August—September) well-water is useful and in *aśvina* (September—October) the water of *cuṇḍa* (big well without any border wall) is useful. In *kārtika* (October—November) and *mārgaśīrṣa* (November—December) all types of water are useful.

**अथ जलोद्धरणकाल :**

भौमानामम्भसां प्रायो ग्रहणं प्रातरिष्यते ।
शीतलं[58] निर्मलत्वं च यतस्तेषां परो[59] गुणाः ॥ ६१ ॥

**Time of Collection**

All types of water available on the ground should be collected in the early morning because during this time they are extremely cold and clean.

60 अत्यम्बुपानान्नविपच्यतेऽन्नमनम्बुपानाच्च स एव दोषः ।

61 तस्मान्नरो वह्निविवर्द्धनाय मुहुर्मुहुर्वारि पिबेदभूरि ॥६२॥'

[भावप्रकाशः वारिवर्ग १३ : ६१-६६]

**Mode of intake**

Taking water in excess or not taking any water—both affect the process of digestion of food. Therefore, with a view to promoting the power of digestion, a person should take water in small quantities very frequently.

चन्द्रकान्तोद्भवं रूक्षं विषपित्तज्वरापहम् ।

[माधवद्रव्यगुणः तोयवर्ग १५ : ११]

*Candrakānta* **water**

The water collected by moon stone (*candrakānta*) is un-unctuous. It cures *viṣa* (poisoning), aggravation of *pitta* and *jvara* (fever).

सामुद्रमुदकं विस्रं लवणं सर्वदोषकृत् ॥ ६३ ॥

**Sea-water**

The water of the sea is *visra* (foul smelling) and saline. It aggravates all the *doṣas*.

62 नद्यः पाषाणविच्छिन्नक्षुभिताभिहतोदकाः ।

63 मलयप्रभवा याश्च तासामम्भोऽमृतोपमम् ॥ ६४ ॥

**River water**

The rivers which pass in a strong current through stones and those whose source is in the Malaya mountain—their water is like ambrosia.

पश्चिमाभिमुखा याश्च पथ्यास्ता निर्मलोदकाः ।

64 प्रायो मृदुवहा गुर्व्यो याश्च पूर्वसमुद्रगाः ॥ ६५ ॥

पारिजात्रभवा[65] याश्च विन्ध्यसह्यभवाश्च याः ।

शिरोहृद्रोगकुष्ठानां हेतवः श्लीपदस्य च ।। ६६ ।।

The rivers which flow towards the west generally carry clean water. Those flowing towards the sea of the east are generally of slow current and their water is heavy. Rivers originating from *Parijātra*, *Vindhya* and *Sahya* mountains carry water which causes *śiraroga* (diseases of head), *hṛdroga* (diseases of heart), *kuṣṭha* (obstinate skin diseases including leprosy) and *ślīpada* (filariasis).

चन्द्रार्ककरसस्पृष्टं[66] वायुना स्फालितं च[67] यत् ।

पर्वतोपरि यद्वारि सम पौरंदरेण तत्' ।। ६७ ।।

[माधवद्रव्यगुणः तोयवर्ग १५ : १८-२३]

The water at the top of a mountain which is exposed to the rays of the sun and the moon, and strong currents of wind is like ambrosia (lit. suitable for Indra).

कीटमूत्रपुरीषाण्डशावकादिप्रदूषितम् ।

तृणपर्णोत्करैर्युक्तं कलुषं विषदूषितम् ।। ६८ ।।

योऽवगाहेत वर्षासु पिवेद्वापि नवं जलम् ।

वाह्याम्यन्तरतोरोगान् लभतेऽसौ न संशयः ।। ६९ ।।

**Polluted water**

The water which is mixed with the urine, stool, egg or embryo of insects, grass, leaves and poisons, and which is freshly collected on the ground should not be used either for a bath or for drinking. By doing so, the person falls a victim to a number of diseases—both external and internal. There is no doubt about it.

'मूर्च्छापित्तोष्म[68]दाहेषु विषे रक्ते मदात्यये ।

भ्रमे श्रमे विदग्धेऽन्ने तमके वमयोः तथा ।

ऊर्ध्वगे रक्तपित्ते च शीतमम्भः प्रशस्यते ॥ ७० ॥

**Cold water**

Cold water is useful in *mūrchā* (fainting), vitiation of *pitta*, *usmā* (excessive hot feeling), *dāha* (burning syndrome), *viṣa* (poisoning), vitiation of blood, *madātyaya* (alcoholism), *bhrama* (giddiness), *śrama* (physical fatigue), after digestion of food, in *tamaka* (asthma), *vami* (vomiting) and in *urdhvaga rakta pitta* (bleeding through various orifices in the head).

**अथ तन्निषेधः**

पार्श्वशूले प्रतिश्याये वातरोगे गलग्रहे[69] ।

आध्माने स्तिमिते कोष्ठे सद्यःशुद्धौ नवज्वरे ॥ ७१ ॥

अरुचिग्रहणीगुल्मश्वासकासेषु[70] विद्रधौ ।

हिक्कायां स्नेहपीते[71] च शीताम्बु परिवर्जयेत् ॥ ७२ ॥

**Prohibition**

Cold water should not be used in *pārśva śūla* (pain in the sides of the chest), *pratiśyāya* (cold), diseases of *vāyu*, *gala graha* (obstruction in the throat), *ādhmāna* (flatulence), *stimita koṣṭha* (absence of peristaltic movement in the intestine), *sadya śuddhi* (immediately after the purification therapy), *nava jvara* (beginning stage of fever), *aruci* (anorexia), *grahaṇī* (sprue syndrome), *gulma* (phantom tumour), *śvāsa* (asthma), *kāsa* (bronchitis), *vidradhi* (abscess), *hikkā* (hiccup) and *snehapāna* (immediately after oleation therapy).

आरोचके प्रतिश्याये प्रसेके[72] श्वयथौ क्षये ।

मंदाग्नावुदरे[73] कुष्ठे ज्वरे नेत्रामये तथा ॥ ७३ ॥

व्रणे च मधुमेहे च पानीयं[74] मन्दमाचरेत् ।

In *arocaka* (anorexia), *pratiśyāya* (cold), *praseka* (salivation), *śvayathu* (oedema), *kṣaya* (consumption), *agnimāndya* (indigestion), *udara* (obstinate abdominal diseases including ascitis), *kuṣṭha* (obstinate skin diseases including leprosy), *jvara* (fever), *netrāmaya* (eye disease), *vraṇa* (ulcer) and *madhumeha* (diabetes mellitus) one should take less quantity of water.

जीवनं जीविनां जीवो जगत्सर्वं तु तन्मयम् ।
अतोऽत्यन्तं[75] तृषायां[76] झैर्न क्वचिद्वारि वार्यते' ।। ७४ ।।

[भावप्रकाशः वारिवर्ग १३ : ७०-७४]

'तृषितो मोहमायाति मोहात्प्राणान्विमुञ्चति ।
अतः सर्वास्ववस्थासु न क्वचिद्वारि वार्यते[77] ।।[78] ७५ ।।'

[भावप्रकाशः वारिवर्ग १३ : ७६]

Water is the life of all living creatures and the entire world is pervaded by water. Therefore, when a person is extremely thirsty then giving water is not prohibited. If water is not given, then the thirsty person becomes unconscious and succumbs to death. Therefore in all circumstances water is never prohibited.

'यत्क्वाथ्यमानं[79] निर्वेगं निःफेनं निर्मलं भवेत्[80] ।'

[माधवद्रव्यगुणः तोयवर्ग १५ : ४१]

तत्तोयं दोषहृत्सर्वं दीपनं पाचनं लघु ।

**Boiled water**

The water which is boiled and when the boiling is over and the foam subsides, it is cleaned, then it alleviates all the *doṣas*. It is digestive stimulant, carminative and light.

तत्पादहीनं वातघ्नमर्द्धहीनं[81] तु पित्तनुत् ।। ७६ ।।

[माधवद्रव्यगुणः तोयवर्ग १५ : ४२]

त्रिपादहीनं श्लेष्मघ्नं संग्राह्यग्निप्रदं लघु ।

When it is reduced to three-fourth after boiling, it alleviates *vāyu.* When it is reduced to half by boiling, it alleviates *pitta.* When it is reduced to one-fourth after boiling, it alleviates *kapha* and it becomes constipative, digestive stimulant and light.

‘अर्द्धावशिष्टं[82] यत्तोयं तदुष्णोदकमुच्यते ।।’ ७७ ।।

[माधवद्रव्यगुणः तोयवर्ग १५ : ४१]

उष्णोदकं सदा पथ्यं श्वासकासज्वरार्तिजित् ।

कफवातामदोषघ्नं पित्तघ्नं बस्तिशोधनम् ।। ७८ ।।

‘भिनत्ति श्लेष्मसंघातं मारुतं चापकर्षति’ ।

अजीर्णं जरयत्याशु पीतमुष्णोदकं[83] निशि’ ।। ७९ ।।

**Hot water**

The water which is reduced to half after boiling and which is hot is called *uṣṇodaka.* This hot water is always wholesome and it cures *śvāsa* (asthma), *kāsa* (bronchitis), *jvara* (fever), aggravation of *kapha* and *vāyu, āma* and aggravation of *pitta.* It cleanses the urinary bladder and gets detached the adhered *kapha.* It helps in the elimination of *vāyu.* When hot water is taken at night, it removes indigestion.

पादशेषं तु तत्तोयं **आरोग्याम्बु** तदुच्यते ।

आरोगयम्बु सदा पथ्य श्वासकासकफापहम् ।। ८० ।।

सद्यो ज्वरहरं भेदी दीपनं पाचनं लघु ।

[84]आनाहपांडुशूलार्शो—गुल्मशोथोदरापहम् ।। ८१ ।।

*Ārogyāmbu*

When the water is boiled and reduced to one-fourth, it is called *ārogyāmbu* (healthy water). It is always wholesome. It cures *śvāsa* (asthma), *kāsa* (bronchitis) and aggravation of *kapha.* It instantaneously reduces fever. It is purgative, digestive stimulant, carminative and light. It cures *ānāha* (flatulence), *pāṇḍu* (anemia), *śūla* (colic pain), *arśas* (piles), *gulma* (phantom tumour), *śotha* (oedema) and *udara* (obstinate abdominal diseases including ascitis).

[85]
उष्णं तदग्निजननं लघ्वलं वस्तिशोधनम् ।
पार्श्वरुक् पीतं साध्मानं हिक्कानिलकफापहम् ॥८२॥
शस्तं तृष्णामशूलेषु तदशुद्धौ नवज्वरे ।

When the *ārogyāmbu* is hot, it stimulates digestive power. It is extremely light. It cleanses the urinary bladder. It cures *parśvaruk* (pain in the sides of the chest), *adhmāna* (flatulence), *hikkā* (hiccup) and aggravation of *vāyu* and *kapha*. It is useful in *tṛṣā* (morbid thirst), *āma*, *śūla* (colic pain), *aṣuddhi* (when the purificatory therapy has not acted properly) and *nava jvara* (beginning stage of fever).

दाहातीसारपित्तासृक्— मूर्च्छामद्यविषार्तिषु ॥ ८३ ॥
कफजे बातजे रोगे तृष्णाच्छर्दिभ्रमादिषु ।
[86]
'मद्यपानसमुद्भूते रोगे पित्तोच्छ्रिते तथा ।
[87]
सन्निपातसमुत्थे च शृतं शीतं प्रशस्यते ॥' ८४ ॥

[माधवद्रव्यगुणः तोयवर्ग १५ : ३३-३४]

When the *ārogyāmbu* becomes cold, it is called *śṛta śīta*. This cold water is useful in *dāha* (burning syndrome), *atisāra* (diarrhoea), vitiation of *pitta* and blood, *mūrcchā* (fainting), *madya* (alcoholism), *viṣa* (poisoning), diseases caused by *kapha* and *vāyu*, *tṛṣṇā* (morbid thirst), *chardi* (vomiting), *bhrama* (giddiness), diseases caused by excessive intake of alcohol, excessive vitiation of *pitta* and *sannipāta* (when all the three *doṣas* are vitiated simultaneously).

[88]
शृताम्बु तत् त्रिदोषघ्नं यदन्तर्वाष्पशीतलम् ।
अरूक्षमनभिष्यन्दि कृमितृड्ज्वरहृल्लघु ।

The boiled water which is cooled along with its steam alleviates all the three *doṣas*. It is not un-unctuous and it does not obstruct the channels of circulation. It cures *kṛmi* (parasitic infection), *tṛṭ* (morbid thirst) and *jvara* (fever). It is light.

'धाराशीतेन विष्टम्भी दुर्जरं पवनाहतम् ॥' ८५ ॥

[माधवद्रव्यगुण: तोयवर्ग १५ : ४३]

When the boiled water is cooled by pouring over another container, it becomes constipative and difficult of digestion because during this process the water comes in contact with a lot of air.

'दिवाश्रृतं तु यत्तोयं रात्रौ तद् गुरुतां व्रजेत् ।

89

रात्रौ श्रृतं दिवा तद्वद्गुरुत्वमधिगच्छति ॥' ८६ ॥

[माधवद्रव्यगुण: तोयवर्ग १५ : ४४]

If the water is boiled during the day time and kept overnight, it becomes heavy. Similarly, if water is boiled at night and kept till the day time, then it becomes heavy.

पानीयं न तु पानीयं पानीयेऽन्यप्रदेशजे ।

अजीर्णे क्वथितं चामे पक्वे जीर्णे च नेतरत् ॥ ८७ ॥

Water of another place should not be taken when there is indigestion and formation of *āma*. It should be taken only when it is properly boiled and not otherwise.

'स्निग्धं स्वादु हिम हृद्यं दीपनं बस्तिशोधनम् ।

90

रक्तपित्तपिपासाघ्नं **नालिकेरोदकं** गुरु ।

**Coconut water**

The water of tender coconuts is unctuous, delicious, cooling, cardiac tonic and digestive stimulant. It cleanses the urinary bladder and cures *raktapitta* (a disease characterised by bleeding from different parts of the body) and *pipāsā* (morbid thirst). It is heavy.

तदेव जीर्णं विष्टम्भि गुरु पित्तकरं स्मृतम् ।।' ८८ ।।

[माधवद्रव्यगुणः तोयवर्ग १५ : ४९-५०]

The water of the matured coconut causes wind formation in stomach. It is heavy and it aggravates *pitta*.

भक्तादौ सलिलं पीतं कासमन्दाग्निदोषकृत् ।

मध्ये तु दीपनं श्रेष्ठमन्ते स्थौल्यकर परम् ।। ८९ ।।

**Time of taking water**

Water taken before eating food causes *kāsa* (bronchitis) and *agnimāndya* (suppression of the power of digestion). When it is taken during the process of eating, it stimulates the power of digestion. If, however, it is taken after the completion of the process of eating, then it causes *sthaulya* (adiposity).

अजीर्णे भेषजं वारि जीर्णेऽन्ने च बलप्रदम् ।

अमृतं भोजनार्द्धे तु भोजनोपरि तद्विषम् ।। ९० ।।

If there is indigestion water works as a medicine. When there is proper digestion, intake of water promotes strength. When taken in the middle of a meal it works like ambrosia and when taken after a meal, water works like a poison.

"अत्यम्बुपानान्न विपच्यतेऽन्नमनम्बुपानाच्च स एव दोषः ।
91
तस्मान्नरो वह्निविवर्धनाय मुहुर्मुहुर्वारि पिबेदभूरि ।।९१।।"

[माधवद्रव्यगुणः तोयवर्ग १५ : ५३]

If water is taken in excess or if water is not taken at all, then it hampers the process of digestion. Therefore with a view to promoting the power of digestion, a person should take small quantities of water very frequently.

यत्तु व्यापन्नं [तत्] न ग्राह्यम् ।। ९२ ।।

**Water pollution**

Polluted water should not be used.

**तस्य लक्षणानि—**

92
'यत्पंकशैवालतृणपद्मपत्रप्रभृतिभिरवच्छन्नं रविशशि-

किरणानिलैर्नाभिजुष्टं गन्धवर्णरसोपसृष्टं तद् व्यापन्नम्' ॥९३॥

[सुश्रुत:सूत्र ४५ : ११]

The signs and symptoms of polluted water are as below :

The water which is mixed with mud, moss, grass, lotus leaf etc., which is not exposed to the rays of the sun and the moon and wind and which has manifested smell, colour and taste, is called polluted.

अनार्त्तवं वार्षिकमपि प्रथमं तच्च भूमिगम् ।

व्याप-मिति जानीयात्सर्वदोषप्रकोपणम् ॥ ९४ ॥

The water collected of unseasonal rain or the water collected from the ground immediately after rain is also polluted. It aggravates all the *doṣas.*

93
'तस्य स्पर्शरूपरसगन्धवीर्यविपाकदोषा: संभवन्ति ।

94
तत्र खरता पैच्छिल्यमौष्ण्यं दन्तग्राहिता च स्पर्शदोषा: ।

पंकसिकताशैवालवहुवर्णता रूपदोषा: ।

Polluted water has defects of touch, colour, taste, smell, *vīrya* (potency) and *vipāka* (taste after digestion).

Roughness, sliminess, heat and sticking to teeth—these are the defects in touch. The appearance of mud, sand and moss, and variegated colour are the defects in colour.

व्यक्तरसता रसदोष: । अनिष्टगन्धता गन्धदोष: । यदुप-

95
युक्तं चिराद्विपच्यते तृष्णागौरवशूलकफप्रसेकानापाद-

यति सवीर्यदोष:। यदुपयुक्तं चिराद्विपच्यते विष्टंभयति

वाशनं [स विपाकदोष इति] । यस्तु व्यापन्नं पिबति

स नानाविकारानाप्नोति ॥ ९५ ॥

Manifestation of taste is the defect in taste.

The presence of a foul smell is the defect in smell.

When water is taken, if it gets digested after a long time and if it produces thirst, heaviness, colic pain and slivation, then these are the defects in potency.

If water gets digested very late and causes fermentation of the food, then it should be determined that the water has the defect of *vipāka*.

A person who takes defective water succumbs to many diseases.

सप्त कलुषस्य प्रसादनानि भवन्ति—कतकगोमेदविसग्र-

न्थिशैवालमूलवस्त्राणि मुक्तामणिश्चेति ॥

शीतलीकरणानि प्रवातस्थापनमुदकप्रक्षेपणं यष्टिका-

भ्रामणम् वीजनं वस्त्रोद्धरणं च वालुकाप्रक्षेपणम्

96

शिक्यावलम्बनं चेति ॥ ९६ ॥

[सुश्रुतः सूत्र ४५ : ११, १७, १९]

Water pollution can be corrected by seven items, viz., (1) *kataka*, (2) *gomeda*, (3) *visa granthi*, (4) *śaivāla mūla*, (5) *vastra* (cloth), (6) *muktā* (pearl) and (7) *maṇi* (jewel).

For cooling the water, the container should be kept in an airy place, water should be cooled over the container, the water should be stirred with the help of a stick, it should be fanned, the container should be covered with a piece of cloth, sand should be poured over water and the container should be kept hanging on a *śikya*.

पादावशेषं सलिलं ग्रीष्मे शरदि शस्यते ।'
हिमेऽर्द्धशेषं शिशिरे तथा वर्षावसन्तयोः ॥ ९७ ॥

**Boiling in different seasons**

During summer and autumn seasons, water which is boiled and reduced to one-fourth is useful. During the remaining seasons, viz., *hemanta* (early winter), *śiśira* (later part of winter), rainy season and spring season, water boiled and reduced to half is useful.

**कश्चित्तु** :

वसुगन्धेषु वाणेषु वेदेषु त्रिषु पक्षयोः ।
एकभागावशेषं स्यादम्बु वर्षादिषु क्रमात् ॥ ९८ ॥

**Another view**

During the rainy season, autumn, *hemanta* (early winter), *śiśira* (later part of winter), spring and summer, water to be used should be boiled and reduced to 6/8 (*vasu*), 5/8 (*vāṇa*), 4/8 (*veda*), 3/8 (*tri*), 2/8 (*pakṣa*) and 1/8 (*ekabhāga*) respectively.

अत्र यथा दोषाणां हीनता प्रौढता तथा व्यवस्था कल्पनीया ॥ ९९ ॥

In this context, however; the exact nature of processing should be determined on the basis of the diminution and aggravation of the *doṣas*.

**अथ निर्दोषीकरणानि** :

व्यापन्नमपि पानीयं क्वथितं सूर्यतापितम् ।
सुवर्णं रजतं लोहं पाषाणं सिकता मृदम् ॥ १०० ॥
भृशं संताप्य निर्वाप्य सप्तधा साधितं तथा ।
कर्पूरजातीपुन्नागपाटलादिषु वासितम् ॥ १०१ ॥
सुचि सान्द्रपटे स्राव्यं क्षुद्रजन्तु[97]भिरक्षितम् ।
स्वच्छं कतक[98]मुक्ताद्यैः शुद्धं दोषा[99]पहं भवेत् ॥ १०२ ॥

**Removal of pollution**

For the removal of pollution, the boiled water should be exposed to the sun's rays and in this water hot pieces of gold, silver, iron, stone, sand or clod of earth should be immersed seven times. To this water fragrant things like *karpūra, jātī, punnāga, pāṭalā* etc. should be added. This should then be filtered with the help of a clean and compact piece of cloth. It should be protected from small insects. In the vessel containing this clean water, *kataka,* pearl etc. should be added. This process corrects pollution.

आमं जलं जीर्यति याममात्रं तदर्द्धमात्रं श्रृतशीतलं च ।

तदर्धमात्रं तु श्रृतं कदुष्णं पयः प्रपाके त्रय एव कालाः ॥१०३॥

**Time taken for digestion**

Unboiled water gets digested in one *yāma* (three hours). The water which is boiled and cooled takes one and a half hours for digestion. The water which is boiled and warm gets digested in forty five minutes. These are the three different times for digestion of water.

॥ इति वारिवर्गः ॥

Thus end the groups dealing with different types of water.

## NOTES AND REFERENCES

1. द्रष्टव्यम् भावप्रकाशः वारिवर्ग 13 : 2।
2. चतुर्धा इति द्वितीयपुस्तके पाठः ।
3. यावत्पति इति द्वितीयपुस्तके पाठः ।
4. नो इति द्वितीय पुस्तके पाठः ।
5. आकाशगङ्गासम्बन्धि इति श्राकरे पाठः ।

6. प्रायो वर्षति वारिदः इति आकरे पाठः ।
7. सर्वथा इति आकरे पाठः ।
8. तथैव इति आकरे पाठः ।
9. स्थापिते इति आकरे पाठः ।
10. द्रष्टव्यम् भावप्रकाशः वारिवर्ग 13 : 14 ।
11. दिव्यमण्याश्विनं विना इति आकरे पाठः ।
12. दिव्यवाय्वग्निसंयोगात्संहताः इति आकरे पाठः ।
13. पाषाणखण्डवच्चापस्ताः इति आकरे पाठः ।
14. करकाजं इति आकरे पाठः ।
15. दारुणं इति आकरे पाठः ।
16. अपि नद्याः इति आकरे पाठः ।
17. वह्निरापस्तदुद्भवाः इति आकरे पाठः ।
18. रापश्चतद्भवाः इति द्वितीय पुस्तके पाठः ।
19. ताः इति आकरे पाठः ।
20. स्मृताः इति आकरे पाठः ।
21. तुषाराम्बु हिमं रूक्षं स्यादुवातलपित्तलम् इति आकरे पाठः ।
22. कफोरुस्तम्भकण्ठाग्निमेहगण्डादिरोगनुत् इति आकरे पाठः ।
23. हिमाम्बु शीतं पित्तघ्नं गुरु वातविवर्द्धनम् इति आकरे पाठः ।
24. और्वानलधूमेरितमम्बु इति आकरे पाठः ।
25. कथ्यते सद्भिः इति आकरे पाठः ।
26. द्रष्टव्यम् भावप्रकाशः वारिवर्ग 13 : 24 ।
27. द्वैविध्यमायातम् इति द्वितीयपुस्तके पाठः ।
28. दोषगुणान्वितम् इति आकरे पाठः ।
29. घनं इति आकरे पाठः ।
30. वह्निहृत्कफकृद्हृद्यं इति आकरे पाठः ।
31. रोचनं तृष्णादाहदोषत्रयप्रणुत् इति आकरे आकरे पाठः ।
32. कफपित्तनुत् इति आकरे पाठः ।
33. वदन्तीति महर्षयः इति आकरे पाठः ।
34. झरः इति आकरे पाठः ।

35. स तु प्रस्रवणश्चापि तत्रत्यं नैर्झरं जलम् इति आकरे पाठः ।

36. स्यादपित्तलम् इति आकरे पाठः ।
च न पित्तकृत् इति षष्ठपुस्तके पाठः ।

37. बद्धमूत्रबलं इति षष्ठपुस्तके पाठः ।

38. स्याद्यचन्द्रर्क्षगेरवौ इति द्वितीयपुस्तके पाठः ।

39. स्वादुपाकि इति षष्ठपुस्तके पाठः ।

40. कफकरं इति षष्ठपुस्तके पाठः ।

41. द्रष्टव्यम् भावप्रकाश वारिवर्ग १३ : ४६-४८ ।

42. केदारः इति आकरे पाठः ।

43. स्मृतम् इति आकरे पाठः ।

44. भूमिस्थमहितं इति आकरे पाठः ।

44. तोयं इति आकरे पाठः ।

46. वाहितं स्मृतम् इति आकरे पाठः ।

47. हेमन्ते विहितं तोयं शिशिरेऽपि प्रशस्यते इति आकरे पाठः ।

48. कौपं इति आकरे पाठः ।

49. विषवद्वनवृक्षाणां पत्राद्यैर्दूषितं यतः इति आकरे पाठः ।

50. औद्भिदं वाऽन्तरीक्षं वा कौपं वा प्रावृषि स्मृतम् इति आकरे पाठः ।

51. रविकरैर्जुष्टं इति आकरे पाठः ।

52. स्वच्छमुदयादगस्त्यस्याखिलं इति आकरे पाठः ।

53. फाल्गुणे इति द्वितीयपुस्तके पाठः ।

54. चौञ्ज्यं इति आकरे पाठः ।

55. तथोद्भिदम् इति आकरे पाठः ।

56. चौञ्ज्यमेव इति आकरे पाठः ।

57. जलमात्रं इति आकरे पाठः ।

58. शीतत्वं इति आकरे पाठः ।

59. मतोगुणः इति आकरे पाठः ।

60. अत्यम्बुपानान्नविपच्यतेऽन्नं निरम्बुपानाच्च इति आकरे पाठः ।

61. वह्निविवर्धनाय इति द्वितीयपुस्तके पाठः ।

62. पाषाणविच्छिन्ना क्षुभिताभिहतोदकाः इति आकरे पाठः ।

63. मलयप्रभवाः याश्च इति आकरे पाठः ।
64. मृदुरवहा इति षष्ठपुस्तके पाठः ।
65. पारियात्रभवा इति आकरे च षष्ठपुस्तकयोः पाठः ।
66. चन्द्रार्ककरसंस्पृष्टं इति आकरे पाठः ।
67. मुहुः इति आकरे पाठः ।
68. मूर्च्छापित्तोष्णदाहेषु इति आकरे पाठः ।
69. लघु ग्रहे इति आदर्शपुस्तिकासु पाठः ।
70. अरुचिग्रहणीगुल्मश्वासकासे च इति षष्ठपुस्तके पाठः ।
71. स्नेहपाने च इति आकरे पाठः ।
72. मन्देऽग्नौ जठरे इति आकरे पाठः ।
73. मुखप्रसेके जठरे कुष्ठे नेत्रामये ज्वरे इति आकरे पाठः ।
74. पिबेत्पानीयमल्पकम् इति आकरे पाठः ।
75. नातोऽत्यन्तनिषेधे न कदाचिद्वारि वार्य्यते इति आकरे पाठः ।
76. सुधासु इति आदर्श पुस्तकेसु पाठः । तथा इति द्वितीयपुस्तके पाठः ।
77. तृषितो........वार्यते पाठोऽयं षष्ठपुस्तके नोपलभ्यते ।
78. वारयेत् इति आकरे पाठः ।
79. तत्क्वाथ्यमानं इति आदर्शपुस्तिकासु पाठः ।
80. च यत् इति आकरे पाठः ।
81. वातघ्नमर्धहीनं इति द्वितीयपुस्तके पाठः ।
वातघ्नमर्धहीनं च पित्तजित इति आकरे पाठः ।
82. भवति इति आकरे पाठः ।
83. द्रष्टव्यम् माधवद्रव्यगुणः तोयवर्ग १५ : ३२-३३ ।
84. आनाहपांडुशोफार्शो इति षष्ठपुस्तके पाठः ।
85. लघवं इति षष्ठपुस्तके पाठः ।
86. पित्तोत्थिते इति षष्ठपुस्तके पाठः ।
87. हितं पयः इति आकरे पाठः ।
88. शृतशीतं त्रिदोषघ्नं बाष्पान्तर्भाविशीतलम् इति आकरे पाठः ।
89. तु दिवसे गुरुत्वमधिगच्छति इति आकरे पाठः ।
90. वृत्तं पित्तपिपासघ्नं इति द्वितीयपुस्तके पाठः ।
वृष्यं पित्तपिपासघ्नं इति आकरे पाठः ।

91. द्रष्टव्यम्—श्लोक-६२।
92. हठ इति आकरे अधिकं पाठः।
93. षट् इति आकरे अधिकं पाठः।
94. स्पर्शदोषः इति आकरे पाठः।
95. पाठोऽयं सुश्रुते नोपलभ्यते।
96. वसुप्यङ्गेषु इति द्वितीयपुस्तके पाठः।
97. क्षुद्रजन्तुविवर्जितं इति षष्ठपुस्तके पाठः।
98. कनकमुद्गाद्यैः इति षष्ठपुस्तके पाठः।
99. दोषापगं इति द्वितीयपुस्तके पाठः।

# CHAPTER 15

**रक्तशालिस्त्रिदोषघ्नश्चक्षुष्यः शुक्रमूत्रलं ।**
**तृष्णौजोबलकृत्स्वर्यो हृद्यस्तदनु चापरम् ॥ १ ॥**

*Rakta śāli* **(Oriza sativa Linn.)**

The red variety of *śāli* rice alleviates all the three *doṣas*. It promotes eyesight and semen. It is diuretic. It causes thirst and promotes *ojas*, strength and voice. It is a cardiac tonic.

**शीतो लघुस्त्रिदोषघ्नो मधुरो गौरषष्टिकः ।**

*Gaura ṣaṣṭika* **(a variety of Oriza sativa Linn.)**

The white variety of *ṣaṣṭika* rice is cooling and light. It alleviates all the three *doṣas* and it is sweet.

**किञ्चिद्धीनो गुरुस्तस्मादपरो[1] रसपाकतः ॥ २ ॥**

There is another variety of it which is slightly inferior in taste and *vipāka* and which is heavier than the former.

**महाशालिः परं वृष्यः कलमः[2] श्लेष्मपित्तहा ।**

### *Mahā śāli* and *Kalama*

*Mahā śāli* type of rice is exceedingly aphrodisiac. *Kalama* variety of rice alleviates *kapha* and *pitta*.

मधुरश्चाम्लपाकश्च व्रीहिः पित्तकरो गुरुः ॥ ३ ॥

### *Vrīhi* (a variety of Oryza sativa Linn.)

The *vrīhi* type of rice is sweet. It produces acidity during digestion. It aggravates *pitta* and is heavy.

अत्युष्णो बह्वभिष्यन्दि पाटलस्तु त्रिदोषकृत् ।

### *Pāṭala*

The *pāṭala* type of rice is very hot and is exceedingly *abhiṣyandi* (which obstructs the channels of circulation). It aggravates all the three *doṣas*.

वापितं गुरु तद्धान्यं किञ्चिद्धीनमवापितम् ।

रोपितं तु नवं वृष्यं पुराणं च लघु स्मृतम् ॥ ४ ॥

**Sowing and transplantation**

The rice which is cultivated by sowing is heavy; otherwise it is slightly inferior in quality. The rice which is cultivated by transplantation is aphrodisiac when freshly harvested. When preserved for a long time, it becomes light.

[3]दग्धीयामवनौ जाताः शालयो लघुपाकिनः ।

कषाया [4]बद्धविण्मूत्राः [5]रूक्षा श्लेष्मापकर्षणः ॥ ५ ॥

**Cultivation**

The *śāli* rice which is cultivated in a forest land after setting fire to the vegetation is light for digestion. It is astringent. It causes retention of stool and urine. It is un-unctuous and alleviator of *kapha*.

स्थलजाः कफपित्तघ्नाः कषायाः [6]कटुकान्विताः ।

किञ्चित्सतिक्तमधुराः पवनानलवर्द्धनाः[7] ।। ६ ।।

The *śāli* rice which is cultivated on plain ground alleviates *kapha* and *pitta*. It is astringent, pungent, slightly bitter and sweet. It aggravates *vāyu* and stimulates the power of digestion.

केदारा मधुरा वृष्या बल्याः पित्तनिबर्हणाः ।
ईषत्कषायाल्पमला[8] गुरवः कफशुक्रलाः ।। ७ ।।

The rice which is cultivated in the rice field is sweet, aphrodisiac, strength promoting and alleviator of *pitta*. It is slightly astringent and it produces less excreta. It is heavy. It produces more of *kapha* and semen.

रोप्यातिरोप्या लघवः शीघ्रपाका गुणोत्तराः ।
अदाहिनो[9] दोषहरा बल्या मूत्रविवर्धनाः ।। ८ ।।

The rice which is cultivated by repeated transplantation is light. It gets digested easily and is superior in quality. It does not cause burning sensation. It alleviates *doṣas*. It promotes strength. It is diuretic.

शालयः छिन्नरूढा ये रूक्षास्ते बद्धवर्चसः ।
तिक्ताः कषायाः पित्तघ्नाः लघुपाकाः कफापहाः ।।९।।

[माधवद्रव्यगुणः शालिवर्ग १६ : १-९]

The rice which is grown after cutting the plant, is unctuous. It causes retention of stool. It is bitter and astringent. It alleviates *pitta*. It is light for digestion. It also alleviates *kapha*.

।। इति शालयः ।।

Thus ends the group dealing with various types of rice.

## NOTES AND REFERENCES

1. रसस्तस्मादपरो इति षष्ठपुस्तके पाठः ।
2. कमलः इति द्वितीयपुस्तके पाठः ।
3. दग्धायामवनौ इति आकरे द्वितीयपुस्तके च पाठः ।
4. बद्धविण्मूत्रा इति आकरे पाठः ।
5. रूक्षाः इति आकरे पाठः ।
6. कटुकाश्रयाः इति आकरे पाठः ।
7. पवनानलवर्धना इति द्वितीयपुस्तके पाठः ।
8. ईषत्कषायाल्पबला इति षष्ठपुस्तके पाठः ।
9. विदाहिनो इति आकरे पाठः ।

# CHAPTER 16

श्यामाकः शोषणो रूक्षो वातलः श्लेष्मपित्तहा ।

*Śyāmāka* **(Echinochloa frumentacea Linn.)**

*Śyāmāka* is *śoṣaṇa* (drying) and un-unctuous. It aggravates *vāta* and alleviates *kapha* and *pitta*.

तद्वत्[1] प्रियंगुनीवारकोरदूषाः प्रकीर्तिता ॥ १ ॥

*Priyaṅgu* **(Setaria italica Beauv.)**, *Nīvāra* **(a type of paddy) &** *Koradūṣā* **(Paspalum scorbiculatum Linn.)**

*Priyaṅgu, nīvāra* and *koradūṣa* share the properties of *śyāmāka*.

रूक्षः शीतो गुरुः स्वादुः सरो विड्वातकृद्यवः ।

वृष्यः स्थैर्यकरो मूत्रमेदःपित्तकफान् जयेत् ॥ २ ॥

पीनसश्वासकासोरुस्तम्भ[2]कंठासृगामयान् ।

*Yava* **(Hordeum vulgare Linn.)**

*Yava* is un-unctuous, cooling, heavy, sweet, laxative, producer of more of stool and flatus and aphrodisiac. It produces *sthairya* (steadiness) and reduces urine, fat, *pitta* and *kapha*. It cures *pīnasa* (chronic rhinitis), *śvāsa* (asthma), *kāsa* (bronchitis), *urustambha* (which produces immobility of thigh) and diseases of the throat and blood.

न्यूनो यवादनुयवो[3] रूक्षोष्णो वंशजो[4] **यव**: ।। ३ ।।

*Anuyava* & *Vaṁśaja yava*

The *anuyava* is slightly inferior in quality in comparison to *yava*. The *yava* (fruit) of *vaṁśa* (bamboo) is un-unctuous and hot.

[5]वृष्यशीतो गुरुः स्निग्धो जीवनो वातपित्तहा ।
[6]संधानकारी मधुरो **गोधूमः** स्थैर्यकृत्सरः ।।' ४ ।।

[माधवद्रव्यगुणः कुधान्यवर्ग १७ : २-५]

**Godhūma (Triticum aestivum Linn.)**

*Godhūma* (wheat) is aphrodisiac, cooling, heavy, unctuous and life giver. It alleviates *vāta* and *pitta*, and helps in the union of broken tissues. It is sweet. It produces steadiness. It is also a laxative.

गोधूम उक्तो मधुरो गुरुश्च बल्यः स्थिरः शुक्ररुचिप्रदश्च ।
स्निग्धो [शीतश्चा] निलपित्तहारी सवातकृत् [?] श्लेष्मकरः सरश्च ।।५।।

**Another view**

*Godhūma* is sweet, heavy, promoter of strength, steadiness and semen, appetiser, unctuous and cold. It alleviates *vāyu* and *pitta* and produces flatus (*vāta* ? ) and *kapha*. It is laxative.

'ईषत्कषायो मधुरः सतिक्तः संग्राहकः पित्तकरस्तथोष्णः ।
[7]तिलो विपाके मधुरो बलिष्ठ स्निग्धो व्रणालेपन पथ्य[8] उक्तः ।। ६ ।।
[9]दन्त्योऽग्निमेधाजननोऽल्पमूत्रस्त्वच्योऽथ केश्योऽनिलहा गुरुश्च ।

### *Tila* (Sesamum indicum Linn.)

*Tila* is slightly astringent, sweet, bitter, constipative, aggravator of *pitta*, hot, sweet in *vipāka*, promoter of strength and unctuous. It is useful for application over ulcers and for teeth. It is a promoter of digestive power and intellect. It reduces the quantity of urine. It is useful for the skin and the hair. It alleviates *vāyu* and is heavy.

तिलेषु सर्वेष्वसितः प्रधानो मध्यः सितो हीनतरास्तथान्ये[10] ॥ ७ ॥

[माधवद्रव्यगुणः कुधान्यवर्ग १७ : २-७], [सुश्रुतः सूत्र ४६ : ३९-४०]

Among the different types of *tila*, the black variety is the best, the white variety is middling and other varieties are inferior in quality.

**कृष्णमुद्गा महामुद्गा गौरा हरितपीतकाः ।**

**श्वेता रक्ताश्च** निर्दिष्टा लघवः पूर्वपूर्वतः ॥ ८ ॥

### *Mudga* (Phaseolus radiatus Linn.)

**Variety**

*Kṛṣṇa mudga*, *mahā mudga*, white, green, yellow, white and red—these are the different varieties of *mudga*. The former ones are lighter than the latter ones.

सुश्रुतेन पुनः प्रोक्ता प्रधाना हरिता गुणैः[11] ।

According to *Suśruta*, the green variety is the best among the *mudgas*.

कफपित्तास्रजिन्मुद्गः कषायो मधुरो लघुः ।

ग्राही शीतः कटुः पाके चक्षुष्यो नातिवातलः ॥ ९ ॥

**Property**

*Mudga* alleviates *kapha*, *pitta* and blood. It is astringent, sweet, light, constipative, cooling and pungent in *vipāka*. It promotes eye sight and does not aggravate *vāyu* in excess.

[12]
प्रधानाचरितास्तद्वद्वन्यमुद्गाः समाः स्मृताः ।

*Vanya mudga*

Different varieties of *vanya* (wild variety) *mudga* share all the properties of cultivated varieties of *mudga*.

[13] [14]
**मसूरो** मधुरो रुच्यः संग्राही कफपित्तहा ॥ १० ॥

*Masūra* **(Lens culinaris Medic.)**

*Masūra* is sweet, appetiser and constipative. It alleviates *kapha* and *pitta*.

[15]
रक्तपित्तज्वरोन्माथि शीतो ग्राही **मकुष्ठकः** ।

*Makuṣṭha* **(Phaseolus aconitifolius Jacq.)**

*Makuṣṭhaka* alleviates *rakta pitta* (a disease characterised by bleeding from different parts of the body) and *jvara* (fever). It is constipative.

कफासृक् पित्तपुंस्त्वघ्नाश्**चणका** वातला हिमाः ॥११॥
[माधवद्रव्यगुणः शिम्बिधान्यवर्ग १९-१-५]

*Caṇaka* **(Cicer arietinum Linn.)**

*Caṇaka* alleviates *kapha*, blood and *pitta*. It causes impotency and aggravates *vāyu*. It is cooling.

**हरेणवः** **सतीनाश्च** विज्ञेया बद्धवर्चसः ।
[सुश्रुतः सूत्र ४६ : ३३]

*Hareṇu* & *Satīna*
**(Pisum arvens Linn. & Pisum sativum Linn.)**

*Hareṇu* and *satīna* cause constipation.

[16] [17]
**आढक्य** कफपित्तघ्न्यः कषायाश्चातिवातलाः ॥ १२ ॥
ता एव घृतसंयुक्तास्त्रिदोषशमनाः मता ।

### *Āḍhakī* (Cajanus cajan Millsp.)

*Āḍhakī* alleviates *kapha* and *pitta*. It is astringent. It aggravates *vāyu* in excess. When added with ghee, it alleviates all the three *doṣas*.

उष्णः कुलत्थो रसतः कषायः कटुर्विपाके कफमारुतघ्नः ॥१३॥

### *Kulattha* (Dolichos biflorus Linn.)

*Kulattha* is hot, astringent in taste, pungent in *vipāka* and alleviator of *kapha* as well as *vāyu*.

[18] शुक्राश्मरीगुल्मनिषूदनश्च संग्राहकः पीनसकासहन्ता ।

आनाहमेदोगुदकीलहिक्काश्वासापहः [19] शोणितपित्तकृच्च ॥१४॥

It cures *śukrāśmarī* (stone in the seminal tract) and *gulma* (phantom tumour). It is constipative. It also cures *pīnasa* (chronic rhinitis), *kāsa* (bronchitis), *ānāha* (flatulence), *medas* (adiposity), *guda kīla* (piles), *hikkā* (hiccup) and *śvāsa* (asthma). It vitiates blood and *pitta*.

[20] बलासहन्ता पवनामयघ्नो विशेषतो वन्यकुलत्थकस्तु ।

### *Vanya Kulattha*

The wild variety of *kulattha* specifically alleviates *kapha* and cures diseases caused by *vāyu*.

स्निग्धोष्णो मधुरो वृष्यो मेदोमांसकफप्रदः ।

वातनुद् बृंहणो बल्यो माषो बहुमलो गुरुः ॥' १५ ॥

[माधवद्रव्यगुणः शिम्बिधान्यवर्ग १८ : १-६]

### *Māṣa* (Phaseolus mungo Linn.)

*Māṣa* is unctuous, hot, sweet and aphrodisiac. It produces more of fat, flesh and *kapha*. It alleviates *vāyu*, promotes nourishment and strength and produces more of stool. It is heavy.

21

'माषो गुरुर्भिन्नपुरीषमूत्रः स्निग्धो वृष्यो मधुरोऽनिलघ्नः ।

22

संतर्पणः स्तन्यकरो विशेषाद्बलप्रदः पित्तकफावहश्च ॥ १६ ॥

**Another view**

*Māṣa* is heavy, laxative, diuretic, unctuous, aphrodisiac, sweet, alleviator of *vāyu*, refreshing and promoter of lactation. It has the specific property of promoting strength and aggravating *pitta* as well as *kapha*.

माषैः समानं फल**मात्मगुप्तमुक्तं** च **काकाण्डफलं** तथैव च ।

The fruits of *ātmaguptā* and *kākāṇḍa* have properties similar to those of *māṣa*.

23

**अरण्यमाषा** गुणतः प्रदिष्टा रूक्षाः कषायाश्च विदाहिनश्च' ॥१७॥

[सुश्रुतः सूत्र ४६ : ३४, ३६]

*Araṇya māṣa*

The wild variety of *māṣa* is un-unctuous and astringent. It causes burning sensation.

**'राजमाषः** सरो रुच्यः कफशुक्राम्लपित्तनुत् ।

सुस्वादुर्वातलो रूक्षः कषायो विशदो गुरुः ॥ १८ ॥

*Rāja māṣa* **(Vigna cylindrica Skeels)**

*Rāja māṣa* is laxative and appetiser. It reduces *kapha* and semen, and cures *amla pitta* (hyper acidity in stomach). It is delicious, aggravator of *vāyu*, un-unctuous, astringent, *viśada* (non-slimy) and heavy.

गुरूष्णं स्निग्धमधुरं **काकाण्डं चात्मगुप्तजम्** ।

फलं वृष्यं च बल्यं च बृहणं वातजित्परम् ॥ १९ ॥

*Kākāṇḍa* (?) & *Ātmaguptā* **(Mucuna pruriens DC.)**

The fruits of *kākāṇḍa* and *ātma guptā* are heavy, hot,

unctuous, sweet, aphrodisiac, strength promoting and nourishing. They are excellent alleviators of *vāyu.*

स्निग्धा[24]**तसी**[25] स्वादुतिक्ता कफपित्तकरा गुरुः ।
दृक्शुक्रहृत्कटुः पाके तद्वद्बीजं **कुसुम्भजम्** ॥ २० ॥

*Atasī* **& *Kusumbha***
**(Linum usitatissimum Linn. & Carthamus tinctorius Linn.)**

*Atasī* is unctuous, sweet, bitter, aggravator of *kapha* as well as *pitta* and heavy. It reduces eye sight and semen. It is pungent in *vipāka.*

Seed of *kusumbha* shares properties of *atasī.*

वातपित्तकरा रूक्षा **निष्पावाः** श्लेष्मशोषणाः ।

*Niṣpāva* **(Dolichos lablab Linn.)**

Different types of *niṣpāva* are aggravaters of *vāyu* and *pitta* and un-unctuous. They dry up *kapha.*

बलघ्नाः[26] कफनाशिन्यो विरूक्षाः स्वादु शीतलाः ।
विष्टम्भिन्योऽग्निशमना निर्दिष्टाः **शिबिजातयः** ॥२१॥
[माधवद्रव्यगुणः शिम्बिधान्यवर्ग १८ : १०-१३]

*Śiṁbi* **(a type of Dolichos lablab Linn.)**

Different types of *śimbi* reduce strength and alleviate *kapha.* They are exceedingly un-unctuous, sweet, cooling and constipative. They reduce the power of digestion.

'रूक्षः कषायो बलकृद्विदाही बलासदृष्टिक्षयकृत्कषायः[27] ।
कटुर्विपाके मधुरश्च[28] **शिबः** प्रभिन्नविण्मारुतपित्तलश्च ॥२२॥

*Śiṁba* **(a type of Dolichos lablab Linn.)**

*Śiṁba* is un-unctuous, astringent and promoter of

strength. It causes burning sensation and reduces *kapha* and eye sight. It is pungent in *vipāka* and sweet. It eliminates stool as well as *vāyu* and aggravates *pitta.*

सितासिताः पीतकरक्तवर्णाः[29] भवन्ति येनैकरसाश्च[30] शिबाः ।
यथोदितास्तद्गुणतः[31] प्रधाना ज्ञेयाः कटूष्णा रसपाकतश्च[32] ।।२३।।'

[सुश्रुतः सूत्रस्थान ४६ : ४४-४६]

It has several varieties viz., white, black, yellow and red. They have different tastes but all of them share the properties described above. They are predominantly pungent in taste as well as *vipāka* and hot.

विदाहवन्त्यश्च भृशं[33] च रूक्षा विष्टंभ्यवीर्यमनिलप्रदाश्च[34] ।
सुदुर्जराश्चैवरुचिप्रदाश्च सर्वे[35] स्मृता वैदलिकाश्च शिबाः ।।२४।।

[सुश्रुतः सूत्रस्थान ४६ : ४७-४८]

अनलश्लेष्मपित्तघ्नो[36] बद्धविण्मूत्रवातलः ।

### *Vaidalikas* & *Siṁbas*

Pulses having dicotyledons and different type of *siṁba*—all produce burning sensation. They are exceedingly un-unctuous and constipative. They aggravate *vāyu* and are extremely difficult of digestion and are appetisers.

They reduce the power of digestion, alleviate *kapha* as well as *pitta* and cause retention of stool, urine and flatus.

'कफवातहरस्तीक्ष्णः **सिद्धार्थो** रक्तपित्तकृत् ।। २५ ।।
स्निग्धोष्णः क्रिमिकुष्ठघ्नः कटुको रसपाकतः ।

### *Siddhārtha*

*Śiddhārtha* alleviates *kapha* and *vāta*. It is sharp. It causes *raktapitta* (a disease characterised by bleeding from different parts of the body). It is unctuous and hot. It cures *kṛmi* (parasitic infection) and *kuṣṭha* (obstinate skin diseases including leprosy). It is pungent both in taste and *vipāka*.

तद्गुणा **राजिका** रुच्या तद्गुणोऽन्योऽपि **सर्षपः** ।।२६।।

*Rājikā* **&** *Sarṣapa* **(Brassica campestris Linn.)**

*Rājikā* and *sarṣapa* share the properties of *siddhārtha*. In addition *rājikā* is an appetiser.

शूकधान्यं शिंबिधान्यं [37] परिसंवत्सरोषितम् ।
लघुपथ्यतमं प्रोक्तं गुर्वपथ्यतमं नवम् ।
यद्यदागच्छति क्षिप्रं तत्तल्लघुतरं स्मृतम् ।। २७ ।।

**Property in preservation**

*Śūka dhānya* and *śiṁbī dhānya* which are preserved for one year before use, are the lightest and most wholesome. Freshly harvested ones are heavy and extremely unwholesome. The earlier they ripen, the lighter they are.

यवगोधूममाषाश्च तिलश्चापि नवा हिताः ।
पुराणा विरसा [38] रूक्षा न तथा बलकारिणः ।।' २८ ।।

[माधवद्रव्यगुणः शिम्बिधान्यवर्ग १८ : १४-१७]

*Yava*, *godhūma*, *māṣa* and *tila* are useful when they are freshly harvested. When preserved for a long time, they become tasteless and un-unctuous. They do not promote strength to the same extent as the fresh ones do.

विदाहि गुरु विष्टम्भि विरूढं दृष्टिदूषणम् ।

[माधवद्रव्यगुणः शिम्बिधान्यवर्ग १८ : १९]

**Other defects**

The germinated corns cause burning sensation. They are heavy and constipative. They cause impairment of eye sight.

अनार्त्तवं व्याधिकरमपर्यागतमेव च ॥ २९ ॥

अभूमिजं नवं वापि न धान्यं गुणवत्स्मृतम् ।

नवं धान्यमभिष्यन्दि लघु संवत्सरोषितम् ॥ ३० ॥

[माधवद्रव्यगुण: शिम्बिधान्यवर्ग १८ : १८-१९]

Unseasonal and immature corns cause many diseases. Those which are not grown on the ground and which are freshly harvested do not possess the prescribed properties. Freshly harvested corns are *abhiṣyandi* (which obstruct the channels of circulation) and they become light after preservation for one year.

॥ इति धान्यवर्गः ॥

Thus ends the group dealing with different type of corns.

## NOTES AND REFERENCES

1. तद्वच्च कंगुनीवारकोरदूषाः इति आकरे पाठः ।
2. पीनसश्वासकासोरुस्तम्भकंठत्वगामयान् इति आकरे पाठः ।
3. यवादपयवो इति आकरे पाठः ।
4. रुक्षोऽम्लो इति आकरे पाठः ।
5. वृष्यः शीतो इति आकरे पाठः ।
6. संधानो बृंहणो बल्यो गोधूमः स्थैर्यकृत्परम् इति आकरे पाठः
7. तिक्तो इति आकरे पाठः ।
8. एव पथ्यः इति आकरे पाठः ।
9. दन्योऽग्निमेधा इति द्वितीयपुस्तके पाठः ।
   बलाऽग्निमेधा० इति आकरे पाठः ।
10. हीनतरास्तथाऽन्ये इति आकरे पाठः ।
11. द्रष्टव्यम्—सुश्रुतः सूत्र ४६ : २९ ।
12. प्रधानाहृरिता मुद्गा वन्या मुद्गास्तु मुद्गवत् इति आकरे पाठः ।

13. मधुरः इति आकरे पाठः ।
14. शीतः इति आकरे पाठः ।
15. रक्तपित्तज्वरोन्माद शीतो इति आदर्शपुस्तिकासु पाठः ।
16. आढकी कफपित्तघ्नी कलायास्त्वतिवातलाः इति आकरे पाठः ।
17. कफवातघ्न्यः इति द्वितीयपुस्तके पाठः ।
18. शुक्राश्मरीगुल्मनिसूदनश्च इति आकरे पाठः ।
19. शोणितपित्तकर्त्ता इति आकरे पाठः ।
20. कफस्य हन्ता नयनामयघ्नो विशेषतो वन्यकुलत्थ उक्तः इति आकरे पाठः।
21. स्निग्धोष्णवृष्यो इति आकरे पाठः ।
22. शुक्रकफावहश्च इति आकरे पाठः ।
23. कषाया अविदाहिनश्च इति आकरे पाठः ।
24. स्निग्धोमा इति आकरे पाठः ।
25. स्वादुतिक्तोष्णा इति आकरे पाठः ।
26. वातघ्नाः कफशुक्रघ्नाः इति आकरे पाठः ।
27. रूक्षः कषायो विषशोषशुक्रबलासदृष्टिक्षयकृद्विदाही इति आकरे पाठः।
28. मधुरस्तु इति आकरे पाठः ।
29. पीतकरक्तवर्णा इति आकरे पाठः ।
30. येऽनेकविधास्तु इति आकरे पाठः ।
31. यथादितस्ते गुणतः इति आकरे पाठः ।
32. रसपाकयोश्च इति आकरे पाठः ।
33. विरूक्षा इति आकरे पाठः ।
34. विष्टभ्य जीर्यन्त्यनिलप्रदाश्च इति आकरे पाठः ।
35. वैदलिकास्तु इति आकरे पाठः ।
36. जोनलः श्लेष्मपित्तघ्नो इति द्वितीयपुस्तके पाठः ।
37. समातीतं प्रशस्यते इति आकरे पाठः ।
38. तथाऽर्थकराः स्मृताः इति आकरे पाठः ।

# CHAPTER 17

सर्ववातहरं **मांसं** वृष्यं बल्यतमं गुरु ।

तद्रसस्तर्पणो बल्यः स्निग्धः प्राणप्रदो लघुः ।

**Meat**

All types of meat alleviate *vāyu.* They are aphrodisiac, exceedingly strength promoting and heavy. Meat soup is refreshing, strength promoting, unctuous, life giver (*prāṇa prada*) and light.

मांसवर्गो द्विधाज्ञेयो जांगलानूपभेदतः ॥ १ ॥

There are two groups of *māṁsa* (meat) viz., meat of *jāṅgala* animals and the meat of *ānūpa* animals.

**तत्र जांगललक्षणगुणाः**

**जङ्घालं**[1] मांसवर्गेऽत्र [**वि**[2]]लस्थाश्च **गुहाशयाः** ।

तथा **पर्णभृता ज्ञेया विष्किराः प्रतुदा** अपि ॥ २ ॥

[**प्रसहा**[3]**ऽप्यथ च**] **ग्राम्या अष्टौ** जाङ्गलजातयः ।

### *Jāṅgala* (Meat of animals dwelling in dry land forests)

*Jāṅgala* is of eight categories viz., (1) *jaṅghāla*, (2) *vilastha*, (3) *guhāśaya*, (4) *parṇa mṛga*, (5) *viṣkira*, (6) *pratuda*, (7) *prasaha* and (8) *grāmya*.

जांगला मधुरा रूक्षास्तुवरा लघवस्तथा ॥ ३ ॥

बल्या वृष्या बृंहणाश्च दीपना दोषहारिणः ।

मूकतां मिन्मिनत्वं च गद्गदत्वार्दिते तथा ॥ ४ ॥

वाधिर्यमशुचिं च्छर्दि प्रमेहं मुखजान्गदान् ।

गलगण्डं श्लीपदं च नाशयत्यनिलामयान् ॥ ५ ॥

Meat of this variety is sweet, un-unctuous, astringent, light, strength promoting, aphrodisiac, nourishing and digestive stimulant. It alleviates *doṣas* and cures *mūkatā* (dumbness), *minminatva* (stammering), *gadgadatva* (lulling speech), *ardita* (facial paralysis), *vādhirya* (deafness), *aśuci* (sense of impurity), *chardi* (vomiting), *prameha* (obstinate urinary disorders including diabetes), *mukharoga* (diseases of the oral cavity), *gala gaṇḍa* (goitre), *ślīpada* (filariasis) and diseases caused by *vāyu*.

कूलेचराः[4] प्लवाश्चापि कोशस्थाः[5] पादिनस्तथा ।

मत्स्या एतत्ते विख्याताः पञ्चधानूपजातयः ॥ ६ ॥

### *Ānūpa* (Meat of animals inhabiting marshy land)

*Ānūpa* is of five categories viz., (1) *kūlecara*, (2) *plava*, (3) *kośastha*, (4) *pādin* and (5) *matsya*.

आनूपाः मधुराः स्निग्धाः गुरवो वह्निसादनाः ।

श्लेष्मलाः पिच्छिलाश्चैव मांसवृद्धिप्रदाः परम् ।

प्रायोऽभिष्यन्दिनस्ते हि प्रायो[ऽ]पथ्यतमाः मताः ॥७॥

Meat of this variety is sweet, unctuous, heavy, suppresser of the power of digestion, alleviator of *kapha* and slimy. It increases muscle tissue considerably. It is generally *abhiṣyandin* (which obstructs the channels of circulation) and unwholesome.

**अथ जांगललक्षणम्, विशिष्टगुणा :**

**हरिणैणकुरंगार्क्षवातायुमृगमातृकाः** ।
**राजीवः पृषतश्चापि**[6] **श्वदंष्ट्रः शरभादयः** ॥ ८ ॥
**जङ्घालसं**ज्ञिताः एते तेषां चिह्नं पृथक् शृणु ।
**हरिण**स्ताम्र उद्दिष्टः **एणः** कृष्णतनुर्मतः ॥ ९ ॥
**कुरंग**स्ताम्रवर्णः स्याद्धरिणाकृतिको महान् ।
**ऋष्यो** नीलांडुको लोके सरोरु इति भण्यते ॥ १० ॥
**वातायुस्तु** किशोराभो मृगः स्वल्पः प्रकीर्तितः ।
स्वल्पः पृथूदरो ज्ञेयः[7] शशाभो **मृगमातृकः** ॥ ११ ॥
**कस्तूरीहरिणं** चैके वदंति मृगमातृकम् ।
**राजीवस्तु** मृगो ज्ञेयो राजीभिः परितो वृतः ॥ १२ ॥
**पृषत**श्चन्द्रविन्दुः स्याद्धरिणात्किञ्चिदल्पकः ।
**श्वदंष्ट्रः** सम्मतो यस्तु काश्मीरे कर्कटाभिधः ॥ १३ ॥
काश्मीरदेशे **शरभो**ऽष्टपात्स्यादुत्साहयुक्तश्चतुरूर्ध्वपादः ।
उष्ट्रप्रमाणः समहाविषाणः ख्यातो नवस्थः स महामृगाख्यः ॥ १४ ॥

**Different types of *Jāṅgala* meat**

*Hariṇa*, *eṇa*, *kuraṅga*, *ṛkṣa*, *vātāyu*, *mṛga mātṛkā*, *rājīva*, *pṛṣat*, *śvadaṁṣṭra*, *śarabha*—these animals are called *jaṅghāla*. Their characteristic features are given below:

*Hariṇa* is of coppery colour. *Eṇa* has a black body.

*Kuraṅga* is of coppery colour. It looks like *hariṇa* but it is bigger in size. *Ṛṣya* (*ṛkṣa*) is commonly called *nīlāṇḍuka* or *saroru*. *Vātāyu* is like a deer calf and it is small in size. *Mṛga mātṛka* is like a rabbit. It is small in size and it has a bulging abdomen. Some people, however, take musk deer as *mṛga mātṛka*. *Rājīva* has a spotted body. *Pṛṣat* is dotted like the moon in its body and it looks like a *hariṇa* of small size. *Śvadaṁṣṭra* is called *karkaṭa* in Kashmir. *Śarabha* is found in Kashmir. It has eight legs, four of which are upwards. It is like a camel in size and it has big horns. This animal, which is also known as *mahā mṛga* is locally called *navastha* (?).

**‘कृतमालो वप्रचुरः विश्रुतो विन्दुचित्रकः[8] ।’**

‘जांगलाः[9] प्रायशः सर्वे[10] पित्तश्लेष्महरा मताः[11] ॥ १५ ॥
किञ्चिद्वातकरा[12] ज्ञेया लघवो बलवर्धनाः ।

*Kṛtamāla*, *vapracura*, *viśruta* and *vindu citraka*—these animals also come under the *jaṅghāla* category.

The meat of all these animals generally alleviates *pitta* and *kapha*. It slightly aggravates *vāyu*. It is light and promoter of strength,

**गोधाशशभुजंगाखुशल्लक्याद्या[13] विलेशयाः ॥ १६ ॥**

*Vileśaya* **(Meat of animals which live in burrows in the earth)**

*Godhā*, *śaśa*, *bhujaṅga*, *ākhu*, *śallaki* etc., are called *vileśaya* animals.

बिलेशया वातहरा मधुरा रसपाकयोः ।
बृंहणा बद्धविण्मूत्राः[14] वीर्योष्णाश्च प्रकीर्तिताः ॥ १७ ॥

The meat of these animals alleviates *vāyu*. It is sweet both in taste and *vipāka*. It is nourishing and it causes retention of stool and urine. It is hot in potency.

[15]सिंहव्याघ्रवृकाक्षर्क्षतरक्षु[16]द्वीपिनस्तथा ।

बभ्रुजम्बुकमार्जारा इत्याद्या स्युर्गुहाशयाः ॥ १८ ॥'

[भावप्रकाशः मांसवर्ग ११ : १४-१६]

### *Guhāśaya* (Meat of animals that dwell in caves)

*Simha, vyāghra, vṛka, akṣa, ṛkṣa, tarakṣu, dvīpin, babhru, jambuka, mārjāra* etc., are called *guhāśaya* animals.

तरक्षुः हडहा इति लोके । द्वीपिः चित्रः व्याघ्रः ।

स्थुलपुच्छो रक्तनेत्रो बभ्रुभेदः स नकुलः ॥ १९ ॥

*Tarakṣu* is commonly known as *haḍahā*. *Dvīpin* is the tiger with a spotted body. A variety of *babhru* which has a thick tail and red eyes is called *nakula*.

'गुहाशया वातहरा गुरूष्णा मधुराश्च ते ।

स्निग्धा बल्या हिता नित्यं नेत्रगुह्यविकारिणाम् ।

The meat of these animals alleviates *vāyu*. It is heavy, hot, sweet, unctuous and promoter of strength. It is always wholesome for patients suffering from the diseases of the eye and the anus.

[17]वनौका वृक्षमार्जारवृक्षमर्कटिकाऽऽदयः ॥ २० ॥'

[भावप्रकाशः मांसवर्ग ११ : १७-१८]

'स्मृताः पर्णमृगा वृष्याश्चक्षुष्याः शोणिते हिताः ।

श्वास।र्शः कासशमनाः सृष्टमूत्रपुरीषकाः ॥२१॥'

[भावप्रकाशः मांसवर्ग ११ : १९]

### *Parṇa mṛga*

***Vanaukā, vṛkṣa mārjāra, vṛkṣa markatikā*** etc., are called ***parṇa mṛga*** animals.

The meat of these animals is aphrodisiac, promoter of eye sight and useful in the correction of the vitiation of blood. It cures *śvāsa* (asthma), *arśas* (piles) and *kāsa* (bronchitis). It helps in the elimination of urine and stool.

**वर्तिकालावविकिरकपिंजलकतित्तिराः[18]** ।
**चकोरक्रकराद्याश्च[19] विष्किराः** समुदाहृताः ॥ २२ ॥

### *Viṣkira* (Meat of gallinacious birds)

*Vartikā, lāva, vikira, kapiñjalaka tittira, cakora, krakara,* etc., are called *viṣkira* animals.

विकीर्य भक्षयन्त्येते यस्मात्तस्माद्धि विष्किराः ।

They eat by tearing (*vikīrya*) the food because of which they are called *viṣkira.*

कपिंजल इति ख्यातो[20] लोके **कपिशतित्तिरः** ।

[भावप्रकाशः मांसवर्ग ११ : २०-२१]

चकोरः प्रसिद्धः । क्रकरः कथर इति लोके ॥ २३ ॥

The gray coloured *tittira* (*kapiśa tittira*) is called *kapiñjala. Cakora* is a well known bird. *Krakara* is locally called *kathara.*

'विष्किरा मधुराः शीता कषायाः कटुपाकिनः ।
बल्या वृष्यास्त्रिदोषघ्नाः[21] पथ्याश्च लघवो मताः ॥२४॥'

[भावप्रकाशः मांसवर्ग ११ : २२]

The meat of these animals is sweet, cooling, astringent in taste, pungent in *vipāka,* strength promoting and aphrodisiac. It alleviates all the three *doṣas.* It is wholesome and light.

**'कालकंठकहारीतकपोतशतपत्रकाः** ।
**सारिका[22] खंजरीटश्च** पिकाद्या **प्रतुदा मताः** ।

*Pratuda* **(Meat of packer birds)**

*Kālakaṇṭhaka, hārīta, kapota, śatapatra, sārikā, khañjariṭa, pika* etc., are called *pratuda* animals.

[23] प्रत्युद्य भक्षयन्त्येते तुण्डेन प्रतुदास्ततः ॥ २५ ॥'

[भावप्रकाशः मांसवर्ग ११ : २३]

They eat by picking (*pratudya*) the food because of which they are called *pratuda*.

कालकंठकगौडादौ गौरै अडागके इति प्रसिद्धः ॥२६॥

In the country of *gauḍa*, *kālakaṇṭhaka* is popularly called *gaurai* and *aḍāgake*.

हारीता हारिला इति लोके ॥ २७ ॥

*Hāritā* is called *hārilā* in the local vernacular.

कपोतो धवलः पाण्डु शतपत्रो बृहच्छुकः ।

*Kapota* is white and yellowish (*pāṇḍu*). *Śatapatra* is the bigger variety of *śuka*.

'प्रतुदा मधुराः पित्तकफघ्नास्तुवरा हिमाः ।
लघवो बद्धवर्चस्का किञ्चिद्वातप्रकोपनाः[24] ॥ २८ ॥

The meat of these animals is sweet. It alleviates *pitta* and *kapha*. It is astringent, cooling and light. It causes retention of stool and it slightly aggravates *vāyu*.

काको गृध्र उलूकाश्च चिल्लुश्च[25] शशघातिनः[26] ।

चाषो भासश्च कुरर इत्याद्याः प्रसहाः स्मृताः ॥२९॥'

[भावप्रकाशः मांसवर्ग ११ : २३-२५]

*Prasaha* **(Meat of animals & birds who eat by snatching)**

*Kāka, gṛdhra, ulūka, cillu, śaśaghātin, cāṣa, bhāṣa, kurara* etc., are called *prasaha* animals.

'प्रसहाः कीर्तिता एते प्रसह्यान्नाद्यभक्षणाः[27] ।

These animals eat by snatching (*prasahya*) their food because of which they are called *prasaha*.

वीर्योष्णाः[28] प्रसहाः सर्वे तन्मांसं चाहरन्ति ये ॥ ३० ॥'

[भावप्रकाशः मांसवर्ग ११ : २६-२७]

ते शोषभस्मकोन्मादरेतक्षीणा[29] भवन्ति हि ।

The meat of all these animals is hot in potency. Persons who eat their meat suffer from *śoṣa* (consumption), *bhasmaka* (gluttonous appetite), *unmāda* (insanity) and reduction in semen.

**छागमेषवृषाश्वाद्या[30] ग्राम्याः** प्रोक्ता महर्षिभिः ॥३१॥

## *Grāmya* (Meat of domesticated animals)

*Chāga, meṣa, vṛṣa, aśva* etc., are called *grāmya* animals by the great sages.

ग्राम्या[31] वातहराः सर्वे दीपनाः कफपित्तलाः ।

मधुरा रसपाकाभ्यां बृंहणा बलवर्धनाः ॥३२॥

The meat of all these animals alleviates *vāyu*, stimulates digestion and aggravates *kapha* and *pitta*. It is sweet both in taste and *vipāka*, nourishing and strength promoting.

**लुलायगण्डवाराहचमरीवारणादयः** ।

एते **कूलेचराः**[32] प्रोक्ता यस्मात् कूले चरन्त्यपाम् ॥३३॥

## *Kūlecara* (Meat of animals who live near water)

*Lulāya, gaṇḍa, vārāha, camarī, vāraṇa,* etc., are called *kūlecara* animals.

These animals graze (reside) by the side of water (*kūla*) because of which they are called *kūlecara*.

लुलायो महिषः। गण्डः खड्गः। चमरी चमरपुच्छो गौः ॥३४॥

*Lulāya is mahiṣa* (buffalo), *gaṇḍa* is ***Khaḍga*** (rhinoceros) and *camarī* is a *type of cow* having a chowrie tail.

कुलेचरा मरुत्पित्तहरा वृष्या बलावहाः ।
मधुराः शीतलाः स्निग्धाः मूत्रलाः श्लेष्मवर्धनाः ॥३५॥

The meat of *kūlecara* animals like *lalāya*, *mahiṣa*, ***gaṇḍa***, *khadga*, *camarī*, *camara puccha* and *go* alleviate *vāyu* **and** ***pitta***. It is aphrodisiac, promoter of strength, sweet, cooling, unctuous and diuretic. It aggravates *kapha*.

**[33] हंससारसकाचाक्षबककौञ्चससारिकाः ।**
**नंदीमुखी सकादम्ब बलाकाद्याः प्लवा** मताः[34] ।
[35] प्लवन्ते सलिले यस्मादेते तस्मात्प्लवाः स्मृता ॥३६॥

*Plava* **(Meat of animals who swim in water)**

*Haṁsa*, *sārasa*, *kācākṣa*, *baka*, *krauñca*, *sasārikā*, ***nandī*** *mukhī*, *kādamba*, *balākā* etc., are called *plava* animals.

काचाक्षः[36] कर्दिकाक्षो[37] बृहद्बकः[38] । क्रौञ्चः शरद्विहङ्ग[39] स्यात् टेंक
इति लोके । ससरिका[40] सिंधु[41] इति लोके ॥ ३७ ॥

*Kācākṣa* is also known as *karditākṣa or bṛhadbaka*. *Krauñca* is also called *śarad vihaṅga* and in folk language it is called *teṅka*. *Sasārikā* is called *sindhu* in folk language.

स्थूला कठोरा वृत्ता च यस्याश्चञ्चूपरिस्थिता ।
गुटिका[42] जम्बु सदृशी ज्ञेया[43] नन्दीमुखीति सा ॥ ३८ ॥
कादंबः[44] कयंवा इति लोके । बलाका लघुवकः[45] बगुली इति लोके ॥३९॥

*Nandī mukhi* has, above its bill, a projection which is big in size, hard to touch and round in shape. *Kādamba* is called

*Kayaṁbā* in folk lore. *Balākā* is the small variety of *vaka*, which in folk lore is called *bagulī*.

प्लवाः पित्तहराः स्निग्धाः मधुरा गुरवो हिमाः ।
वातश्लेष्मप्रदाश्चैव[46] बलशुक्रकराः सराः ॥ ४० ॥

The meat of these animals alleviates *pitta*. It is unctuous, sweet, heavy and cooling. It aggravates *vāyu* and *kapha* and promotes strength as well as semen. It is laxative.

शशक[47]विणकश्चैव शुक्तिशंबूकभल्लुकाः ।
जीवा[48]श्चैवंविधाः सर्वे कोशस्थाः परिकीर्तिताः ॥४१॥

*Kośastha* **(Meat of animals that dwell in shells)**

*Śaśaka, viṇaka, śukti, śaṁbūka, bhalluka* etc., are called *kośastha* animals.

कोशस्थाः मधुराः स्निग्धा पित्तवातहरा हिमाः ।
बृंहणा[49]श्च तथा वृष्याः वर्चस्याः कफवर्धनाः ॥ ४२ ॥

The meat of these animals is sweet, unctuous, alleviator of *pitta* as well as *vāyu*, cooling, nourishing and aphrodisiac. It increases the quantity of stool and *kapha*.

कुम्भीरकूर्मनक्राश्च कर्कटः[50] कृष्णकर्कटः ।
घण्टिका[51] शिशुमारश्चेत्यादयः पादिनः स्मृताः ॥ ४३ ॥

*Pādin*

*Kumbhīra, kūrma, nakra, karkaṭa, kṛṣṇa karkaṭa, ghaṇṭikā, śiśumāra* etc., are called *pādin* animals.

कुम्भीरो[52] जलजन्तु विशेषः । कूर्म[53] कच्छप इति लोके ।
नक्रः[54] नाक इति लोके शरंघादि नद्यां बहुलः ॥ ४४ ॥

[55] ‘कर्कटः कंकडा इति लोके । कृष्णकर्कटस्तद्भेदः[56] । घंटिका

घडियाल इति लोके । शिशुमारः सूसि इति लोके ॥ ४५ ॥

*Kumbhīra* is a type of aquatic animal. *Kūrma* is known as *kacchapa* in folk lore. *Nakra* is called *nāka* in folk lore; they are found in large numbers in rivers like *Saranghā*. *Karkaṭa* is known as *keṁkaḍā* in the folk language. *Kṛṣṇa karkaṭa* is a variety of *karkata*. *Śiśumāra* is called *sūsi* in the folk lore.

पादिनोऽपि च ये ते तु कोशस्थानां गुणैः समाः’।’

[भावप्रकाशः मांसवर्ग ११ : २७-३७]

The meat of these animals shares the properties of the meat of *kośastha* animals.

‘**रोहिताद्यास्तु** ये जीवास्ते **मत्स्याः** परिकीर्त्तिताः ।

*Matsya* (**fish**)

Living creatures like *rohita* etc., are called *matsya* (fish).

मत्स्याः स्निग्धोष्णमधुरा गुरवः कफपित्तलाः ॥४६॥

[भावप्रकाशः मांसवर्ग ११ : ३८]

बल्याभिष्यन्दिनो वृष्याः बृंहणाः पवनापहाः ।

व्यवायाध्वरतानां च दीप्ताग्नीनां च पूजिताः ॥४७॥

Fish is unctuous, hot, sweet and heavy. It aggravates *kapha* and *pitta* and promotes strength. It is *abhiṣyandi* (which obstructs the channels of circulation), aphrodisiac, nourishing and alleviator of *vāyu*. It is useful for those indulging in sex and walking and for those who have a strong power of digestion.

**अथ जांगलादीनां कतिपयानां विशिष्टानां गुणा :**

‘**हरिणः** शीतलो बद्धविण्मूत्रो दीपनो लघुः ।

रसेपाके च मधुरः[57] सुगन्धि सन्निपातहा ॥ ४८ ॥

**Property of the meat of individual animals**

### *Hariṇa* (Red deer)

The meat of *hariṇa* is cooling. It causes retention of the stool and urine. It is digestive stimulant and light. In taste and *vipāka* it is sweet. It has a good smell and it alleviates all the three *doṣas*.

[58] कषायो मधुरो हृद्यः पित्तासृक्कफवातजित् ।
संग्राही रोचनो [59] "बल्यस्तेषामेणो ज्वरापहः ॥ ४६ ॥'
[भावप्रकाशः मांसवर्ग ११ : ४१-४२]

### *Eṇa* (Black buck)

The meat of *eṇa* is astringent, sweet and a cardiac tonic. It alleviates *pitta*, blood, *kapha* and *vāta*. It is constipative and appetiser. It cures fever.

मधुरो मधुरः पाके दोषघ्नोऽनलदीपनः ।
'पृषतस्तु भवेत्स्वादु [60] ग्राहकः शीतलो लघुः ।
दीपनो रोचनः" [61] श्वासज्वरदोषत्रयास्रजित् ॥ ५० ॥'
[भावप्रकाशः मांसवर्ग ११ : ४५]

### *Pṛṣat* (Spotted deer)

The meat of *pṛṣat* is sweet both in taste and *vipāka*. It alleviates *doṣas* and is digestive stimulant. It is delicious, constipative, cooling and light. It is an appetiser. It cures *śvāsa* (asthma) and *jvara* (fever). It alleviates all the three *doṣas* as well as the vitiated blood.

'मुण्डिनी ज्वरकासास्रक्षयश्वासापहा हिमा ।'

### *Muṇḍinī*

The meat of *muṇḍinī* cures *jvara* (fever), *kāsa* (bronchitis), vitiation of blood, *kṣaya* (consumption) and *śvāsa* (asthma). It is cooling.

'न्यङ्कुः स्वादुर्लघुर्बल्यो वृष्यो दोषत्रयापहः ॥५१॥'

[भावप्रकाशः मांसवर्ग ११ : ४६]

### *Nyaṅku* (Antelope)

The meat of *nyaṅku* is sweet, light, strength promoting and aphrodisiac. It alleviates all three *doṣas*.

ऋष्यस्तु मधुरो वृष्यः स्निग्धोष्णः कफपित्तलः ।

### *Ṛṣya*

The meat of *ṛṣya* is sweet, aphrodisiac, unctuous and hot. It aggravates *kapha* and *pitta*.

'शशः शीतो लघुर्ग्राही रूक्षः स्वादु सदा हितः ॥५२॥

62

वह्निकृत्कफपित्तघ्नो वातसाधारणः स्मृतः ।

63

ज्वरातिसारशोषास्रश्वसनार्शोहरश्च सः ।

### *Śaśa* (Hare)

The meat of *śaśa* is light, constipative, un-unctuous, sweet and always wholesome. It stimulates digestion and alleviates *kapha* as well as *pitta*. It is neutral for *vāyu*. It cures *jvara* (fever), *atisāra* (diarrhoea), *śoṣa* (consumption), vitiation of blood, *śvasana* (asthma) and *arśas* (piles).

शल्यकः श्वासकासास्रशोषदोषत्रयापहः ॥' ५३ ॥

[भावप्रकाशः मांसवर्ग ११ : ५०-५१]

॥ गुहाशयाः ॥

### *Śalyaka*

The meat of *śalyaka* cures *śvāsa* (asthma), *kāsa* (bronchitis), vitiation of blood and *śoṣa* (consumption). It alleviates all the three *doṣas*.

64

'लावा विष्किरवर्गे स्युस्ते चतुर्धा मता बुधैः ।

[65]**पांसुलो** [66]**गौरकाश्चापि पौण्ड्रको दर्भरस्तथा** ॥' ५४ ॥

[भावप्रकाशः मांसवर्ग ११ : ५४-५५]

## *Lāva* (Common quail)

*Lāva*, which is included in the *viṣkira* group, is of four types viz., (1) *pāṁsula*, (2) *gauraka*, (3) *pauṇḍraka* and (4) *darbhara*.

[67]'लावा हृद्या हिमा स्निग्धा ग्राहिणो वह्निदीपनाः' ।

The meat of *lāva* in general is a cardiac tonic, cooling, unctuous, constipative and digestive stimulant.

[68]**पांशुलः** श्लेष्मलस्तेषां वीर्योष्णानिलनाशनः ॥ ५५ ॥

The meat of the *pāṁśula* type of *lāva* aggravates *kapha*. It is hot in potency. It alleviates *vāta*.

**गौरो** लघुतरो रूक्षो वह्निकारी त्रिदोषजित् ।

The meat of the *gaura* type of *lāva* is lighter, un-unctuous and stimulant of digestion. It alleviates all the three *doṣas*.

**पौण्ड्रकः** पित्तकृत्किञ्चिल्लघुर्वातकफापहः ॥ ५६ ॥

The meat of *pauṇḍraka* type of *lāva* aggravates *pitta*. It is slightly light. It alleviates *vāyu* and *kapha*.

**दर्भरो** रक्तपित्तघ्नो हृदामयहरो हिमः ।

The meat of *darbhara* type of *lāva* cures *rakta pitta* (a disease characterised by bleeding from different parts of the body) and *hṛdāmaya* (heart disease). It is cooling.

[69]**वर्त्तीको** मधुरः शीतो [70]**रूक्षश्च** कफपित्तनुत् ॥ ५७ ॥

[भावप्रकाशः मांसवर्ग ११ : ५६-५७, ५८]

### *Vartika* (Gray partridge)

The meat of *vartika* is sweet, cooling and un-unctuous. It alleviates *kapha* and *pitta*.

[71] '**चटकः** शीतलः स्निग्धो स्वादुः शुक्रकफप्रदः ।

### *Caṭaka* (Tree sparrow)

The meat of *caṭaka* is cooling, unctuous and sweet. It increases semen and *kapha*.

सन्निपातहरो **वेश्मचटक**स्त्वतिशुक्रलः ॥ ५८ ॥'

[भावप्रकाशः मांसवर्ग ११ : ६१]

### *Veśma caṭaka* (House sparrow)

The meat of *veśma caṭaka* alleviates *sannipāta* (a condition caused by the vitiation of all the three *doṣas*). It increases semen in excess.

**वर्तको**ऽग्निधमः [?] शीतो ज्वरदोषत्रयापहः ।

सुरुच्यः शुक्रदो बल्यो [72] **वर्तिका**ल्पगुणा ततः ॥ ५९ ॥

### *Vartaka* and *Vartikā* (Male bustard and female bustard)

The meat of *vartaka* is cooling. It cures *jvara* and alleviates all three *doṣas*. It is delicious and promoter of semen as well as strength.

The meat of *vartikā* is slightly inferior in quality.

[73] '**तित्तिरि**र्वर्णदो ग्राही हिक्कादोषत्रयापहः ।

[74] श्वासकासहरः पथ्यस्तमा**द्गौरो**ऽधिको गुणैः ॥' ६० ॥

[भावप्रकाशः मांसवर्ग ११ : ५९]

### *Tittiri* (Partridge) & *Gaura*

The meat of *tittiri* promotes complexion. It is constipative. It cures *hikkā* (hiccup). It alleviates all the three *doṣas.* It cures *śvāsa* (asthma) and *kāsa* (bronchitis). It is wholesome.

The meat of *gaura* is better in quality.

**‘कुक्कुटो** बृंहणः स्निग्धो वीर्योष्णोऽ[75]निलजिद्गुरुः ।
चक्षुष्यः शुक्रकफकृत् बल्यो वृष्यः[76] कषायकः ॥ ६१ ॥

### *Kukkuṭa* (Cock)

The meat of *kukkuṭa* is nourishing, unctuous, hot in potency, alleviator of *vāyu* and heavy. It promotes eyesight. It increases semen and *kapha.* It is strength promoting, aphrodisiac and astringent.

**पानीयकुक्कुटः**[77] स्निग्धो बृंहणः श्लेष्मलो गुरुः ।
वातपित्तक्षय[78]कृमीविषमज्वरनाशनः ॥ ६२ ॥

### *Pānīya Kukkuṭa* (Water cock)

The meat of *pānīya kukkuṭa* is unctuous, nourishing, aggravator of *kapha*, heavy and alleviator of *vāyu* and *pitta.* It cures *kṣaya* (consumption), *kṛmi* (parasitic infection) and *viṣama jvara* (irregular fever).

**अथ प्रतुदाः**

**हारीतः**[79] उष्णो रूक्षश्च रक्तपित्तकफापहः ।
स्वेद[80]स्वरकरः प्रोक्त ईषद्वातकरश्च सः ॥ ६३ ॥'

[भावप्रकाशः मांसवर्ग ११ : ६३-६५]

### *Hārita*

The meat of *hārita* is hot and un-unctuous. It alleviates

vitiation of blood, *pitta* and *kapha*. It promotes sweating and good voice. It slightly aggravates *vāyu*.

**पाण्डुकः** कफवातघ्नो ग्रहणीदोषनाशनः ।
रक्तपित्तहरः शीतो मधुरो रसपाकयोः ॥ ६४ ॥

*Pāṇḍuka*

The meat of *pāṇḍuka* alleviates *kapha* and *vāyu*. It cures *grahaṇī doṣa* (sprue syndrome), *rakta pitta* (a disease characterised by bleeding from different parts of the body). It is cooling and sweet both in taste and *vipāka*.

संग्राही वातशमनः **कपोतः** परिकीर्त्तितः ।
कपोत इति विज्ञेयो लोके धवलपाण्डुकः ।

*Kapota* **(Dove)**

The meat of *kapota* is constipative and alleviator of *vāyu*. This bird is white and yellowish in colour.

'**पारावतो** गुरु स्निग्धो रक्तपित्तानिलापहः ॥' ६५ ॥

[भावप्रकाशः मांसवर्ग ११ : ७१]

संग्राही शुक्रलः शीतः कपोतोऽपि समोऽमुना ।

*Pārāvata* **(Pigeon)**

The meat of *pārāvata* is heavy and unctuous. It cures *rakta pitta* (a disease characterised by bleeding from different parts of the body) and vitiation of *vāyu*. It is constipative, promoter of semen and cooling. It shares the properties of *kapota*.

'नातिस्निग्धानि बृष्याणि स्वादुपाकरसानि च ।'

81

वातघ्नान्यतिशुक्राणि गुरुण्यण्डानि पक्षिणाम्' ॥६६॥

[भानप्रकाशः मांसवर्ग ११ : ७२]

## Egg

Eggs of birds are not very unctuous. They are aphrodisiac, sweet in *vipāka* and taste, alleviator of *vāyu*, promoter of semen in excess and heavy.

**अथ ग्राम्याः**

'छागमांसं लघु स्निग्धं स्वादुपाकं त्रिदोषजित्[82] ।
नातिशीतमदाहित्वात्[83] स्वादु पीनसनाशनम् ॥ ६७ ॥
परं बलकरं रुच्यं बृंहणं धातुवर्द्धनम्[84] ।

### *Chāga* (Goat)

The meat of the goat is light, unctuous, sweet in *vipāka* and alleviator of all the three *doṣas*. It is not very cold and it does not cause burning sensation. It is sweet. It cures *pīnasa* (chronic rhinitis). It is an excellent promoter of strength. It is appetiser and nourishing. It promotes tissue elements.

अजायास्तु[85] प्रसूताया मांसं पीनसनाशनम् ॥ ६८ ॥
शुष्ककासेऽरुचौ शोथे[86] हितमग्नेश्च दीपनम् ।

The meat of a recently delivered she-goat cures *pīnasa* (chronic rhinitis). It is useful in *śuṣka kāsa* (dry cough), *aruci* (anorexia) and *śotha* (oedema). It stimulates the power of digestion.

अजासुतस्य बालस्य मांसं लघुतरं भवेत्[87] ॥ ६९ ॥
हृद्यं[88] ज्वरहरं श्रेष्ठं सुस्वादु[89] बलदं भृशम् ।

The meat of a male calf of the goat is lighter. It is cardiac tonic. It is an excellent curative of *jvara* (fever). It is exceedingly delicious and promoter of strength.

मांसं निष्कासिताण्डस्य[90] छागस्य कफकृद्गुरु ॥ ७० ॥

स्रोतःशुद्धिकरं बल्यं मांसदं वातपित्तनुत् ।

The meat of the castrated goat aggravates *kapha*. It is heavy. It cleanses the channels of circulation. It promotes strength and muscle tissue. It alleviates *vāyu* and *pitta*.

91

वृद्धस्य वातलं रूक्षं व्याधितस्य मृतस्य च ।

The meat of an old-goat aggravates *vāyu*. It is unctuous. The meat of diseased and dead goat shares these properties also.

ऊर्ध्वजत्रुविकारघ्नं **छागमुंडं** रुचिप्रदम् ॥' ७१ ।

[भावप्रकाशः मांसवर्ग ११ : ७४-७६]

The meat from the head of the goat cures diseases of head and neck and is delicious.

92

**मेषस्य** बृंहणं मांसं पित्तश्लेष्मकरं गुरु ।

*Meṣa* **(Sheep)**

The meat of the sheep is nourishing. It aggravates *pitta* and *kapha*. It is heavy.

93

ततो वृषणहीनस्य मांसं किञ्चिल्लघु स्मृतम् ॥ ७२ ॥

The meat of a castrated sheep is slightly lighter.

मेदः [?] पुच्छोद्भवं मांसं हृद्यं वृष्यं श्रमापहम् ।

पित्तश्लेष्मकरं किंचिद्वातव्याधिविनाशनम् ॥ ७३ ॥'

[भावप्रकाशः मांसवर्ग ११ : ८१, ८३]

The fat and the meat of the tail of the sheep are cardiac tonic, aphrodisiac and alleviator of fatigue. They aggravate *pitta* and *kapha* and alleviate to some extent diseases caused by *vāyu*.

94

**गोमांसं** गुर्वपथ्यं च पित्तश्लेष्मविवर्धनम् ।

स्निग्धं वातहरं बल्यं बृहणं पीनसं प्रणुत् ॥ ७४ ॥

*Go* **(Cow)**

Beef is heavy and unwholesome. It aggravates *pitta* and *kapha.* It is unctuous, alleviator of *vāyu*, strength promoting and nourishing. It cures *pīnasa* (chronic rhinitis).

95

'**अश्वमांसं** सलवणं वह्निकृत्कफपित्तलम् ।

वातहृद्बृंहणं बल्यं चक्षुष्यं मधुरं लघु ॥ ७५ ॥'

[भावप्रकाशः मांसवर्ग ११ : ८७]

*Aśva* **(Horse)**

The meat of the horse is saline and stimulant of the power of digestion. It aggravates *kapha* and *pitta.* It alleviates *vāyu.* It is nourishing, promoter of strength as well as eye sight, sweet and light.

**अथ कुलेचराः**

**माहिषं** मधुरं मांसं स्निग्धोष्णं वातनाशनम् ।

निद्रारेतोबलस्तन्यतनुदीर्घकरं लघु (?) ॥ ७६ ॥

*Mahiṣa* **(Buffalo)**

The meat of the buffalo is sweet, unctuous, hot and alleviator of *vāyu.* It increases sleep, semen, strength, lactation and size of the body. It is light (?).

**अथ प्लवाः**

96

'**कादंबकं चक्रांगं** च मांसं स्निग्धं हिमं गुरु ।

वृष्यं च सृष्टविण्मूत्रं वातपित्तास्रनाशनम् ॥ ७७ ॥'

[भावप्रकाशः मांसवर्ग ११ : ९०]

### *Kadambaka* and *Cakrāṅga*

The meat of *kadambaka* and *cakrāṅga* is unctuous, cooling, heavy and aphrodisiac. It helps in the elimination of stool and urine. It alleviates *vāyu*, *pitta* and vitiation of blood.

**अथ कोशस्थाः**

'**कच्छपो** बलदो वातपित्तजित्पुंस्त्वकारकः [97] ।'

[भावप्रकाशः मांसवर्ग ११ : ६२]

### *Kacchapa* (Tortise)

The meat of *kacchapa* is promoter of strength. It alleviates *vāyu* and *pitta* and promotes potency.

विरूक्षणो लेखनश्च वीर्यौजःपित्तदूषणः ॥ ७८ ॥

स्वाद्वम्ललवणस्तेषां **गज**श्लेष्मानिलापहः ।

### *Gaja* (Elephant)

The meat of *gaja* is un-unctuous and depleting. It vitiates semen, *ojas* and *pitta*. It is sweet, sour and saline. It alleviates *kapha* and *vāyu*.

'स्नेहनं बृंहणं वृष्यं [98] ''श्रमघ्नमनिलापहम् ।

**वाराहं** [99] पिशितं बल्यं रोचनं स्वाददं गुरु ॥ ७९ ॥'

[माधवद्रव्यगुणः मांसवर्ग १९ : ११-१२]

### *Varāha* (Hog)

The meat of *varāha* is unctuous, nourishing, aphrodisiac, alleviator of fatigue and *vāyu*, promoter of strength, appetiser, delicious and heavy.

**स्निग्धं** समधुरं वृष्यं'' गुर्वभिष्यन्दि शीतलम् ।

वातपित्तहरं **हृद्यं सौकरं चर्मचित्रितम्** ॥ ८० ॥

### *Carmacitrita sukara*

The meat of *sukara* who has a spotted skin is unctuous, sweet, aphrodisiac, heavy, *abhiṣyandi* (which obstructs the channels of circulation), cooling, alleviator of *vāyu* as well as *pitta* and cardiac tonic.

'कफघ्नं **खड्गि**पिशितं कषायमनिलापहम् ।
पित्र्यं पवित्रमायुष्यं बद्धमूत्रं विरूक्षणम् ॥ ८१ ॥'

[माधवद्रव्यगुणः मांसवर्ग १९ : १२-१३]

### *Khaḍga* (Rhinoceros)

The meat of *khaḍga* alleviates *kapha*. It is astringent and alleviator of *vāyu*. It is *pitrya* (liked by *pitṛs* or dead ancestors), sacred and promoter of longevity. It causes retention of urine and is un-unctuous.

[100]'**बर्ही** हिततमो बल्यो वातघ्नो मांसशुक्रदः ।'

[माधवद्रव्यगुणः मांसवर्ग १९ : १७]

### *Barhī* (Peacock)

The meat of *barhī* is most wholesome. It promotes strength, alleviates *vāyu* and increases muscle tissue as well as semen.

[101]'कषायमधुराः शीता रक्तपित्तनिबर्हणाः ॥ ८२ ॥
विपाके मधुराश्चैव [102]**कपोताः गृहवासिनः** ।

### *Kapota* (Dove ?)

The meat of various types of *kapota* residing in houses is astringent and sweet in taste and cooling. It cures *rakta pitta* (a disease characterised by bleeding from different parts of the body). It is sweet in *vipāka*.

तेभ्यो लघुतराः किंचित् **कपोताः वनवासिनः** ॥ ८३ ॥

शीताः संग्राहिणश्चैव स्वल्पमूत्रकराश्च ते ।

The meat of those residing in forests is slightly lighter. It is cooling and constipative. It produces less of urine.

किञ्चिल्लघुतरा रूक्षा ग्राहिणः श्लेष्मपित्तलाः ।

हितास्ते पाण्डु चित्रांगा हारीता वनवासिनः ॥८४॥'

[माधवद्रव्यगुणः मांसवर्ग १९ : १९-२२]

The meat of *kapotas* which are yellowish, spotted or green in colour and which reside in the forests, is slightly lighter, un-unctuous and constipative. It aggravates *kapha* and *pitta*, and it is wholesome.

103

'**चक्षुष्या मधुराः पाके सर्पा मेधकराः स्मृताः ।**

### *Sarpa* (Snake)

The meat of *sarpa* is promoter of eye sight, sweet in *vipāka* and promoter of intellect.

**दर्वीकरा दीप्यकाश्च** तेषूक्ताः कटुपाकिनः ॥ ८५ ॥

मधुरात्यर्थचक्षुष्याः सृष्टविण्मूत्रमारुताः ।

Of them, *darvīkara* and *dīpyaka* are pungent in *vipāka*. They are sweet in taste and excellent promoter of eye sight. They help in the elimination of stool, urine and flatus.

104

**शंखकूर्मा**दयः स्वादुरसपाका बलावहाः ॥ ८६ ॥

105 106

शीताः स्निग्धा हिताः पित्ते चक्षुष्याः शुक्रवर्द्धनाः ।

### *Śaṅkha*, *Kūrma* etc., (Conch shell, tortoise etc.)

The meat of *śaṅkha*, *kūrma* etc., is sweet both in taste and in *vipāka*. It is strength promoting, cooling, unctuous, useful for *pitta* and promoter of eye sight as well as semen.

**कृष्णकर्कटक**स्तेषां बल्यः कोष्णोऽनिलापहः ।

107
शुक्रसंधानकृत्सृष्टविण्मूत्रोऽनिलपित्तहा ॥ ८७ ॥'

[माधवद्रव्यगुणः मांसवर्ग १९ : २७-३०]

*Kṛṣṇa Karkaṭa* **(Block crab)**

The meat of the black variety of *karkaṭa* is strength promoting and slightly hot. It alleviates *vāyu.* It promotes semen and healing. It helps in the elimination of stool and urine. It alleviates *vāyu* and *pitta*.

**'हंसो** वातहरो वृष्यो स्वर्यो मांसबलप्रदः ।

*Haṁsa* **(Swan)**

**The meat of *haṁsa* alleviates *vāyu.* It is aphrodisiac. It is promoter of good voice, muscle tissue and strength.**

108
**चक्रवाकस्तथाठेंकश्चटको** वातनाशनः ॥ ८८ ॥

*Cakravāka, Theṅka* **and** *Caṭaka*

The meat of *cakravāka, ṭheṅka* and *caṭaka* alleviates *vāyu.*

109
**सारिकाबककादम्बलावकाः** पवनापहाः ।

स्निग्धाः सृष्टमेला वृष्या रक्तपित्तहरा हिमाः ॥८९॥'

*Sārikā, Baka, Kadamba* **and** *Lāvaka* **(Shama thrush, Common crane, Whistling teal & Common quail)**

The meat of *sārikā, baka, kadamba* and *lāva* alleviates *vāyu.* It is unctuous. It helps in the elimination of stool. It is aphrodisiac. It cures *rakta pitta* (a disease characterised by bleeding from different parts of the body). It is cooling.

कासश्वासक्षयहरी **गोधा** मधुरशीतला ।

*Godhā* **(Inguana)**

The meat of *godhā* cures *kāsa* (bronchitis), *śvāsa* (asthma) and *kṣaya* (consumption). It is sweet and cooling.

110

मूषको मधुरः स्निग्धो कफशुक्रविवर्द्धनः ।

दुर्नामानिलदोषघ्नः कृमिदूषीविषापहः ॥ ९० ॥'

[माधवद्रव्यगुणः मांसवर्ग १९ : २४-२७]

*Mūṣaka* **(Mouse)**

The meat of ***mūṣaka*** is sweet and unctuous. It increases ***kapha*** and semen. It cures *durnāman* (piles), aggravation of *vāyu*, ***kṛmi*** (parasitic infection) and *dūṣī viṣa* (artificial poisoning).

रोचनं बृंहणं चारुकरीरैः सह जांगलम् ।

रक्तपित्तविसर्पे च कुष्ठे मेहे विषे हितम् ॥ ९१ ॥

**Combinations**

Along with *cāru karira*, the meat of *jāṅgala* type of animals is appetiser and nourishing. It cures *raktapitta* (a disease characterised by bleeding from different parts of the body), *visarpa* (erysipelas), *kuṣṭha* (obstinate skin diseases including leprosy), *meha* (obstinate urinary disorders including diabetes) and *viṣa* (poisoning).

रोचनं दीपनं हृद्यं घंटोलैः सह जांगलम् ।

Along with *ghaṇṭola*, the meat of *jāṅgala* type of animals works as appetiser, digestive stimulant and cardiac tonic.

111

'वातश्लेष्मविकारघ्नं दीपनं चानुलोमनं ॥ ९२ ॥

ह्लादनीयं विशेषेण वीताग्नेः सह जांगलं ।'

Along with *vītāgni*, the meat of *jāṅgala* type of animals cures diseases caused by *vāyu* and *kapha*. It is digestive stimulant and laxative. It is very delicious.

शुष्कमूलकसंसिद्धं मांसं यक्ष्महरं नृणाम् ॥ ९३ ॥

The meat prepared with dry radish cures *yakṣmā* (tuberculosis).

स्नेहनं दीपनं हृद्यं मांसं दधिकमुच्यते ।

The meat prepared with curd is unctuous, digestive stimulant and cardiac tonic.

बल्यं स्वर्यं च चक्षुष्यं ताडोगैः सह साधितम् ॥६४॥

The meat prepared with *tāḍoga* promotes strength, good voice and eyesight.

'दूरे[112] जलान्तनिलया दूरे पानीयगोचराः ।
ये मृगाश्च विहंगाश्च[113] तेऽल्पाभिष्यन्दिनो मताः ॥६५॥
अतीव[114] ते बलीयांसः समीपोदकगोचराः ।
ये मृगाश्च विहंगाश्च महाभिष्यन्दिनो मताः ॥६६॥

**Habitat**

The meat of animals and birds residing and grazing far away from water is less *abhiṣyandi* (which obstructs the channels of circulation). The meat of animals which graze near water is an excellent promoter of strength. Such animals and birds are extremely *abhiṣyandi* (which obstructs the channels of circulation).

॥ इति मांसवर्गः ॥

Thus ends the group dealing with various types of meat.

## NOTES AND REFERENCES

1. जंगला इति षष्ठपुस्तके पाठः ।
2. चिलस्थाश्च इति द्वितीयपुस्तके पाठः ।

3. प्रमहा अप्पथ इति षष्ठपुस्तके पाठः ।
सहा अथ च इति द्वितीयपुस्तके पाठः ।
4. अथानूपाः इति षष्ठपुस्तके अधिको पाठः ।
5. पल्वाद्यश्च इति षष्ठपुस्तके पाठः ।
6. राजीवतृषतश्चापि इति द्वितीयपुस्तके पाठः ।
7. शषाभों इति द्वितीयपुस्तके पाठः ।
8. "कृत........चित्रकः" पाठोऽयं द्वितीयपुस्तके नोपलभ्यते ।
9. जाङ्गलाः इति आकरे पाठः ।
10. सत्वपित्तश्लेष्महरा इति षष्ठपुस्तके पाठः ।
11. स्मृताः इति आकरे पाठः ।
12. किञ्चिद्वाकराश्चापि इति आकरे पाठः ।
13. गोधाशशभुजंगाखुसल्लक्याद्या इति आकरे पाठः ।
14. बद्धविण्मूत्रा इति आकरे पाठः ।
15. सिहव्याघ्रवृका ऋक्षतरक्षुद्वीपिनस्तथा इति आकरे पाठः ।
16. द्विपिनस्तथा इति षष्ठपुस्तके पाठः ।
17. "वनौको वृक्षमार्जारो वृक्षमर्कटिका रुखी इति लोके" इति आदर्शपुस्तके पाठः ।
18. वर्त्तका लाववर्त्तीरकपिञ्जलकतित्तिराः इति आकरे पाठः ।
19. कुलिङ्गकुक्कुटाद्याश्च इति आकरे पाठः ।
20. प्राज्ञैः कथितो गौरतित्तिरिः इति आकरे पाठः ।
21. पथ्यास्ते लचवः स्मृताः इति आकरे पाठः ।
22. पारावतः खञ्जरीटः पिकाद्याः प्रतुदाः स्मृताः इति आकरे पाठः ।
23. प्रतुद्य इति आकरे पाठः ।
24. किञ्चिद्वातकराः स्मृताः इति आकरे पाठः ।
25. चिल्लश्च इति आकरे पाठः ।
26. शशघातकः इति आकरे पाठः ।
27. प्रसह्याच्छिद्य भक्षणात् इते ति आकरे पाठः ।
28. प्रसहाः खलु वीर्योष्णास्तन्मांसं भक्षयन्ति ते इति आकरे पाठः ।
29. शोषभस्मकोत्साद इति आदर्शपुस्तकेषु पाठः ।
30. छागमेषबृषाद्याश्वाः इति द्वितीयपुस्तके पाठः ।
31. ग्राम्यासु वातला इति षष्ठपुस्तके पाठः ।

32. यतः इति आकरे पाठः ।
33. हंससारसकारण्डवकक्रौञ्चशरारिकाः आकरे पाठः ।
34. स्मृताः इति आकरे पाठः ।
35. प्लवन्ति इति आकरे पाठ ।
36. कारण्ड इति आकरे पाठः ।
37. कपर्दिकाख्यो इति आकरे पाठः ।
38. बृहद्धंसभेदः इति आकरे पाठः ।
39. धारवि इति षष्ठपुस्तके पाठः ।
40. शरारिका इति आकरे पाठः ।
41. सिन्धू इति आकरे पाठः ।
42. चञ्चुसदृशी इति आदर्शपुस्तकेषु पाठः ।
43. प्रोक्त इति आकरे पाठः ।
44. करवा इति आकरे पाठः ।
45. पाठोऽयं आकरे नोपलभ्यते ।
46. वातश्लेष्मप्रदाश्चापि इति आकरे पाठः ।
47. शङ्खःनखश्चापि शुक्तिशम्बूककर्कटाः इति आकरे पाठः ।
48. जीवा एवं विधाश्चान्ये कोशस्याः परिकीर्त्तिता इति आकरे पाठः ।
49. बृंहणा बहुवर्चस्का वृष्याश्च बलबर्द्धनाः इति आकरे पाठः ।
50. गोधामकरशङ्कवः इति आकरे पाठः ।
51. घण्टिकः इति आकरे पाठः ।
52. मारको जलजन्तुः इति आकरे पाठः ।
53. कासव इति आदर्शपुस्तकेषु पाठः ।
54. सरय्वादिनदीषु इति आकरे पाठः ।
55. "कर्कटः........स्तद्भेदः" पाठोऽयं आकरे नोपलभ्यते ।
56. सूस इति आकरे पाठः ।
57. सुगन्धिः इति आकरे पाठः ।
58. एणः कषायो मधुरः पित्तासृक्कफवातहृत् इति आकरे पाठः ।
59. बल्यो ज्वरप्रशमनः स्मृतः इति आकरे पाठः ।
60. भवेत्स्वादुर्ग्राहकः इति आकरे पाठः ।
61. "बल्य········रोचकः" पाठोऽयं षष्ठपुस्तके नोपलभ्यते ।
62. वातसाधारणैः इति आकरे पाठः ।

63. ज्वरातीसारशोषास्रश्वासामयहरश्च सः इति आकरे पाठः ।
64. विष्किरवर्गेषु ते इति आकरे पाठः ।
65. पांशुलो इति आकरे वा षष्ठपुस्तकयोः पाठः ।
66. गौरकोऽन्यस्तु इति आकरे पाठः ।
67. लावा वह्निकराः स्निग्धागरघ्ना ग्राहका हिताः इति आकरे पाठः ।
68. श्लेष्मलस्तेषु वीर्योष्णोऽनिलनाशनः इति आकरे पाठः ।
69. लावका इति षष्ठपुस्तके पाठः ।
70. कफपित्तकृत् इति आकरे पाठः ।
71. कुलिङ्गः इति आकरे पाठः ।
72. मतः इति षष्ठपुस्तके पाठः ।
73. तित्तिरोर्वर्णदो इति षष्ठपुस्तके पाठः ।
तित्तिरिर्बलदो इति आकरे पाठः ।
74. श्वासकासज्वरहरस्तस्माद्गौरोऽधिको गुणैः इति आकरे पाठः ।
75. वीर्योष्णेऽनिलहृद्गुरुः इति आकरे पाठः ।
76. रुक्षः इति आदर्शपुस्तकेषु पाठः ।
77. आरण्यकुक्कुटः इति आकरे पाठः ।
पानीयकुक्कुटः स्निग्धो वीर्योष्णोऽनिलजित् इति षष्ठपुस्तके पाठः ।
78. वातपित्तक्षयवमिविषमज्वरनाशनः इति आकरे पाठः ।
79. हारीतो रूक्ष उष्णश्च इति आकरे पाठः ।
80. स्वेदः स्वरकरः इति आदर्शपुस्तकेषु पाठः ।
81. शुक्राणि इति आकरे पाठः ।
82. त्रिदोषनुत् इति आकरे पाठः ।
83. अदाहिस्यात्स्वादु इति आकरे पाठः ।
महाहिस्या स्वादु इति द्वितीयपुस्तके पाठः ।
84. वीर्यबर्द्धनम् इति आकरे पाठः ।
85. अजायास्त्वप्रसूताया इति आकरे पाठः ।
86. शोषे इति आकरे पाठः ।
87. स्मृतम् इति आकरे पाठः ।
88. लघुतरं इति आदर्शपुस्तकेषु पाठः ।
89. सुखदं बलदं इति आकरे पाठः ।
90. निष्काशिताण्डस्य इति आदर्शपुस्तकेषु पाठः ।

91. तथा व्याधिमृतस्य च इति आकरे पाठः ।
92. मांसं पुष्टौ स्थात्पित्तश्लेष्मकरं गुरु इति आकरे पाठः ।
93. तस्यैवाण्डविहीनस्य इति आकरे पाठः ।
94. गुणपथ्यं इति षष्ठपुस्तके पाठः ।
95. अश्वमांसन्तु तुवरं इति आकरे पाठः ।
96. कदंवक चाक्रारि मासं इति आकरे पाठः ।
97. वातपित्तनुत्पुंस्त्वकारकः इति आकरे पाठः ।
98. श्रमघ्नमनिलापहम्.......वृष्यं पाठोऽयं द्वितीयपुस्तके नोपलभ्यते ।
99. स्वेदनं रोचनं गुरु इति आकरे पाठः ।
100. वह्ने: इति षष्ठपुस्तके पाठः ।
वह्नी इति द्वितीयपुस्तके पाठः ।
101. कषाया मधुराः शीताः इति आकरे पाठः ।
102. कपोता इति आकरे पाठः ।
103. सर्पाः मेधाग्निवर्द्धनाः इति आकरे पाठः ।
104. शंखाः कूर्मादयः इति आकरे पाठः ।
105. हिता इति आकरे पाठः ।
106. शुक्रवर्धना इति आकरे च द्वितीयपुस्तके पाठः ।
107. शुक्र्यः संधानकृत् इति आकरे पाठः ।
108. "चक्र ......वातनाशनः" पाठोऽयं आकरे नोपलभ्यते ।
109. सारिकाकाककादम्बबलाकाः इति आकरे पाठः ।
110. व्यवायी शुक्रवर्धनः इति आकरे पाठः ।
कफशुक्रविवर्धनः इति द्वितीयपुस्तके पाठः ।
111. "वातश्लेष्मविकारघ्नं......सहजांगलं" पाठोऽयं द्वितीयपुस्तके नोपलभ्यते ।
112. जनान्तनिलयाद् दूरे इति आकरे पाठः ।
113. बलाभिष्यंदिनो इति आकरे पाठः ।
114. अतीवासन्ननिलयाः इति आकरे पाठः ।

# CHAPTER 18

स्निग्धोष्णाः[1] स्वादुगुरवः सृष्टविण्मूत्रमारुताः ।
महाभिष्यन्दिनो वृष्याः[2] बल्या वातहराः परम् ॥ १ ॥

### *Matsya* (**Fish**)

Fish is unctuous, hot, sweet and heavy. It helps in the elimination of stool, urine and flatus. It is aphrodisiac. It promotes strength and alleviates *vāyu.*

कफपित्तकरा[3] मत्स्याः[4] बलोपचयवर्द्धनाः[5] ।
व्यायामाध्वरतानां च दीप्ताग्नीनां च पूजिताः ॥२॥

It aggravates *kapha* and *pitta* and promotes strength as well as plumpness. It is exceedingly useful for persons who indulge in exercise and walk in excess and also for those who have a strong power of digestion.

कषायानुरसः स्वादुर्वातघ्नो नातिपित्तकृत् ।
**रोहितः** सर्वमत्स्यानां वरो वृष्योर्दितार्तिजित्[6] ॥ ३ ॥

### *Rohita*

*Rohita* fish is astringent in *anurasa* (subsidiary taste) and sweet. It alleviates *vāyu* and does not aggravate *pitta* in excess. It is the best among all the types of fish. It is aphrodisiac and it cures *ardita* (facial paralysis).

कषायमधुरो रूक्षो विशदो रोचनो लघुः ।
ग्राही तु नन्दिकावर्त्तस्तस्यानु शकुलः स्मृतः ॥ ४ ॥
[माधवद्रव्यगुण : मत्स्यवर्ग २० : १-४]

### *Nandikāvarta* and *Śakula*

*Nandikāvarta* fish is astringent, sweet, un-unctuous, *viśada* (non-slimy), appetiser, light and constipative.

The *śakula* type of fish is slightly inferior.

'पाठीनः[7] श्लेष्मलो[8] वृष्यो निद्रालुः पिशिताशिनः ।
दूषयेद्रक्तपित्तं[9] च कुष्ठरोगं करोत्यसौ ॥ ५ ॥'
[भावप्रकाशः मत्स्याः मांसवर्ग ११ : १०९]

### *Pāṭhīna*

The *pāṭhīna* fish aggravates *kapha* and is aphrodisiac. It resorts to sleep in excess and eats the meat of other animals. It causes *raktapitta* (a disease characterised by bleeding from different parts of the body) and *kuṣṭha* (obstinate skin diseases including leprosy).

'श्रृंगी समुद्गरः[10] शंकु गोमत्स्यालित्रिकण्टकाः ।
कंटकैः सविषा ज्ञेया भक्ष्यमाणास्तु निर्विषा ॥ ६ ॥

### *Śṛṅgī* etc.

*Śṛṅgī*, *madgura*, *śaṅku*, *gomatsya*, *āli* and *trikaṇṭaka*—all these type of fish have spikes. These spikes are poisonous. But the fish when eaten is non-poisonous.

**भृङ्गी** तु वातशमनी स्निग्धा श्लेष्मप्रकोपिणी ।
[11]कषायाः तिक्तभावाच्च तेभ्यो लघुतरास्मृताः ॥ ७ ॥

*Śṛṅgī*

*Śṛṅgī* fish alleviates *vāyu.* It is unctuous, aggravator of *kapha*, astringent and bitter. Therefore, it is lighter than others in this group.

विपाके मधुरो वृष्यो वातघ्नो **मद्गुरो** गुरुः ।

*Madgura*

The *madgura* fish is sweet in *vipāka*. It is aphrodisiac, alleviator of *vāyu* and heavy.

**कृष्णमत्स्यो** गुरुः स्निग्धो वातजित् श्लेष्मकोपनः ॥८॥'

[माधवद्रव्यगुणः मत्स्यवर्ग २० : ५-७]

*Kṛṣṇa matsya*

*Kṛṣṇa matsya* is heavy and un-unctuous. It alleviates *vāyu* and aggravates *kapha.*

[12]'**अलिर्मत्स्यो** गुरुः स्निग्धो कटुको रूक्ष [?] एव च ।

*Ali*

The *ali* fish is heavy, unctuous and pungent.

[13]**पृयुर्मत्स्यो** गुरुस्निग्धश्लेष्मलो वातनाशनः ॥ ९ ॥

*Pṛyu*

The *pṛyu* type of fish is heavy and unctuous. It aggravates *kapha* and alleviates *vāyu.*

[14]**इल्लिशो** मधुरः स्निग्धः पित्तकृत् श्लेष्मकोपनः ।
**नृणां व्यवायनित्यानां** [15]हितोऽग्नेरतिवर्धनः ।

*Illiśa*

The *illiśa* type of fish is sweet and unctuous. It aggravates *pitta* as well as *kapha.* It is useful for persons who indulge in sex in excess. It excessively stimulates the power of digestion.

16
**बलंग**: स्निग्धमधुरो विष्टंभी लघु शीतलः ॥ १० ॥'

[माधवद्रव्यगुणः मत्स्यवर्ग २० : ८-१०]

*Balaṅga*

The *balaṅga* type of fish is unctuous, sweet, wind forming, light and cooling.

**प्रोष्टिका** मधुरा वृष्या महती वातनाशिनी ।

*Proṣṭikā*

The *proṣṭikā* type of fish is sweet and aphrodisiac. It is an excellent alleviator of *vāyu.*

17
**नंदीवर्तो** गुरुः स्निग्धो वातजित्श्लेष्मवर्द्धनः ॥११॥

कषायमधुरः प्रोक्तस्तद्गुणो **दीर्घतुण्डकः** ।

*Nandīvarta* **and** *Dīrgha tuṇḍaka*

The *nandīvarta* type of fish is heavy and unctuous. It alleviates *vāyu* and aggravates *kapha.* It is astringent and sweet.

The *dīrgha tuṇḍaka* type of fish shares the properties of *nandīvarta.*

**भास्करो** मधुरो रूक्षो मारुतस्य प्रकोपनः ॥ १२ ॥

*Bhāskara*

The *bhāskara* type of fish is sweet and un-unctuous. It aggravates *vāyu.*

**शकुलो** गुरु रूक्षोऽथ मारुतस्य प्रकोपनः ।

*Śakula*

The *śakula* type of fish is heavy and un-unctuous. It aggravates *vāyu*.

**शैलीन्धुः** श्लेष्मलो वृष्यो विपाके मधुरो गुरुः ॥१३॥

*Sailīndhu*

The *sailīndhu* type of fish is aggravator of *kapha*, aphrodisiac, sweet in *vipāka* and heavy.

**गर्गभो** मधुरः स्निग्धो वातजित् श्लेष्मकोपनः ।

*Gargabha*

The *gargabha* type of fish is sweet and unctuous. It alleviates *vāyu* and aggravates *kapha*.

**इंवाकस्त्व**नभिष्यन्दि तेषां पीनसनाशनः ॥ १४ ॥

*Iṁvāka*

The *iṁvāka* type of fish does not obstruct the channels of circulation and it cures *pīnasa* (chronic rhinitis).

अनभिष्यन्दि मधुरा **इंबिका** रसवर्धिनी ।

*Iṁbikā*

The *iṁbikā* type of fish does not obstruct the channels of circulation. It is sweet and it increases plasma.

लघवः **क्षुद्रमत्स्यास्तु** ग्राहिणो ग्रहणीहिताः ॥ १५ ॥

**Small fish**

Different types of small fish are light and constipative. They are useful in *grahaṇī* (sprue syndrome).

**मत्स्यकूर्मखगाण्डानि** स्वादु बाजीकराणि च ।

### Eggs

The eggs of fish, tortoise and birds are sweet and aphrodisiac.

समत्स्यगर्भः खगाण्डः स्निग्धः स्थौल्यकरो गुरुः ।

'कफमेदःप्रदो बल्यो ग्लानिकृन्मेहनाशनः ॥ १६ ॥'

[भावप्रकाशः मांसवर्ग ११ : १२५]

If the egg of birds is prepared along with egg of fish, then it becomes unctuous, promoter of corpulence and heavy. It increases *kapha* and fat, promotes strength, produces fatigue and cures *meha* (obstinate urinary disorders including diabetes).

विष्टंभिनः **शुष्कमत्स्या** अबल्या दुर्जरामताः ।

### Dry fish

The dry fish produces wind in the colon. It does not promote strength and it is difficult of digestion.

**पूतिमत्स्या** अभक्षाः स्युः सर्वदोषप्रकोपणाः ।

### Putrified fish

The fish which is putrified should not be eaten. It aggravates all the *doṣas*.

18
'**दग्धमत्स्यो** गुणैः श्रेष्ठः पुष्टिकृद्बलवर्द्धनः ॥ १७ ॥'

[भावप्रकाशः मांसवर्ग ११ : १२७]

### Burnt fish

The burnt fish is excellent in property. It is nourishing and strength promoting.

19
'**नादेया** मधुरा मत्स्या गुरवो मारुतापहाः ।

रक्तपित्तहराः सोष्णा वृष्या स्निग्धाल्पवर्चसः ।

कषायानुरसस्तेषां शष्पशैवालभोजनः ॥ १८ ॥'

[सुश्रुतः सूत्रस्थान ४६ : ११४-११५]

**River fish**

The fish collected from river is sweet and heavy. It alleviates *vāyu* and cures *rakta pitta* (a disease characterised by bleeding from different parts of the body). It is hot, aphrodisiac and unctuous. It produces less of stool. It is astringent in *anurasa* (subsidiary taste). The river fish feed on grass and moss.

'**सरस्तडागसंभूताः** स्निग्धाः स्वादुरसाः स्मृताः ।'

[सुश्रुतः सूत्रस्थान ४६ : ११७]

**Pond fish**

The fish collected from big and small ponds is unctuous and sweet in taste.

**सामुद्राः** गुरवः स्निग्धा मधुरा नातिपित्तला ॥ १९ ॥

20

उष्णा वातहरा वृष्याः वर्चस्याः शुक्रवर्धनाः ।

बलावहा विशेषेण मांसाशित्वात्समुद्रजाः ॥ २० ॥

**Sea fish**

The fish collected from sea is heavy, unctuous and sweet. It does not aggravate *pitta* in excess. It is hot, alleviator of *vāyu* and aphrodisiac. It increases stool and semen. It is an excellent promoter of strength because the sea fish feed on the meat of other animals.

समुद्रजेभ्यो नादेया बृंहणास्तद्गुणोत्तराः ।

In comparison to sea fish, the river fish is more nourishing and better in quality.

तेभ्योऽतीवानिलघ्नत्वा**च्चौण्डयकौप्यौ** गुणोत्तरौ ।

स्निग्धत्वात्स्वादुपाकत्वात्तयोर्वाप्या गुणोत्तराः ॥२१॥

[सुश्रुतः सूत्र ४६ : ११९-१२१]

**Well fish**

The fish of *cuṇḍa* (a big well without boundary wall) and well is better than the sea fish and river fish because the former is a strong alleviator of *vāyu.* The fish of *vāpi* (a big well with a boundary wall and a stair case) is better than the fish of *cuṇḍa* and *kūpa* because the former is unctuous and sweet in *vipāka.*

'हेमन्ते कूपजा मत्स्याः शिशिरे सारसाः हिताः ।'

[भावप्रकाशः मांसवर्ग ११ : १२९]

मधौ नदीभवाः श्रेष्ठाः ग्रीष्मे ह्रदसमुद्भवाः ।

तडागजाता वर्षासु पथ्याः शरदि नैर्झराः ॥ २२ ॥

**Fish in different seasons**

In *hemanta* (early winter), fish from a well is useful and in *śiśira* (later part of winter) fish from big ponds is useful. In the spring season, river fish is most useful and in summer season, fish collected from lake is useful. In rainy season, fish collected from small ponds is wholesome and in autumn, fish from springs is useful.

नादेया गुरवो मध्ये यस्मात्पुच्छास्य चारिणः ।

सरस्तडागजानां तु विशेषेण शिरो गुरुः ॥ २३ ॥

**Different parts of fish**

The river fish is heavy in the middle of its body because it moves with the help of the tail and the mouth. In the case of fish from the big and small ponds, the head is heavy.

21

अदूरगोचराम्भस्थास्तेभ्यो दोषवहाः स्मृताः ।

किंचिन्मुक्त्वा शिरोदेशमत्यर्थं गुरवस्तु ते ॥ २४ ॥

The fish which does not travel long distances inside the

water is harmful. Leaving a small portion behind the head, this fish is very heavy.

> अधस्ताद्गुरवो ज्ञेया मत्स्याः सरसि[22] संभवाः ।
> उरोविचरणं[23] तेषां पूर्वमंगं लघु स्मृतम् ॥ २५ ॥
> [सुश्रुतः सूत्रस्थान ४६ : १२२-१२४]

The lower part of the pond fish is heavy. Because it moves through the help of its chest, its front portion is light.

> 'महाप्रमाणगुरवः[24] क्रियावद्भ्योऽल्पचेष्टिनः ।
> युवभ्यः[25] स्थविरा ये स्युः स्त्रीभ्यश्च[26] पुरुषाश्च ये ॥२६॥
> मृदुभ्यः[27] स्थिरगात्राश्च खेचरेभ्यश्च[28] भूचराः ।
> गुरुरूक्षा[29] बहुभुजो ये चोपचितमेदसः ॥ २७ ॥'
> [माधवद्रव्यगुणः मत्स्यवर्ग २० : १२-१३]

**Heaviness**

The fish of a big size is generally heavy. In comparison to the fish which is very active, the one with a sluggish movement is heavy. In comparison to the young ones, the old fish is heavier. The male fish is heavier than the female. In comparison to the fish having a soft body, the one having a compact body is heavier. In comparison to the birds .which move in the sky, the animals which move on the ground are heavier. Those which feed on heavy and on un-unctuous articles in large quantities and those having accumulated fat are heavier.

> विहङ्गेषु पुमान् श्रेष्ठः स्त्रीः चतुष्पदजातिषु ।
> परार्धं लघु पुंसः स्यात्स्त्रीणां पूर्वार्द्धमादिशेत् ॥ २८ ॥
> देहमध्यं गुरु प्रायः सर्वेषां प्राणिनां मतम् ।
> पक्षोत्क्षेपाद्विहंगानां तदेव वरमुच्यते[30] ॥ २९ ॥

**Male and female animals**

Among birds the males are the best. Among quadrupeds the females are the best. The hind portion of the body of the males is light. The front portion of the body of female animals is light. The middle portion of the body of animals is generally heavy. In the case of birds, their middle portion is better because the feathers attached to it help in its movement.

'सर्वेषां च शिरःस्कन्धप्लीहचर्मयकृद्गुदम् ।
पादमस्तिष्कपुच्छांत्रमुष्कक्रोडाः समीरणाः[31] ।
धातवः शोणिताद्याश्च गुरवः स्युर्यथोत्तरम्[32] ॥ ३० ॥'

[माधवद्रव्यगुणः मत्स्यवर्ग २० : १४-१५]

**Different parts**

In all animals the head, neck, spleen, skin, liver, anus, feet, brain, tail, colon, testicles, pelvic region (*kroḍa*), airy portion (*samīraṇa*) and tissue elements like blood are progressively heavier.

लघु वातहरं मांसं खगानां धन्वचारिणाम्[33] ।
मत्स्याशिनां पित्तकरं वातघ्नं गुरु कीर्तितम् ॥ ३१ ॥
जलाशिनां श्लेष्महरं लघु रूक्षमुदीरितम् ।
बृंहणं गुरु वातघ्नं तेषामेव पलाशिनाम् ॥ ३२ ॥

**Habitat**

The meat of birds inhabiting deserts is light and alleviator of *vāyu*. The meat of birds which feed on fish aggravates *pitta* and alleviates *vāyu*. It is heavy. The meat of birds which live on water is alleviator of *kapha*, light and ununctuous. The meat of birds which eat the meat of other animals is nourishing, heavy and alleviator of *vāyu*.

॥ इति मत्स्यवर्गः ॥

Thus ends the group dealing with various types of meat and fish.

## NOTES AND REFERENCES

1. निग्धोष्णाः इति आकरे पाठः ।
2. वृष्या इति आकरे पाठः ।
3. कफपित्तहरा इति षष्ठपुस्तके पाठः ।
4. मत्स्या इति आकरे पाठः ।
5. कालोपचयवर्धमाः इति षष्ठपुस्तके पाठः ।
6. वृष्योऽर्दितार्तिषु इति आकरे पाठः ।
7. पानीनः इति षष्ठपुस्तके पाठः ।
8. बल्या इति आकरे पाठः ।
9. दूष्येद्रुधिरं पित्तं कुष्ठरोगं करोति च इति आकरे पाठः ।
10. मद्गुरुशंकू च इति आकरे पाठः ।
11. कषयाः⋯⋯लघुतरास्मृताः पाठोऽयं आकरे नोपलभ्यते ।
12. अलिमत्स्यो गुरुः स्निग्धः कषायो रूक्ष एव च इति आकरे पाठः ।
13. गुरुमत्स्यो गुरु स्निग्धः श्लेष्मलो वातनाशनः इति आकरे पाठः
14. इल्लिसो मधुरः स्निग्धः पित्तहृत् श्लेष्मकोपनः इति आकरे पाठः ।
15. वह्निविवर्धनः इति आकरे पाठः ।
16. चडंगः स्निग्धमधुरो गुर्विष्टंभिशीतलः इति आकरे पाठः ।
17. नंद्या इति षष्ठपुस्तके पाठः ।
18. पुष्टिकृद्बलवर्धनः इति द्वितीयपुस्तके पाठः ।
19. नादेया बृंहणा मत्स्या गुरवोऽनिलनाशनाः ।
    रक्तपित्तकरा वृष्याः स्निग्धोष्णाः स्वल्पवर्चसः इति भावप्रकाशे पाठः ।
20. श्लेष्मवर्धनाः इति आकरे पाठः ।
21. अदूरगोचरा यस्मात्तस्मादुत्सोदपानजाः इति आकरे पाठः ।
    अदूरगोचराः मत्स्या स्तेभ्यो इति षष्ठपुस्तके पाठः ।

22. सागरसंभवाः इति आकरे पाठः ।
23. उरो विचरणात् तेषां इति आकरे पाठः ।
24. महाप्रमाणाः गुरवः क्रियावन्तोऽल्पचेष्टिताः इति आकरे पाठः ।
25. युवत्यः इति आकरे पाठः ।
26. स्त्रियश्च इति आकरे पाठः ।
27. कठिनेभ्यो मृदुभ्यश्च स्थिरगात्राश्च भूचराः इति षष्ठ पुस्तके पाठः ।
28. खेचरेभ्योऽपि इति आकरे पाठः ।
29. गुरुरूक्षाः इति आकरे पाठः ।
30. बलमुच्यते इति आकरे पाठः ।
31. समीरिणाः इति आकरे पाठः ।
32. गुरवस्तूत्तरोत्तराः इति आकरे पाठः ।
33. वातचारिणाम् इति षष्ठपुस्तके पाठः ।

# CHAPTER 19

'अम्लं[1] कषायं मधुरं वातघ्नं ग्राहि दीपनम् ।
स्निग्धोष्णं **दाडिमं** हृद्यं कफपित्ताविरोधि च ॥ १ ॥

### *Dāḍima* (Pomegranate)

*Dāḍima* is sour, astringent, sweet, alleviator of *vāyu*, constipative, stimulant of digestion, unctuous, hot and cardiac tonic. It does not aggravate *kapha* and *pitta*.

द्विविधं तत्तु विज्ञेयं मधुरं चाम्लमेव च ।
त्रिदोषघ्नं तु मधुरमम्लं वातकफापहम् ॥ २ ॥'

[माधवद्रव्यगुण: फलवर्ग २१ : १-२]

It is of two types viz., sweet and sour. The sweet variety alleviates all the three *doṣas* and the sour variety alleviates *vāyu* as well as *kapha*.

**'नीपं**[2] **सवालुकं पीलु तृणशून्यं विकंकतम्** ।
**प्राचीनामलकं**[3] चैव दोषघ्नं गरहारि च ॥ ३ ॥

### *Nīpa* etc.,

*Nīpa, vāluka, pīlu, tṛṇaśūnya, vikaṅkata* and *prācīnāmalaka* alleviate *doṣas* and cure *viṣa* (poisoning).

कर्कन्धुकोलबदरमम्लं वातकफापहम् ।

### *Karkandhu, Kola* & *Badara* (Jujuba fruit)

*Karkandhu, kola* and *badara* are sour and they alleviate *vāyu* as well as *kapha*.

पक्वं पित्तानिलहरं स्निग्धं समधुरं सरम् ॥ ४ ॥

Ripe fruits alleviate *pitta* and *vāyu*. They are unctuous, sweet and laxative.

पुराणं तृट्प्रशमनं श्रमघ्नं लघु दीपनम् ।

Dry fruits (*purāṇa*) alleviate *tṛṭ* (morbid thirst) and *śrama* (physical fatigue). They are light and digestive stimulant.

रक्तपित्तकरं बालं[4] पित्तकृद्बद्धकं सरम् ॥ ५ ॥

Tender fruits cause *rakta pitta* (a disease characterised by bleeding from different parts of the body). They vitiate *pitta*. The matured fruits are laxative.

हृद्यं वर्णकरं[5] रुच्यमाम्रशुक्रबलप्रदम् ।
पित्ताविरोधि वातघ्नं पक्वमाम्रं सरं गुरु ॥ ६ ॥'
[माधवद्रव्यगुणः फलवर्ग २१ : १०-१३]

'कषायानुरसं वह्निश्लेष्मशुक्रविवर्द्धनम् ।

### *Āmra* (Mango)

*Āmra* is cardiac tonic. It promotes complexion, appetite, semen and strength. It does not aggravate *pitta* and alleviates *vāyu*.

The ripe *āmra* is laxative and heavy. It is astringent in

*auurasa* (subsidiary taste). It increases digestive power, *kapha* and semen.

तदेव वृक्षके[6] पक्वं गुरु वातहरं परम् ॥ ७ ॥
मधुराम्लं सरं किञ्चिद्भवेत्पित्तप्रकोपणम् ।

*Āmra* which has become ripe in the tree itself is heavy and it is an excellent alleviator of *vāyu*. It is sweet, sour and slightly laxative. It slightly aggravates *pitta*.

आम्रं[7] कृत्रिमपक्वं[8] यत्तद्भवेत्पित्तनाशनम् ॥ ८ ॥'

[भावप्रकाशः आम्रादिफलवर्ग ७ : ५-७]

*Āmra* which is ripened by artificial means alleviates *pitta*.

'शुष्काम्रं सकषायाम्लं भेदनं कफवातकृत् ।'

[माधवद्रव्यगुणः फलवर्ग २१ : १५]

Dry mango is astringent, sour and purgative. It aggravates *kapha* and *vāyu*.

"चूषितं[9] तत्परं रुच्यं बलवीर्यकरं लघु ।
शीतलं शीघ्रपाकि स्याद्वातपित्तहरं सरम् ॥ ९ ॥

If ripe *āmra* is taken by sucking (*coṣaṇa*), then it is appetiser, promoter of strength and energy, light and cooling. It gets digested early. It alleviates *vāyu* and *pitta*. It is laxative.

तद्रसो गालितो बल्यो गुरुर्वातहरः सरः ।
अहृद्यस्तर्पणोऽतीव बृंहणः कफवर्द्धनः[10] ॥ १० ॥

The juice extracted out of it is a promoter of strength, heavy, alleviator of *vāyu*, laxative, *ahṛdya* (which is not cardiac tonic), exceedingly *tarpaṇa* (refreshing), nourishing and aggravator of *kapha*.

तत्सखण्डं गुरुपरं रोचनं चिरपाकि च ।

मधुरं बृंहणं बल्यं शीतलं वातनाशनम् ॥ ११ ॥

Along with sugar, the mango juice becomes very heavy. It is an appetiser. It gets digested very late. It is sweet, nourishing, strength promoting, cooling and alleviator of *vāyu*.

'वातपित्तहरं रुच्यं बृंहणं बलवर्द्धनम् ।

वृष्यं वर्णकरं स्वादु दुग्धाम्र गुरु शीतलम् ॥ १२ ॥'

[माधवद्रव्यगुणः फलवर्ग २१ : १४]

Along with milk, the mango juice alleviates *vāyu* and *pitta*. It is appetiser, nourishing, strength promoting, aphrodisiac, promotor of complexion, delicious, heavy and cooling.

11

मन्दानलत्वं विषमज्वरं च रक्तामयं बद्धगुदोदरं च ।

आम्रातियोगो नयनामयं वा करोति तस्मादति तानि नाद्यात् ॥१३॥

12

एतदम्लाम्रविषयं मधुराम्रपरं न तु ।

13

मधुरस्य परं नेत्रहितत्वाद्या गुणा यतः ॥ १४ ॥"

[भावप्रकाशः आम्रादिफलवर्ग ७ : ८-१३]

Mango used in large quantities causes *mandānala* (suppression of the power of digestion), *viṣama jvara* (irregular fever), *raktāmaya* (diseases of blood) *baddhagudodara* (obstinate type of abdominal disease caused by obstruction in the rectum) and eye diseases. Therefore, one should not consume mango in excess. This description relates to sour variety of mango and does not apply to sweet variety of mango because the latter is exceedingly useful for eyes and in similar other conditions.

14

'अतोदुग्धानुपानं स्यादाम्राणामतिभक्षणे

जीरकं वा प्रयोक्तव्यं सहसौवर्चलेन च ।। १५ ।।

If mango is to be used in excess then milk should be used after it as *anupāna*. It can also be taken with *jīraka* or *sauvarcala* type of salt.

पक्वस्य सहकारस्य कटे[15] विस्तारितो रसः ।

घर्मशुष्को मुहुर्दत्त **आम्रावर्त** इतिस्मृतः ।। १६ ।।

*Āmrāvarta*

If the juice of ripe mango is spread over a thick piece of cloth and made to dry in sun by repeatedly adding additional quantity of juice, then this is called *āmrāvarta*.

आम्रावर्तस्तृषा[16]च्छर्दिवातपित्तहरः सरः ।

रुच्यः सूर्यांशुभिः पाकी[17] लघुश्च परिकीर्तितः[18] ।। १७ ।।

It alleviates *tṛṣā* (morbid thirst), *chardi* (vomiting), *vāyu* and *pitta*. It is laxative and appetiser. If it is dried in the sun's rays, then it becomes light.

**आम्रबीजं** कषायं स्याच्छर्द्यतीसारनाशनम् ।

ईषदम्लं च मधुरं तथा हृदयदाहनुत् ।। १८ ।।'

[भावप्रकाशः आम्रादिफलवर्ग ७ : १४-१७]

*Āmra bīja*

The seed of mango is astringent. It cures *chardi* (vomiting) and *atisāra* (diarrhoea). It is slightly sour and sweet. It cures *hṛdaya dāha* (burning sensation in the chest).

'**आम्रातमम्लं** वातघ्नं गुरूष्णं रुचिकृत्सरम् ।

### *Āmrātaka* (Hog plum)

**Āmrāta** is sour, alleviator of *vāyu*, heavy, hot, appetiser and laxative.

पक्वं तु तुवरं स्वादुरसपाकं[19] हिमं मतम्[20] ।। १९ ।।
तर्पणं [श्लेष्मलं][21] स्निग्धं वृष्यं विष्टम्भि बृंहणम् ।
गुरु बल्यं मरुत्पित्तक्षतदाहक्षयास्रजित् ।। २० ।।'

[भावप्रकाशः आम्रादिफलवर्ग ७ : १९-२०]

The ripe fruit is astringent, sweet in taste and *vipāka*, cooling, refreshing, aggravator of *kapha*, unctuous, aphrodisiac, constipative, nourishing, heavy and strength promoting. It alleviates *vāyu* and *pitta*. It cures *kṣata* (phthisis), *dāha* (burning syndrome), *kṣaya* (consumption) and vitiation of blood.

'गुरु विष्टम्भि **लकुचं** दोषलं[22] शुक्रदूषणम् ।

### *Lakuca* (Monkey fruit)

*Lakuca* is heavy, wind forming in the stomach and aggravator of *doṣas*. It vitiates semen.

अम्लं तृष्णाहरं[23] रुच्यं पित्तकृत्**करमर्दकम्** ।। २१ ।।'

[माधवद्रव्यगुणः फलवर्ग २१ : १९]

### *Karamardaka* (Carissa carandus Linn.)

*Karamardaka* is sour and it cures *tṛṣā* (morbid thirst). It is appetiser and it aggravates *pitta*.

'**अम्लवेतस**मत्यम्लं तीक्ष्णं स्निग्धं च दीपनम् ।'

[माधवद्रव्यगुणः फलवर्ग २१ : प्रक्षिप्तपाठः]

### *Amlavetasa* (Garcinia pedunculata Roxb.)

*Amlavetasa* is exceedingly sour. It is sharp, unctuous and digestive stimulant.

वातापहं **तिन्तिडीकं** आमपित्तबलासकृत् ।। २२ ।।

### *Tintiḍīka* (Rhus parviflora Roxb.)

*Tintiḍīka* alleviates *vāyu* and produces *āma*, *pitta* as well as *kapha*.

24

ग्राह्युष्णं दीपनं हृद्यं सुपक्वं कफवातनुत् ।

Fully matured fruit of it is constipative, hot, digestive stimulant, cardiac tonic and alleviator of *kapha* as well as *vāyu*.

**अम्लिकायाः** फलं पक्वं तद्वद्भेदि तु केवलम् ।

तस्मादल्पान्तरगुणं **कोशाम्रफलमुच्यते** ॥ २३ ॥'

[माधवद्रव्यगुणः फलवर्ग २१ : २०-२१]

### *Amlikā* and *Kośāmra* (Tamarindus indica Linn. & Schleichera oleossa Merr.)

The ripe fruit of *amlikā* has all the properties of ***tintiḍika***. In addition, it is a purgative.

*Kośāmra* is slightly inferior in quality.

'**ऐरावतं दंतशठमम्लं** शोणितपित्तकृत् ।

### *Airāvata* and *Dantaśaṭha*

*Airāvata* and *dantaśaṭha* are sour and they cause ***śoṇita** pitta* (a disease characterised by bleeding from different parts of the body).

सुगन्धि मधुरं चाम्लं विशदं भक्तरोचनम् ।

दुर्जरं वातशमनं **नारंगस्यफलं** गुरु ॥ २४ ॥'

[माधवद्रव्यगुणः फलवर्ग २१ : २३-२४]

### *Nāraṅga* (Orange)

The fruit of *nāraṅga* is fragrant, sweet, sour, ***viśada*** (non-slimy), appetiser, difficult of digestion, alleviator of ***vāyu*** and **heavy.**

'**निंबूकमम्लं** वातघ्नं पाचनं दीपनं लघु ।

### *Nimbūka* (Lime fruit)

*Nimbūka* is sour, alleviator of *vāyu*, carminative, digestive stimulant and light.

**राजनिंबूफलं** स्वादु गुरु पित्तसमीरजित् ।
25
तृष्णाशूलकफोत्क्लेशच्छर्दिश्वासनिवारणम् ॥ २५ ॥

### *Rāja nimbū*

The fruit of *rājanimbū* is sweet and heavy. It alleviates *pitta* and *vāyu*. It cures *tṛṣṇā* (morbid thirst), *śūla* (colic pain), *kaphotkleśa* (salivation), *chardi* (vomiting) and *śvāsa* (asthma).

वातश्लेष्मविबन्धघ्नं **जंबीरं** गुरु पित्तकृत् ।'

[माधवद्रव्यगुणः फलवर्ग २१ : ३२-३३]

### *Jambīra* (Citrus limon Linn. Burm. f.)

*Jambīra* alleviates *vāyu* and *kapha* and relieves constipation. It is heavy and it aggravates *pitta*.

**करुणं** कफवातामदोषघ्नं पित्तकोपनम् ॥ २६ ॥

[माधवद्रव्यगुणः फलवर्ग २१ : ३७]

### *Karuṇa*

*Karuna* alleviates *kapha*, *vāyu* and *āmadoṣa*. It aggravates *pitta*.

कासश्वासारुचिहरं तृष्णाहृत्कण्ठशोधनम् ।

लघ्वम्लदीपनं हृद्यं **मातुलुंगमुदाहृतम्** ॥ २७ ॥

### *Mātuluṅga* (Citron)

*Mātuluṅga* cures *kāsa* (bronchitis), *śvāsa* (asthma), *aruci* (anorexia) and *tṛṣṇā* (morbid thirst). It cleanses the throat. It is light, sour, digestive stimulant and cardiac tonic.

**त्वक्तिक्ता** दुर्जरा तस्य वातकृमिविषापहा ।
स्वादु शीतं गुरु हिममामं मारुतपित्तजित् ॥ २८ ॥

*Tvaktiktā*

*Tvaktikā* is difficult to digest. It alleviates *vāyu* and cures *kṛmi* (parasitic infection) as well as *viṣa* (poisoning). It is sweet, cooling and heavy.

The unripe fruit of it is cooling and it alleviates *vāyu* and *pitta.*

मेध्यं शूलानिलछर्दिकफारोचकनाशनम् ।
दीपनं लघु संग्राहि गुल्मार्शोघ्नं तु **केशरम्** ॥ २९ ॥

*Keśara*

*Keśara* promotes intellect. It cures *śūla* (colic pain), vitiation of *vāyu*, *chardi* (vomiting) vitiation of *kapha* and *arocaka* (anorexia). It is digestive stimulant, light and constipative. It cures *gulma* (phantom tumour) and *arśas* (piles).

एवं प्रकारा विज्ञेया वृष्या च **मधुकर्कटी** ।
शूलाजीर्णविबन्धेषु मन्देऽग्नौ कफमारुते ॥ ३० ॥

*Madhu karkaṭī* **(Sweet lime)**

*Madhu karkaṭī* shares the properties of *kesara.* In addition, it is aphrodisiac. It cures *śūla* (colic pain), *ajīrna* (indigestion) and *vibandha* (constipation). It is useful in suppression of the power of digestion and in vitiation of *kapha* as well as *vāyu.*

अरुचिश्वासकासेषु रसस्तस्योपदिश्यते ।

Its juice is indicated in *aruci* (anorexia), *śvāśa* (asthma) and *kāsa* (bronchitis).

'कषायं मधुरं पाके श्लेष्मलं गुरु शीतलम् ॥३१ ॥

**कपित्थमामं** कण्ठघ्नं विशदं ग्राहि वातलम् ।

27

मधुराम्लकषायत्वात्सौगन्ध्याच्च रुचिप्रदम् ॥ ३२॥

Kapittha (Wood apple)

The unripe fruit of *kapittha* is astringent, sweet in *vipāka*, aggravator of *kapha*, heavy and cooling. It causes impairment of the throat. It is *viśada* (non-slimy), constipative and aggravator of *vāyu*. In view of its sweet, sour and astringent tastes and fragrance, it is an appetiser.

तदेव पक्वं दोषघ्नं विशदं ग्राहि गुर्वपि ।'

[माधवद्रव्यगुण: फलवर्ग २१ : ४०-४२]

The ripe fruit of *kapittha* alleviates *doṣas*. It is *viśada* (non-slimy), constipative and heavy.

**जांबवं** वातलं रूक्षं ग्राहि पित्तकफापहम् ॥ ३३ ॥

*Jaṁbu* (**Jamun fruit**)

*Jaṁbu* aggravates *vāyu*. It is un-unctuous and constipative. It alleviates *pitta* and *kapha*.

28

कषायं **तिन्दुकं** स्वादु गुरु पित्तकफावहम् ।

*Tinduka* (**Diospyros tomentosa Roxb.**)

*Tinduka* is astringent, sweet and heavy. It aggravates *pitta* and *kapha*.

वातपित्तहरं वृष्यं **प्रियालं** गुरु शीतलम् ॥ ३४ ॥

*Priyāla* (**Buchanania lanzan Spreng.**)

*Priyāla* alleviates *vāyu* and *pitta*. It is aphrodisiac, heavy and cooling.

29

'कषायमधुरं साम्लं नातिमारुतकोपनम् ।'

वातलं [?] कफपित्तघ्नं विद्यात्**पर्पटिकं** फलम् ॥३५॥'

*Parpaṭika* **(Physalis minima Linn.)**

The fruit of *parpaṭika* is astringent, sweet and sour. It aggravates *vāyu* but not in excess. It also aggravates *kapha* and *piita*.

30

'**क्षिरीवृक्षफलं** तेषां गुरु विष्टम्भि शीतलम् ।

कषायमधुरं साम्लं नातिमारुतकोपनम् ॥ ३६ ॥'

[सुश्रुत: सूत्र ४६ : १६५]

*Kṣirī*

The fruit of *kṣirī* tree is heavy, wind forming in stomach and cooling. It is astringent, sweet and sour. It does not aggravate *vāyu* in excess.

31

'विष्टंभि मधुरं स्निग्धं **फल्गु** संतर्पणं गुरु ।'

[सुश्रुत: सूत्र ४६ : १७१]

*Phalgu* **(Ficus hispida Linn. f.)**

*Phalgu* is wind forming, sweet, unctuous, refreshing and heavy.

**बिंबीफलं** च पित्तासृक्कासश्वासक्षयापहम् ॥ ३७ ॥

*Bimbī* **(Coccinia indica W. & A.)**

The fruit of *bimbī* alleviates *pitta* as well as blood and cures *kāsa* (bronchitis), *śvāsa* (asthma) and *kṣaya* (consumption).

**शमीफलं** गुरु स्वादु रूक्षोष्णं केशनाशनम् ।

*Śamī* **(Prosopis spicigera Linn.)**

The fruit of *śamī* is heavy, delicious, un-unctuous and hot. It causes the hair to fall.

'**मृद्वीका** मधुरा स्निग्धा शीता वृष्यानुलोमनी ॥३८॥

रक्तपित्तज्वरश्वासतृष्णादाहक्षयापहा ।'

**Mṛdvīkā (Vitis vinifera Linn.)**

*Mṛdvīkā* is sweet, unctuous, cooling, aphrodisiac and laxative. It cures *rakta pitta* (a disease characterised by bleeding from different parts of the body), *jvara* (fever), *śvāsa* (asthma), *tṛṣṇā* (morbid thirst), *dāha* (burning syndrome) and *kṣaya* (consumption).

द्राक्षा गोस्तनिका तद्वद्गुर्वी वृष्या[32] कफापहा ।।'३९।।

[माधवद्रव्यगुणः फलवर्ग २१ : ३५-३६]

The *gostani* type of *drākṣā* shares all the above mentioned properties. In addition, it is heavy, aphrodisiac and alleviator of *kapha*.

निर्वीजान्या स्वल्पतरा गोस्तनी सदृशीगुणैः ।

It has another variety which is without seeds. This is smaller in size. It shares all the properties of *gostani* type of *drākṣā*.

द्राक्षा पर्वतजा लघ्वी साम्ला श्लेष्माम्लपित्तकृत्[33] ।।४०।।

*Drākṣā* which grows on hills is light and sour. It produces *kapha* and causes *amla pitta* (hyperacidity in stomach).

'श्रामास्तु[34] सर्वा द्राक्षाः स्युः पित्तश्लेष्मप्रकोपणाः[35] ।

All green *drākṣās* aggravate *pitta* and *kapha*.

द्राक्षाकरीरकर्कन्धुबदराण्यारुकानि[36] च ।। ४१ ।।

परुषकानि[37] चाम्लानि कफपित्तकराणि च ।

स्वादुपाकानि यान्येषां तानि पित्तहराणि च ।। ४२ ।।'

[माधवद्रव्यगुणः फलवर्ग २१ : ३७,३८-३९]

### *Drākṣā, Karīra* etc.,

The sour variety of *drākṣā, karīra, karkandhu, badara, āruka* and *paruṣaka* aggravate *kapha* and *pitta*. The sweet variety among them alleviates *pitta*.

**कदल्या** मधुरं शीतं विष्टंभि कफकृद्गुरु ।
स्निग्धं पित्तास्रतृट्दाहक्षतक्षयसमीरजित् ।। ४३ ।।
[माधवद्रव्यगुणः फलवर्ग २१ : ५२]

### *Kadalī* (Musa paradisiaca Linn.)

*Kadalī* is sweet, cooling and wind forming. It aggravates *kapha*. It is unctuous. It alleviates *pitta* and blood. It cures *dāha* (burning syndrome), *kṣata* (phthisis) and *kṣaya* (consumption). It alleviates *vāyu*.

रूक्षं गुरु हिमं पक्वं स्वादुपित्तानिलापहम् ।

The unripe *kadalī* is un-unctuous, heavy and cooling. The ripe *kadalī* is sweet and it alleviates *pitta* and *vāyu*.

"हृद्यं[38] मूत्रविबन्धघ्नं पित्तासृग्वातनाशनम् ।
केश्यं रसायनं मेध्यं **काश्मर्यफल**मुच्यते ।। ४४ ।।'
[माधवद्रव्यगुणः फलवर्ग २१ : ५५-५६]

### *Kāśmarya* (Gmelina arborea Linn.)

The fruit of *kāśmarya* is cardiac tonic. It relieves retention of urine. It alleviates *pitta*, blood and *vāyu*. It is promoter of good hair, rejuvenating and promoter of intellect.

'क्षतक्षयापहं हृद्यं बृंहणं[39] तर्पणं गुरु ।"
[सुश्रुतः सूत्र ४६ : १८४-१८५]

स्निग्धं वृष्यं[40] च मधुरं **खर्जूरं**[41] रक्तपित्तजित् ।। ४५ ।।'
[माधवद्रव्यगुणः फलवर्ग २१ : ४५]

### *Kharjūra* (Phoenix Sylvestris Roxb.)

*Kharjūra* cures *kṣata* (phthisis) and *kṣaya* (consumption). It is cardiac tonic, nourishing, refreshing, heavy, unctuous, aphrodisiac and sweet. It cures *rakta pitta* (a disease characterised by bleeding from different parts of the body).

खर्जूरी गोस्तनाकारा [42]परावाराद्दिहागता ।

[भावप्रकाश: आम्रादिफवर्ग ७ : ११६]

[43]'साखरीकेतिविख्याता देशे भवति पश्चिमे ॥ ४६ ॥

### *Kharjūrī* (Phoenix dactylifer Linn.)

*Kharjūrī* is like the *udder* of a cow. It has come to this country from other islands. In the western part of this country it is called *sākharīkā*.

[44]पिण्डखर्जूरीका त्वन्या सापि [45]तत्रैव जायते ।'

ततोऽन्यथा भवेत्स्वल्पा सा तु सर्वत्र जायते ॥ ४७ ॥

Another variety of it is called *piṇḍa kharjūrīkā* and it grows in that country also. The third variety is very small in size and it grows everywhere.

'खर्जूरीत्रितयं शीतं मधुरं रसपाकयो: ।

स्निग्धं रुचिकरं हृद्यं क्षतक्षयहरं गुरु ॥ ४८ ॥

तर्पणं रक्तपित्तघ्नं पुष्टिविष्टम्भशुक्रदम् ।

कोष्ठमारुतकृ[46]द्बल्यं [47]वाह्यवातकफापहम् ॥ ४९ ॥

ज्वराभिघातक्षु[48]त्तृष्णा [49]कासश्वासनिवारणम् ।

मदमू[50]र्च्छामरुतिपत्तमदात्ययगदास्रजित् ॥ ५० ॥

All these three varieties of *kharjūrī* are cooling and sweet both in taste and *vipāka*. They are unctuous, appetiser and cardiac tonic. They cure *kṣata* (phthisis) and *kṣaya* (consumption). They are heavy and nourishing. They cure *rakta pitta*-

(a disease characterised by bleeding from different parts of the body). They cause corpulence and wind formation in the stomach. They produce more of semen, wind in the colon and strength. They alleviate external *vāyu* and *kapha*. They cure *jvara* (fever), *abhighāta* (injury), *kṣut* (morbid hunger), *tṛṣṇā* (morbid thirst), *kāsa* (bronchitis), *śvāsa* (asthma) *mada* (intoxication), *mūrchā* (fainting), vitiation of *vāyu* as well as *pitta*, *madātyaya* (alcoholism) and vitiation of blood.

[51]ताभ्यामल्पगुणं ज्ञेयमल्पखर्जूरिकाफलम् ।

The fruit of *kharjūrīkā* which is smaller in size is inferior in quality in comparison with others.

**[52]खर्जूरिकावृक्षतोयं** मदपित्तकरं [53]मतम् ।
वातश्लेष्महरं रुच्यं दीपनं बलशुक्रकृत्' ॥ ५१ ॥

[भावप्रकाश: आम्रादिफलवर्ग ७ : ११७-१२१]

The juice of the tree of *kharjūrikā* causes *mada* (intoxication) and aggravation of *pitta*. It alleviates *vāyu* and *kapha*. It is appetiser, digestive stimulant and promoter of strength and semen.

तन्मज्जामूर्द्धजःशीतो वृष्यः पित्तास्रदाहजित् ।

The pith (*majjā*) of this tree from the top of the trunk is cooling, aphrodisiac and alleviator of *pitta* as well as blood. It cures *dāha* (burning syndrome).

'**मधूकपुष्पं** मधुरं शीतलं गुरु बृंहणम् ।
बलशुक्रकरं प्रोक्तं [54]पित्तमारुतनाशनम् ॥ ५२ ॥

*Madhūka* **(Madhuca indica J.F. Gmel.)**

The flower of *madhūka* is sweet, cooling, heavy and nourishing. It promotes strength and semen and alleviates *pitta* as well as *vāyu*.

फलं शीतं गुरु स्वादुः शुक्रलं[55] वातपित्तजित् ।

अहृद्यं[56] हन्ति तृषास्रदाहश्वासक्षतक्षयान् ॥ ५३ ॥'

[भावप्रकाशः आम्रादिफलवर्ग ७ : ९६-९७]

Its fruit is cooling, heavy and sweet. It increases semen and alleviates *vāyu* as well as *pitta*. It is not good for the heart. It cures *tṛṣā* (morbid thirst), vitiation of blood, *dāha* (burning syndrome), *śvāsa* (asthma), *kṣata* (phthisis) and *kṣaya* (consumption).

'अत्यम्लमीषन्मधुरं कषायानुरसं लघु ।

वातघ्नं पित्तजननमामं विद्यात्**परूषकम्** ॥ ५४ ॥

### *Parūṣaka* (Grewia asiatica Linn.)

The unripe *parūṣaka* is extremely sour, slightly sweet, astringent in *anurasa* (subsidiary taste) and light. It alleviates *vāyu* and aggravates *pitta*.

तदेवपक्वं मधुरं वातपित्तनिबर्हणम् ।'

[सुश्रुतः सूत्र ४६ : १७१-१७२]

The ripe *parūṣaka* is sweet and it alleviates *vāyu* as well as *pitta*.

वातहा पित्तहा वृष्यः क्रिमिहा कुष्ठनाशनः ।

रक्तपित्तहरः स्वादुस्तालः सप्तगुणः स्मृतः ।

### *Tāla* (Borassus flabellifer Linn.)

*Tāla* alleviates *vāyu* and *pitta*. It is aphrodisiac. It cures *kṛmi* (parasitic infection), *kuṣṭha* (obstinate skin diseases including leprosy) and *rakta pitta* (a disease characterised by bleeding from different parts of the body). It is sweet. These are its seven attributes.

'तद्बीजं स्वादुपाकं च मूत्रलं वातपित्तजित्[57] ॥ ५५ ॥'

[सुश्रुतः सूत्र ४६ : १७९]

The seed of *tāla* is sweet in *vipāka*. It is diuretic and it alleviates *vāyu* and *pitta*.

'पक्वं तालफलं पित्तरक्तश्लेष्मविवर्द्धनम्[58] ।
दुर्जरं बहुमूत्रं च तन्द्राभिष्यन्दशुक्रदम्[59] ॥ ५६ ॥

The ripe *tāla* fruit aggravates *pitta*, blood and *kapha*. It is difficult of digestion and is exceedingly diuretic. It causes *tandrā* (drowsiness) and *abhiṣyanda* (obstruction to the channels of circulation). It produces more of semen.

तालमज्जा तु तरुणः किञ्चिन्मदकरो लघुः[60] ।
श्लेष्मलो वातपित्तघ्नः सस्नेहो मधुरः सरः ॥ ५७ ॥

The pulp of tender *tāla* is slightly intoxicating and light. It aggravates *kapha* and alleviates *vāyu* and *pitta*. It is unctuous, sweet and laxative.

तालजं तरुणं तोयमतीव मदकृन्मतम् ।
अम्लीभूतं[61] यदा तत्स्यात्पित्तकृद्वातदोषनुत् ॥ ५८ ॥'

[भावप्रकाशः आम्रादिफलवर्ग ७ : ५३-५५]

The water of the tender *tāla* is exceedingly intoxicating. When it becomes sour, then it aggravates *pitta* and alleviates *vāyu*.

तालस्य मस्तकं स्वादुः वस्तिशुद्धिकरं परम् ।

The head of the trunk of this tree is sweet and it cleanses the urinary bladder..

'नालिकेरफलं शीतं दुर्जरं वस्तिशोधनम् ।

[62]
विष्टम्भिबृंहणं बल्यं वातपित्तास्रदाहजित् ॥ ५९ ॥'

[भावप्रकाशः आम्रादिफलवर्ग ७ :३९]

*Nārikela* (**Coconut**)

The fruit of *nārikela* is cooling and difficult of digestion. It cleanses the urinary bladder and causes wind formation in the stomach. It is nourishing and strength promoting. It alleviates *vāyu, pitta* and blood. It cures *dāha* (burning syndrome).

बालस्य नालिकेरस्य जलं प्रायो विरेचनम् ।

नालिकेराम्बु तरुणं तृष्णाघ्नं पित्तनाशनम् ॥६०॥

The water of the tender coconut is generally purgative. It cures *tṛṣṇā* (morbid thirst) and alleviates *pitta*.

'**पनसं** शीतलं पक्वं स्निग्धं पित्तानिलापहम् ।

तर्पणं बृंहणं स्वादु मांसलं श्लेष्मलं भृशम् ।

बल्यं शुक्रप्रदं हन्ति [63]रक्तपित्तक्षतक्षयान् ॥ ६१ ॥

*Panasa* (**Jack fruit**)

The ripe fruit of *panasa* is cooling and unctuous. It alleviates *pitta* and *vāyu*. It is refreshing, nourishing, delicious and promoter of muscle tissue. It aggravates *kapha* in excess. It promotes strength and semen and cures *rakta pitta* (a disease characterised by bleeding from different parts of the body), *kṣta* (phthisis) and *kṣaya* (consumption).

आमं तदेव विष्टम्भि वातलं तुवरं गुरु ।

[64]दाहकृन्मधुरं बल्यं कफमेदो[65]विवर्द्धनम् ॥ ६२ ॥

The unripe fruit of *panasa* is wind forming, aggravator of *vāyu*, astringent and heavy. It causes burning sensation. It is sweet and strength promoting. It increases *kapha* and fat.

पनसोत्थानि[66] बीजानि वृष्याणि मधुराणि च ।
गुरूणि वद्धवर्चांसि[67] सृष्टमूत्रानिलानि च ॥ ६३ ॥'

[भावप्रकाशः आम्रादिफलवर्ग ७ : २५-२८]

The seeds of *panasa* are aphrodisiac, sweet and heavy. It causes retention of stool and helps in the elimination of urine and flatus.

'मज्जा तस्यापि पित्तघ्नो वृष्यः श्लेष्मानिलापहः ।
विशेषात्पनसं वर्ज्यं गुल्मिभिः दुर्बलाग्निभिः[68] ॥ ६४ ॥'

Its pulp alleviates *pitta.* It is aphrodisiac. It also alleviates *kapha* and *vāyu.* Persons who are suffering from *gulma* (phantom tumour) and those having poor power of digestion should specifically avoid *panasa.*

'**मोचं** स्वादुरसं प्रोक्तं कषायं नातिशीतलम् ।
रक्तपित्तहरं वृष्यं रुच्यं श्लेष्मकरं गुरु ॥ ६५ ॥'

[माधवद्रव्यगुणः फलवर्ग २१ : ५१]

*Moca* **(Musa paradisiaca Linn. Var. sapientum Kuntze)**

*Moca* is sweet in taste and astringent. It is not cooling in excess. It cures *rakta pitta* (a disease characterised by bleeding from different parts of the body). It is aphrodisiac, appetiser, aggravator of *kapha* and heavy.

'श्लेष्मलं मधुरं शीतं[69] **श्लेष्मातकफलं** गुरु ।'

[माधवद्रव्यगुणः फलवर्ग २१ : ५३]

*Śleṣmātaka* **(Cordia myxa Roxb.)**

The fruit of *śleṣmātaka* is aggravator of *kapha,* sweet, cooling and heavy.

70
'**पौष्करं** स्वादु विष्टम्भि बल्यं कफकरं गुरु ।'

[माधवद्रव्य गुणः फलवर्ग २१ : ५५]

*Puṣkara* **(Lotus fruit)**

The fruit of *puṣkara* is sweet, wind forming, strength promoting, aggravator of *kapha* and heavy.

71
**उदुम्बर**फलं ग्राहि वातपित्तनिवर्हणम् ॥ ६६ ॥

[माधवद्रव्यगुणः फलवर्ग २१ : ५८]

*Udumbara* **(Ficus racemosa Linn.)**

The fruit of *udumbara* is constipative and it alleviates *vāyu* as well as *pitta*.

"मधुरं च कषायं च स्निग्धं संग्राहि **वालुकम्** ।

'स्थिरीकरं च दन्तानां विशदं फलमुच्यते ॥ ६७ ॥"

[सुश्रुतः सूत्र ४६ : १६६]

विपाके मधुरं वृष्यं रक्तपित्तप्रसादनम् ।'

[माधवद्रव्यगुणः फलवर्ग २१ : ५४]

*Vāluka*

*Vāluka* is sweet, astringent, unctuous and constipative. It produces sturdiness of teeth and it is *viśada* (non-slimy). It is sweet in *vipāka* and aphrodisiac. It cures *rakta pitta* (a disease characterised by bleeding from different parts of the body).

कषायं **तिन्दुकं** स्वादु गुरु पित्तकफापहम् ॥६८॥

*Tinduka* **(Diospyrus tomentosa Roxb.)**

*Tinduka* is astringent, delicious and heavy. It alleviates *pitta* and *kapha*.

72
'**प्रियालमज्जा** मधुरो वृष्यः पित्तानिलापहः ।

*Priyāla* (**Buchanania lanzan Spreng.**)

The pulp of *priyāla* is sweet and aphrodisiac. **It** alleviates ***pitta*** and ***vāyu.***

[73]**विभीतको** मदकरः कफमारुतनाशनः ॥ ६९ ॥

*Vibhītaka* (**Terminalia belerica Roxb**.)

The pulp of the seed of *vibhītaka* produces intoxicating effect and it alleviates *kapha* as well as *vāyu*.

कषायमधुरो **मज्जा कोलानां** पित्तनाशनः ।

*Kola* (**Zizyphus jujuba Lam.**)

The pulp of the seed of different types of *kola* is astringent and sweet. It alleviates *pitta*.

[74]तृष्णाछर्द्यनिलघ्नश्च **तद्वदामलकस्य** च ॥ ७० ॥

*Āmalaka* (**Emblica officinalis Gaertn.**)

The pulp of the seed of *āmalaka* cures *tṛṣṇā* (morbid thirst), *chardi* (vomiting) and vitiation of *vāyu*.

**बीजपूरकशम्पाकमज्जा कोशाम्रसंभवः** ।

स्वादुः पाकेऽग्निबलदः स्निग्धः पित्तानिलापहः ॥७१॥'

[माधवद्रव्यगुणः फलवर्ग २१ : ५८-६१]

*Bījapūraka*, *Śampāka* **and** *Kośāmra*

The pulp of the seed of *bījapūraka*, *śampāka* and *kośāmra* is sweet in *vipāka*. It produces digestive power and strength. It is unctuous and it alleviates *pitta* and *vāyu*.

[75]**'वादाममुष्णं** सुस्निग्धं वातघ्नं गुरुशुक्रकृत् ।

*Vādāma* (**Almond**)

*Vādāma* is hot, exceedingly unctuous, alleviator **of** *vāyu* and heavy. It promotes semen formation.

**वादाममज्जा** मधुरो वृष्यः पित्तानिलापहः ।। ७२ ।।'

स्निग्धोष्णः कफकृन्नेष्टो[76] रक्तपित्तविकारिणाम् ।

बृंहणो गुरुरुद्दिष्टः सुस्निग्धो रुचिवर्धनः ।। ७३ ।।

The pulp of the seed of *vādāma* is sweet, aphrodisiac, alleviator of *pitta* and *vāyu*, unctuous, hot and aggravator of *kapha*. It should not be given to patients suffering from *rakta pitta* (a disease characterised by bleeding from different parts of the body). It is nourishing, heavy and appetiser.

'यस्य यस्य फलस्येह वीर्यो[77] भवति यादृशम् ।

तस्य तस्यैव वीर्येण मज्जानमपि निर्दिशेत् ।। ७४ ।।

**Pulp in general**

The pulp of the seeds generally follow the properties of their respective fruits.

व्याधितं कृमियुष्टं[78] च पाकातीतमकालजम्[79] ।

वर्जनीयं फलं सर्वमपर्यागतमेव[80] च ।। ७५ ।।'

[माधवद्रव्यगुणः फलवर्ग २१ : ६५, ६५]

[सुश्रुतः सूत्र ४६ : २०८-२१०]

**Bad fruits**

Fruits afflicted with diseases and *kṛmi* (parasitic infection), fruits which are over ripened and which are unseasonal and fruits which are not fully matured should be rejected.

।। इति फलवर्गः ।।

Thus ends the group dealing with different types of fruits.

## NOTES AND REFERENCES

1. कषामधुरं इति आकरे पाठः ।
2. शतालुकं इति आकरे पाठः ।
3. गरघाति इति आकरे पाठः ।
4. पित्तमारुतकृद्बालं पित्तलं लघु दीपनम् इति आकरे पाठः ।
5. रुच्यं मांसशुक्रबलप्रदम् इति आकरे पाठः ।
6. वृक्षसम्पक्वं इति षष्ठपुस्तके पाठः ।
7. (क) कृत्रिमपक्वञ्च इति आकरे पाठः ।
   (ख) भक्षितं पक्वं इति षष्ठपुस्तके पाठः ।
8. तद्भवेत्पित्तनाशनम् इति आकरे पाठः ।
9. उषितं इति आकरे पाठः ।
10. कफवर्धनः इति द्वितीयपुस्तके पाठः ।
11. मन्दानिलत्वं इति आदर्शपुस्तके पाठः ।
12. मधुराम्लपरं इति आकरे पाठः ।
13. नेत्रहितं त्वाद्या इति आकरे पाठः ।
14. शुण्ठम्भसोऽनुपानं इति आकरे पाठः ।
15. पटे इति आकरे पाठः ।
16. आम्रावर्त्तस्तृषाच्छर्दिवातपित्तहरः इति आकरे पाठः ।
17. पाकाल्लघुश्च इति आकरे पाठः ।
18. स हि कीर्त्तितः इति आकरे पाठः ।
19. रसे पाके इति आकरे पाठः ।
20. स्मृतम् इति आकरे पाठः ।
21. श्लेम्लं इति द्वितीयपुस्तके पाठः ।
22. त्रिदोषं इति आकरे पाठः ।
23. तृष्णापहं इति आकरे पाठः ।
24. रूक्षं इति आकरे पाठः ।
25. तृष्णाशूलकफोत्क्लेशच्छर्दिश्वासनिवारणम् इति आकरे पाठः ।
26. विषदं इति द्वितीयपुस्तके पाठः ।
27. मधुराम्लकषायञ्च सौगन्ध्याच्च इति आकरे पाठः ।
28. पित्तकफापहम् इति षष्ठपुस्तके पाठः ।

29. 'कषायं.......कोपनम्' पाठोऽयं द्वितीयपुस्तके नोपलभ्यते।
30. क्षीरवृक्षफलं इति द्वितीयपुस्तके पाठः।
31. फल्गुजं इति आकरे पाठः।
32. वृष्यतमा मता इति आकरे पाठः।
33. श्लेष्माम्लपित्तनुत् इति षष्ठपुस्तके पाठः।
34. सर्वाः इति आकरे पाठः।
35. पित्तश्लेष्मप्रकोपणाः इति आकरे पाठः।
36. द्राक्षाकरीरकर्कन्धुबदराण्यारुकाणि इति आकरे पाठः।
37. परूषकाणि इति आकरे पाठः।
38. मूत्रविबन्धजं इति माधवद्रव्यगुणे पाठः।
39. शीतलं इति आकरे पाठः।
40. समधुरं इति आकरे पाठः।
41. खार्जूरं इति आकरे पाठः।
42. परद्वीपादिहागता इति आकरे पाठः।
43. साखरिकेति इति षष्ठपुस्तके पाठः।
44. पिंडखजूरिका इति द्वितीयपुस्तके पाठः।
45. द्रष्टव्यम् — भावप्रकाशः आम्रादिफलवर्ग ७ : ११६।
46. कोष्ठमारुतहृद्बल्यं इति आकरे पाठः।
47. वान्तिवातकफापहम् इति आकरे पाठः।
48. ज्वरातिसारक्षुत्तृष्णा इति आकरे पाठः।
49. कासश्वासनिवारकम् इति आकरे पाठः।
50. मदमूर्च्छामरुत्पित्तमद्यादभूतगदान्तकृत् इति आकरे पाठः।
51. महतीभ्यां गुणैरल्पा स्वल्पखर्जूरिका स्मृता इति आकरे पाठः।
52. खर्जूरीतरुतोयं इति आकरे पाठः।
53. भवेत् इति आकरे पाठः।
54. वातपित्तविनाशनम् इति आकरे पाठः।
55. वातपित्तनुत् इति आकरे पाठः।
56. तृष्णाऽस्रदाहश्वासक्षतक्षयान् इति आकरे पाठः।
57. तु इति आकरे पाठः।
58. पित्तश्लेष्मपित्तवर्द्धनम् इति आदर्शपुस्तके पाठः।
59. तन्द्राऽभिष्यन्दशुक्रदम् इति आकरे पाठः।

60. किञ्चमदकरो इति आकरे पाठः ।
61. तदा तु स्यात्पित्तकृद्वातदोषहृत् इति आकरे पाठः ।
62. विष्टम्भिर्दुर्जरं इति आदर्शपुस्तकेषु पाठः ।
63. रक्तपित्तक्षतव्रणान् इति आकरे पाठः ।
64. दाहहृन्मधुरं इति आदर्शपुस्तके पाठः ।
65. विवर्धनम् इति द्वितीयपुस्तके पाठः ।
66. पनसोद्भूतबीजानि इति आकरे पाठः ।
67. बद्धबिट्कानि इति आकरे पाठः ।
68. द्रष्टव्यम्—भावप्रकाशः आम्रादिफलवर्ग ७ : २६ ।
69. वृष्यं इति आकरे पाठः ।
70. कफहरं फलम् इति आकरे पाठः ।
71. औदुम्बरं फलं ग्राहि इति आकरे पाठः ।
72. पियालमज्जा इति आकरे षष्ठपुस्तके च पाठः ।
73. वैभीतको इति आकरे पाठः ।
74. तृष्णाच्छर्द्यनिलघ्नश्च इति आकरे पाठः ।
75. 'वादाममुष्णं·······पित्तानिलापहः' पाठोऽयं षष्ठपुस्तके नोपलभ्यते ।
76. 'कफकृन्नेष्टो·······रुचिवर्धनः' पाठोऽयं षष्ठपुस्तके नोपलभ्यते ।
77. वीर्यं भवति इति आकरे पाठः।
78. क्रिमिजुष्टं इति आकरे पाठः ।
79. प्रतिनीलमकालजम् इति आदर्शपुस्तके पाठः ।
80. सर्वमपर्यागतमेव इति आकरे पाठः ।

# CHAPTER 20

[1]'पत्रं पुष्पं फलं नालं कंदं संस्वेदजं तथा ।
शाकं षड्विधमुद्दिष्टं[2] गुरु विद्याद्यथोतरम् ॥ १ ॥

### *Śāka* (Vegetables)

*Śāka* is of seven types, viz., leaf, flower, fruit, stalk, rhizome and *saṁsvedaja* (those produced by moist heat). These are progressively heavy.

प्राय: सर्वाणि शाकानि विष्टम्भीनि गुरूणि च ।
रूक्षाणि वहुवर्चांसि सृष्टविण्मारुतानि च ॥ २ ॥

Generally all types of *śāka* are wind forming, heavy and un-unctuous. They produce more of stool and help in the elimination of stool and flatus.

चक्षुष्या सर्वदोषघ्नी जीवन्ती मधुरा हिमा ।

### *Jīvantī* (Leptadenia reticulata W. & A.)

*Jīvantī* promotes eyesight and alleviates all *doṣas.* It is sweet in taste and cooling.

[3]

स्वादुपाकमभिष्यन्दि विषघ्नं **तण्डुलीयकम्** ॥ ३ ॥

*Taṇḍulīyaka* **(Amaranthus spinosus Linn.)**

*Taṇḍulīyaka* is sweet in *vipāka* and *abhiṣyandi* (which obstructs the channels of circulation). It cures *viṣa* (poisoning).

'लघुर्विपाके कृमिहा मेधाग्निबलवर्द्धनः[4] ।

सक्षारः सर्वदोषघ्नो **वास्तुको** रोचनः सरः ॥ ४ ॥

*Vāstuka* **(Chenopodium murale Linn.)**

*Vāstuka* is light for digestion. It cures *kṛmi* (parasitic infection). It promotes intellect, power of digestion and strength. It is alkaline. It alleviates all *doṣas* and it is appetiser and laxative.

[5]**चिल्लिर्वास्तुकवज्ज्ञेयाः** **पालंक्या** तण्डुलीयवत् ।

वातकृद्बद्धविण्मूत्रा रूक्षा पित्तकफे[6] हिता ॥' ५ ॥

[सुश्रुतः सूत्र ४६ : २६०-२६१]

*Cili* **and** *Pālaṅkya* **(Chenopodium album Linn. and Spinacea oleracea Linn.)**

*Cili* shares the properties of *Vāstuka*. *Pālaṅkya* shares the properties of *taṇḍulīyaka*. In addition it aggravates *vāyu* and causes retention of stool and urine. It is un-unctuous and is useful in the aggravation of *pitta* and *kapha*.

[7]'मधुरः कफवातघ्नः पाचनः कण्ठशोधनः ।

विशेषतः पित्तहरः सतिक्तः **कासमर्दकः** ॥ ६ ॥'

[माधवद्रव्यगुणः शाकवर्ग २२ : १-६]

*Kāsamardaka* **(Cassia occidentalis Linn.)**

*Kāsamardaka* is sweet, alleviator of *kapha* and *vāta* and carminative. It cleanses the throat. It specially alleviates *pitta* and it is bitter in taste.

8

'**काकजंघा** विषं हन्ति रक्तपित्तभ्रमज्वरान् ।

*Kākajaṅghā* **(Peristrophe bicalyculata Nees.)**

*Kākajaṅghā* cures *viṣa* (poisoning), *rakta pitta* (a disease characterised by bleeding from different parts of the body), *bhrama* (giddiness) and *jvara* (fever).

पथ्या सरा त्रिदोषघ्नी **मेथिका** वातनाशिनी ॥ ७ ॥'

[माधवद्रव्यगुणः शाकवर्ग २२ : ८-९]

*Methikā* **(Trigonella foecum-graecum Linn.)**

*Methikā* is wholesome, laxative and alleviator of all the three *doṣas*. It specifically alleviates *vāyu*.

'त्रिदोषशमनी वृष्या **काकमाची** रसायनी ।

[माधवद्रव्यगुणः शाकवर्ग २२ : ७]

'नात्युष्णा शीतवीर्या च भेदिनी कुष्ठनाशिनी ॥८॥'

[माधवद्रव्यगुणः शाकवर्ग २२ : ८]

*Kākamācī* **(Solanum nigrum Linn.)**

*Kākamācī* alleviates all the three *doṣas*. It is aphrodisiac and rejuvenating. It is not very hot and is cold in potency. It is purgative and it cures *kuṣṭha* (obstinate skin diseases including leprosy).

9

'ईषत्तिक्तं त्रिदोषघ्नं शाकं कटु **सतीनजम्** ।

*Satīna* **(Pisum sativum Linn.)**

The *śāka* of *satīna* is slightly bitter. It alleviates all the three *doṣas* and it is pungent.

स्वादुपाकरसं शाकं दुर्जरं **हरिमन्थजम्** ॥ ९ ॥

*Harimantha*

The *śāka* of *harimantha* is sweet in *vipāka* as well as in taste. It is difficult of digestion.

भेदनं रूक्षमधुरं **कालाय**मतिवातलम् ।

*Kalāya* **(Lathyrus sativus Linn.)**

*Kalāya* is purgative, un-unctuous and sweet. It aggravates *vāyu* in excess.

**राजक्षवक**शाकं तु त्रिदोषशमनं लघु ॥ १० ॥

ग्राहि शस्तं विशेषेण ग्रहण्यर्शोविकारिणाम् ।

*Rājakṣavaka*

The *śāka* of *rājakṣavaka* alleviates all the three *doṣas*. It is light and constipative. It is specifically useful for patients suffering from *grahaṇī* (sprue syndrome) and *arśas* (piles).

10

कषायावहिता पित्ते स्वादुतिक्तरसा हिमा ॥ ११ ॥

लघ्वी **मण्डूकपर्णी** च तद्वद्**गोजिह्वका** मता ।

*Maṇḍūkaparni* **and** *Gojihvakā* **(Centella asiatica Urban and Launaea asplenifolia Hook. f.)**

*Maṇḍūkaparni* is astringent and useful in *pitta*. It is delicious, bitter in taste, cooling and light.

*Gojihvakā* has similar properties.

अविदाही त्रिदोषघ्नः संग्राही **सुनिषण्णकः** ॥ १२ ॥

*Suniṣaṇṇaka* **(Marsilia minuta Linn.)**

*Suniṣaṇṇaka* does not produce burning sensation and it alleviates all the three *doṣas*. It is constipative,

ग्रहण्यर्शोविकारघ्नी साम्ला[11] वातकफे हिता ।
उष्णा कषायमधुरा **चांगेरी** चाग्निदीपनी ॥ १३ ॥

### *Cāṅgerī* (Oxalis corniculata Linn.)

*Cāṅgerī* cures *grahaṇī* (sprue syndrome) and *arśas* (piles). It is sour and useful in the aggravation of *vāyu* as well as *kapha*. It is hot, astringent, sweet and digestive stimulant.

रक्तपित्तानिलहरं सतिक्तं **कंचटं** मतम् ।

### *Kaṁcaṭa*

*Kaṁcaṭa* alleviates vitiation of blood, *pitta* and *vāyu*. It is bitter.

कफवातहरं ग्राहि[12] **मौदकं**[13] तत्प्रकीर्तितम् ॥ १४ ॥

### *Modaka*

*Modaka* alleviates *kapha* and *vāyu* and it is constipative.

कफापहं शाकमुक्तं **वरुणप्रपुन्नाटयोः** ।
रूक्षं लघु च शातं च वातपित्तप्रकोपणम् ॥ १५ ॥

### *Varuṇa* and *Prapunnāṭa* (Crataeva nurvala Buch.—Ham. and Cassia tora Linn.)

The *śāka* of *varuṇa* and *prapunnāṭa* alleviates *kapha*. It is un-unctuous, light, cooling and aggravator of *vāyu* as well as *pitta*.

**वत्सादनी बिल्वपत्रं श्रेयसी तिलपर्ण्यपि** ।
**गण्डीरश्चित्रकश्चेति** शस्यते कफमारुते ॥ १६ ॥

### *Vatsādanī* etc.

The *śāka* of *vatsādanī*, leaf of *bilva*, *śreyasī*, *tilaparṇī*, *gaṇḍīra* and *ciṭraka* is useful in the aggravation of *kapha* and *vāyu.*

कालशाकं गरश्लेष्मशोथघ्नं दीपनं कटु ।

**Kālaśāka (Corchorus capsularis Linn.)**

*Kālaśāka* cures *gara* (a type of poisoning), aggravation of *kapha* and *śotha* (oedema). It is digestive stimulant and pungent.

वर्षाभ्वौ[14] कफवातघ्नौ हितौ शोथोदरार्शसि[15] ॥ १७ ॥

**Varṣābhū (Trianthema portulacastrum Linn.)**

Both the type of *varṣābhū* alleviate *kapha* and *vāyu* and they are useful in *śotha* (oedema), *udara* (obstinate abdominal diseases including ascitis) and *arśas* (piles).

दीपनाः कफवातघ्नाश्चिरबिल्वांकुरासनाः[16] ।

**Cirabilva, Aṅkura and Asana**

The *śāka* of *cirabilva*, *aṅkura* and *asana* is digestive stimulant and it alleviates *kapha* as well as *vāyu.*

वातपित्तकरा रूक्षा कटुका[17] रसपाकतः ॥ १८ ॥

वेणोः करीरा[18] श्लेष्मघ्नाः कषायाश्च[19] विदाहिनः ।

**Veṇu Karīra (Bambusa arundinacea Willd.)**

The *karīra* of *veṇu* aggravates *vāyu* and *pitta.* It is unctuous and pungent both in taste and *vipāka.* It alleviates *kapha.* It is astringent and it produces burning sensation.

तथा नव्यांकुराश्चापि[20] श्लेष्मपित्तहराः स्मृताः ॥१९॥

Freshly sprouted *karīra* is known to alleviate *kapha* and *pitta.*

**आटरूषकवेत्राग्रगुडूचीनिम्बपर्पटाः ।**

**किराततिक्त**[21]सहिता रक्तपित्तकफापहा[22]: ॥ २० ॥'

[माधवद्रव्यगुणः शाकवर्ग २२ : ६-२१]

### *Āṭarūṣaka* etc.

*Āṭarūṣaka, vetrāgra, guḍūcī, nimba, parpaṭa* and *kirātatikta* alleviate the vitiation of blood, *pitta* and *kapha*.

'**वार्ताकं** कटु तीक्ष्णोष्णं मधुरं कफवातजित् ।

सक्षारमग्निजननं हृद्यं रुच्यमपित्तलम् ॥ २१ ॥

### *Vārtāka* (Solanum melongena Linn.)

*Vārtāka* is pungent, sharp, hot, sweet, alleviator of *kapha* as well as *vāyu*, alkaline, digestive stimulant, cardiac tonic and appetiser. It does not aggravate *pitta*.

तद्बालं कफपित्तघ्नं पक्वं सक्षारपित्तलम् ।

तद्वृद्धं[23] गुरु[24] संशुष्कं कफवातामयापहम् ॥ २२ ॥

The tender *vārtāka* alleviates *kapha* and *pitta*. The matured *vārtāka* is alkaline and aggravator of *pitta*. When over matured (*bṛddha*) it is heavy. The dried *vārtāka* cures the diseases caused by *kapha* and *vāyu*.

कफमेदोऽनिलहरमत्यल्पं[25] लघु दीपनम् ।

वार्ताकं पित्तलं किञ्चिदंगारपरिपाचितम् ।

तदेवं[26] तु गुरु स्निग्धं सतैललवणान्वितम् ॥ २३ ॥

*Vārtāka* burnt over charcoal reduces *kapha*, fat and *vāyu*. It is very slightly light and digestive stimulant. It aggravates *pitta*. When mixed with oil and salt it becomes heavy and unctuous.

अग्निप्रदा मारुतनाशिनी[27] च शुक्रप्रदा शोणितवर्द्धिनी च ।
वलासकासक्षयनाशिनी[28] च **वार्ताकुरेषा**[29] गुणसम्प्रयुक्ता ॥ २४ ॥

*Vārtāku*

*Vārtāku* stimulates digestion, alleviates *vāyu*, promotes semen and blood and cures aggravation of *kapha*, *kāsa* (bronchitis) and *kṣaya* (consumption).

कंडूकुष्ठक्रिमिघ्नानि कफपित्तहराणि च ।
फलानि **बृहतीनां**[30] च कटुतिक्तलघूनि च ॥ २५ ॥

*Bṛhatī* **(Solanum indicum Linn.)**

The fruit of *bṛhatī* cures *kaṇḍū* (itching), *kuṣṭha* (obstinate skin diseases including leprosy) and *kṛmi* (parasitic infection). It alleviates *kapha* and *pitta*. It is pungent, bitter and light.

**पटोलपत्रं** पित्तघ्नं नालं तस्य कफापहम् ।
**फलं**[31] तस्य त्रिदोषघ्नं मूलं तस्य विरेचनम् ॥ २६ ॥

*Paṭola* **(Trichosanthes dioica Roxb.)**

The leaf of *paṭola* alleviates *pitta*. Its stem alleviates *kapha*. Its fruit alleviates all the three *doṣas* and its root is purgative.

रोचनं कफपित्तघ्नमवृष्यं **कारवेल्लकम्** ।

*Kāravellaka* **(Momordica charantia Linn.)**

*Kāravellaka* is an appetiser. It alleviates *kapha* and *pitta*. It reduces virility.

कारवेल्लकवज्ज्ञेयं[32] फलं **कर्कोटिकस्य** च ॥ २७ ॥
**हस्तिकर्कोटिकं** तद्वद्गुणैस्तच्च[33] बृहत्फलम् ।

*Karkoṭika* **and** *Hastikarkoṭika*

The fruit of *karkoṭika* shares the properties of *kāravellaka*.

*Hasti karkoṭika* has similar properties but its fruits are bigger in size.

34
विषघ्नं **वन्ध्याकर्कोटि केवुकं** कफपित्तजित् ॥२८॥'

[माधवद्रव्यगुणः शाकवर्ग २२ : २३-३१]

### *Vandhyā karkoṭi* and *Kevuka*

*Vandhyākarkoṭi* and *kevuka* cure *viṣa* (poisoning) and alleviate *kapha* as well as *pitta*.

35
'**कूष्माण्डकं** च **कालिंगकर्कोटैर्वारुडिंडिसम्** ।
36
तथा **त्रपुसचीनाकं** विष्टम्भि कफवातजित् ॥ २९ ॥

भेदि विष्टम्भ्यभिष्यन्दि स्वादुपाकरसं गुरु ।

### *Kūṣmāṇḍaka* etc.

*Kūṣmāṇḍaka, kāliṅga, karkoṭi, ervāru, ḍiṅḍisa, trapusa* and *cīnāka* are wind forming, alleviator of *kapha* and *vāyu*, purgative, *abhiṣyandi* (which obstructs the channels of circulation), sweet in *vipāka* and taste and heavy.

पित्तनुत्तेषु **कूष्माण्डं** बालं मध्यं कफापहम् ॥ ३० ॥'

[माधवद्रव्यगुणः शाकवर्ग २२ : ३५-३६]

पक्वं लघूष्णं सक्षारदीपनं बस्तिशोधनम् ।

सर्वदोषहरं हृद्यं पथ्यं चेतोविकारिणाम् ॥ ३१ ॥

### *Kūṣmāṇḍa* (Cucurbita pepo F.I.)

The tender *kūṣmāṇḍa* alleviates *pitta*. The mature *kūṣmāṇḍa* alleviates *kapha*. The ripe *kūṣmāṇḍa* is light, hot, alkaline and digestive stimulant. It cleanses the urinary bladder and alleviates all *doṣas*. It is cardiac tonic and wholesome for patients suffering from mental diseases.

37
'वर्चोभेदीन्यलाबूनि रूक्षशीतगुरुणि च ।

Alābū (Lagenaria siceraria Standl.)

Different types of *alābū* are purgative, un-unctuous, cooling and heavy.

कटुतुंबी हिमा हृद्या पित्तकासविषापहा ॥ ३२ ॥

*Kaṭu tumbī*

*Kaṭu tumbī* is cooling and cardiac tonic. It alleviates *pitta* and cures *kāsa* (bronchitis) and *viṣa* (poisoning).

38
त्रपुसैर्वारुककारु गुरु विष्टम्भि शीतलम् ।
39
मुख्यं रूक्षं च त्रपुसं मूत्रलं त्वतिमारुतम् ॥ ३३ ॥
40
सनीलं त्रपुसं तेषां कफपित्तहरं स्मृतम् ।

तत्पाण्डु कफकृज्जीर्णमम्लं वातकफापहम् ॥ ३४ ॥

*Trapusa, Ervāru & Kakāru*

*Trapusa, ervāru* and *kakāru* are heavy, wind forming, cooling, delicious and un-unctuous.

Trapusa (Cucumis sativus Linn.)

*Trapusa* is diuretic and it exceedingly aggravates *vāyu*. *Trapusa* when it is green alleviates *kapha* and *pitta*. When it becomes yellowish in colour, it aggravates *kapha*. When over matured, it becomes sour and it alleviates *vāta* as well as *kapha*.

41
एर्वारुकं तु सम्पक्वं दाहतृष्णाश्रमार्त्तिनुत् ।

सक्षारपित्तलं तेषु शीर्णवृन्तं कफापहम् ॥ ३५ ॥
42
भेदनं दीपनं हृद्यमानाहप्लीहनुल्लघ ।

### *Ervāruka* (Cucumis utilissimus Roxb.)

The ripe *ervāruka* cures *dāha* (burning syndrome), *tṛṣṇā* (morbid thirst) and *śrama* (physical fatigue). It is alkaline and aggravator of *pitta.*

*Ervāruka* whose stalk is dried up alleviates *kapha.* It is purgative, digestive stimulant and cardiac tonic. It cures *ānāha* (flatulence) and *plīhan* (splenic disorder). It is light.

सक्षारमधुरा रुच्या [43]रूक्षा वातकफापहा ॥ ३६ ॥
[44]अश्मरी भेदनी गुर्वी **नाडी कूष्माण्डसंभवा** ।

*Kūṣmāṇḍa nāḍī*

The stalk of *knṣmāṇḍa* is alkaline, sweet, appetiser and un-unctuous. It alleviates *vāta* as well as *kapha* and removes *aśmarī* (stone in the urinary tract). It is heavy.

**अलाबुनालिका** गुर्वी मधुरा पित्तनाशिनी ।
वातश्लेष्मकरी रूक्षा शीतला मलभेदिनी ॥ ३७ ॥'

[माधवद्रव्यगुणः शाकवर्ग २३ : ३७-४३]

*Alābu nālikā*

The stalk of *Alābu* is heavy and sweet. It alleviates *pitta* and aggravates *vāyu* as well as *kapha.* It is un-unctuous, cooling and purgative.

[45]'विड्भेदि मधुरास्निग्धा प्रायो विष्टंभि वातला ।
कफापहा शीततरारुच्यपहा **पटोलिका** ॥ ३८ ॥'

### *Paṭolikā* (Trichosanthes cucumerina Roxb.)

*Paṭolikā* is purgative, sweet, unctuous and mostly wind forming. It aggravates *vāyu* and alleviates *kapha.* It is cooler and it cures *aruci* (anorexia).

‘स्वादुपाकरसा वृष्या रक्तपित्तमदापहा ।
उपोदिका[46] सरा स्निग्धा बल्या श्लेष्मकरी हिमा ।।३९।।’

[माधवद्रव्यगुण: शाकवर्ग २२ : ४३]

### *Upodikā* (Basella rubra Linn.)

*Upodikā* is sweet in *vipāka* and taste and aphrodisiac. It cures *rakta pitta* (a disease characterised by bleeding from different parts of the body). It is laxative, strength promoting, aggravator of *kapha* and cooling.

‘आरुकस्य[47] च सक्षारं शाकं श्लेष्मकरं गुरु ।’

[माधवद्रव्यगुण शाकवर्ग २२ : ४५]

### *Āruka* (Prunus domestica Linn.)

*Āruka* is alkaline, aggravator of *kapha* and heavy.

‘स्वभावात्पिच्छल:[48] शीतो विष्टम्भी वातकोपक: ।।४०।।
रक्तपित्तहर: स्वादु नीरीच:[49] परिकीर्तित: ।

### *Nīrīca*

*Nīrīca* is slimy by nature, cooling, wind forming and aggravator of *vāyu.* It cures *rakta pitta* (a disease characterised by bleeding from different parts of the body) and is delicious.

मारुसो[50] मधुर: शीतो विष्टम्भी गुरु[51] पित्तकृत् ।।४१।।
रक्तनीलादयश्चैव[52] तज्जातीयाश्च तद्गुणा: ।

### *Mārusa*

*Mārusa* is sweet, cooling, wind forming, heavy and aggravator of *pitta*. It has many varieties, viz., red, blue etc. and all of them have the same properties.

स्तन्यकृच्छीतगुर्वी[53] च सकषाया कलंवुका[54] ।। ४२ ।।

### *Kalaṁbuka* (Ipomoea reptans Poir.)

*Kalaṁbuka* promotes lactation. It is cooling, heavy and astringent.

भेबिनी कफपित्तघ्नी कुष्ठघ्नी **हिलमोचिका** ।

### *Hilamocikā* (Enhydra fluctuans Lour.)

*Halamocikā* is purgative. It alleviates *kapha* and *pitta* and cures *kuṣṭha* (obstinate skin diseases including leprosy).

कफपित्तहरस्तिक्तो रोचनो **ग्रीष्मसुन्दरः** ॥ ४३ ॥

### *Grīṣma sundara*

*Grīṣma sundara* alleviates *kapha* and *pitta*. It is bitter and appetiser.

[55]कटुतिक्तरसा हृद्या रोचनी वह्निदीपनी ।
[56]सर्वदोषहरा लघ्वी कंठ्या **मूलकपोतिका** ॥ ४४ ॥

### *Mūla kapotikā*

*Mūla kapotikā* is pungent and bitter in taste, cardiac tonic, appetiser, digestive stimulant, alleviator of all *doṣas*, light and promoter of good voice.

**मूलकं** गुरु विष्टंभी तीक्ष्णमामत्रिदोषकृत् ।
[57][स्नेहसिद्धं] तदेव स्याद्दोषत्रयविनाशनम् ।
[58]तत्फलं कफपित्तघ्नं तत्पुष्पं कफवातजित् ॥ ४५ ॥'

[माधवद्रव्यगुणः शाकवर्ग २२ : ५०-५६]

### *Mūlaka* (Raphanus sativus Linn.)

*Mūlaka* is heavy, wind forming and sharp. It produces *āma* and aggravates all the three *doṣas*. When prepared along with fat, it alleviates all the three *doṣas*. Its fruit alleviates *kapha* and *pitta* and its flower alleviates *kapha* and *vāta*.

विष्टम्भि वातलं शाकं शुष्कमन्यत्तु मूलकात् ।

All types of *śāka*, when dried cause wind formation and aggravate *vāyu*. *Mūlaka*, however, is an exception.

59
त्रिदोषघ्नमभिष्यन्दि **शाकं सर्षपजं** गुरु ॥ ४६ ॥

*Sarṣapa* **(Brassica compestris Boiss)**

The *śāka* of *sarṣapa* alleviates all the three *doṣas* (?). It is *abhiṣyandi* (which obstructs the channels of circulation) and heavy.

60
तथैव **राजिका** तिक्ता तीक्ष्णा **पञ्चांगुलः** सरः ।

*Rājikā* **and** *Pañcāṅgula* **(Brassica nigra Koch. and Ricinus communis Linn.)**

*Rājikā* shares the properties of *sarṣapa śāka*. In addition it is bitter and sharp.

The *śāka* of *pañcāṅgula* is laxative.

सरूक्षमुष्णं **कौसुम्भं** पित्तकृत्कफवातजित् ॥ ४७ ॥

*Kusuṁbha* **(Carthamus tinctorius Linn.)**

*Kusuṁbha* is un-unctuous and hot. It aggravates *pitta* and alleviates *kapha* as well as *vāta*.

61
ईषतिक्तं समधुरं **माषपत्रं** तु शुक्रलम् ।

*Māṣa* **(Phaseolus mungo Linn.)**

The leaves of *māṣa* are slightly bitter, sweet and promoter of semen.

62 63
**आहस्तिनी सपत्तूरा** मूत्रलाश्मरिनाशिनी ॥ ४८ ॥

*Āhastinī* **and** *Pattūrā*

*Āhastinī* and *pattūrā* are diuretics. They cure *aśmari* **(stone** in the urinary tract).

न्यग्रोधोदुम्बराश्वत्थप्लक्षपद्मादिपल्लवाः ।
कषायाः स्तम्भनाः[64] शीता हिताः पित्तातिसारिणाम् ॥४९॥

*Nyagrodha* etc.

The leaf of *nyagrodha*, *udumbara*, *aśvattha*, *plakṣa*, *padma* etc. is astringent, constipative and cooling. It is useful for patients suffering from *paittika* type of *atisāra* (diarrhoea).

'छात्रकास्तु पला[65][लि]क्षुकरीषक्षितिवेणुजाः[66] ।
सर्वे संस्वेदजाः शीताः कषायाः स्वादुपिच्छिलाः ॥५०॥

*Saṁsvedaja* (Mushroom)

Mushrooms which grow on *palāla* (straw), *ikṣu* (sugarcane), *karīṣa* (cow dung), *kṣiti* (ground) and *veṇu* (bamboo) are called *saṁsvedaja*. All of them are cooling, astringent, delicious and slimy.

गुरवश्छर्द्यतीसारज्वरश्लेष्मामयप्रदाः ।
स्वादुपाकरसा रूक्षा दोषलास्ते पलालयाः[67] ॥ ५१ ॥

Mushrooms which grow on straw are heavy. They produce *chardi* (vomiting), *atisāra* (diarrhoea), *jvara* (fever) and diseases caused by *kapha*. They are sweet in *vipāka* as well as taste and un-unctuous. They aggravate *doṣas*.

श्वेताः शुचि[68]स्थलीकाष्ठवंश[69]गोव्रजसंभवाः ।
'[नातिदोषकरा[70] ज्ञेयाः] शेषास्तेभ्यो विगर्हिताः ॥५२॥

Mushrooms which are white in colour, which grow in clean places or on wood, bamboo and cattle shed are not very injurious. Remaining types of mushrooms should not be used.

[71]तद्विकल्पोऽल्पदोषश्च [72]स्थलीगोव्रजसंभवः ।

खुखुंडक इति ख्यातो वृष्यो बल्योऽथ बृंहणः ।

Another variety of mushroom is called *khukhuṇḍaka.* It is less injurious and it grows on the ground and in a cattle shed. It is aphrodisiac, strength promoting and nourishing.

विष्टम्भिनः स्मृताः [73]सर्वे छत्राका वातकोपनाः ॥५३॥

[माधवद्रव्यगुणः शाकवर्ग २२ : ५७-६४]

All the mushrooms are known to be wind forming and they aggravate *vāyu.*

[74]पिनाकिर्वातला [75]सार्द्रा रुचिष्यानिलदीपनी ।

*Pinākī*

*Pinākī* aggravates *vāyu.* When it is green it is an appetiser and stimulant of digestion.

विदारी वातपित्तघ्नी वृष्या बल्या रसायनी ॥५४॥

*Vidārī* **(Ipomoea paniculata R. Br.)**

*Vidārī* alleviates *vāyu* and *pitta.* It is aphrodisiac, strength promoting and rejuvenating.

[76]शतावरी महाबल्या चक्षुष्या वातपित्तनुत् ।

*Śatāvarī* **(Asparagus racemosus Willd.)**

*Śatāvarī* is an excellent promoter of strength and eyesight. It alleviates *vāyu* and *pitta.*

[77]महती चैव हृद्या च मेधाग्निबलवर्धिनी ॥ ५५ ॥

ग्रहण्यर्शोविकारघ्नी वृष्या बल्या रसायनी ।

The bigger variety is a cardiac tonic and promoter of

intellect, power of digestion and strength. It cures *grahaṇī* (sprue syndrome) and *arśas* (piles). It is aphrodisiac, strength promoting and rejuvenating.

कासपित्तहरास्तिक्तास्तस्या[78] **एवांकुरा** मता[79] ।। ५६ ।।

Its sprouts cure *kāsa* (bronchitis) and alleviate *pitta*. They are bitter.

सरूक्षं[80] **विसशालूकं** **क्रौञ्चादनं** **कसेरुकम्** ।

**शृंगाटकं** **गलोड्यं** च गुरु विष्टंभि शीतलम् ।।५७।।

*Visaśālūka* **etc.**

*Visaśālūka*, *krauñcādana*, *kaseruka*, *sṛṅgāṭaka* and *galoḍhya* are un-unctuous, heavy, wind forming and cooling.

**पौष्करं** तु भवेद्बीजं रक्तपित्तज्वरापहम् ।

*Pauṣkara* **(Lotus seed)**

The seed of *puṣkara* cures *rakta pitta* (a disease characterised by bleeding from different parts of the body) and *jvara* (fever).

तथा **तालप्रलंबं** च उरःक्षतरुजापहम् ।। ५८ ।।

*Tāla pralamba* **(Borassus flabellifer Linn.)**

The inflorescence of *tāla* cures *uraḥkṣata* (phthisis).

पित्तानिलहरो[81] हृद्यः[82] स्वादुः **मुंजातकः**[83] स्मृतः ।

*Muñjātaka* **(Orchis latifolia Linn.)**

*Muñjātaka* alleviates *pitta* and *vāyu*. It is a cardiac tonic and delicious.

**शंखहस्तीकरक्तांयं**[84] **मधुपिण्डकशुंगकम्** ।। ५९ ।।

शंखाद्यान्यालुकानीह[85] रक्तपित्तहराणि च ।
गुरूणि स्वादुशीतानि स्तन्यशुक्रकराणि च ॥ ६० ॥

*Āluka* **(Dioscorea Sp.)**

*Śaṅkha*, *hastīka*, *raktāṅga*, *madhupiṇḍaka* and *śuṅgaka*—these are the different types of *āluka*. They cure *rakta pitta* (a disease characterised by bleeding from different parts of the body). They are heavy, delicious and cooling. They promote lactation and semen.

पिंडारुकं[86] कफकरं गुरु वातप्रकोपणम् ।

*Piṇḍāruka* **(Colocasia esculenta Schott)**

*Piṇḍāruka* aggravates *kapha*. It is heavy. It also aggravates *vāyu*.

सुरेन्द्रकन्दः श्लेष्मघ्नो विपाके कटु[87] पित्तकृत् ॥ ६१ ॥

*Surendra kanda* **(Amorphophalus sylvaticus Kunth)**

*Surendra kanda* alleviates *kapha*. It is pungent in *vipāka* and it aggravates *pitta*.

'बल्यः कदल्याः कंदस्तु वातपित्तहरः[88] सदा[89] ।'

*Kadali kanda* **(Musa paradisica Linn.)**

The rhizome of *kadalī* promotes strength and it alleviates *vāyu* and *pitta*.

माणकं स्वादु शीतं[90] च गुरु चापि प्रकीर्तितम् ॥६२॥

*Mānaka* **(Alocasia indica Schott.)**

Māṇaka is sweet, cooling and heavy.

दीपनः **सूरणो** रुच्यः कफघ्नो विशदो लघुः ।
'विशेषादर्शसां पथ्यो, **भूकन्द**स्त्वतिदोषलः ॥ ६३ ॥

### *Sūraṇa* and *Bhūkanda*

*Sūraṇa* is digestive stimulant, appetiser, alleviator of *kapha, viśada* (non slimy) and light. It is specifically useful for *arśas* (piles).

*Bhū kanda* is exceedingly harmful.

**अम्लिकायाः** स्मृतः कन्दो ग्रहण्यर्शोहितो[91] लघुः[92] ।
नात्युष्णः कफवातघ्नो ग्राही शस्तो मदात्यये ॥६४॥

### *Amlikā kanda*

The rhizome of *amlikā* is useful in *grahaṇī* (sprue syndrome) and *arśas* (piles). It is light and not very hot. It alleviates *kapha* and *vāyu*. It is constipative and is useful in *madātyaya* (alcoholism).

**कुमुदोत्पलपद्मानां** कंदा मारुतकोपनाः[93] ।
कषायाः पित्तशमना विपाके मधुरा[94] हिमाः ॥ ६५ ॥

### *Kumuda kanda* etc.

The rhizome of *kumuda*, *utpala* and *padma* aggravates *vāyu*. It is astringent, alleviator of *pitta*, sweet in *vipāka* and cooling.

**मुसली**[95] बृंहणी वृष्या वीर्योष्णा[96]र्शोऽनिला[97]पहा ।

### *Muśalī* (Chlorophytum tuberosum Baker)

*Múśalī* is nourishing, aphrodisiac and hot in potency. It cures *arśas* (piles) and vitiation of *vāyu*.

**वाराहकन्दः**[98] श्लेष्मघ्नः कटुको रसपाकतः ।। ६६ ।।
कुष्ठकृमिहरो[99] वृष्यो बलवर्णविवर्धनः[100] ।

### *Vārāha kanda* (Tacca aspera Roxb.)

*Vārāha kanda* alleviates *kapha*. It is pungent in taste and *vipāka*. It cures *kuṣṭha* (obstinate skin diseases including leprosy) and *kṛmi* (parasitic infection). It is aphrodisiac and it promotes strength as well as complexion.

**तालस्य**[101] **नालिकेरस्य खर्जूरस्य शिरांसि च** ।। ६७ ।।
कषायस्निग्धमधुरं बृंहणानि गुरूणि च ।
सृष्टमूत्राणि वृष्याणि जीवनीयप्रदानि[102] च ।। ६८ ।।
बलपुंस्त्वक्षये कासे[103] रक्तपित्तेऽनिले विषे ।
प्रशस्तानि सदा पुंसां शीतानि[104] रुचिराणि[105] च ।।६९।।

### *Tāla śiras* etc.

The top portion of the trunk of *tāla*, *nārikela* and *kharjūra* is astringent, unctuous, sweet, nourishing and heavy. It helps in the elimination of urine. It is aphrodisiac and vitalising. It is always useful for persons who have lost their strength and potency. It cures *kāsa* (bronchitis), *rakta pitta* (a disease characterised by bleeding from different parts of the body), vitiation of *vāyu* and *viṣa* (poisoning). It is cooling and delicious.

बालं[106] ह्यनार्त्तवं जीर्णं व्याधितं कृमिभक्षितम् ।
कंदं विवर्जयेत्सर्वं यो वा सम्यक् न रोहति ।। ७० ।।

**Bad quality**

All rhizomes which are immature, unseasonal, old, diseased, eaten away by parasites and which are not properly grown should not be used.

धान्येषु मांसेषु फलेषु चैव शाकेषु चानुक्तमिह प्रमोहात्[107] ।
आस्वादतो भूतगुणैर्गृहीत्वा[108] तदादिशेद्द्रव्यमनल्पबुद्धिः ॥७१॥

**Miscellaneous**

The description of the properties of different type of *dhānyas* (corns and cereals), *māṁsa* (meat), *phala* (fruits) and *śāka* (vegetables) which is omitted here by mistake should be determind by the Wise by examining the taste and attributes of *mahābhūtas* in them.

॥ इति शाकवर्गः ॥

**Thus ends the group dealing with different types of vegetables.**

## NOTES AND REFERENCES

1. 'श्री गणेशाय नमः' पाठोऽयं चतुर्थपुस्तके उपलभ्यते ।
2. षड्विधं शाकमुद्दिष्टं इति आकरे पाठः ।
3. स्वादुपाकमसृक्पित्तविषनुत् इति आकरे पाठः ।
4. मेधाग्निबलवर्धनः इति आकरे द्वितीयपुस्तके च पाठः ।
5. चिल्ली वास्तूकवज्ज्ञेया इति आकरे पाठः ।
6. पित्तकफापहा इति आकरे पाठः ।
7. मधूरा इति द्वितीयपुस्तके पाठः ।
8. रक्तपित्तविषज्वरान् इति आदर्शपुस्तकेषु पाठः ।
9. सतीनकम् इति आकरे पाठः ।
10. कषायानु हिता इति आकरे पाठः ।
11. चाम्ला इति आकरे पाठः ।
12. संग्राहकं वातकरं इति आकरे पाठः ।
13. त्वादकं इति चतुर्थपुस्तके पाठः ।
14. वर्षाम्भ्वौ इति आदर्शपुस्तकेषु पाठः ।

15. हितौ शोथोदरार्शसाम् इति आकरे पाठः ।
16. कफवातघ्नाश्चिरबिल्वांकुराः सराः इति आकरे पाठः ।
17. रूक्षाः इति आकरे पाठः -
18. करीराः इति आकरे पाठः ।
19. सकषाया इति आकरे पाठः ।
20. नालांकुराश्चान्ये इति आकरे पाठः ।
21. किराततिक्तसहिताः इति आकरे पाठः ।
22. सर्वे पित्तकफापहाः इति आकरे पाठः ।
23. तद्वदेव इति आकरे पाठः ।
24. तु इति आकरे पाठः ।
25. कफमेदोनिलहरमत्यर्थं इति आकरे चतुर्थपुस्तके च पाठः ।
26. तदेकं इति आदर्शपुस्तके पाठः ।
27. मारुतनाशनी इति आकरे पाठः ।
28. बलासकासक्षयनाशनी इति आकरे पाठः ।
29. वार्ताकिरेषां इति आकरे पाठः ।
30. फलीनि इति चतुर्थपुस्तके पाठः ।
31. पाठोऽयं आकरे नोपलभ्यते ।
32. कारवेल्लकवद्ज्ञेयं इति आकरे पाठः ।
33. तद्वद् गुणैस्तत्तु इति आकरे पाठः ।
34. वंध्यकर्कोटं केवुकं इति आकरे पाठः ।
वन्धिकार्कोटि केबुं इति द्वितीयपुस्तके पाठः ।
35. कूष्मांडतुम्बकालिंगकर्कोटैर्वारुडिंडिसम् इति आकरे पाठः ।
36. तथा त्रपुसबीजं तु रुचिदं कफवातजित् इति आकरे पाठः ।
तथा त्रपुसचानाकर्चिमिटं कफवातकृत् इति चतुर्थपुस्तके पाठः ।
37. वर्च्योभेदीन्यलावूनि इति चतुर्थपुस्तके पाठः ।
38. त्रपुसैर्वारुकं स्वादु इति आकरे पाठः ।
39. मुखप्रियं च रूक्षं च मूत्रलं त्रपुसं त्वति इति आकरे चतुर्थपुस्तके च पाठः ।
40. बालं सनीलं त्रपुसं तेषां पित्तहरं स्मृतम् इति आकरे पाठः ।
41. दाहतृष्णाक्लमार्त्तिनुत् इति आकरे पाठः ।
42. ह्रियमानाहाष्ठीलनुल्लघु इति आकरे पाठः ।
43. शीर्णवृन्तं लघु स्वादु भेद्युक्तं वह्निपित्तकृत् ।

सक्षारमधुरा रुच्या वातपित्तकफापहा ॥ इति आकरे पाठः ।
(माधवद्रव्यगुणः शाकवर्ग २२ : ४१-४२)

44. स्थिराविभेदिनी इति द्वितीयपुस्तके पाठः ।
45. 'विड्भेदमधुरास्निग्धा''''पटोलिका' पाठोऽयं चतुर्थपुस्तके अधिकमुपलभ्यते ।
46. उपोदका इति द्वितीयपुस्तके पाठः ।
47. विषमस्य यवक्षारं सार्षश्लेष्मकरं गुरु [?] इति द्वितीयपुस्तके पाठः ।
48. स्वभावपिच्छिलः इति आकरे पाठः ।
49. स्वादुर्नाडीचः इति चतुर्थपुस्तके आकरे च पाठः ।
50. मातुसो इति चतुर्थपुस्तके पाठः ।
51. पित्तनुद् गुरुः इति आकरे पाठः ।
52. रक्तनालादयश्चान्ये इति आकरे पाठः ।
53. स्तन्यवृष्या च गुर्वी च चतुर्थपुस्तके पाठः ।
स्तन्या वृष्या च इतिं आकरे पाठः ।
54. करंबुका इति चतुर्थपुस्तके पाठः ।
55. कटुतिक्ता सरा इति आकरे पाठः ।
कटुतिक्तसहा हृद्या इति द्वितीयपुस्तके पाठः ।
56. सर्वदोषहरी इति आकरे पाठः ।
57. स्निग्धसिद्धिं इति द्वितीयपुस्तके पाठः ।
58. 'तत्फलं''''''''कफवातजित्' पाठोऽयं द्वितीयपुस्तके नोपलभ्यते ।
59. त्रिदोषं बह्वभिष्यन्दि इति आकरे पाठः ।
60. तीक्ष्णा तिक्तः इति आकरे पाठः ।
61. माषपर्णन्तु इति आकरे पाठ. ।
62. श्रीहस्तिनी इति आकरे चतुर्थतुस्तके च पाठः ।
63. मूत्रलाश्मरीभेदनी इति आकरे चतुर्थपुस्तके च पाठः ।
64. शीताः इति आकरे पाठः ।
65. पलाशेक्षुकरीषक्षितिवेणुजाः इति चतुर्थपुस्तके पाठः ।
66. 'छत्रकास्तु''''''''स्वादुपिच्छिला' पाठोऽयं द्वितीयपुस्तके नोपलभ्यते ।
67. पलालजाः इति आकरे पाठः ।
68. शुंद्धस्थली इति आकरे पाठः ।
69. काष्ठवंशग्रोव्रजसंभवाः इति आदर्शपुस्तकेषु पाठः ।
70. पाठोऽयं चतुर्थपुस्तके नोपलभ्यते ।
71. तद्विकल्पोऽल्पदोषाश्च इति आकरे पाठः ।

72. 'नातिदोषकरा···:स्थलीगोव्रजसंभवः' पाठोऽयं द्वितीयपुस्तके नोपलभ्यते ।
73. छत्रका इति आकरे पाठः ।
74. पिण्याकी वातला इति आकरे पाठः।
75. सान्द्रा इति आकरे पाठः ।
76. वृष्या शतावरी बल्या इति आकरे पाठः ।
77. सैव इति आकरे पाठः ।
78. कफपित्तहरास्तिक्तास्तस्या इति आकरे पाठः ।
79. स्मृताः इति आकरे पाठः ।
80. तरूढबिसशालूकक्रौंचादनकसेरुकम् इति आकरे पाठः।
81. पित्तानिलकरो इति द्वितीयपुस्तके पाठः ।
82. वृष्यः इति आकरे चतुर्थपुस्तके च पाठः ।
83. स्वादुर्मुञ्जातकः इति आकरे पाठः ।
84. शंखहस्तिकरक्तांगमधुपिण्डकश्रृंगकम् इति आकरे पाठः ।
85. षडद्यात्पाण्डुकानाह इति आदर्शपुस्तकेषु पाठः ।
86. पिण्डालुकं इति आकरे पाठः ।
87. कटुः इति आकरे पाठः ।
88. वातपित्तहरश्च इति आकरे पाठः ।
89. 'बल्यः····सदा' पाठोऽयं चतुर्थपुस्तके नोपलभ्यते ।
90. पित्तं इति आदर्शपुस्तकेषु पाठः ।
91. लघुः इति आकरे पाठः ।
92. 'विंशेषादर्शसां····लघु' पाठोऽयं चतुर्थपुस्तके नोपलभ्यते ।
93. मारुतकोपनाः इति आकरे पाठः ।
94. मधुराः इति आकरे पाठः ।
95. मुशली इति आकरे चतुर्थपुस्तके च पाठः ।
96. वीर्योष्णाऽर्शोऽनिलापहा इति आकरे पाठः ।
97. अस्य श्लोकस्यानन्तरम् 'नातिश्लेष्मघ्नः पित्तदूषणः ।' पाठोऽयं द्वितीयपुस्तके अधिकं उपलभ्यते ।
98. वराहकंदः इति आकरे पाठः ।
99. कुष्ठमेहक्रिमिहरो वृष्योष्णः पित्तवर्द्धनः इति आकरे चतुर्थपुस्तके च पाठः।
100. अस्य श्लोकस्यानन्तरम् 'कंदो हलिन्याः श्लेष्मघ्नः पित्तलो गर्भपातनः' पाठोऽयं चतुर्थपुस्तके अधिकमुपलभ्यते ।

101. वालस्य इति द्वितीयपुस्तके पाठः ।
102. जीवन प्रीणनानि च इति आकरे पाठः ।
103. कार्श्ये इति चतुर्थपुस्तके पाठः ।
104. रुचिदानि इति आकरे पाठः ।
105. द्वितीयचतुर्थपुस्तकयोः अत्रैव "इति शाकवर्गः" इति पठितं । अस्य श्लोकस्यानन्तरम् '·····परिजीर्णं च कांमेजुष्टमदेशजं । वर्ज्जयेत्पत्रशाकं च यदकाले प्ररोहि च' पाठोऽयं चतुर्थपुस्तके अधिकं उपलभ्यते ।
106. बालं अनार्त्तवं इति चतुर्थपुस्तके पाठः ।
107. प्रमादात् इति आकरे पाठः ।
108. समादिशेद् द्रव्यमनल्पबुद्धिः इति आकरे पाठ ।

# CHAPTER 21

'षष्टिका यवगोधूमा लोहिता ये च शालयः ।
मुद्गाढकीमसूराश्च **धान्येषु** प्रवराः स्मृताः ॥ १ ॥

*Dhānya* **(Corns and Cereals)**

Among the corns and cereals, *ṣaṣṭika*, *yava*, *godhūma*. red variety of *śāli*, *mudga*, *āḍhakī* and *masūra* are the best.

एणः कुरंगो [1]हरिणस्तित्तिरिर्लाव एव च ।
मयूर[2]वर्गिकूर्माश्च श्रेष्ठा [3]**मांस**गुणेषु च ॥ २ ॥

*Māṁsa* **(Meat)**

Among different types of meat, the meat of *eṇa*, *kuraṅga*, *hariṇa*, *tittiri*, *lāva*, *mayūra*, *vargi* (?) and *kūrma* are the best.

दाडिमामलकं द्राक्षा खर्जूरं सपरूषकम् ।
राजादनं मातुलुंग[4]**फलवर्गे** प्रशस्यते ॥ ३ ॥

*Phala* **(Fruits)**

Among different types of fruits *dāḍima*, *āmalaka*, *drākṣā*, *kharjūra*, *paruṣaka*, *rājādana* and *mātuluṅga* are the best.

चंचूसतीनवास्तूकचिल्लमूलकपोतिका[5] ।
मण्डूकपर्णी जीवन्ती शाकवर्गे[6] प्रशस्यते ।। ४ ।।

### *Śāka* (Vegetables)

Among vegetables, *caṅcū*, *satīna*, *vāstūka*, *cilla*, *mūlakapotikā*, *maṇḍūkaparṇī* and *jīvantī* are the best.

गव्यं क्षीरघृतं[7] श्रेष्ठं सैन्धवं लवणेषु च ।

### *Kṣīra*, *Ghṛta* and *Lavaṇa*

Among milk and ghee, those derived from the cow are the best.

Among salts, rock salt is the best.

धात्री दाडिमम्लेषु पिप्पलीनागरे[8] कटौ ।। ५ ।।

### Sour and Pungent articles

Among sour things, *dhātrī* and *dāḍima* are the best.

Among pungent things *pippalī* and *nāgara* are the best.

तिक्ते पटोलकं[9] श्रेष्ठं मधुरे घृतमुच्यते ।

### Bitter and Sweet articles

Among bitter things *paṭola* is the best.

Among sweet things ghee is the best.

क्षौद्रं[10] पूगफलं श्रेष्ठं कषाये सपरूषकम् ।। ६ ।।

### Astringent things

Among astringent things, honey, *pūgaphala* and *parūṣaka* are the best.

शर्करेक्षुविकारेषु पानजातौ[11] सुरासवौ ।

**Sugarcane products and Drinks**

Among sugar cane products, *śarkarā* is the best.

Among different types of drinks, *surā* and *āsava* are the best.

परिसंवत्सरं धान्यं मांसं वयसि मध्यमे ॥ ७ ॥
अपर्युषितमन्नं[12] तु संस्कृतं मात्रया शुभम् ।
फलं पर्यागतं शाकमशुष्कं तरुणं नवम् ॥' ८ ॥

[माधवद्रव्यगुणः श्रेष्ठवर्ग २३ : १-८]

**Miscellaneous**

Among different types of *dhānya* (corns and cereals), those preserved for one year are the best. The meat of animals in their middle age is the best. Food which is not stale, which is properly prepared and which is taken in proper quantity is the best. Fruit which is matured is the best. The vegetable which is not dried, which is tender and fresh is the best.

'रसेसु मधुरः श्रेष्ठः कंदशाकेषु सूरणः ।
जलेषु दिव्यं मत्स्येषु रोहितः प्रवरो मतः ।
तैलेषु तिलजं तैलं श्रेष्ठं प्रोक्तं[13] मनीषिभिः ॥ ९ ॥

Among different types of tastes, the sweet taste is the best. Among the rhizomes *sūraṇa* is the best. Among the different types of water, *divya* (which is directly collected from the sky) is the best. Among different types of fish, *rohita* is the best. Among the different types of oil, *til* oil is the best.

॥ इति श्रेष्ठवर्गः ॥

Thus ends the section dealing with different types of best articles.

## NOTES AND REFERENCES

1. हरिणः तितिरार्लाव इति आकरे पाठः ।
2. मयूखर्मिकूर्माश्च इति आकरे पाठः ।
3. मांसगणेषु इति आकरे पाठः ।
4. मातुलुङ्गं फलवर्गे इति आकरे पाठः ।
5. चंचूसतीनवास्तूक-चिल्लीमूलकपोतिकाः इति आकरे पाठः।
6. शाकवर्गेषु शस्यते इति द्वितीयपुस्तके पाठः ।
7. क्षीरं घृतं इति आकरे पाठः ।
8. नागरं इति आकरे पाठः ।
9. पटोलवार्ताके इति आकरे पाठः ।
10. खर्जूर इति द्वितीयपुस्तके पाठः ।
11. पानकादी इति चतुर्थपुस्तके पाठः ।
12. अपर्युषितमम्लं इति आदर्शपुस्तकेषु पाठः ।
13. रसेषु....मनीषिभिः पाठोऽयं द्वितीयपुस्तके नोपलभ्यते ।

# CHAPTER 22

'चक्षुष्यः प्रीणनो वृष्यो बृंहणो रक्तपित्तजित् ।
रसायनो गुरुः शीतः स्निग्धश्च मधुरो रसः ॥ १ ॥

### Sweet Taste

Sweet taste is a promoter of eyesight, pleasing, aphrodisiac and nourishing. It cures *rakta pitta* (a disease characterised by bleeding from different parts of the body). It is rejuvenating, heavy, cooling and unctuous.

[पक्ता][1] हृद्योऽग्निरुचिकृत्क्लेदनस्तर्पणो मृदुः[2] ।
स्निग्धोष्णो[ऽ]म्लो लघु[र्वापि][3] वातहा रक्तनाशनः ॥२॥
क्लेदी तीक्ष्णः सरः शुक्रविबंधानाहदृष्टिहा[4] ।

### Sour taste

Sour taste is unctuous, hot, light and alleviator of *vāyu* and vitiation of blood. It produces stickiness. It is sharp and laxative. It reduces semen, constipation and eye sight.

भेदी पक्ताग्निरुचिकृत्स्निग्धोष्णो [5]**लवणो** गुरुः ॥३॥

**Saline taste**

Saline taste is purgative, promoter of digestive power, appetiser, unctuous, hot and heavy.

**कर्षणो** लघुरुक्षोष्णः कृमिशुक्रकफापहा ।
[6]रुच्योऽग्निपित्तकृच्छेदि तीक्ष्णः शोषप्रदः **कटुः** ॥४॥

**Pungent taste**

Pungent taste is *karṣaṇa* (which eliminates by force), light, un-unctuous and hot. It cures *kṛmi* (parasitic infection) and reduces semen as well as *kapha*. It is an appetiser, stimulant of digestion, aggravator of *pitta*, *chedi* (which has the power to penetrate by incision), sharp and producer of dryness (*śoṣa*).

[7]कफपित्तविषक्लेदकंडूकुष्ठज्वरापहः ।
रूक्षः शीतो [8]लघु**स्तिक्तः** शोषणः कृमिहाऽग्निकृत् ॥५॥

**Bitter taste**

Bitter taste alleviates *kapha* as well as *pitta*. It cures *viṣa* (poisoning), stickiness (*kleda*), *kaṇḍū* (itching), *kuṣṭha* (obstinate skin diseases including leprosy) and *jvara* (fever). It is un-unctuous, cooling, light and drying (*śoṣaṇa*). It cures *kṛmi* (parasitic infection) and stimulates the power of digestion.

**कषायः** [9]शोषणः स्तम्भी ग्राही [10]रोपणपीडनः ।

कफशोणितपित्तघ्नो रूक्षः शीतो गुरुस्तथा ॥ ६ ॥

[माधवद्रव्यगुणः रसवर्ग २४ : १-६]

**Astringent taste**

Astringent taste is drying, *stambhana* (which causes retention), constipative, healing and *pīḍana* (which causes pain). It

**alleviates vitiation of *kapha*, blood and *pitta*. It is un-unctuous, cooling and heavy.**

॥ इति षड्रसाः ॥

Thus ends the section dealing with the attributes of the six tastes.

## NOTES AND REFERENCES

1. पक्त्वा इति द्वितीयपुस्तके पाठः ।
2. परः इति द्वितीयपुस्तके पाठः ।
3. लघुर्व्यापी इति द्वितीयपुस्तके पाठः ।
4. शुक्लः विबंधानाहदृष्टिहा इति द्वितीयपुस्तके पाठः ।
5. रसः इति आकरे पाठः ।
6. रुच्योऽग्निपित्तकृच्छेत्ता तीक्ष्णः शोषी कटुः कटुः इति आकरे पाठः ।
7. कफपित्तविषक्लेदिकंडूकुष्ठज्वरापहः इति आदर्शपुस्तके पाठः ।
8. शीतो लघुस्तिक्तः इति आकरे पाठः ।
   शीतलघु स्निग्धः इति चतुर्थपुस्तके पाठः ।
9. स्तम्भनः शोषी ग्राही इति आकरे पाठः ।
10. रोपणप्रीणनः इति चतुर्थपुस्तके पाठः ।

# CHAPTER 23

'मंडस्तु त्रिविधो ज्ञेय एकद्वित्रिपरिश्रुतः[1] ।

*Maṇḍa*

*Maṇḍa* is prepared by filtering once, twice or three times. Thus, it is of three types.

लाजैर्भृष्टैरभृष्टैश्च तण्डुलैः परिसंस्कृतैः[2] ॥ १ ॥
चतुस्त्रिद्विगुणाम्भः स्यात् पूर्वः[3] पूर्वो लघुर्हितः ।

*Lāja maṇḍa*

*Lāja maṇda* is prepared either after frying or without frying the *lājā* (fried paddy). Before preparing *lājā*, the rice should be made clean. Thereafter, for its preparation water is added four, three or two times. The former varieties are lighter than the latter ones.

**लाजमण्डो** विशुद्धानां पथ्यः पाचनदीपनः ॥ २ ॥

*Lāja maṇḍa* is wholesome for a person whose body is cleaned by the administration of elimination therapy. It is

**carminative and a digestive stimulant.**

वातानुलोमनो हृद्यः पिप्पलीनागरैर्युतः[4] ।

When added with *pippalī* and *nāgara* it helps in the elimination of *vāyu* through the downward tract. It is a cardiac tonic.

पाचनो दीपनश्चैव पित्तश्लेष्मानिलापहः ॥ ३ ॥
शूलांनाहविबन्धघ्नो **धान्यमण्डः**[5] प्रकीर्तितः ।

*Dhānya maṇḍa*

*Dhānya maṇḍa* is carminative, digestive stimulant and alleviator of *pitta*, *kapha* and *vāyu.* It cures *śūla* (colic pain), *ānāha* (flatulence) and *vibandha* (constipation).

वाते[6] वा सकफे पित्ते सामे वा तरुणज्वरे ॥ ४ ॥
**वाट्यमंडं** प्रशंसन्ति पटोलमगधान्वितम् ।
[वाट्यमंडो यवैर्भृष्टैर्लाजमंडस्तु शालिभिः][7] ॥ ५ ॥

*Vāṭya maṇḍa*

*Vāṭya maṇḍa* mixed with *paṭola* and *magadhā* is useful in the aggravation of *vāyu, kapha* and *pitta,* in *āma* and in the beginning stage of *jvara* (fever).

*Vāṭya maṇḍa* is prepared by fried barley and *lāja maṇḍa* is prepared by fried *śāli*.

रक्तशाल्यादिभिर्धान्यैर्मण्डो[8] मधुरशीतलः ।
श्रेष्ठो[9] संतर्पणो बल्यो रक्तपित्तप्रसादनः[10] ॥ ६ ॥

***Raktaśāli maṇḍa***

The *maṇḍa* prepared of red variety of *śāli* etc., is sweet and cooling. It is the most wholesome, refreshing and strength promoting. It alleviates *rakta pitta* (a disease characterised by bleeding from different parts of the body).

सुतण्डुलानां प्रसृतिद्वयं च तदर्द्धमुद्गाः कटुकत्रयं च ।
11
कुस्तुम्बरीसैन्धवहिंगुतैलमेभिश्च सर्वैः क्रियते च मण्डः ॥७॥
क्षुद्बोधनो बस्तिविशोधनश्च प्राणप्रदः शोणितवर्धनश्च ।
ज्वरापहारी कफपित्तहंता वायुं जयेदष्टगुणो हि मण्डः ॥८॥

*Aṣṭaguṇa maṇḍa*

The *maṇḍa* prepared of two *prasṛti* of good quality rice and half in quantity of *mudga* mixed with *kaṭutraya* (*śuṇṭhī*, *pippalī* and *marica*), *kustumbarī*, *saindhava*, *hiṅgu* and oil is called *aṣṭaguṇa maṇḍa*.

It promotes appetite and cleanses the urinary bladder. It promotes vitality and blood formation. It cures *jvara* (fever) and aggravation of *kapha*, *pitta* as well as *vāyu*.

हस्तवस्त्रकृतो मंडः सैन्धवेनावचूर्णितः ।
12
रक्तपित्तहरो ग्राही ज्वरातीसारनाशनः ॥ ९ ॥

**Miscellaneous**

The *maṇḍa* prepared with the help of the hands and a piece of cloth and sprinkled with the powder of *saindhava* cures *rakta pitta* (a disease characterised by bleeding from different parts of the body). It is constipative and cures *jvara* (fever) and *atisāra* (diarrhoea).

मंडस्तु दीपयत्यग्निं वातं चाप्यनुलोमयेत् ।
मृदुकरोति स्रोतांसि स्वेदं संजनयत्यपि ॥ १० ॥

*Maṇḍa* stimulates the power of digestion and helps in the elimination of *vāyu* through the downward tract. It softens the channels of circulation and produces sweating.

13
लंघितानां विरिक्तानां जीर्णे स्नेहे च तृष्यताम् ।

दीपनत्वाल्लघुत्वाच्च मंडः स्यात्प्राणधारणः ॥११॥'

[माधवद्रव्यगुणः मण्डवर्ग २५ : १-११]

After fasting, purgation, and digestion of the potion given for oleation therapy, if the patient feels thirsty, then *maṇḍa* helps in the sustenance of his life because it is a digestive stimulant as well as light.

॥ इति मण्डवर्गः ॥

Thus ends the group dealing with different types of *maṇḍa*.

## NOTES AND REFERENCES

1. एकद्वित्रिपरिस्रुतः इति आकरे चतुर्थपुस्तके च पाठः ।
2. परिसंस्कृतः इति आकरे पाठः ।
3. पूर्वपूर्वो इति आकरे पाठः ।
4. पिप्पलीनागरान्वितः इति आकरे पाठः ।
5. वाट्यमंडः इति आकरे पाठः ।
6. वातकफे इति आकरे पाठः ।
7. 'वाट्यमंडो····शालिभिः' पाठोऽयं द्वितीयचतुर्थपुस्तकयोर्नोपलभ्यते ।
8. रक्तशाल्यादिभिर्धान्यैर्मण्डा इति आकरे पाठः ।
9. श्रेष्ठाः संतर्पणा बल्या रक्तपित्तप्रसादनः इति चतुर्थपुस्तके पाठः ।
10. रक्तपित्त प्रसादनाः इति आकरे पाठः ।
11. हि इति आकरे पाठः ।
    स इति चतुर्थपुस्तके पाठः ।
12. ज्वरातीसारवारणः इति आकरे चतुर्थपुस्तके च पाठः ।
13. तृष्यती इति आदर्षपुस्तकेषु पाठः ।

# CHAPTER 24

"क्षुत्तृष्णानिलदौर्बल्यकुक्षिरोगविनाशिनी[1] ।
स्वेदाग्निजननी **पेया** वातवर्चोऽनुलोमनी ॥ १ ॥

*Peyā*

*Peyā* cures *kṣut* (morbid hunger), *tṛṣā* (morbid thirst), vitiation of *vāyu*, weakness and diseases of the pelvic region. It causes sweating, stimulates the power of degestion and helps in the elimination of *vāyu* and stool through the downward tract.

'**विलेपी** तर्पणी हृद्या ग्राहिणी बलवर्धिनी ।
पथ्या स्वादुरसा लघ्वी दीपनी क्षुत्तृषापहा ॥ २ ॥'

[सुश्रुतः सूत्र ४६ : ३४२-३४३]

*Vilepī*

*Vilepī* is refreshing, a cardiac tonic, constipative, strength promoting, wholesome, sweet in taste, light and a digestive stimulant. It cures *kṣut* (morbid hunger) and *tṛṣā* (morbid thirst).

तृष्णापनयनी लघ्वी दीपनी बस्तिशोधनी ।

ज्वरे चैवातिसारे च **यवागूः** सर्वदा हिता ।।" ३ ।।

[माधवद्रव्यगुणः अन्नवर्ग २६ : १-३]

*Yavāgū*

*Yavāgū* cures *tṛṣṇā* (morbid thirst). It is light and a digestive stimulant. It cleanses the urinary bladder. In *jvara* (fever) and *atisāra* (diarrhoea), *yavāgū* is always useful.

यवागुनामपि भेदः [**पायस**][2]**कृशरादयः** ।

**क्षैरेयः पायसः क्षीरापरमान्नमुदाहृतम्** ।। ४ ।।

**Variety**

*Pāyasa*, *kṛśarā* etc., are the different varieties of *yavāgū*. *Pāyasa* is also called *kṣaireya*, *ksīrā* and *paramānna*.

"यैर्यैरेवौषधगुणैर्यवागूः साधु साधिता ।

तांस्तानेवौषधगुणान्पुष्णाति विधियोजिता ।। ५ ।।

*Yavāgū* is prepared by adding different drugs and when properly prepared *yavāgū* enhances the properties of these drugs.

विष्टम्भी **पायसो** बल्यो मेदःकफकरो गुरुः ।

*Pāyasa*

*Pāyasa* is wind forming and strength promoting. It increases fat and *kapha*. It is heavy.

कफपित्तकरी बल्या **कृशरा**निलनाशिनी ।। ६ ।।

*Kṛṣarā*

*Kṛśarā* aggravates *kapha* and *pitta*. It promotes strength and alleviates *vāyu*.

सौमनस्यं बलं पुष्टिमुत्साहं तर्पणं सुखम् ।
स्वादु संजनयत्यन्नमस्वादु[3] च विपर्ययम् ॥ ७ ॥

*Anna*

Delicious variety of *anna* promotes pleasure, strength, corpulence, enthusiasm, refreshment and happiness.

The *anna* which is not delicious acts other wise.

सुधौततंडुलः[4] स्विन्नः[5] प्रस्रुतो विशदो लघुः ।

If the rice is washed well, boiled and after boiling the residual water is removed then it becomes *viśada* (non-slimy) and light.

सोष्णश्चैवौदनः पथ्यो विपरीतस्तु दोषकृत् ॥ ८ ॥

The *odana*, which is hot, is wholesome; otherwise it is harmful.

भृष्टतण्डुलकश्चैकद्विस्त्रिर्वापि[6] परिस्रुतः ।
यथोत्तरं[7] लघुर्वह्निमोदनो[8] दीपयत्यपि ॥ ९ ॥

If the fried rice is washed once twice or thrice, then the *odana* becomes progressively lighter and more stimulant of digestion.

स्नेहैर्मांसैः फलैः कंदैर्विदलाम्लैश्च संस्कृताः ।
गुरवो बृंहणा वृष्या ये च क्षीरोपसाधिताः ॥ १० ॥

If the *anna* is prepared with fat, meat, fruit, rhizome, pulse, sour thing or milk, then it becomes heavy, nourishing and aphrodisiac.

अत्युष्णानि[9] बलं घ्नन्ति[10] शीतं शुष्कं च दुर्जरम् ।
अतिविलन्नं ग्लानिकरं दुर्जरं तण्डुलान्वितम् ॥ ११ ॥

*Anna*, which is exceedingly hot, reduces strength. If it is cold or dry then it becomes difficult of digestion. If it is exceedingly sticky, then it produces *glāni* (tiredness). If it contains unboiled rice then it is difficult of digestion.

शीतलं मधुरं साम्लं अर्शोघ्नं दीपनं परम् ।
श्रमघ्नं तर्पणं हृद्यं **घोलभक्तं** रुचिप्रदम् ॥ १२ ॥

*Ghola bhakta*

*Ghola bhakta* (curd mixed rice) is cooling, sweet and sour. It cures *arśas* (piles). It is an excellent stimulant of digestion. It cures *śrama* (physical fatigue). It is refreshing, a cardiac tonic and appetiser.

शीतलं मधुरं रूक्षं श्रमघ्नं तर्पणं परम् ।
लघु द्रुतविपाकं च सद्योन्नं[11] वारिभावितम् ॥ १३ ॥

*Vāryanna*

Freshly prepared rice soaked in water is cooling, sweet, un-unctuous, alleviator of fatigue, refreshing *par excellence*, light and easily digestible.

त्रिदोषकोपनं रूक्षं मलकृन्मूत्रलं परम् ।
स्वेदमेद[12]:कफोत्क्लेदि वार्यन्नं निशि संस्थितम् ॥१४॥"

[माधवद्रव्यगुण: अन्नवर्ग २६ : ४-१३]

If this prepared rice is soaked in water and kept over night, then it aggravates all the three *doṣas*. It is un-unctuous. It produces more of stool. It is a diuretic *par excellence*. It increases sweating, fat and *kapha*.

[13]
॥ इति पेयादिवर्ग: ॥

Thus, ends the group dealing with various types of *peyā* and allied preparations.

## NOTES AND REFERENCES

1. क्षुत्तृष्णाग्लानिदौर्बल्यकुक्षिरोगविनाशिनी इति आकरे पाठः ।
2. पाकक्रसरादयः इति द्वितीयपुस्तके पाठः ।
3. संजनयत्यम्लमस्वादु इति आदर्शपुस्तके पाठः ।
4. विशुद्धतंडुलः इति द्वितीयपुस्तके पाठः ।
5. स्निग्धः इति द्वितीयपुस्तके आकरे च पाठः ।
6. भृष्टतण्डुलश्चैव द्विस्त्रिर्वापि इति आदर्शपुस्तके पाठः ।
7. यथोत्तरलघुवह्निमोदते इति आदर्शपुस्तकेषु पाठः ।
8. लघुर्बह्निमोदनी इति चतुर्थपुस्तके पाठः ।
9. अत्युष्णान्नं इति चतुर्थपुस्तके आकरे च पाठः ।
10. हन्ति इति चतुर्थपुस्तके आकरे च पाठः ।
11. सद्योऽन्नं इति आकरे पाठः ।
12. स्वेदभेदः इति आदर्शपुस्तकेषु पाठः ।
13. मण्डादिः इति द्वितीयपुस्तके पाठः ।
    इति अन्नवर्गः इति आकरे पाठः ।

# CHAPTER 25

"सुस्विन्नो निस्तुषो भृष्टः ईषत्सूपो[1] लघुर्हितः ।

'स्विन्नं[2] निःपीडितं शाकं हितं स्यात्स्नेहसंस्कृतम् ॥१॥"

[माधवद्रव्यगुणः पानभक्ष्यवर्ग २७-१]

## *Sūpa*

The *sūpa* prepared of corn which is well steamed, dehusked and fried, is light and useful. If it is mixed with the juice extracted from steamed vegetables and with fat then also it is useful.

अस्विन्नस्नेहलवणमपीडितमतोन्यथा ।

If the *sūpa* is prepared of corn which is not steamed and which is not mixed with fat, salt and juice of vegetables, then it is not useful.

निस्तुषैर्भर्जितैः सम्यक् यवै सचणकैः कृताः ।

**सक्तवः** शर्करासर्पिःयुक्ता ग्रीष्मेतिपूजिता ॥ २ ॥

*Yava saktu & Caṇaka saktu*

*Saktu* prepared of fried *yava* or *caṇaka* along with their husk is very useful in summer if taken along with sugar and ghee.

**सक्तवः शालिसंभूता** वह्निदा लघवो हिमाः ।
मधु[राः][3] ग्राहिणो हृद्याः कषाया रुचिशुक्रदाः[4] ॥३॥'

*Śāli saktu*

*Saktu* prepared of *śāli* is digestive stimulant, light, cooling, sweet, constipative, cardiac tonic, astringent, appetiser and promoter of semen.

मधुराः[5] लघवः शीताः सक्तवः शालिसंभवाः ।
ग्राहिणो रक्तपित्तघ्नास्तृष्णाछर्दि[6]ज्वरापहाः ॥ ४ ॥

**Another view**

*Saktu* prepared of *śāli* is sweet, light, cooling and constipative. It cures *rakta pitta* (a disease characterised by bleeding from different parts of the body) *tṛṣṇā* (morbid thirst), *chardi* (vomiting) and *jvara* (fever).

छर्द्यतीसारतृट्दाहविषमूर्च्छाज्वरापहाः
**लाजानां सक्तवः** क्षौद्रसितायुक्ता विशेषतः ॥ ५ ॥

*Lāja saktu*

The *saktu* of *lājā* cures *chardi* (vomiting), *atīsāra* (diarrhoea), *tṛṭ* (morbid thirst), *dāha* (burning syndrome), *viṣa* (poisoning), *mūrchā* (fainting) and *jvara* (fever). It becomes more effective in these conditions when this *saktu* is mixed with honey and sugar.

लेखना दीपना रूक्षा वातला **यवसक्तवः** ।
कफामयप्रशमनाः वातवर्चोनुलोमनाः ॥ ६ ॥

### *Yava saktu*

The *saktu* of *yava* is depleting, digestive stimulant and un-unctuous. It aggravates *vāyu* and cures diseases caused by *kapha*. It helps in the elimination of *vāyu* and stool through the downward tract.

पीताः संतर्पणा हृद्याः सद्यो[7] हि बलवर्धनाः ।
वातातपाध्वव्यायामकर्शितानां श्रमापहाः ॥ ७ ॥

When used as a drink, *yava saktu* is refreshing and a cardiac tonic. It promotes strength instantaneously. It alleviates the fatigue of persons who are emaciated by exposure to wind, sun, walking and exercise in excess.

गुर्वी पिंडी खरात्यर्थं लघ्वी सैव विपर्ययात् ।

If it is used in the form of a bolus (*piṇḍī*) then it is very heavy and un-unctuous (*khara*); otherwise it is light.

सक्तूनामाशु जीर्येत मृदुत्वादवलेहिका ॥ ८ ॥

### *Avalehikā*

*Avalehikā* prepared of *saktu* gets digested early because of its softness.

सक्तवः सर्पिषाभ्यक्ता शीतवारिपरिप्लुताः ।
नातिद्रवो[8] नातिसान्द्रो[9] मंथ इत्यभिधीयते ॥ ९ ॥

### *Mantha*

*Saktu* kneaded with ghee and mixed with water is called *mantha*. It is neither very thick nor very thin.

मंथः सद्योबलकरः पिपासादाहनाशनः ।
साम्लस्नेहगुडो[10] मूत्रकृच्छ्रोदावर्तनाशनः ॥ १० ॥

शर्करेक्षुमधुद्राक्षायुक्तः पित्तविकारनुत् ।

द्राक्षामधुसमायुक्तः कफरोगहरः स्मृतः ॥ ११ ॥

वर्गत्रयेणोपहितो मलदोषानुलोमनः ।

*Mantha* promotes strength instantaneously and cures *pipāsā* (morbid thirst) and *dāha* (burning syndrome). Along with sour things, fat and *guḍa*, it cures *mūtra kṛcchra* (dysuria) and *udāvarta* (flatulence). Along with sugar, sugarcane juice, honey and *drākṣā*, it cures diseases caused by *pitta*. Along with *drākṣā* and honey, it cures diseases caused by *kapha*. Along with the three groups of drugs, it helps in the elimination of stool and *doṣas* through the downward tract.

**धानोलंबाः** सुलघवः कफमेदोविशोषिणः ॥ १२ ॥

*Dhānolamba*

*Dhānolamba* is very light and it reduces *kapha* as well as fat.

**लाजा** तृट्छर्द्यतीसारमेदोमेहकफच्छिदः ।

[11] कासपित्तप्रशमना दीपना लघवो हिमाः ॥ १३ ॥

*Lājā*

*Lājā* cures *tṛṭ* (morbid thirst), *chardi* (vomiting), *atīsāra* (diarrhoea), adiposity, *meha* (obstinate urinary disorders including diabetes) and aggravation of *kapha*. It cures *kāsa* (bronchitis) and alleviates *pitta*. It is a digestive stimulant, light and cooling.

**पृथुका** गुरवः स्निग्धा बृंहणाः कफवर्धनाः ।

[12] बल्या सक्षीरभावित्वाद्वातघ्ना भिन्नवर्चसः ॥ १४ ॥

***Pṛthukā***

***Pṛthukā*** **is heavy, unctuous and nourishing. It aggravates *kapha* and promotes strength. When impregnated with milk, it alleviates *vāyu* and works as a laxative.**

**धाना** विष्टंभिनी रूक्षा तर्पणी लेखनी गुरुः ।

*Dhānā*

*Dhānā* is wind forming, un-unctuous, refreshing, depleting and heavy.

विष्टंभी दुर्जरं रूक्षं शीतलं वातकोपनम् ।
वद्धवर्चस्करं चैव भृष्टं **निष्पावजं फलम्** ।। १५ ।।

*Niṣpāva*

The fried fruit of *niṣpāva* is wind forming, difficult of digestion, un-unctuous, cooling, aggravator of *vāyu* and constipative.

संधानकृत्पिष्टमात्रं[13] **तंडुलः** कृमिमेहकृत् ।

*Taṇḍula piṣṭa*

All types of pastries prepared of *taṇḍula* cause *sandhāna* (union of tissue elements), *kṛmi* (parasitic infection) and *meha* (obstinate urinary disorders including diabetes).

सुदुर्जरः[14] स्वादुरसो बृंहणस्तण्डुलो नवः ।। १६ ।।

If freshly harvested *taṇḍula* is used for this purpose, then it is extremely difficult of digestion. It is sweet in taste and nourishing.

[इति सूपादिवर्गः]

Thus ends the group dealing with different types of *sūpa* and allied preparations.

## NOTES AND REFERENCES

1. भृष्ट इति आकरे पाठः ।
2. अन्नभिः पिष्टितं इति चतुर्थ पुस्तके पाठः ।

3. मधु इति चतुर्थपुस्तके पाठः ।
4. स्विन्नं····रुचि शुक्रदा पाठोऽयं द्वितीयपुस्तके नोपलभ्यते ।
5. मधुरा लघवः इति आदर्शपुस्तके पाठः ।
6. रक्तपित्तघ्नास्तृष्णाच्छर्दिज्वरापहाः इति आकरे पाठः ।
7. सद्योबलविवर्धनाः इति आकरे पाठः ।
8. नातिद्रवा इति आकरे पाठः ।
9. नातिसान्द्रा इति आकरे पाठः ।
10. सान्द्रस्नेहगुडो इति द्वितीयपुस्तके पाठः ।
11. कासपित्तोपशमना इति आकरे पाठः ।
12. बल्याः सक्षीरभावात्त वातघ्ना इति आकरे पाठः ।
13. संधानकृत्पिष्टमाषं इति चतुर्थपुस्तके पाठः ।
संधानकृत्पिष्टमामं इति आकरे पाठः ।
14. स्वादुरच्छो इति आकरे पाठः ।

# CHAPTER 26

स्नेहगोरसधान्याम्लफलाम्लकटुकैः सह ।
सिद्धं[1] **मांसं** हितं बल्यं बृंहणं रोचनं लघु ॥ १ ॥

*Māṁsa*

Meat boiled with fat, milk, *dhānyāmla*, *phalāmla* and *kaṭuka* (spices having pungent taste) is useful, strength promoting, nourishing, appetiser and light.

तदेव गोरसादानं[2] सुरभिद्रव्यसंस्कृतम् ।
विद्यात्पित्तकफोत्क्लेदि बलमांसाग्निवर्धनम् ॥ २ ॥

If meat is prepared with milk and added with fragrant spices, then it reduces (?) *pitta* as well as *kapha* and increases strength, muscle tissue and the power of digestion.

**परिशुष्कं** स्थिरं स्निग्धं तर्पणं प्रीणनं गुरु[3] ।
रोचनं बलमेधाग्निमांसौजःशुक्रवर्धनम् ॥ ३ ॥

Dried meat is *sthira* (which produces stability), unctuous, refreshing, pleasing, heavy and appetiser. It promotes strength, intellect, digestive power, muscle tissue, *ojas* and semen.

[4] तदेव लुप्तभृष्टस्वादुलाप्तमिति पावकाः ।
परिशुष्कं गुणैर्युक्तं वह्नेः पथ्यतमं मतम् ॥ ४ ॥

If the meat is burnt on the fire and then fried, then it is called *ulāpta*. It shares all the properties of dried meat. In addition, it is the most wholesome as a promoter of digestion.

तदेव शूलिकं प्रोक्तमंगारपरिपाचितम् ।
ज्ञेयं गुरुतरं [5] किञ्चित्प्रदिष्टं गुरुपाकतः ॥ ५ ॥

If the meat is burnt over charcoal then it is called *śūlika*. It is heavier because it gets excessively burnt.

[6] उत्प्लुष्टं भर्जितं पिष्टं प्रतप्त कटुपाचितम् ।
परिशुष्कं प्रदिग्धं च शूल्यं यच्चान्यदीदृशम् ॥ ६ ॥
'दीप्ताग्नीनां सदा पथ्यं खानिष्कं तु परं गुरु ।

Different preparations of meat viz., *utpluṣṭa* (burnt), *bharjita* (fried), *piṣṭa* (made to a paste), *pratapta* (heated), *kaṭu-pācita* (boiled with pungent spices), *pariśuṣka* (dried), *pradigdha* (excessively burnt), *śūlya* (burnt over charcoal) and similar other preparations are always wholesome for persons having strong digestive power. *Khaniṣka* type of meat preparation is exceedingly heavy.

मांसं यत्तैलसिद्धं तु वीर्योष्णं [7] पित्तकृद्गुरु ॥ ७ ॥'

Meat prepared in oil is hot in potency, aggravator of *pitta* and heavy.

लघ्वग्निदीपनं हृद्यं रुच्यं दृष्टिप्रसादनम् ।
अनुष्णवीर्यं पित्तघ्नं [8] मनोज्ञं घृतसाधितम् ॥ ८ ॥

Meat prepared in ghee is light, digestive stimulant, cardiac tonic, appetiser and promoter of eyesight. It is not hot in potency. It alleviates *pitta* and is pleasing to the mind.

प्रीणनः सर्वधातूनां विशेषान्मुखशोषिणाम् ।

9 10 11

क्षुत्तृष्णापहरः श्रेष्ठः **सौरावः** स्वादुशीतलः ॥ ९ ॥

*Saurāva* type of meat nourishes all the tissue elements. It is specially useful for patients having *mukhaśoṣa* (dryness of mouth). It is an excellent curative for *kṣut* (morbid hunger) and *tṛṣṇā* (morbid thirst). It is delicious and cooling.

12

प्रीणनः प्राणजननः श्वासकासक्षयापहः ।

वातपित्तश्रमहरो हृद्यो **मांसरसो** मतः ॥ १० ॥

*Māṁsa rasa*

Meat soup is refreshing and vitalizing. It cures *śvāsa* (asthma), *kāsa* (bronchitis) and *kṣaya* (consumption). It alleviates *vāyu, pitta* and fatigue. It is cardiac tonic.

स्मृत्योजःस्वरहीनानां ज्वरक्षीणक्षतौजसाम् ।

भग्नविश्लिष्टसंधीनां कृशानामल्परेतसाम् ॥ ११ ॥

आप्यायनः संहननः शुक्रदो बलवर्धनः ।

It is useful for persons having less of memory and *ojas*, imperfect voice, *jvara* (fever), *kṣīṇa* (emaciation), *kṣata* (phthisis) and broken and dislocated joints. It is also useful for thin persons and those having less of semen. It causes nourishment, *saṁhanana* (joining of tissues) and promotes semen as well as strength.

सदाडिमयुतो वृष्यः संस्कृतो दोषनाशनः ॥ १२ ॥

The meat soup prepared along with *dāḍima* is aphrodisiac and alleviator of *doṣas*.

यन्मांसमुद्घृतरसं न तत्पुष्टिबलप्रदम् ।

विष्टम्भि दुर्जरं रूक्षं विरसं मारुतावहम्[13] ।। १३ ।।

[माधवद्रव्यगुण: पानभक्ष्यवर्ग २७ : २१-२६]

The meat, from which juice is extracted, does not produce nourishment and strength. It is wind forming, difficult of digestion, ununctuous and aggravater of *vāyu*.

दीप्ताग्नीनां सदा शस्तमामिषं[14] परमं गुरु[15] ।

Meat is always useful for persons having a strong power of digestion. It is very heavy.

मांसं निरस्थि[16] सुस्विन्नं[17] पुनर्दृषदि चूर्णितम् ।। १४ ।।

पिप्पलीमरिचशुण्ठी[18]हिंगुसर्पि:समन्वितम् ।

ऐकध्यं[19] साधयेत् सम्यक् तत् सोराव[20]मिति स्मृतत् ।।१५।।

*Sorāva*

The meat which is free from bones, which is triturated in a pastle and mortar after proper boiling and which is prepared by boiling together with *pippalī*, *marica*, *śuṇṭhī*, *hiṅgu* and ghee is called *sorāva*.

।। इति मांसादिप्रकार: ।।

Thus ends the group dealing with various types of meat and their different preparations.

## NOTES AND REFERENCES

1. स्निग्धं इति आकरे पाठ: ।
   सिक्तं इति द्वितीयपुस्तके पाठ: ।

2. गोरसान्तं तु इति आकरे पाठः ।
3. अस्य श्लोकस्यानन्तरम् 'सुरभिद्रव्यसंस्कृतं विद्यात्पित्तकफोत्क्लेदि बलगुरु' पाठोऽयं चतुर्थपुस्तके अधिकं उपलभ्यते ।
4. तदेवोलुप्तपिष्टत्वादुलुप्तमिति इति आकरे पाठः ।
5. किंचित् प्रदिग्धं इति आकरे पाठः ।
6. उलुप्तं इति आकरे पाठः ।
7. दीप्ताग्नीनां···पित्तकृद्गुरु पाठोऽयं द्वितीयपुस्तके नोपलभ्यते ।
8. अस्य श्लोकस्यानन्तरं 'अथ मांसप्रकारा :—

तलितं भर्जितं स्विन्नं प्रलेहस्रवितं रसः ।
[पोषितं] च तथा शूल्यं पूरणं पुटपाकजं ।
अमीप्रकाराः मांसस्य संक्षेपात्परिकीर्तिताः ।
तलितं मांसं हि बल्यं रुच्यं पूरणं पित्तानिलापहं ।
सुस्वादु मधुरं पाके किंचित्कफकरं गुरु ।
भर्जितं तत्सुधातुल्यं [रुच्यं] वह्निकरं लघु ।
स्विन्नं मांसं बलं बीर्यं विदधाति रुचिमनाक् ।
वातं पित्तं कफं हंति प्रदीपयति चानलं ।
प्रलेहस्रावितं बल्यं रोचनं दीपनं गुरु ।
मांसाग्निवर्द्धनं पित्तकफोद्रेकि विशेषतः ।
पेषितं पाचितं मांसं सुस्वादु लघु दीपनम् ।
बल्यं सुरुचिकृत्प्राणप्रदं दोषत्रयापहं ।
तत्रापि जांगलं श्रेष्ठं श्रेष्ठं तत्रापि पक्षीणाम् ।
उष्णे स्नेहो निशाहिंगुलवंगकैला [धान्यक-]
जीरार्द्रकनागराणि अम्लोषणं सैंधवचूर्ण युक्तां ।
उपस्कराः संस्कृता ये फलस्य ।
एलालवंगकर्पूरमरिचादि विनिर्मितं ।
[वर्ण] मुद्धलनायोक्तं पाचकर्मविचक्षणैः ।
अस्य वर्णस्य करणे कुंकुमं रक्तचन्दनम् ।
चूर्णं च यत्र यद्युक्तं तत्र तत्संप्रयोजयेत् ।
धुयोऽगुरु कृतो यः किंवा रामठशलाकाग्रथितं शुद्धं पललं साज्यसैन्धवम् ।
वह्नौ विधूमसे संपक्वं शूल्यमुक्तं मनीषिभिः ।
शूल्यं बल्यं सुधातुल्यं पलं वह्निकरं लघु ।

कफपित्तहरं प्रोक्तं विशेषाद्रुचिकारकं ।
मांसंस्विन्नं सूक्ष्मकृतं पिष्ट्वा सदुपस्करां धत्ते ।
तप्तेन्धनभृष्टं पूरणं प्रोच्यते बुधैः ।
मांसपूरणकं रुच्यं बल्यं पुष्टिकरं परम् ।
वातपित्तहरं वृष्यं वह्निमांद्यकफप्रणुत् ।
सूक्ष्मकृतं पलं पत्रैः छादितं वेष्टितं मृदा ।
पक्वं सोपस्करं यत्र विज्ञेयं पुटपाकजं ।
पुटपाकेन यत्कृतं तन्मांसं पाचकं परं ।
सोष्मं तद्गुणवद्वेद्यं शीतं शूष्कं च दुर्ज्जरं ।
समितानिर्मितं पूर्णं पूरणे तद्घृते पुनः ।
भृष्टं शृंगाटकाकारं तत्स्यात्पूरणपूरितं ।
चक्षुष्यं बृंहणं वृष्यं वातपित्तहरं गुरु ।
अतीव रुचिकृत् बल्यं भवेत्पूरणपूरितं' ।
वहुप्रमादपूर्णः पाठोऽयं चतुर्थपुस्तके अधिकं उपलभ्यते ।

9. क्षुत्तृष्णापहः इति आकरे पाठः ।
10. शान्तः इति द्वितीयपुस्तके पाठः ।
11. शौरावः इति आदर्शपुस्तके पाठः ।
12. अस्य श्लोकस्यानन्तरम् कफघ्नो दीपनो हृद्यः शुद्धानां व्रणनाशनः पाठोऽयं माधवद्रव्यगुणें अधिकमुपलम्यते ।
13. मारुतापहम् इति आकरे पाठः ।
14. शस्तास्वाणिस्तु इति द्वितीयपुस्तके पाठः ।
15. दीप्ताग्नीनां ······गुरुः पाठोऽयं चतुर्थपुस्तके नोपलभ्यते ।
16. चास्थि च इति द्वितीयपुस्तके पाठः ।
17. सुस्निग्धं इति द्वितीयपुस्तके पाठः ।
18. शुण्ठिहिंगुजीरसमन्वितम् इति द्वितीयपुस्तके पाठः ।
    शुण्ठिसैंधवेनसमन्वितम् इति चतुर्थपुस्तके पाठः ।
19. एकत्र इति द्वितीयपुस्तके पाठः ।
    एकस्थं इति चतुर्थपुस्तके पाठः ।
20. सौरावमिति इति द्वितीयपुस्तके पाठः ।

# CHAPTER 27

'कफघ्नो दीपनो हृद्यः शुद्धानामपि[1] दोषहृत् ।
उक्तः पथ्यतमश्चापि **मुद्गयूषः**[2] कृताकृतः ॥ १ ॥

*Mudga yūṣa*

*Mudga yūṣa* alleviates *kapha*, stimulates digestion and tones up the heart. It helps in the elimination of *doṣas* even for persons whose bodies are free from *doṣas* by the administration of elimination therapies (?). It is wholesome par excellence. It is of two types viz., *kṛta* (which is fried with ghee etc.,) and *akṛta* (which is not fried with ghee etc.,).

स तु दाडिममृद्वीकायुक्तः **स्याद्रागषाडवः** ।
स वृष्यो[3] लघुपाकश्च दोषाणामविरोधकृत्[4] ॥ २ ॥'

[माधवद्रव्यगुणः पानभक्ष्यवर्ग २७ : २९-३१]

*Rāga ṣāḍava*

If *mudga yūṣa* is added with *dāḍima* and *mṛdvīkā* then it is called *rāga ṣāḍava*. It is aphrodisiac and light for digestion. It does not aggravate *doṣas*.

[5]

'मसूरमुद्गगोधूमकुलत्थलवणैः कृतः ।
कफपित्ताविरोधी स्याद्वातव्याधौ प्रशस्यते ॥ ३ ॥

The *rāga ṣāḍava* prepared of *masūra, mudga, godhūma, kulattha* and salt does not aggravate *kapha* and *pitta.* It is extremely useful in diseases caused by *vāyu.*

मृद्वीकादाडिमयुतः स चाप्युक्तोऽनिलार्दितः[6] ।
रोचनो दीपनो हृद्यो लघुपाक्युपदिश्यते ॥ ४ ॥

The *rāga ṣāḍava* prepared of *mṛdvīkā* and *dāḍima* also alleviates *vāyu*. It is appetiser, digestive stimulant, cardiac tonic and *laghu pāki* (which is easy for digestion).

**पटोलनिम्बूयूषौ** तु कफमेदोविशधनौ ।
पित्तघ्नौ दीपनौ हृद्यौ क्रिमिकुष्ठज्वरापहौ ॥ ५ ॥

*Paṭola yūṣa* **and** *Nimbū yūṣa*

The *yūṣa* prepared of *paṭola* and *nimbū* cleanses *kapha* and *medas* (fat). It alleviates *pitta*. It is digestive stimulant and cardiac tonic. It cures *krimi* (parasitic infection), *kuṣṭha* (obstinate skin diseases including leprosy) and *jvara* (fever).

श्वासकासप्रतिश्यायप्रसेकारोचकज्वरान् ।
हन्ति **मुलकयूषस्तु** कफमेदोगलग्रहान् ॥ ६ ॥

*Mūlaka yūṣa*

The *yūṣa* of *mūlaka* cures *śvāsa* (asthma), *kāsa* (bronchitis), *pratiśyāya* (chronic rhinitis), *praseka* (excessive salivation), *arocaka* (anorexia) and *jvara* (fever). It reduces *kapha* and *medas* (fat). It also cures *gala graha* (obstruction in throat).

**कुलत्थयूषो**ऽनिलहा शर्कराश्मरिनाशनः ।
तूनीप्रतूनीकासार्शोगुल्ममेहकफापहः ॥ ७ ॥

### *Kulattha yūṣa*

The *yūṣa* of *kulattha* alleviates *vāyu*. It cures *śarkarā* (gravels in the urine), *aśmari* (stone in urinary tract), *tūnī* (a disease characterised by acute pain in intestine, anus and phallus), *pratūnī* (a variety of *tūnī* in which pain starts from anus and moves to the intestine), *kāsa* (bronchitis), *arśas* (piles), *gulma* (phantom tumour), *meha* (obstinate urinary disorders including diabetes) and aggravation of *kapha*.

यवकोलकुलत्थानां मुद्गमूलकशुंठयोः ।
[7] एकैकमुष्टिमादाय पचेदष्टगुणे जले ॥ ८ ॥
**पञ्चमुष्टिक** इत्येष [8] वातपित्तकफापहः ।
शस्यते [9] गुल्मशूले सा कासे श्वासे ज्वरे क्षये ॥ ९ ॥

### *Pañca muṣṭika yūṣa*

*Pañca muṣṭika yūṣa* is prepared by taking one *muṣṭi* (handful) of each of *yava*, *kola*, *kulattha*, *mudga*, *mūlaka* and *śuṇṭhī* (instead of five, six items are included in the text) and boiling them in eight times of water. It alleviates *vāyu*, *pitta* and *kapha* and is useful in *gulma* (phantom tumour), *śūla* (colic pain), *kāsa* (bronchitis), *śvāsa* (asthma), *jvara* (fever) and *kṣaya* consumption).

मुद्गामलाभ्यां यवदाडिमाभ्यां कर्कन्धुना मूलकशुंठकेन [?] ।
शुण्ठीकणाभ्यां च कुलत्थकेन [10] **यूषो नवांगो** कफरोगहन्ता ॥ १० ॥

### *Navāṅga yūṣa*

*Navāṅga yūsa* is prepared of *mudga*, *āmalaka*, *yava*, *dāḍima*, *karkandhu*, *mūlaka*, *śuṇṭhī*, *kaṇā* and *kulattha*. This cures diseases caused by *kapha*.

दाडिमामलकैर्यूषो हृद्यः संशमनो लघुः ।
प्राणाग्निजननो मूर्च्छागेदोघ्नः [11] पित्तवातजित् ॥११॥

**Other varieties**

The *yūṣa* prepared of *dāḍima* and *āmalaka* is cardiac tonic, alleviator of *doṣas*, light, vitalising and digestive stimulant. It cures *mūrcchā* (fainting) and *medas* (adiposity). It specifically alleviates *pitta* and *vāta*.

[12] मुद्गामलकयूषश्च भेदी पित्तकफापहः ।

The *yūṣa* prepared of *mudga* and *āmalaka* is purgative and it alleviates *pitta* as well as *kapha.*

पंचकोलकुलत्थानां यूषः कंठ्योऽनिलापहः ॥ १२ ॥

The *yūṣa* prepared of *pañcakola* (*pippalī, pippalī mūla, cavya, citraka* and *nāgara*) and *kulattha* is a promoter of good voice and alleviator of *vāyu.*

यवमंडस्तु कथितो वातपित्तकफापहः ।

[13] पाचनो दीपनश्चैव शूलानाहविबन्धनुत् ॥ १३ ॥

*Yava maṇḍa*

*Yava maṇḍa* alleviates *vāyu, pitta* and *kapha*. It is carminative and digestive stimulant. It cures *śūla* (colic pain), *ānāha* (flatulence) and *vibandha* (constipation).

सर्वधान्यकृतस्तद्वत् बृंहणः प्राणवर्धनः ।

*Sarva dhānya maṇḍa*

The *maṇḍa* prepared of all the types of *dhānya* is nourishing and vitalising.

[14] खडकाम्बलिकौ हृद्यौ छर्दिवातकफे हितौ ॥ १४ ॥

*Khaḍa* and *Kāmbalika*

*Khaḍa* and *kāmbalika* are cardiac tonic. They are useful in *chardi* (vomiting) and aggravation of *vāyu* as well as *kapha.*

दधिमत्स्याम्लसिद्धस्तु यूषः काम्बलिकः स्मृतः ।

The *yūṣa* which is prepared by adding *dadhi*, *matsya* and articles having sour taste is called *kāmbalika*.

बल्यः कफानिलौ[15] हन्ति **दाडिमाम्लो**ऽग्निदीपनः ॥१५॥

*Dāḍimāmla*

*Dāḍimāmla* promotes strength, alleviates *kapha* and *vāyu* and stimulates digestion.

**धान्याम्लो** दीपनो हृद्यः पित्तकृद्वातनाशनः ।

*Dhānyāmla*

*Dhānyāmla* is digestive stimulant, cardiac tonic, aggravator of *pitta* and alleviator of *vāyu*.

**दध्यम्लः** श्लेष्मलो बल्यः स्निग्धो वातहरो गुरुः ॥१६॥

*Dadhyamla*

*Dadhyamla* aggravates *kapha* and promotes strength. It is unctuous, alleviator of *vāyu* and heavy.

**तक्राम्लः** पित्तकृत्प्रोक्तो विषरक्तप्रदूषणः ।

*Takrāmla*

*Takrāmla* aggravates *pitta* and *viṣa* (poisoning). It vitiates blood.

अस्नेहलवणं[16] सर्व**मकृतं** कटुकैर्विना ॥ १७ ॥

विज्ञेयं कटुकस्नेहलवणैः संस्कृतं[17] **कृतम्** ।

*Kṛta* **and** *Akṛta yūṣa*

The *yūṣa* which is not mixed with fat, salt and pungent spices is called *akṛta*. *Kṛta yūṣa*, on the other hand, is prepared of pungent spices, fat and salt.

अथ गोरसधान्याम्लफलाम्लै रचितं च यत्[18] ॥ १८ ॥

यथोत्तरं लघु हितं संस्कृतासंस्कृतं तथा ।

**Other varieties**

The *yūṣas* prepared of milk, *dhānyāmla* and the *yūṣa* of sour fruits are progressively lighter. Whether fried or not they are useful.

तिलपिण्याकविकृतिः शुष्कशाकं विरूढकम् ।

19

शंडाकीनि गुरूणि स्युः पित्तश्लेष्मकराणि च ॥१६॥'

[माधवद्रव्यगुणः पानभक्ष्यवर्ग २७ : ३३-४६]

*Śaṇḍākī*

*Śaṇḍākī* is prepared of oil cake, dry vegetables and germinated corns and cereals. They are heavy and they aggravate *pitta* as well as *kapha*.

लघवो बृंहणा वृष्या हृद्या रोचनदीपनाः ।

भ्रममृत्युतृषाछर्दिश्रमघ्ना **रागषाण्डवा** ॥ २० ॥

*Rāga ṣāṇḍava*

*Rāga ṣāṇḍava* is light, nourishing, aphrodisiac, cardiac tonic, appetiser and digestive stimulant. It cures *bhrama* (giddiness), *mṛtyu* (apprehension of death ?), *tṛṣā* (morbid thirst), *chardi* (vomiting) and *śrama* (physical fatigue).

20

'**रसाला** रोचनी बल्या स्निग्धा वृष्या सुबृंहणी ।

*Rasālā*

*Rasālā* is an appetiser, strength promoting, unctuous, aphrodisiac and extremely nourishing. It causes oleation of the body.

21

स्नेहनं गुडसंयुक्तं हृद्यं दध्यनिलापहम् ॥ २१ ॥

If prepared by adding *guḍa* and curd, then it is cardiac tonic and alleviator of *vāyu*.

गौडमम्लमनम्लं च[22] पानकं गुरु मूत्रलम् ।

### *Pānaka*

*Pānaka* of *guḍa* (whether added with sour things or not) is heavy and diuretic.

तदेव खण्डमृद्वीकाशर्करासहितं पुनः ॥ २२ ॥
साम्लं सुतीक्ष्णं सहिमं[23] पानकं स्यान्निरत्ययम् ।

*Pānaka* prepared of *khaṇḍa*, *mṛdvīkā*, *śarkarā* and sour things is extremely sharp and cooling. It is not harmful.

मार्द्वीकं तु श्रमहरं मूर्च्छादाहज्वरापहम् ॥ २३ ॥

*Pānaka* prepared of *mṛdvīkā* alleviates *śrama* (physical fatigue) and cures *mūrchā* (fainting), *dāha* (burning syndrome) and *jvara* (fever).

परूषकाणां कोलानां हृद्यं विष्टम्भि पानकम् ।

The *pānaka* prepared of *parūṣaka* and *kola* is cardiac tonic and wind forming.

द्रव्यसंयोगसंस्कारान्[24] ज्ञात्वा मात्रां च सर्वशः ।
पानकानां यथायोग्यं[25] गुरुलाघवमादिशेत् ॥ २४ ॥

Depending upon the ingredients and the method of preparation, the heaviness and lightness of a *pānaka* should be ascertained and their dose should be determined accordingly.

भक्ष्याः क्षीरकृता बल्या वृष्या[हृद्याः][26]सुगन्धिनः ।
अदाहिनः पुष्टिकरा[27] दीपना[28] वातनाशनाः[29] ॥ २५ ॥

### *Bhakṣya*

Different types of *bhakṣya* prepared of milk is strength promoting, aphrodisiac, cardiac tonic, fragrant, *adāhin* (which does not produce burning sensation), digestive stimulant and alleviator of *vāyu.*

सद्यःप्राणकराः हृद्याः घृतपूराः[30] कफावहाः ।
वातपित्तहरा वृष्या गुरवो[31] रक्तमांसदाः ॥ २६ ॥'

[माधवद्रव्यगुणः पानभक्ष्यवर्ग २७ : ५०-५५]

*Ghṛta pūra*

*Ghṛta pūra* is instantaneously vitalising and a cardiac tonic. It aggravates *kapha* and alleviates *vāyu* as well as *pitta.* It is aphrodisiac, heavy and promoter of blood as well as muscle tissue.

[32]'वृष्यास्ते **गौडिका** भक्ष्या गुरवोऽनिलनाशनाः ।
विदाहिनः पित्तकरा[33] बृंहणाः कफवर्द्धनाः ॥ २७ ॥

*Guḍa bhakṣya*

The *bhakṣya* prepared of *guḍa* is aphrodisiac, heavy and alleviator of *vāyu.* It causes burning sensation and aggravates *pitta.* It is nourishing and aggravator of *kapha.*

**मधुशीर्षक**[34]**संयावाः** **पूपा** ह्येते विशेषतः ।
गुरवो बृंहणाश्चैव **मोदका**[35]श्चापि दुर्जराः[36] ॥ २८ ॥

*Madhu śīrṣaka* etc.

*Madhu śīrṣaka, saṁyāva* and *pūpa* are specially heavy and nourishing.

*Modaka* is difficult for digestion.

रोचनो दीपनः स्वर्यः[37] पित्तघ्नः पवनापहः ।
गुरुर्मिष्टतमश्चैव **सट्टकः** प्राणवर्धनः ॥ २९ ॥

### Saṭṭaka

*Saṭṭaka* is appetiser, digestive stimulant, promoter of good voice, alleviator of *pitta* as well as *vāyu*, heavy, extremely delicious and vitalising.

हृद्यः सुगन्धिर्मधुरः स्निग्धः श्लेष्मकरो गुरुः ।
पित्तापहस्तृप्तिकरो[38] बल्योऽ**भिष्यन्द** उच्यते ।। ३० ।।'
[माधवद्रव्यगुणः पानभक्ष्यवर्ग २७ : ५७-६०]

### Abhiṣyanda

*Abhiṣyanda* is cardiac tonic, fragrant, sweet, unctuous, aggravator of *kapha*, heavy, alleviator of *pitta*, *tṛptikara* (which causes satisfaction) and promoter of strength.

'बृंहणा वातपित्तघ्नाः बल्याः[39] वृष्यास्तु[40] शालिजाः[41] ।
हृद्याः पथ्यतमास्तेषां लघवः **फेनकादयः** ।। ३१ ।।'
[सुश्रुतः सूत्र ४६ : ३९८-३९९]

### Phenaka

*Phenka* etc. prepared of *śāli* rice are nourishing, alleviator of *vāyu* as well as *pitta*, strength promoting, aphrodisiac, cardiac tonic, extremely wholesome and light.

'मुद्गादिवेसवारैस्तु पूर्णा विष्टम्भिनो मताः ।
वेसवारैस्तु पिशितैः सम्पूर्णा[42] गुरुबृंहणाः ।। ३२ ।।'

*Phenaka* prepared by filling with *vesavāra* of *mudga* etc. is wind forming. If it is filled with the *vesavāra* of meat, then it is heavy and nourishing,

**वेसवारो** गुरु स्निग्धो बलोपचयवर्धनः[43][44] ।

### Vesavāra

*Vesavāra* is heavy, unctuous and promoter of strength as

well as plumpness.

45
पललाः श्लेषमजनना **शष्कुल्यः** कफपित्तलाः ॥ ३३ ॥

*Palala* **and** *Śaṣkulī*

*Palala* aggravates *kapha*. *Śaṣkulī* aggravates *kapha* as well as *pitta*.

46
**पर्पटा** लघवो रुच्याः लघिष्ठाः **क्षीरपर्पटी** ।

*Parpaṭa* **and** *Kṣīra parpaṭī*

*Parpaṭa* is light and appetiser. *Kṣīra parpaṭī* is light par excellence.

47
वीर्योष्णाः पैष्टिका **भक्ष्याः** कषाया सृष्टमारुताः ॥३४॥'

[माधवद्रव्यगुणः पानभक्ष्यवर्ग २७ : ६३-६६]

'विष्टम्भिनः पित्तकराः श्लेष्मघ्ना भिन्नवर्चसः ।

*Paiṣṭika bhakṣya*

The *bhakṣya* prepared of pastes is hot in potency and astringent. It produces more of wind and causes flatulence. It aggravates *pitta* and alleviates *kapha*. It is laxative.

48 49
**विरूढककृता भक्ष्या** गुरवोऽनिलपित्तलाः ॥ ३५ ॥'

50
विदाहोत्क्लेदजनना रूक्षा दृष्टिप्रदूषणाः ।

*Virūḍhaka bhakṣya*

The *bhakṣya* prepared of germinated grains is heavy. It aggravates *vāyu* as well as *pitta* and produces a burning sensation as well as stickiness in the body. It is ununctuous and it vitiates eyesight.

51
फलमांसवसाशाकपललक्षौद्रसंयुताः ॥ ३६ ॥

भक्ष्या[52] हृद्याश्च बल्याश्च गुरवो बृंहणात्मकाः[53] ।

**Another variety**

The *bhakṣya* prepared of fruit, meat, *vasā* (muscle fat), vegetables, oil cake and honey is a cardiac tonic, strength promoting, heavy and nourishing.

गुरवस्तर्पणा[54] हृद्याः क्षीरेक्षुरसपूपकाः[55] ॥ ३७ ॥

*Pūpaka*

*Pūpaka* prepared of milk and sugar cane juice is heavy, refreshing and cardiac tonic.

सगुडाः सतिलाश्चैव[56] सक्षीरक्षौद्रशर्कराः[57] ।
भक्ष्या बल्याश्च वृष्याश्च परं तु गुरवः स्मृताः[58] ॥३८॥

**Other varieties of *bhakṣya***

The *bhakṣya* prepared of *guḍa*, *tila*, milk, honey and sugar is strength promoting, aphrodisiac and extremely heavy.

हृद्याः सुगन्धिनो वृष्या[59] लघवो घृतपाचिताः ।
वातपित्तहरा बल्या वर्णदृष्टिप्रसादनाः ॥ ३९ ॥

The *bhakṣya* prepared by frying with ghee is cardiac tonic, fragrant, aphrodisiac, light, alleviator of *vāyu* as well as *pitta* and promoter of strength, complexion as well as eyesight.

विदाह्निनस्तैलकृताः गुरवः कटुपाकिनः ।
ऊष्णा[60] मारुतदृष्टिघ्नाः पित्तरक्तप्रदूषणाः[61] ॥ ४० ॥

The *bhakṣya* prepared by frying with oil produces burning sensation. It is heavy, pungent in *vipāka* and hot. It reduces *vāyu* and eyesight and vitiates *pitta* as well as *rakta*.

फलमांसेक्षुविकृतितिलमाषेण संस्कृताः[62] ।

भक्ष्या बल्यास्तु गुरवो बृंहणा हृदयप्रियाः ॥ ४१ ॥

The *bhakṣya* prepared by adding fruit, meat, sugarcane products, *tila* and *māṣa* is strength promoting, heavy, nourishing and pleasing to the heart.

खर्परांगारपक्वास्तु[63] लघवो वातकोपनाः ।

The *bhakṣya* prepared by frying on a piece of earthen pot over charcoal is light and aggravator of *vāyu*.

सकिलाटादयो[64] भक्ष्या[65] गुरवः कफवर्धनाः ॥ ४२ ॥

The *bhakṣya* prepared of *kilāṭa* (a milk product) is heavy and aggravator of *kapha*.

कुल्माषा वातला रूक्षाः[66] गुरवो भिन्नवर्चसः[67] ।

*Kulmāṣa*

*Kulmāṣa* aggravates *vāyu*. It is ununctuous, heavy and laxative.

द्रव्येण यद्गुणेनेह[68] यद्वीर्येणेह[69] साधिताः ।
तद्वीर्यास्तद्गुणाश्चैव भक्ष्याः ज्ञेयाः[70] चिकित्सकैः ॥४३॥'

[माधवद्रव्यगुणः पानभक्ष्यवर्ग २७ : ६७-७६]

**Miscellaneous**

A physician should know that the attributes and the potency of a type of *bhakṣya* is based on the attributes and potency of the ingredients by which it is prepared.

॥ इति यूषादिकः[71] ॥

Thus ends the group dealing with various types of *yūṣa* and allied food preparations.

## NOTES AND REFERENCES

1. शुष्कानामपि इति द्वितीयपुस्तके पाठः।
   शुद्धानां व्रणिनामपि इति आकरे पाठः।
2. अस्य श्लोकस्यानन्तरम् 'प्रीणनः प्राणजननः श्वासकासक्षयापहः' पाठोऽयं माधवद्रव्यगुणे अधिकमुपलभ्यते।
3. रुचिष्यो इति आकरे पाठः।
4. दोषाणामपि रोधकृद् इति आदर्शपुस्तकेषु पाठः।
5. मसूरमुद्गगोधूमकुलत्थचणकैः इति आकरे पाठः।
6. चाप्युक्तोऽनिलार्दिते इति आकरे पाठः।
7. एकैकां इति आकरे पाठः।
8. वातपित्तकफे हितः इति आकरे पाठः।
9. गुल्मशूलेषु इति आकरे पाठः।
10. नवांगः इति आकरे पाठः।
11. कफवातजित् इति आकरे पाठः।
12. मुद्गामलकयूषस्तु इति आकरे पाठः।
13. शूलाध्मानविवंधनुत् इति चतुर्थपुस्तके पाठः।
14. खलकाम्वलिकौ आकरे चतुर्थपुस्तके च पाठः।
15. कफानलौ इति आकरे पाठः।
16. सस्नेहलवणं इति आदर्शपुस्तकेषु पाठः।
17. संयुतं इति आकरे पाठः।
18. रंधितं इति आकरे पाठः।
19. संडकिनी इति चतुर्थपुस्तके पाठः।
20. च बृंहणी इति आकरे चतुर्थपुस्तके च पाठः।
21. स्नेहं इति आकरे पाठः।
22. वा इति आकरे पाठः।
23. सुहिमं इति आकरे पाठः।
24. द्रव्यसंयोगसंस्कारात् इति आकरे पाठः।
25. यथायोगं इति आकरे पाठः।
26. वृष्यावल्याः इति द्वितीयपुस्तके पाठः।
27. पुष्टिकराः इति आकरे पाठः।

28. दीपनाः इति आकरे पाठः ।
29. पित्तनाशनाः इति आकरे पाठः ।
30. कफावहाः इति आदर्शपुस्तकेषु पाठः ।
31. रक्तमांसला इति आकरे चतुर्थपुस्तके च पाठः ।
32. बृंहणा गौडिकाः भक्ष्याः गुरवोऽनिलनाशनाः इति आकरे पाठः ।
33. पित्तवहा इति आकरे पाठः ।
34. मधुशीर्षकसंयाव इति आकरे पाठः ।
35. मोदकास्तु इति आकरे पाठः ।
36. सुदुर्जराः इति आकरे पाठः ।
37. कफघ्नः इति द्वितीयपुस्तके पाठः ।
38. पित्तप्लीहार्तृप्तिकरो इति द्वितीयपुस्तके पाठः ।
39. भक्ष्यास्तु इति आकरे पाठः ।
40. सामिताः इति आकरे चतुर्थपुस्तके च पाठः ।
41. बृंहणा वातपित्तघ्ना भक्ष्या बल्यास्तु सामिताः इति आकरे पाठः ।
42. 'मुद्गादिवेशवारैस्तु……गुरुबृंहणाः' पाठोऽयं द्वितीयपुस्तके नोपलभ्यते ।
43. बलोपचयबृंहणः इति आदर्शपुस्तकेषु पाठः ।
44. अस्य श्लोकस्यानन्तरम् 'मांसनिरस्थिसुस्विन्नं पुनर्दृषदिचूर्णितं ।
पिप्पलीमरिचशुण्ठीगुडसर्पिः समन्वितं ।
एवं विपाचयेत्सम्यक् वेसवार इति स्मृतः ।' पाठोऽयं चतुर्थपुस्तके अधिकमुपलभ्यते ।
45. श्लेष्मजननाः इति आकरे पाठः ।
46. रुच्या विशेयाः शालिसंभवाः इति आकरे पाठः ।
47. पौष्टिका भक्ष्याः कफपित्तप्रकोपणाः इति आकरे पाठः ।
48. विरूढकक्कताः इति आकरे पाठः ।
49. विष्टम्भिनः……गुरवोऽनिलपित्तलाः पाठोऽयं चतुर्थपुस्तके नोपलभ्यते ।
50. रूक्षाः इति आकरे पाठः ।
51. फलमांसवसाशाकपटोलक्षौद्रसंयुताः इति आदर्शपुस्तकेषु पाठः ।
52. भक्ष्याः इति आकरे पाठः ।
53. बृंहणास्तथा इति आकरे पाठः ।
बृंहणात्मता इति चतुर्थपुस्तके पाठः ।

54. गुरवस्तर्पणाः इति आकरे पाठः ।
55. क्षीरेक्षुरसपयसा इति चतुर्थपुस्तके पाठः ।
56. खलिलाश्चैव इति द्वितीयपुस्तके पाठः ।
57. सक्षारक्षौद्रशर्कराः इति आकरे पाठः ।
58. गुरवो मताः इति आकरे पाठः ।
59. वृष्याः इति आकरे पाठः।
60. उष्णाः इति आकरे पाठः ।
61. पित्तलासृक्प्रदूषणाः इति माधवद्रव्यगुणे पाठः ।
62. मांसेक्षुवसाचैव तिलमाषेणसंस्कृताः इति द्वितीयपुस्तके पाठः, फलमांसेक्षुविकृतितिलमाषोपसंस्कृताः इति आकरे पाठः ।
63. कर्पराङ्गारपक्तास्तु इति द्वितीयपुस्तके पाठः ।
64. सकिलाटादयो इति आकरे पाठः ।
65. भक्ष्याः इति आकरे पाठः ।
66. रूक्षाः इति आकरे पाठः ।
67. अस्यश्लोकस्यानन्तरम् 'लोहचक्रेसु प्रतप्रेयाचिताचक्रचतुंलाः।
भूयाः संस्वेदितांगारे गोधूमान्योनिका भवेत् ।
पोलिका कफकृद्बल्यापित्तला वातनुद्गुरुः ।
सात्युष्णारुचिकृत्पथ्या शीता सुगुरुरुच्यते ।
समिता निर्मितः ख्यातो मंडको विस्तृतस्तनुः ।
हस्तलालनयासिद्धः खर्परे मृदुवह्निना ।
मंडका शुक्रलो ग्राही लघुर्दोषत्रयापहः ।
शुद्धगोधूमचूर्णस्य स्थूला जलविनिर्मिता ।
एतद् धूमानले पक्वा विज्ञेयांगारकर्कटी ।
अंगारकर्कटी बल्या बृंहणी शुक्रला लघुः ।
दीपनी कफहृद्रोगपीनसश्वासकासजित् ।
माषादी पिष्टिका मध्या पोलिका वेष्टनी मता ।
वेष्टनिका वृष्या स्वादुः स्निग्धा [पित्ता]निलापहः ।
'उष्णा संतर्पणी बल्या शुक्रला बृंहणी परम् ।
भिन्नमूत्रमलास्तन्यमेदःपित्तकफप्रदाः ।
गुदकीलार्दितश्वासयकृच्छूलविनाशिनी ।'
[भावप्रकाशः कृतान्नवर्ग १२ : ४२-४३]

चमसीनवितापोली कथिता बलमद्रिका ।
किंचिद् हीनगुणा प्रोक्ता वेष्टनी गुणतो बुधैः ।
धूमसी रचिता सैव ख्याता कर्करिका बुधैः ।
कर्करीकातु पित्तघ्नी किंचिद्वातहरी मता ।
पूरिका तैलसंपक्वता रुच्या बलकरी गुरु ।
चक्षुस्तेजोहरा चोष्णा वातहृत् पित्तरक्तकृत् ।
घृतपक्वाऽपि तद्वत्स्यात् चक्षुष्या रक्तपित्तहृत ।
प्रोक्ता मुद्गवटी रुच्या बलकृद्रोगिणे हिता ।
मुद्गसूपगुणाः ये तु तष्टवात्राधिका मताः ।
माषस्य वटिका हृद्या बल्या पुष्टिप्रदायिनी ।
वातहृत् शुक्रला मोक्रा तलितापि प्रलेहिता ।
वटी कुष्मांडसंयुक्तमाषपिष्टिकया कृता ।
अम्लपित्तकरी ज्ञेया यकृद्वातविनाशिनी ।
चणकस्यापि वटिका व्यंजनेषु वरा भवेत् ।
रुच्या विष्टम्भजननी बल्या पुष्टिविवर्द्धिनी ।
तक्रादिक्वाथसंसिद्धा क्वथिका कथिता बुधैः ।
क्वथिका पाचनी हृद्या रुच्या वह्निप्रदा लघु ।
कफानिल विबंधघ्नी किंचित्पित्तप्रकोपिणी ।
जीरैर्हिंगु इवेणोषणलवणयुतै राईकैः ।
पूर्णगर्भश्चक्राकारः सुपुष्टः प्रचुरपरिमल कोमलः ।
कुंकुमाभः प्राप्ते दंतान्तरालं मुरूमुरूः खणः स्वच्छा ।
तैले सुपक्वो धन्यानामास्यदेशं प्रविशति ।
चठको भीमभोगायसिद्धाः ।
वटः शुष्को वातहरो बल्यो विष्टम्भपित्तकृत् ।
ग्राह्लादजनकः प्रोक्तो दाहकरी तृषाकरः ।
सष्टवद्योलमग्रश्वेद्रुव्यः शुक्रकरो गुरुः ।
बल्यो विष्टंभकारी च विदाही पवनापहः ।
कांजिके वटको रुच्यो वातजित्कफकारकः ।
पित्तरक्तकरश्चोक्तो न हितो नेत्ररोगिणां ।
सामेतावत्तिर्काः कृत्वा सुसूक्ष्मा यवसंनिभाः ।
शुष्का पायसवत्साध्या भोज्याः खडघृतान्विताः ।

सेविका तृप्ति जननी रुचिपित्तानिलापहा ।
संधानकृद्ग्राहिणी च सा सेव्या स्तोकमात्रया ।
शुभ्रेऽर्धसाधिते दुग्धे घृताक्तांस्तंदुलान्क्षिपेत् ।
सुसिद्धा खंडसंयुक्तां चंद्राभा क्षीरिका भवेत् ।
क्षीरिकार्दुर्ज्जरा बल्या धातुपुष्टिप्रदा गुरुः ।
विष्टम्भिनी हरेत्पित्तं रक्तपित्ताग्निमारुतान् ।
गोसिका गुरवो भक्ष्या वातघ्ना कफशुक्रलाः ।
पोलिका घृतसंपक्वा सूक्ष्मा सोहालिका मता ।
सौहाली शुक्रला रुच्या वातपित्तहरा गुरुः ।
पुटैरनेकैः संयुक्ता सोमाली फेनिका भवेत् ।
फेनिकं मधुरा शीता वृष्या गुर्वी मनोहरा ।
वातपित्तहरी बल्या किंचित्कफकरी सरा ।
चक्राकाराः सुपुष्टाश्चससर्पिसम्मिता कृताः ।
घृते सिद्धाः पक्वखंडमंडिता मधुशीर्षकाः ।
समितां सर्पिषा भृष्टा सितामरिचमिश्रिता ।
एलालंवगकर्पूरचूर्णादि परिसंस्कृतां ।
क्षिप्ताऽन्यसंमिता लपुटे सर्पिषि संपचेत् ।
तरुः खंडेतिपक्वेन संयावोऽयमुदाहृतः ।
संयावमवि जानीयान्मधुशीर्षकवद्गुणैः ।
संमिता सेविकाः कृत्वा वर्त्तिवत्पाचिता घृतैः ।
मिश्रिताः पक्वखण्डेन ताभिर्भवति मोदकः ।
सेविका लड्डुका बल्या गुरवो मधुरा हिमाः ।
वातपित्तहराः स्निग्धाः शुक्रलाः श्लेष्मकारिणः ।
कृताकर्करपात्रेण पिष्टिका विंदवो घृते मर्दिताः ।
पक्वखंडेन लड्डुर्कविधायते ।
मोदको मुद्गसिद्धः प्रणिनो वातपित्तहृत् ।
रुचिकृद्बलकृत्सद्यः किंचित्कफकरो हिमः ।
स चेच्चणकसंसिद्धो विशेषाद्वातलो मतः ।
समिता संधिता क्षिप्ता सच्छिद्रे भाजनांतरे ।
परिभ्राम्यपरिभ्राम्य पतिता तप्तसर्पिषि ।
द्विशः वृत्या त्रिरावृत्या विहिता कंकणा कृतिः ।

सिताद्रवे मज्जिता च रसगर्भेति सोच्यते ।
रसगर्भा परं रुच्या पुष्टिकाऽतिबलप्रदा ।
धातुवृद्धिकरी गुर्वी तर्पणी वातपित्तहृत् ।
आममाम्रफलं खंड इव पक्वं घृतान्वितं ।
एलामरिचसंयुक्तं ज्ञातव्यं स च खाडवः ।
खंडाम्रखाडवः स्निग्धो मधुरोऽष्णो गुरुस्तथा ।
परं रुचिकरो बल्यस्तुष्टिपुष्टिप्रदो मतः ।
समिता सर्पिषा भृष्टा शुभ्रशर्क्करया युता ।
युता क्षीरेण संपक्वा लप्सिका मरिचान्विता ।
लप्सिका बृंहणी वृष्या वातपित्तहरा गुरुः ।
मेहः कफकरी स्निग्धा रुच्या तृप्तिप्रदायिनी ।
एलालंवगकर्पूरमरिचैः सहशर्क्करा ।
अम्लीका फलसंभूतं पानकं वातनाशनं ।
कफपित्तकरं किंचित्सुरुच्यं वह्निबोधनं ।
अपक्वाम्लफलोद्भुतं पानकं वातनाशनं ।
कफपित्तकरं चाम्लं रुच्यं पक्वाम्रसंभवं ।
तत्तु स्वाद्रष्टं च गुरुपित्तहृत् ।
विदंश्लेष्मलबल्यं चूर्णं वृष्यवमे नाशयेत् ।
निंबूजं पानं पाचनं वातनाशनं ।
धान्यकल्कसिताजातं पानकं शशिवासितम् ।
शीतं परं पित्तहरं मूत्रकृच्छ्रविनाशनं ।
अपक्वभृष्टो गोधूमो वुधैरुवीति कथ्यते ।
उंदी कफप्रदा बल्या लघ्वी पित्तानिलापहा ।
शिबीधान्यैर्वृद्धपक्वैर्सुभृष्टैर्होलको मतः ।
होलको वातलो मेदकफदोषश्रमापहः ।' बहुप्रमादपर्णः पाठोऽयं चतुर्थपुस्तके अधिकमुपलभ्यते ।

68. यद्गुणेनेह इति आकरे पाठः ।

69. यद्वीर्येण च इति आकरे पाठः ।

70. भक्ष्याश्चिकित्सकैः इति आकरे पाठः ।

71. इति पानभक्ष्यवर्गः इति आकरे पाठः ।
इति यूषादिक्रमः इति चतुर्थपुस्तके पाठः ।

# CHAPTER 28

**'शीतोष्णतोयासवमद्ययूषफलाम्लधान्याम्लपयोरसानाम् ।**

**यस्यानुपानं तु हितं भवेद्यत्तस्मै प्रदेयं तु हि मात्रया वै ॥१॥**

व्याधिं कालं च विभाव्य धीरैर्द्रव्याणि योज्यानि च तानि तानि ।

*Anupāna*

Cold water, hot water, *āsava*, alcohols, *yūṣa*, *phalāmla*, *dhānyāmla*, milk and juice—these are generally used as *anupāna* and these should be used in proper quantity after ascertaining their utility, the nature of the disease and its stage of manifestation.

सर्वानुपानेषु वरं वदन्ति मेध्यं यदम्भः शुचिभाजनस्थम् ॥ २ ॥'

[माधवद्रव्यगुणः अनुपानविधि २८: १-२]

Among all the *anupānas* the water which is kept in a clean pot is the best. It promotes intellect.

'स्निग्धोष्णं मारुते शस्तं पित्ते मधुरशीतलम् ।

कफेऽनुपानं रूक्षोष्णं क्षये मांसरसः परम् ॥ ३ ॥

**उष्णोदकानुपानं तु स्नेहानामथ शस्यते ।**

ऋते भल्लातकस्नेहात्तत्र [7] तोयं सुशीतलम् ॥ ४ ॥

If there is aggravation of *vāyu*, *anupānas* which are unctuous and hot are useful; in *pitta* sweet and cooling *anupānas* are useful and in *kapha* ununctuous and hot *anupānas* are useful. If there is *kṣaya* (consumption) meat soup is the best *anupāna*.

After taking oil, ghee etc. hot water should be used as *anupāna*. The oil of *bhallātaka* is an exception to this rule and cold water should be used after this oil.

अनुपानं च [8] दातव्यं [9] तैलयूषाम्लकांजिकम् ।

शीतोदकं माक्षिकस्य पिष्टान्नस्य च सर्वशः ॥ ५ ॥

[10] दधिपायसमद्यार्त्तिविषयुष्टेस्तथैव ये ।

After honey and pastries (*piṣṭānna*) the *anupāna* should invariably be oil, *yūṣa*, *amla kāñjika* or cold water. Similar types of *anupāna* are useful after the intake of *dadhi*, *pāyasa* and alcohol and in *viṣa* (poisoning).

[11] केचित्पिष्टमये प्राहुरनुपानं सुखोदकम् ॥ ६ ॥

According to some scholars ordinary water should be used as *anupāna* after taking pastries (*piṣṭa*).

पयो [12] मांसरसो वापि [13] शालिमुद्गादिभोजिनाम् ।

Milk and meat soup should be used as *anupāna* for persons taking *śāli*, *mudga* etc.

माषादेरनुपानं तु धान्याम्ल दधिमस्तु वा ॥ ७ ॥

*Dhānyāmla* or *dadhi mastu* is useful as *anupāna* for persons taking *māṣa* etc.

अल्पाग्नीनामनिद्राणां [14] तन्द्राशोषभ्रमक्लमे ।

मद्यमांसोचितानां च मद्यमेवानुशस्यते ॥ ८ ॥

Alcohol is useful as *anupāna* for persons suffering from weak digestive power, sleeplessness, drowsiness, *śoṣa* (consumption), *bhrama* (giddiness) and *klama* (physical fatigue) and also for persons who are habituated to alcohol and meat.

अमद्यपानामुदकं **फलाम्लं** वा प्रशस्यते ।

Persons who are not accustomed to drinking should use water or *phalāmla* as *anupāna*.

उपवासाध्व[15]भाष्यस्त्रीमारुतातपकर्मभिः ॥ ९ ॥

क्लान्तानामनुपानार्थं **पयः** पथ्यं परं[16] स्मृतम् ।

Milk is extremely wholesome for persons who are fatigued because of fast, excessive walking, talking or sexual intercourse and exposure to wind, sun ray or excessive exercise.

सुराकृशाणां स्थूलानामनुपानं **मधूदकम्** ॥ १० ॥

*Madhūdaka* should be used as *anupāna* by persons who are emaciated because of excessive drinking and also for persons who are obese.

निरामयाणां[17] चित्तं [?] तु भुक्तमध्ये प्रकीर्तितम्[18] ।

For healthy persons *anupāna* should be used in the middle of the food.

हितं शोणितपित्तेभ्यः क्षीरमिक्षुरसस्तथा ॥ ११ ॥

Patients suffering from *śoṇita pitta* (a disease characterised by bleeding from different parts of the body) should use milk or sugar cane juice as *anupāna*.

अक्ष[19]शेलुशिरीषाणामासवास्तु विषार्त्तिषु ।

Patients suffering from poisoning should use the *āsava* of *akṣa*, *śelu* and *śirīṣa* as *anupāna*.

[20]
दोषवत् गुरु वा युक्तमतिमात्रमथापि वा ।
[21]
यथोक्तेनानुपानेन सुखमन्नं हि जीर्य्यति ॥ १२ ॥

When *anupāna* is used in excess quantity, then it is injurious and heavy. If *anupāna* is used according to the prescription, then it helps in easy digestion of food.

[22]
'रोचनं बृंहणं वृष्यं दोषसंघातभेदनम्' ।
[23]
तर्पणं मार्दवकरं श्रमक्लमहरं सुखम् ॥ १३ ॥

दीपनं दोषशमनं पिपासाछेदनं परम् ।
[24]
बल्यं वर्णकरं चापि अनुपानं सदोच्यते ॥ १४ ॥

*Anupāna* is invariably appetiser, nourishing and aphrodisiac. It helps in the detachment of all the *doṣas* from the tissue elements. It is refreshing. It produces softness and cures physical as well as mental fatigue. It produces happiness, stimulates digestion, alleviates *doṣas*, reduces thirst and promotes strength as well as complexion.

[25]
तदादौ कर्शयेत्पीतं स्थापयेन्मध्यसेवितम् ।
पश्चात्पीतं बृंहयति तत्समीक्ष्य प्रयोजयेत् ॥ १५ ॥

If *anupāna* is used before food, then it causes emaciation. If it is used in the middle of the food, then it keeps the *doṣas* in their proper positions. If it is used after food, then it produces a nourishing effect. Keeping these facts in view one should administer *anupāna*.

[26]
स्थिरतांगतमक्लिन्नमन्नमद्रवपायिनाम ।
[27]
भवत्यावाधाजननमनुपानमतः पिवेत् ॥ १६ ॥
[28]
न पिबेच्छ्वासकासार्त्तो रोगे वाप्यूर्ध्वजत्रुगे ।
[29] [30]
क्षतोरस्तु प्रसेकी च यस्य [ह्य]पहतः स्वरः ॥१७॥

If food is taken without any drink, then it remains there without undergoing the process of softening. Therefore one should use *anupāna*. It should not be used by patients suffering from *śvāsa* (asthma), *kāsa* (bronchitis), diseases of the head and neck, *uraḥ kṣata* (phthisis), *praseka* (excessive sliva-tion) and impairment of voice.

[31] पानाध्वभाष्याध्ययनं स्वप्नमेतान्न शीलयेत् ।
[32] प्रदूष्यामाशयं तद्धि तस्य कंठोरसि स्थितम् ॥ १८ ॥
[33] स्यादग्निसादछर्द्यादीन् जनयेदामयान्बहून् ।

One should not indulge in drinking, walking, talking, reading and sleeping in excess. By doing so the stomach gets vitiated and the *doṣas* situated in the throat and chest produce indigestion, vomiting and many such diseases.

[34] अनुपाने प्रयोक्तव्यं व्याधौ श्लेष्मभवे पलम्[35] ।
पलद्वयं त्वनिलजे पित्तजे च पलत्रयम् ॥ १९ ॥'

[माधवद्रव्यगुणः अनुपानविधि २८ : ४-२१]

In diseases caused by *kapha* the *anupāna* should be administered in a dose of one *pala* (48 ml.). In diseases caused by *vāyu* its dose is two *palas* (96 ml.). In diseases caused by *pitta* the dose of *anupāna* is three *palas* (144 ml.).

॥ इत्यनुपानविधिः ॥

Thus end the section dealing with the method of administration of different types of *anupāna*.

## NOTES AND REFERENCES

1. भवेद्धितं यत्तस्मै प्रदेयं त्विह मात्रया तत् इति ग्राकरे पाठः ।
2. भवेत्सत्तस्मै इति द्वितीयपुस्तके पाठः ।

3. च इति चतुर्थपुस्तके पाठः ।
4. द्रव्याणि इति द्वितीयपुस्तके पाठः ।
5. विभज्य इति आकरे पाठः ।
6. योग्यानि इति द्वितीयपुस्तके पाठः ।
7. नोष्णं इति द्वितीयपुस्तके पाठः ।
8. अनुपानं वदन्त्येके इति आकरे पाठः ।
9. तैले इति आकरे पाठः ।
10. दधिपायसमद्यार्त्तिविषयुक्ते तथैव च इति आकरे पाठः ।
    दधिपायसमद्यानां विषयुक्तास्तथैव ये इति द्वितीयपुस्तके पाठः ।
11. केचिदिष्टतम इति द्वितीयपुस्तके पाठः ।
12. यूषो मांसरसो इति आकरे चतुर्थपुस्तके च पाठः ।
13. शालिमुद्गादियोजितम् इति आदर्शपुस्तके पाठः ।
    शालिमुद्गादिभोजने इति चतुर्थपुस्तके पाठः ।
14. तंद्राशोकभ्रमक्लमैः इति आकरे पाठः ।
15. उपवासाध्वकार्श्यस्त्री इति द्वितीयपुस्तके पाठः ।
16. तथाऽमृतम् इति आकरे पाठः ।
17. चित्रं इति आकरे पाठः ।
18. प्रशस्यते इति आकरे चतुर्थपुस्तके च पाठः ।
19. अर्कशेलुशिरीषाणां मांसमस्तु विषार्त्तिषु इति आदर्शपुस्तके पाठः ।
20. दोषं च इति आदर्शपुस्तके पाठः ।
21. प्रजीर्यति इति आकरे पाठः ।
22. 'रोचनं·······दोषसंघातभेदनम्' पाठोऽयं चतुर्थपुस्तके नोपलभ्यते ।
23. सर्वक्लमहरं इति द्वितीयपुस्तके पाठः ।
24. त्वनुपानं इति आकरे पाठः ।
25. तर्पयेत्पीतं इति द्वितीयपुस्तके पाठः ।
26. भवत्यबोधजननमनुपानमतः इति आदर्शपुस्तके पाठः ।
27. न रोगे तूर्ध्वजत्रुगे इति आकरे पाठः ।
28. क्षतोरस्कः इति आकरे पाठः ।
29. यः स्याच्चोपहतस्वरः इति आकरे पाठः ।

यस्य ह्यापहतः स्वरम् इति द्वितीयपुस्तके पाठः ।

30. पीत्वाध्वभाष्याध्ययनगेयस्वप्नान्न इति आकरे चतुर्थपुस्तके च पाठः ।

31. प्रदूष्यामाशये इति आदर्शपुस्तके पाठः ।

32. मंदाग्निसादछर्द्यादीन् इति आकरे पाठः ।

अग्निमान्द्यछर्द्यादीन् इति द्वितीयपुस्तके पाठः ।

33. अनुपानं इति आकरे पाठः ।

34. फलम् इति द्वितीयपुस्तके पाठः ।

35. अनुपानाधिकारः इति चतुर्थपुस्तके पाठः ।

# CHAPTER 29

चित्रकाऽभावतो दन्ती क्षारशिखरिजोऽथवा ।

If *citraka* is not available, then in its place *dantī* or the *kṣāra* of *śikhari* should be used.

अभावे पृष्णिपर्ण्याश्च सिंहपुच्छी प्रदीयते ॥ १ ॥

In the case of non-availability of *pṛṣṇī parṇī*, one should use *siṁha pucchī*.

भाङ्गर्यऽभावे तु तालीसं कंटकारीजटाऽथवा ।

If *bhārṅgī* is not available, then *tālīsa* or the root of *kaṇṭakārī* should be used in its place.

अभावे धन्वयासस्य प्रक्षेप्या च दुरालभा ॥ २ ॥

If *dhanvayāsa* is not available, then *durālabhā* should be added in its place.

पुंजातः [मुंजातः?] पश्चिमे ख्यातस्तस्याभावे तु तालविट् ।

In the place of the drug which is known in the western

regions as *puṁjāta*, one should use *tālaviṭ*.

नततगरपाद्याश्च अभावे वेणु निक्षिपेत् ॥ ३ ॥

If *nata* or *tagara pādi* is not available, then in its place *veṇu* should be added.

अभावे तगरस्यापि कुष्ठं तु प्रक्षिपेत्सदा ।

If *tagara* is not available, then *kuṣṭha* should always be added in its place.

क्षिपेत् करिकणाभावादपि कुक्कुटमस्तकम् ॥ ४ ॥

If *karikaṇā* is not available, then one should use in its place *kukkuṭa mastaka*.

अभावेऽभ्रकसत्त्वस्य कांतलौहं प्रयोजयेत् ।

If the *sattva* (essence) of *abhraka* is not available, then in its place *kānta lauha* should be used.

कान्ताभावे तीक्ष्णलौहं योजयेत् वैद्यसत्तमः ॥ ५ ॥

If *kānṭa lauha* is not available, then an expert physician should used *tīkṣṇa lauha* in its place.

मूर्वाभावे त्वचो ग्राह्या ततो जिंगिनिसंभवा ।

If *mūrvā* is not available, then in its place the bark of *jiṅgini* should be used.

अर्कपर्णादिपयसो ह्यभावे तद्रसो मतः ॥ ६ ॥

If the latex of *arka parṇī* etc. is not available, then in its place the *yūṣa* of these plants is recommended.

लाङ्गल्यभावतो वह्नीपत्रं दद्यात् विचक्षणः ।

An expert should use *vahnī patra* in the place of *lāṅgalī* if the latter is not available.

अहिंस्रायाः अभावे तु मानकंदः प्रकीर्त्तितः ॥ ७ ॥

If *ahiṁsrā* is not available, then in its place *māna kanda* is to be used,

लक्ष्मणाया अभावे तु नीलीकंदशिफा मता ।

If *lakṣmaṇā* is not available, then the root of *nīlī kanda* should be used.

यदा न पौष्करं मूलं कुष्ठं योज्यं तदा बुधैः ॥ ८ ॥

If *puṣkara mūla* is not available, then in its place *kuṣṭha* should be used by the Wise.

चविकागजपिप्पल्यौ पिप्पलीमूलवत् स्मृतौ ।

*Cavikā* and *gaja pippalī* have effects like *pippalī mūla*.

भल्लातकासहत्वे तु रक्तचंदनमिष्यते ॥ ९ ॥

If a person is not able to tolerate *bhallātaka*, then he should be given *rakta candana*.

अभावे सोमराज्यास्तु प्रपुन्नाडफलं मतम् ।

If *somarāji* is not available, then in its place the fruit of *prapunnāḍa* is recommended.

यदा न स्यात् दारुनिशा तदा देया निशा बुधैः ॥१०॥

When *dāru niśā* is not available, then the Wise should use *niśā*.

रसांजनस्याभावे तु सम्यक् दार्वीं प्रयोजयेत् ।

If *rasāñjana* is not available, then in its place *dārvī* is used.

सौराष्ट्र्यभावतो देया कटिभी तद्गुणा जनैः ॥११॥

If *saurāṣṭri* is not available, then in its place *kaṭibhī* which has similar properties should be used.

अम्लवेतसकाभावे चुक्रं दातव्यमीरितम् ।

If *amla vetasa* is not available, then in its place *cukra* should be used.

रुचकाभावतो दद्यात् लवणं पांशुपूर्वकम् ।। १२ ।।

If *rucaka* is not available, then in its place *pāṁśu lavaṇa* should be added.

सुवर्णमथवा रूप्यं मृतं यत्र न विद्यते ।
तत्र लोहेन कर्माणि भिषक् कुर्याद् विचक्षणः ।।१३।।

If the *bhasma* of *suvarṇa* or *rūpya* is not available, then in its place an expert physician should give *lauha*.

सुवर्णाभावतो वैद्यो माक्षिकं वापि निःक्षिपेत् ।
माक्षिकस्याप्यभावे तु प्रदद्यात् स्वर्णगैरिकम् ।। १४ ।।

If *suvarṇa* is not available, then in its place the physician should add *mākṣika*. If, however, *mākṣika* is not available, in its place *svarṇa gairika* should be used.

हेममाक्षिकजं सत्त्वं मृतहेमसमं गुणैः ।

The *sattva* (essence) of *hema mākṣika* is similar to *svarṇa bhasma* in properties.

श्वेतं तु माक्षिकं ज्ञेयं ध्रुवं रजतवद् गुणैः ।। १५ ।।

The white variety of *mākṣika* is certainly like *rajata* in property.

वज्राभावे तु वैक्रान्तं मुनयः प्रक्षिपंति च ।

If *vajra* is not available, then the sages use *vaikrānta* in its place.

कर्पूराभावतो देयं ग्रन्थिपर्णं विशेषतः ।। १६ ।।

If *karpūra* is not available, then *granthi parṇa* is used in its place.

श्रीखण्डचंदनाभावे कर्पूरं देयमिष्यते ।

अलाभे त्वेतयोर्वैद्यः प्रक्षिपेद्रक्तचन्दनम् ॥ १७ ॥

रक्तचन्दनकाभावे नवोशीरं विदुर्बुधाः ।

If *śrīkhaṇḍa candana* is not available, then in its place *karpūra* should be added. If both of them are not available, then the Wise should use *rakta candana* in their place. If *rakta candana* is not available, then the freshly collected *uśīra* is used in its place.

तालीसपत्रकाभावे स्वर्णताली प्रशस्यते ॥ १८ ॥

If *tālīsa patra* is not available, then in its place *svarṇa tālī* is useful.

अभावे नागपुष्पस्य पद्मकेसरमुच्यते ।

If *nāga puṣpa* is not available, then *padma keśara* is to be used.

कस्तूर्यभावे कक्कोलं प्रक्षेप्यं तु विदुर्बुधाः ॥ १९ ॥

कक्कोलस्याप्यभावे तु जातीपुष्पं प्रशस्यते ।

If *kastūrī* is not available, then the Wise should add *kakkola* in its place. If *kakkola* is not available, then the flower of *jāti* is useful in its place.

नीलोत्पलस्याभावे तु कुमुदं देयमिष्यते ॥ २० ॥

If *nīlotpala* is not available, then in its place *kumuda* should be used.

जातीपुष्पं न यत्रास्ति लवंगं तत्र दीयते ।

If the flower of *jāti* is not available, then in its place *lavaṅga* is added.

वंधूकाभावतो देयं पुष्पं पुन्नागनामकम् ॥ २१ ॥

If *vandhūka* is not available, then in its place the flower called *punnāga* should be added.

वकुलाभावतो देयं कल्हारोत्पलपंकजम् ।

If *bakula* is not available, then in its place *kalhāra*, *utpala* and *paṅkaja* can be used.

द्राक्षा यदि न लभ्येत प्रदेयं काश्मरीफलम् ॥ २२ ॥

तयोरभावे कुसुमं मधूकस्य मतं बुधैः ।

If *drākṣā* is not available, then in its place the fruit of *kāśmarī* should be added. If both of them are not available, then the flower of *madhūka* should be used.

मेदाजीवककाकोलीऋद्धिद्वन्द्वेऽपि वाऽसति ॥ २३ ॥

यष्टीविदार्यश्वगंधावाराहीं च क्रमात् क्षिपेत् ।

If both the types of each of *medā*, *jīvaka*, *kākolī* and *ṛddhi* are not available, then in their places *yaṣṭī*, *vidāri*, *aśvagandhā* and *vārāhī* should be added respectively.

वाराह्याश्च तथाभावे चर्मकारालुको मतः ॥ २४ ॥

If *vārāhī* is not available, then in its place *carmakārāluka* should be used.

न भवेत् दाडिमं यत्र वृक्षाम्लं तत्र योजयेत् ।

If *dāḍima* is not available, then in its place *vṛkṣāmla* should be used.

क्षीराभावे रसो मौद्गः मासूरो वा प्रदीयते ॥ २५ ॥

If milk is not available, then the juice of *mudga* or *masūra* should be used.

रूचकतैलाभावे तु हितमारुष्करं विदुः ।

If the oil of *rūcaka* is not available, then in its place the oil of *aruṣkara* should be used.

मुक्ताभावे क्षिपेन्नित्यं मुक्ताशुक्ति न संशयः ॥ २६ ॥

If *muktā* is not available, one can undoubtedly use *muktā-śukti* in its place.

मधु यत्र न लभ्येत तत्र जीर्णगुडो मतः ।
अनर्हत्वादभावाद्वा मधुनः शस्यते बुधैः ।। २७ ।।
रम्भापुष्परसश्चापि खांडजलमथापि वा ।

If honey is not available, then in its place old *guḍa* is recommended. If honey is either not available or not suitable for the patient, then in its place the Wise should use the juice of *rambhā puṣpa* or water mixed with *khaṇḍa.*

मत्स्याण्ड्यभावतो दद्यात् भिषग्भि सितशर्करा ।।२८।।

If *matsyāṇḍi* is not available, then in its place a physician can give white variety of *śarkarā*.

सिद्धार्थः सर्षपे योज्याद्वैद्यविद्याविशारदैः ।

A person proficient in medical science should use *siddhār-tha* in the place of *sarṣapa*.

असंभवे सितायाश्च बुधैः खंडं प्रयुज्यते ।। २९ ।।

If *sitā* is not available, then the Wise should use *khaṇḍa.*

अभावे वेतसाम्लस्य चणकाम्लमपि क्षिपेत् ।
एतयोश्च अभावेऽपि हेमंताम्लं समादिशेत् ।। ३० ।।

If *vetasāmla* is not available, then in its place *caṇakāmla* may be used. If both of them are not available, then in their place, the use of *hemantāmla* is advised.

मुस्ता चातिविषाऽभावे शिवाऽभावे शिव भवेत् ।।३१।।

If *ativiṣā* is not available, then in its place *mustā* should be used. If *śivā* (*harītakī*) is not available, then in its place *śiva* (*āmalaka*) should be used.

अभावे सति पत्राणां रसादौ भावनाविधिः ।

विषमुष्टिकषायेण षड्गुणा भावना भवेत् ।। ३२ ।।

If it is prescribed in the text to give *bhāvanā* (impregnation) by the juice of the leaf *viṣamuṣṭi*, and if it is not available, then in its place the decoction of this drug six times in quantity can be used.

अभावे शालिधान्यस्य षष्टिकादि न्यसेत् बुधैः ।

If *śāli dhānya* is not available, then in its place *ṣaṣṭika* etc. should be added.

मसूराभावतो दद्यात् शशहंसाखुकानपि ।। ३३ ।।

If *masūra* is not available, then in its place the juice of the meat of *śaśa*, *haṁsa* and *ākhu* can be used.

अत्र प्रोक्तानि वस्तूनि यानि यानि च तेषु च ।

योज्यमेकतराभावे परं वैद्येन जानता ।। ३४ ।।

The substitute drugs described in this chapter can be used by a wise physician when the original drugs are not available.

रसवीर्यविपाकाद्यैः समद्रव्यं विचिन्त्य च ।

युंज्यादेवंविधमन्यद्द्रव्यज्ञानविशारदः ।। ३५ ।।

A physician well versed in materia medica should decide substitutes of similar other drugs by taking into consideration their *rasa* (taste), *vīrya* (potency), *vipāka* (taste after digestion) etc.

अन्तःसम्मार्जने मोदास्थाने योज्या यवानिका ।

बहिःसम्मार्जने मोदास्वजमोदैव गृह्यते ।। ३६ ।।

In the place of *modā*, *yavānikā* should be used if the formula is meant for internal cleansing and *ajamodā* should be used if the formula is meant for external cleansing.

अन्तःसम्मार्जने योज्यं वचास्थाने कुलिंजनम् ।
वहिःसम्मार्जने सैव प्रयोज्यात् [?] मरगिर्षिभिः [?] ॥ ३७ ॥

In the place of *vacā*, *kuliñjana* is used if the formula is meant for internal cleansing. For external cleansing, however, *vacā* as such can be used in the formula.

कृष्णजीरकयोगेन कर्तव्ये भक्ष्यभेषजे ।
तस्य स्थाने विधातव्यो जीरकः कुशलो [भिषक्] ॥ ३८ ॥

If any food preparation or medicine is described to be prepared by adding *kṛṣṇa jīraka*, then in its place white variety of *jīraka* should be used by an expert physician.

॥इति अनुकल्यवर्गः॥

Thus ends the chapter dealing with various types of substitutes and allied topics.

# CHAPTER 30

[1]दानशीलदया — सत्यब्रह्मचर्यकृतज्ञता ।

रसायनानि मैत्री च पुण्यायुर्वृद्धिकृद्गणाः ॥ १ ॥

Charity, good conduct, compassion, truthfulness, celibacy, gratefulness, rejuvenation therapy and friendship—these constitute the group which promotes virtue and longevity.

सुश्रुताद्गणान् वक्ष्यामः

उद्देशमात्रमपि लक्षणं प्राग्यदुक्तं व्यक्तं व्यनक्ति

पवनादिगदातुराणां । नृणामदृष्टचरकादि

जडात्मनोऽपि प्रज्ञावतः किमुत कायचिकित्सकस्य ॥२॥

**Description of groups of drugs according to *Suśruta***

What has been described in brief before clearly shows the way for the treatment of patients suffering from diseases caused by *vāyu* etc. even to a less intelligent person who is not acquainted with *Caraka* etc. It is not necessary to describe the usage to which these drugs can be put by an intelligent physician who is specialised in the treatment of internal diseases.

दोषधातुमलमूलमिदं रुग्युक्तमुक्तमृषिभिर्नृशरीरम् ।

तद्विकारमुपलभ्य भिषग्भिर्भेषजैरुपशमः करणीयः ॥ ३ ॥

इतीदमुक्तं यदुदीरितं पुरा समुच्चये सूत्रमविस्तरौषधम् ।

[2] कियद्भिरप्यौषधसंग्रहैर्गणैर्निगद्यते चान्यदतश्चिकित्सितम् ॥ ४ ॥

[3] स्यात्सप्तत्रिंशमेभिर्गणैर्वीक्ष्यवातपित्तकफान् ।

योगा रोगार्त्तानां विभज्य [4] भिषजा प्रकल्पन्ते ॥ ५ ॥

It has been stated by the sages that the human body which suffers from diseases is a conglomeration of *doṣas*, *dhātus* (tissue elements) and *malas* (waste products). If there is morbidity in this body, the physician should alleviate these ailments by the administration of drugs. This has already been stated before in brief. Now some of these drugs are being described by putting them into different groups for the convenience of treatment. These groups are thirty-seven in number. After ascertaining the predominance of either *vāyu*, *pitta* or *kapha* and the nature of the compound, disease and the patient, the physician should administer these drugs after proper selection.

घृततैलचूर्णकल्कप्रलेपसेकावगाहपानानि ।

आस्थापनमनुवासननस्यांजनवर्तिविधा यश्च ॥ ६ ॥

These drugs can be used in the form of medicated ghee, medicated oil, powder, paste, unguent, spray, bath, drink, *āsthāpana* type of enema, *anuvāsana* type of enema, inhalation, collyrium and suppository.

**सुश्रुतः**

समीक्ष्य दोषभेदांश्च [5] गणान्भिन्नान्प्रयोजयेत् ।

पृथङ्मिश्रान्समस्तान्वा गणान्वाच्यस्तु संहतान् ॥७॥

[सुश्रुतः सूत्र ३८ :८२]

*Suśruta*

Depending upon the nature of the *doṣas* involved in the manifestation of the disease, the physician should prescribe drugs described in these groups either separately or jointly. Even drugs of all the groups can be used together.

'तद्यथा—

१. विदारीगन्धा विदारी विश्वदेवा सहदेवा श्वदंष्ट्रा पृथक्पर्णी शृगालविन्ना शतावरी सारिवा जीवकर्षभकौ महासहा क्षुद्रसहा बृहत्यौ पुनर्नवैरण्डो हंसपादी वृश्चिकालीऋषभश्चेति ।। ८ ।।

(1) *Vidārigandhādi gaṇa*

This group includes *vidāri gandhā*, *vidārī*, *viśvadevā*, *sahadevā*, *śvadaṁṣṭrā*, *pṛthakparṇī*, *sṛgāla vinnā*, *śatāvarī*, *sārivā*, *jivaka*, *ṛṣabhaka*, *mahā sahā*, *kṣudra sahā*, *bṛhatī*, *kaṇṭakārī*, *punarnavā*, *eraṇḍa*, *haṁsa pādī*, *vṛścikālī* and *ṛṣabha*.

विदारीगन्धादिरयं गणः पित्तानिलापहः ।
शोषगुल्मांगमर्दोर्ध्वश्वासकासविनाशनः ।। ९ ।।

Drugs of this group alleviate *pitta* and *vāyu*, and cure *śoṣa* (consumption), *gulma* (phantom tumour), *aṅga marda* (malaise), *urdhva śvāsa* (dyspnoea) and *kasā* (bronchitis).

२. आरग्वधमदनगोपघोण्टाकण्टकीकुटजपाठापाटलामूर्वेन्द्रयवसप्तपर्णनिंब-कुरण्टकदासीकुरण्टकगुडूचीचित्रकशार्ङ्गेष्ठापरूषककरंजद्वयपटोलकिराततिक्तकानि सुषवी चेति ।। १० ।।

(2) *Āragvadhādi gaṇa*

This group includes *āragvadha*, *madana*, *gopa ghoṇṭā*, *kaṇṭakī*, *kuṭaja*, *pāṭhā*, *paṭalā*, *mūrvā*, *indrayava*, *saptaparna*, *nimba*, *kuraṇṭaka*, *guḍūcī*, *citraka*, *śārṅgiṣṭhā*, *parūṣaka*, both the types of *karañja*, *paṭola*, *kirāta tikta* and *suṣavī*.

आरग्वधादिरित्येष गणः श्लेष्मविषापहः ।
मेहकुष्ठज्वरवमीकण्डूघ्नो व्रणशोधनः ।। ११ ।।

Drugs of this group alleviate *kapha* and poisoning, and cure *meha* (obstinate urinary disorders including diabetes), *kuṣṭha* (obstinate skin diseases including leprosy), *jvara* (fever), *vamī* (vomiting) and *kaṇḍū* (itching). They also help in the cleansing of ulcers.

३. सालसाराजकर्णखदिरकदरकालस्कन्धक्रमुकभूर्जमेषशृङ्गीतिनिशचंदन-
कुचंदनशिंशिपाशिरीषासनधवार्जुननक्तमालाश्वकर्णशाकगुडूचीकालीय-
कश्चेति ॥ १२ ॥

(3) *Sālasāraādi gaṇa*

This group includes *sālasāra*, *ajakarṇa*, *khadira*, *kadara*, *kāla skandha*, *kramuka*, *bhūrja*, *meṣa śṛṅgī*, *tiniśa*, *candana*, *kucandana*, *śiṁśipā*, *śirīṣa*, *asana*, *dhava*, *arjuna*, *naktamāla*, *aśvakarṇa*, *śāka*, *guḍūcī* and *kālīyaka*.

सालसारादिरित्येष गणः कुष्ठविनाशनः ।
मेहपाण्ड्वामयहरः कफमेदो विशोधनः ॥ १३ ॥

Drugs of this group cure *kuṣṭha* (obstinate skin diseases including leprosy), *meha* (obstinate urinary disorders including diabetes) and *pāṇḍu* (anemia). They also cleanse *kapha* and *medas* (fat).

४. वरुणार्तगलशिग्रुमधुशिग्रुतर्कारीमेषशृङ्गीपूतीकनक्तमालमोरटाग्निमन्थसैरे-[6]
यकद्वयबिम्बीवसुकवसिरचित्रकशतावरीबिल्वाजशृङ्गीदर्भाः बृहतीद्वयं[7]
चेति ॥ १४ ॥

(4) *Varuṇādi gaṇa*

This group includes *varuṇa*, *ārtagala*, *śigru*, *madhu śigru*, *tarkārī*, *meṣaśṛṅgī*, *pūtīka*, *naktamāla*, *moraṭa*, *agnimantha*, both the types of *saireyaka*, *bimbī*, *vasuka*, *vasira*, *citraka*, *śatāvarī*, *bilva*, *ajaśṛṅgī*, *darbha* and both the types of *bṛhatī*.

वरुणादिर्गणो ह्येष कफमेदोनिवारणः ।
विनिहन्ति शिरःशूलगुल्माभ्यन्तरविद्रधीन् ॥ १५ ॥

Drugs of this group alleviate *kapha* and reduce *medas* (fat). They cure *śirahśūla* (headache), *gulma* (phantom tumour) and *ābhyantara vidradhi* (internal abscess).

५. वीरतरुसहचरद्वयदर्भ[8]वृक्षादनीगुन्द्रानलकुशकाशाश्मभेदकाग्निमन्थमोरटा-
वसुकवसिरभल्लूककुरण्टिकेन्दीवरकपोतवङ्काः श्वद्रंष्टा चेति ॥ १६ ॥

(5) *Vīratarvādi gaṇa*

This group includes *vīrataru*, both the types of *sahacara*, *darbha*, *vṛkṣādanī*, *gundrā*, *nala*, *kuśa*, *kāśa* *aśmabhedaka*, *agnimantha*, *moraṭā*, *vasuka*, *vasira*, *bhallūka*, *kuranṭika*, *indīvara*, *kapota vaṇkā* and *svadaṁṣṭrā*.

वीरतर्वादिरित्येष गणो वातविकारनुत् ।
अश्मरीशर्करामूत्रकृच्छ्[9]राघातरुजापहः ॥ १७ ॥

Drugs of this group cure diseases caused by *vāyu*, *aśmarī* (stone in urinary tract), *śarkarā* (gravels in the urinary tract), *mūtra kṛcchra* (dysuria) and *mūtrāghāta* (anuria).

६. [10]रोध्रसावररोध्रपलाशकुटन्नटाशोकफंजीकट्फलैलवालुकसल्लकीजिंगिनी-
कदम्बसालाः कदली चेति ॥ १८ ॥

(6) *Rodhrādi gaṇa*

This group includes *rodhra*, *sāvararodhra*, *palāśa*, *kuṭannaṭa*, *aṣoka*, *phañjī*, *kaṭphala*, *ela vāluka*, *sallakī*, *jiṅginī*, *kadamba*, *sāla* and *kadalī*.

एष रोध्रादिरित्युक्तो मेदःकफहरो गणः ।
योनिदोषहरः स्तम्भी वर्ण्यो विषविनाशनः ॥ १९ ॥

Drugs of this group reduce *medas* (faṭ) and *kapha*. They cure *yonī doṣa* (ailments of female genital tract). They promote the power of retention (*stambhana*) and complexion. They cure *viṣa* (poisoning).

७. अर्कालर्ककरंजद्वयनागदन्तीमयूरकभार्गीरासनेन्द्रपुष्पीक्षुद्रश्वेतामहाश्वेतावृश्चिकाल्यलवणास्तापसवृक्षश्चेति ॥ २० ॥

### (7) *Arkādi gaṇa*

This group includes *arka, alraka,* both the types of *karañja, nāgadantī, mayūraka, bhārgī, rāsanā, indrapuṣpī, kṣudraśvetā, mahā śvetā, vṛścikāli, alavaṇā* and *tāpasa vṛkṣa.*

अर्कादिको गणो ह्येष कफमेदोविषापहः ।
कृमिकुष्ठप्रशमनो विशेषात् व्रणशोधनः ॥ २१ ॥

Drugs of this group reduce *kapha* and *medas* (fat). They cure *viṣa* (poisoning), *kṛmi* (parasitic infection) and *kuṣṭha* (obstinate skin diseases including leprosy). They specially help in the cleansing of ulcers.

८. सुरसाश्वेतसुरसाफणिज्झकार्जकभूस्तृणसुगन्धकसुमुखकालमालकासमर्दक्षवकखरपुष्पविडङ्गकट्फलसुरभीनिर्गुण्डीकुलाहलोन्दुरुकर्णिकाफञ्जीप्राचीगलकाकमाच्यो विषमुष्टिकश्चेति ॥ २२ ॥

### (8) *Śurasādi gaṇa*

This group includes *surasā, śveta, surasā, phaṇijjhaka, arjaka, bhūstṛṇa, sugandhaka, sūmukha, kālmāla, kāsamarda, kṣavaka, kharapuṣpa, viḍaṅga, kaṭphala, surabhī, nirguṇḍī, kulāhala, unduru karnikā, phañjī, prācībala, kākamācī* and *viṣamuṣṭi.*

सुरसादिर्गणो ह्येष कफहृत् क्रमिसूदनः ।
प्रतिश्यायारुचिश्वासकासघ्नो व्रणशोधनः ॥ २३ ॥

Drugs of this group alleviate *kapha* and cure *kṛmi* (parasitic infection), *pratiśyāya* (rhinitis), *arucī* (anorexia), *śvāsa* (asthma) and *kāsa.* They help in the cleansing of ulcers.

९. मुष्ककपलाशधवचित्रकमदनवृक्षकशिंशपावज्रवृक्षास्त्रिफला चेति ॥२४॥

### (9) *Muśkakādi gaṇa*

The group includes *muṣkaka*, *palāśa*, *dhava*, *citraka*, *madama*, *vṛkṣaka*, *śiṁśapā*, *vajra vṛkṣa* and *triphalā*.

मुष्ककादिर्गणो ह्येष मेदोघ्नः शुक्रदोषहृत् ।
मेहार्शः पाण्डुरोगघ्नः शर्कराशनः परः' ॥ २५ ॥

[सुश्रुतः सूत्रः ३८ ८-२१]

Drugs of this group reduce *medas* (adiposity) and correct the vitiation of *śukra* (semen). They cure *meha* (obstinate urinary disorders including diabetes), *arśas* (piles), *pāṇḍu* (anemia), and *śarkarā* (gravels in the urinary tract).

१०. कृष्णाग्रन्थिकचव्यचित्रकविषाविश्वौषधाजाजिभिः ।
पाठारामरेणुकामधुरसासिद्धार्थतिक्तोषणैः ॥ २६ ॥
द्रेक्का शक्रयवाजमोदत्रुटिभिर्भार्गीविडङ्गान्वितैः ।

### (10) *Kṛṣṇādi gaṇa*

This group consists of *kṛṣṇā*, *granthika*, *cavya*, *citraka*, *viṣā*, *viśvauṣadha*, *ajāji*, *pāṭhā*, *rāmaṭha*, *reṇukā*, *madhurasā*, *siddhārtha*, *tiktā*, *uṣaṇa*, *drekkā*, *śakra yava*, *ajamoda*, *tṛti*, *bhārgī* and *viḍaṅga*.

एभिर्दीप्तकरश्च गुल्मशमनः शूलाममुत्पाचनः ।
श्लेष्मघ्नो रुचिकारको ज्वरहरः कृष्णादि रुक्तो गणः' ॥२७॥ [11]

Drugs of this group stimulate the power of digestion. They cure *gulma* (phantom tumour) and *śūla* (colic pain). They help in the *pācana* (metabolic transformation) of *āma*. They alleviate *kapha*, produce appetite and cure *jvara* (fever).

११. 'एलातगरकुष्ठमांसीध्यामकत्वक्पत्रनागपुष्पप्रियङ्गुहरेणुकाव्याघ्रनखशुक्तिचण्डास्थौणेयकश्रीवेष्टकचोचचोरकवालुकगुग्गुलुसर्जरसतुरुष्ककुन्दुरुकागुरुस्पृक्कोशीरभद्रदारुकुंकुमानि पुन्नागकेशरं चेति ॥ २८ ॥

(11) *Elādi gaṇa*

This group consists of *elā*, *tagara*, *kuṣṭha*, *māṁsī*, *dhyāmaka*, *tvak*, *patra*, *nāga puṣpa*, *priyaṅgu*, *hareṇukā*, *vyāghra nakha*, *śukti*, *caṇḍā*, *sthauṇeyaka*, *śrīveṣṭaka*, *coca*, *coraka*, *vāluka*, *guggulu*, *sarja rasa*, *turuṣka*, *kunduruka*, *aguru*, *spṛkkā*, *uśīra*, *bhadra dāru*, *kuṁkuma* and *punnāga keśara*.

एलादिको वातकफौ निहन्याद्विषमेव च ।
वर्णप्रसादनः कण्डूपिडकाकोठनाशनः ॥ २९ ॥

Drugs of this group alleviate *vāyu* and *kapha*, cure *viṣa* (poisoning) and promote complexion. They also cure *kaṇḍū* (itching), *piḍakā* (pimples) and *koṭha* (urticarial rashes).

१२. वचातिविषजीमूतजपादारुसनागरैः ।
१३. हरिद्रे कलशीयष्टि तथा कुटजबीजकैः ॥ ३० ॥

(12) (13) *Vacādi* **and** *Haridrādi gaṇa*

*Vacādi gaṇa* consists of *vacā*. *ativiṣa*, *jīmūta*, *japā*, *dāru* and *śuṇṭhī*.

*Haridrādi gaṇa* consists of *haridrā*, *dāru haridrā*, *kalaśī*, *yaṣṭi* and the seed of *kuṭaja*.

एतौ वचाहरिद्रादिगणौ स्तन्यविशोधनौ ।
आमातिसारशमनौ विशेषाद्दोषपाचनौ ॥ ३१ ॥'

[सुश्रुतः सूत्र ३८ : २४-२८]

Drugs belonging of both these groups help in the purification of the milk and alleviate *āma* as well as *atisāra* (diarrhoea). They specially help in the *pācana* (metabolic transformation) of *doṣas*.

१४. 'काकोलीक्षीरकाकोलीजीवकर्षभकमुद्गपर्णीमाषपर्णीमेदामहामेदाछिन्नरुहाकर्कटशृङ्गीतुगाक्षीरीपद्मकप्रपौण्डरीकऋद्धिवृद्धिमृद्वीकाजीवन्त्यो मधुकं चेति ॥ ३२ ॥

### (14) *Kākolyādi gaṇa*

The group consists of *kākolī*, *kṣīra kākolī*, *jīvaka*, *ṛṣabhaka*, *mudgaparṇī*, *māṣaparṇī*, *medā*, *mahā medā*, *chinnaruhā*, *karkaṭa śṛṅgī*, *tugāksīrī*, *padmaka*, *prapauṇḍarika*, *ṛddhi*, *vṛddhi*, *mṛdvīkā*, *jīvantī* and *madhuka*.

काकोल्यादिरयं पित्तशोणितानिलनाशनः ।
जीवनो बृंहणो वृष्यः स्तन्यश्लेष्मकरस्तथा ॥३३॥

Drugs belonging to this group alleviate *pitta*, blood and *vāyu*. They are vitalizing, nourishing and aphrodisiac. They produce more of milk and *kapha*.

१५. ऊषकसैन्धवशिलाजतुगुग्गुलुकासीसद्वयहिंगूतुत्थकं चेति ॥ ३४ ॥

### (15) *Ūṣakādi gaṇa*

This group consists of *ūṣaka*, *saindhava*, *śilājatu*, *guggulu*, both the types of *kāsīsa*, *hiṅgu* and *tutthaka*.

ऊषकादि कफं हन्ति गणो मेदोविशोषणः ।
अश्मरीशर्करामूत्रकृच्छ्रशूलकगुल्मनुत् ॥ ३५ ॥

Drugs belonging to this group alleviate *kapha* and help in the depletion of fat. They cure *aśmarī* (stone in urinary tract), *śarkarā* (gravels in the urinary tract), *mūtra kṛcchra* (dysuria), *śūlā* (colic pain) and *gulma* (phantom tumour).

१६. सारिवामधुकचन्दनकुचन्दनपद्मककाश्मरीफलमधूकपुष्पाण्युशीरं चेति ॥ ३६ ॥

### (16) *Sārivādi gaṇa*

This group consists of *sārivā*, *madhuka*, *candana*, *kucandana*, *padmaka*, *kāśmarī phala*, *madhuka puṣpa* and *uśīra*.

सारिवादिः पिपासाघ्नो रक्तपित्तहरो गणः ।
पित्तज्वरप्रशमनो विशेषात् दाहनाशनः ॥ ३७ ॥

Drugs belonging to this group cure *pipāsā* (morbid thirst), *rakta pitta* (a disease characterised by bleeding from different parts of the body) and *pitta jvara* (fever caused by *pitta*). They specifically cure *dāha* (burning syndrome).

१७. अञ्जनरसाञ्जननागपुष्पप्रियङ्गुनीलोत्पलनलदनलिनकेशराणि मधुकं चेति ॥ ३८ ॥

(17) *Añjanādi gaṇa*

This group consists of *añjana*, *rasāñjana*, *nāga puṣpa*, *priyaṅgu*, *nīlotpala*, *nalada*, *nalina*, *kesara* and *madhuka*.

अञ्जनादिर्गणो ह्येष रक्तपित्तनिवर्हणः ।
विषोपशमनं दाहं निहन्त्याभ्यन्तरं भृशम् ॥ ३९ ॥

Drugs belonging to this group cure *rakta pitta* (a disease characterised by bleeding from different parts of the body). They cure *viṣa* (poisoning), and acute form of *ābhyantara dāha* (burning sensation inside the body).

१८. परूषकद्राक्षाकट्फलदाडिमराजादनकतकफलशाकफलानि त्रिफला चेति ॥ ४० ॥

(18) *Parūṣakādi gaṇa*

This group consists of *parūṣaka*, *drākṣā*, *kaṭphala* *dāḍima*, *rājādana*, *kataka phala*, *śāka phala* and *triphalā*.

परूषकादिरित्येष गणोऽनिलविनाशनः ।
12
मूत्रदोषहरो हृद्यः पिपासाघ्नो रुचिप्रदः ॥ ४१ ॥'

[सुश्रुतः सूत्र ३८ : ३५-४४]

Drugs belonging to this group alleviate *vāyu* and cure *mūtra doṣa* (urinary disorders). They are cardiac tonic. They cure *pipāsā* (morbid thirst) and produce appetite.

१९. 'बृहतीकण्टकारिकाकुटजफलपाठामधुकं चेति ॥ ४२ ॥

### (19) *Bṛhatyādi gaṇa*

This group consists of *bṛhatī, kaṇṭakārikā, kuṭaja phala, pāṭhā* and *madhuka*.

पाचनीयो बृहत्यादिर्गणः पित्तानिलापहः ।
कफारोचकहृद्रोगमूत्रकृच्छ्ररुजापहः ॥' ४३ ॥
[सुश्रुतः सूत्र ३८ : ३१-३२]

Drugs belonging to this group are carminative. They alleviate *pitta, vāyu* and *kapha*. They cure *arocaka* (anorexia), *hṛdroga* (heart disease) and *mūtra kṛcchra* (dysuria).

**आरोग्यचिन्तामणितः**

२०. 'गुडूची निम्बधान्यकं पद्मकं रक्तचन्दनम् ।

### (20) *Guḍūcyādi gaṇa*

**According to *Ārogya cintāmaṇi***

This group consists of *guḍūcī, nimba, dhānyaka, padmaka* and *rakta candana*.

तृष्णादाहारुचिच्छर्दि पिपासा [?] ज्वरनाशनः ।
13
गुडूच्यादिर्गणो ह्येष दीपनः प्राह सुश्रुतः ॥ ४४ ॥'

According to ***Suśruta*** drugs belonging to this group cure *tṛṣṇā* (morbid thirst), *dāha* (burning syndrome), *aruci* (anorexia), *chardi* (vomiting) and *jvara* (fever). They also stimulate the power of digestion.

२१. वत्सकातिविषामूर्वाभार्ग्येला कटुकोषणैः ।
वचाश्योनाक चोग्रा च पञ्चकोलाजमोदकैः ।
वेल्लाजगन्धासिद्धार्थजीरकद्वयहिङ्गुभिः ॥ ४५ ॥

### (21) *Vatsakādi gaṇa*

This group includes *vatsaka, ativiṣā, mūrvā, bhārgī, elā,*

*kaṭukā, uṣaṇa, vacā, śyonāka, ugrā, pañca kola, ajamodā, vella, ajagandhā, siddhārtha,* both the types *jīraka* and *hiṅgu.*

वत्सकाद्यो मरुत्श्लेष्मगुल्मार्शोज्वरशूलनुत् ।

Drugs belonging to this group alleviate *vāyu* and *kapha,* and cure *gulma* (phantom tumour), *arśas* (piles), *jvara* (fever) and *śūla* (colic pain).

२२. 'मुस्तापाठानिशेतिक्तावचैलारुग्विषाचरा: ॥ ४६ ॥

चापेला वाथ शार्ङ्गीष्ठा गणो मुस्तादिको स्मृत: ।

(22) *Mustādi gaṇa*

The group consists of *mustā, pāṭhā,* both the types of *niśā, tiktā, vacā, elā, ruk, viṣā, cara, āp, elā* and *śārṅgiṣṭhā.*

शोधन: पाचन: स्तन्य: स्तनरोगज्वरापह:[14] ॥ ४७ ॥

Drugs belonging to this group help in cleansing (*śodhana*). They are carminative and galactogogue. They cure *stana roga* (diseases of the breast) and *jvara* (fever),

२३. 'उत्पलं कुमुदं पद्मं कल्हारं लोहितोत्पलम् ।

मधुकं चेति पित्तासृक्विषच्छर्दिदाहरोगण:[15] ॥ ४८ ॥'

(23) *Utpalādi gaṇa*

This group consists of *utpala, kumuda, padma. kalhāra* red variety of *utpala* and *madhuka.*

Drugs belonging to this group alleviate *pitta* and blood and cure *viṣa* (poisoning) and *chardi* (vomiting).

२४. 'हरीतकी चामलकं विभीतकं फलत्रयम् ।

त्रिफला फलमित्युक्त सैव ज्ञेयं फलत्रिकम् ॥ ४९ ॥

एकभागो हरीतक्यात् द्विगुणश्च विभीतक: ।

चतुर्गुणा चामलकी त्रिफलेयं प्रकीर्तिता[16] ॥ ५० ॥'

(24) *Triphalā*

Fruits of three drugs viz., *harītakī*, *āmalakī* and *vibhītakī* taken together are called *triphalā* or *phala trika*. For this purpose, one part of *harītakī*, two parts of *vibhītaka* and four parts of *āmalakī* should be taken.

'त्रिफला कफपित्तघ्नी मेहकुष्ठहरी सरा ।
चक्षुष्या दीपनी चैव विषमज्वरनाशिनी ॥ ५१ ॥'

[सुश्रुत : सूत्र ३८ : ५७]

*Triphalā* alleviates *kapha* as well as *pitta* and cures ***meha*** (obstinate urinary disorders including diabetes) as well as ***kuṣṭha*** (obstinate skin diseases including leprosy). It is laxative, promoter of eye sight and digestive stimulant. It cures *viṣama jvara* (irregular fever).

द्राक्षाखर्जूरकाश्मर्यफलानीति **फलत्रिकम्** ।
इयं प्रोक्ता द्वितीया च त्रिफला चरकादिभिः ॥५२॥
रक्तपित्तादिदोषेषु त्रिफलेयं मता सदा ।

According to some, the fruits of *drākṣā*, *kharjūra* and *kāśmarya* taken together are also called *phala trika*. This second variety of *triphalā* is described by Caraka etc.,. This type of *triphalā* is useful in the treatment of diseases like *rakta pitta* (a disease characterised by bleeding from different parts of the body).

17

२५. 'पिप्पली मरिचं शुंठी त्रयमेतच्च मिश्रितम् ॥ ५३ ॥'
'**त्र्यूषणं** कफमेदोघ्नं मेहकुष्टत्वगामयान् ।
निहन्याद्दीपनं गुल्मपीनसाग्न्यल्पतामपि ॥ ५४ ॥'

[सुश्रुत : सूत्र ३८ : ५६]

(25) *Tryūṣaṇa*

*Pippalī*, *marica* and *śuṇṭhī*—these three drugs mixed together are called *tryūṣaṇa*. It reduces *kapha* and *medas* and cures *meha* (obstinate urinary diseases including diabetes), *kuṣṭha* (obstinate skin diseases including leprosy) and *tvagāmaya* (skin diseases). It is digestive stimulant. It also cures *gulma* (phantom tumour), *pīnasa* (chronic rhinitis) and *mandāgni* (suppression of the power of digestion).

२६. नागरातिविषामुस्तं त्रयमेतत्त्रिकर्षितम् ।
कफपित्तानिलहरं ज्वरघ्नं ग्राहि दीपनम् ॥ ५५ ॥

(26) *Tri karṣita*

*Nāgara*, *ativiṣā* and *musta* – these three drugs taken together are called *tri karṣita*. It alleviates *kapha*, *pitta* and *vāyu* and cures *jvara* (fever). It is constipative and digestive stimulant.

२७. 'आमलक्यभयाकृष्णाचित्रकश्चेत्ययं गणः ।

(27) *Āmalakyādi gaṇa*

This group consists of *āmalakī*, *abhayā*, *kṛṣṇā* and *citraka*.

18

ज्वरघ्नश्चाक्षुषो वृष्यो भेदी चाग्निप्रदीपनः ॥५६॥

Drugs belonging to this group cure *jvara* (fever). They are promoter of eye sight, aphrodisiac, purgative and digestive stimulant.

२८. 'त्रपुसीसताम्ररजतकृष्णलोहसुवर्णानि लोहमलम् ॥५७॥

(28) *Trapvādi gaṇa*

This group consists of *trapu*, *sīsa*, *tāmra*, *rajata*, *kṛṣṇa loha*, *svarṇa* and *loha mala*.

गणस्त्रप्वादिरित्येष रक्तकृमिहरः परः ।
पिपासाविषहृद्रोगपाण्डुमेहहरस्तथा ॥ ५८ ॥

Drugs belonging to this group cure vitiation of blood, *kṛmi* (parasitic infection), *pipāsā* (morbid thirst), *viṣa* (poisoning), *hṛdroga* (heart disease), *pāṇḍu* (anemia) and *meha* (obstinate urinary disorders including diabetes).

२९. लाक्षारेवतकुटजाश्वमारकट्फलहरिद्राद्वयनिम्बसप्तच्छ-
दमालत्यस्त्रायमाणा चेति ॥ ५९ ॥

(29) *Lākṣādi gaṇa*

This group consists of *lākṣā*, *ārevata*, *kuṭaja*, *aśvamāra*, *kaṭphala*, both the types of *haridrā*, *nimba*, *saptacchada*, *mālatī* and *trāyamāṇā*.

कषायतिक्तमधुरः कफपित्तार्तिनाशनः ।
कुष्ठक्रिमिहरश्चैव दुष्टव्रणविशोधनः ॥ ६० ॥'

[सुश्रुतः सूत्र ३८ : ६२-६५]

Drugs belonging to this group are astringent, bitter and sweet. They alleviate vitiation of *kapha* and *pitta*. They cure *kuṣṭha* (obstinate skin diseases including leprosy) and *kṛmi* (parasitic infection). They help in the cleansing of *duṣṭa vraṇa* (suppurated ulcer).

**पंचकान्वक्ष्यामः**

३०. 'पृश्निपर्णी शालिपर्णी बृहतीद्वयगोक्षुरैः ।
बृंहणं वातपित्तघ्नं **कनीयः पञ्चमूलकम्** ॥
कषायतिक्तमधुरं सन्निपातशिरोर्तिनुत् ॥ ६१ ॥

(30) *Kṣudra pañcamūla*

**Groups having five ingredients**

*Pṛśni parṇī*, *śāla parṇī*, both the varieties of *bṛhatī* and *gokṣura*—all these drugs taken together are called *kanīyas pañca mūla*. It is nourishing, alleviator of *vāyu* and *pitta* and astringent, bitter as well as sweet in taste. It cures diseases caused by the simultaneous vitiation of all the three *doṣas* (*sannipāta*) and *śirorti* (headache).

३१. बिल्वोऽग्निमन्थः श्योनाकः काश्मरी पाटला महत ।

दीपनं कफवातघ्नं **पञ्चमूलमिदं महत्** ॥ ६२ ॥

(31) *Mahat pañca mūla*

*Bilva, agnimantha, śyonāka, kāśmarī* and *pāṭalā*—these five drugs taken together, constitute *mahat pañca mūla*. It stimulates digestion and alleviates *kapha* as well as *vāyu*,

प्रायस्त्रिदोषशमनं पवनामयेषु,

श्लेष्मोल्वणेषु च गदेषु भिषग्भिरुक्तम् ।

कासेसु सन्निपतितेषु शिरोरुजायां,

19

श्वासेषु हिक्केषु हितं **दशमूलमेतत्** ॥ ६३ ॥'

*Daśa mūla*

Drugs of both *kṣudra pañca mūla* and *mahat pañca mūla* groups, taken together, constitute *daśa mūla*. It generally alleviates all the three *doṣas* and is effective specially when *vāyu* and *kapha* are aggravated in excess. It is also useful in *kāsa* (bronchitis) caused by the simultaneous aggravation of all the three *doṣas*, *śiroruk* (headache), *śvāsa* (asthma) and *kikkā* (hiccup).

३२. 'विदारी सारिवा छागशृंगी वत्सादनी निशा ।

वृष्यं पित्तानिलं हन्याद्वल्लिजं **पञ्चमूलकम** ॥६४॥

(32) *Vallija pañca mūla*

*Vidārī, sārivā, chāga śṛṅgī, vatsādanī* and *niśā*—these five drugs taken together are called *vallija pañca mūla*.

It is aphrodisiac and it alleviates *pitta* as well as *vāyu*.

३३. करमर्दकसैरीयत्रिकंटकशतावरी ।

तथा गृध्रनखी चेति **पञ्चकंटकसंज्ञकः** ॥ ६५ ॥

रक्तपित्तहरो ह्येष शोफरोगविनाशनः ।

शुक्रमेहहरश्चैव शुक्रदोषहरः परः ॥ ६६ ॥

### (33) *Pañca kaṇṭaka*

*Kara mardaka*, *sairīya*, *tri kaṇṭaka*, *śatāvarī* and *gṛdhra nakhī*—these five drugs taken together are called *pañca kaṇṭaka*. It cures *rakta pitta* (a diseases characterised by bleeding from different parts of the body), *śopha* (oedema), *śukra meha* (spermaturia) and *śukra doṣa* (vitiation of semen).

३४. कुशः काशो नलो दर्भः कांडेक्षुरिति तद्विदः ।

तृणपञ्चमूलं ज्ञेयं दाहप्रशमने हितम् ॥

20

पित्तमूत्रविषार्तानां प्रशस्तं वस्तिशोधनम् ॥ ६७ ॥'

### (34) *Tṛṇa pañca mūla*

*Kuśa*, *kāśa*, *nala*, *darbha* and *kāṇḍekṣu*—the roots of these five drugs taken together are called *tṛṇa pañca mūla*. It is useful in the treatment of *dāha* (burning syndrome), vitiation of *pitta* as well as urine and *viṣa* (poisoning). It cleanses the urinary bladder.

३५. कदम्बवाजिकर्णश्च करंजः क्षवको गुडः ।

वर्गोऽयं कफपाण्डुत्वक्कुष्ठमेहविषापहः ॥ ६८ ॥

### (35) *Kadambādi gaṇa*

The group consists of *kadamba*, *vāji karṇa*, *karañja*, *kṣavaka* and *guḍa*. They cure vitiated *kapha*, *pāṇḍu* (anemia), *tvak roga* (ordinary skin diseases), *kuṣṭha* (obstinate skin diseases including leprosy), *meha* (obstinate urinary disorders including diabetes) and *viṣa* (poisoning).

३६. करंजो वत्ससैरीयसुषवीसप्तपर्णकाः ।

मेहकुष्ठज्वरच्छर्दिविषश्लेष्महरोगणः ॥ ६९ ॥

### (36) *Karañjādi gaṇa*

This group consists of *karañja*, *vatsa*, *sairīya*, *suṣavī* and *sapta parṇa*. They cure *meha* (obstinate urinary disorders including diabetes), *kuṣṭha* (obstinate skin diseases including leprosy), *jvara* (fever), *chardi* (vomiting), *viṣa* (poisoning) and vitiation of *kapha*.

३७. पिप्पलीपिप्पलीमूलचव्यचित्रकनागरैः ।
**दीपनीयः** स्मृतो वर्गः कफानिलगदापहः ॥ ७० ॥

[पञ्चकोलम्]

### (37) *Pañca kola*

This group consists of *pippalī*, *pippalī mūla*, *cavya*, *citraka* and *nāgara*. They stimulate the power of digestion and cure diseases caused by *kapha* and *vāyu*.

समासेन गणाह्येते प्रोक्तास्तेषां च विस्तरम् ।
चिकित्सितेषु वक्ष्यामि ज्ञात्वा दोषबलाबलम् ॥७१॥

In brief these are the various groups of drugs. Keeping in view the strength and otherwise of the *doṣas*, their details will be described in the section dealing with the treatment of diseases.

॥ इति सप्तत्रिंशद्गणोद्देशः सुश्रुतात् ॥

Thus ends the 37 groups of drugs as described in *Suśruta*.

शणमूलकशिग्रूणि फलानि तिलसर्षपाः ।
सक्तवः किण्वमतसी द्रव्याण्युक्तानि **पाचनं** ॥ ७२ ॥

### *Pācana gaṇa*

The fruits of *śaṇa*, *mūlaka* and *śigru*, *tila*, *sarṣapa*, *saktu*, *kiṇva* and *atasī*—these drugs help in suppuration (*pācana*).

चिरबिल्वोऽग्निको दन्ती चित्रको हयमारकः ।
कपोतकंकगृध्राणां पुरीषाणि च **दारणम्** ॥ ७३ ॥

*Dāraṇa gaṇa*

*Cirabilva, agnika, dantī, citraka, haya māraka* and the stool of *kapota, kaṅka* and *gṛdhra*—these drugs help in the incission of the abscess.

द्रव्याणां पिच्छिलानां च त्वग्मूलानि **प्रपीडनं**।
यवगोधूममाषाणां चूर्णानि च समासतः ॥ ७४ ॥

*Prapīḍāna gaṇa*

The bark and root of drugs which are slimy and the powder of *yava, godhūma* and *māṣa* help in *prapīḍana* (which takes out pus by exerting pressure).

शंखिनी कोद सुमनः करवीर सुवर्चला ।
**शोधनानि** कषायाणि वर्गश्चारग्वधादिकः ॥ ७५ ॥

*Śodhana kaṣāya*

*Śaṅkhinī, koda, sumanas, karavīra suvarcalā* and drugs belonging to *āragvadhādi* group—their decoctions help in the cleansing of wounds.

अजगन्धा च शृङ्गी च गवाक्षी लांगलाह्वया ।
पूतीकचित्रकपाठाविडङ्गैलाहरेणवः ॥ ७६ ॥
कटुत्रयं यवक्षारो लवणानि मनःशिला ।
21
कासीसं त्रिफला दन्ती हरितालं सुराष्ट्रजा ॥ ७७ ॥
संशोधनीनां **वर्तीनां** द्रव्याणि तानि निर्दिशेत् ।

*Saṁśodhana varti*

*Ajagandhā, śṛṅgī, gavakṣī, lāṅgala, pūtīka, citraka, pāṭhā, viḍaṅga, elā, hareṇu, trikaṭu, yava kṣāra,* various types of salt, *manaḥśila, kāsiśa, triphalā, dantī, haritāla* and *suraṣṭrajā*—these are the ingredients of the potion of suppository for cleansing of wounds.

एतैरप्यौषधैः कुर्यात्कल्पनापि च शोधने ॥ ७८ ॥

These drugs can also be used through different other pharmaceutical processes for the cleansing of wounds.

गोमूत्रं गोमयं क्षीरं दधि सर्पिस्तथैव च ।

समं संयोजितं ज्ञेयं पञ्चगव्यमिदं बुधैः ॥ ७९ ॥

*Pañca gavya*

The urine, dung, milk, curd and ghee of cow taken together (in equal quantity ?) is called *pañca gavya.*

एवं संयोजयेत्प्राज्ञो पञ्चाजं पञ्चमाहिषम् ।

If these are collected from goat (*ajā*) then the collective term used for them is *pañcāja* and if collected from buffalo (*mahiṣa*) then they are called *pañca māhiṣa.*

कासीसकटुरोहिण्याः जातीकन्दहरिद्रयोः ॥ ८० ॥

पूर्वोद्दिष्टे तु पञ्चाङ्गे कुर्यात्तैलघृतानि वै ।

**Medicated oil & Ghee**

Medicated oil and ghee should be prepared of either *pañca gavya* or *pañcāja* or *pañca māhiṣa* by adding *kāsīsa*, *katu rohiṇī*, root of *jāti* and *haridrā*.

अर्कोत्तमास्नुहीक्षीरं पिष्ट्वा क्षारोत्तमान्यपि ॥८१॥

जातीमूलंहरिद्रे द्वे कासीसं कटुरोहिणी ।

पूर्वोद्दिष्टानि चांगानि कुर्यात् संशोधनं घृतम् ॥८२॥

*Saṁśodhana ghṛta*

The best variety of *arka* should be made to a paste by adding the latex of *snuhī.* To this, the best of alkalies and the root of *jātī*, both the varieties of *haridrā*, *kāsīsa*, *kaṭu rohinī* and *pañca gavya* or *pañcāja* or *pañca māhiṣa* should be added. With these drugs the medicated ghee which is useful in cleansing of ulcers should be prepared.

मयूरको राजवृक्षो निंबकोशातकी तिलाः ।

बृहत्यौ च शिलाले च शोधनानि च शोधने ॥ ८३ ॥

*Śodhana taila*

The medicated oil which is prepared of *mayūraka*, *rāja-vṛkṣa*, *nimba*, *kośātakī*, *tila*, both the types of *bṛhatī*, *śilā* and *āla* is useful for cleansing of ulcers.

तैले द्रव्याणि योज्यानि शेषाणि च तथा शृणु ।

कासीसं सैन्धवं किण्वं वचा च रजनीद्वयम् ।

संशोधनेषु चान्येषु **चूर्णं** कुर्वीत **शोधनम्** ॥ ८४ ॥

*Śodhana cūrṇa*

The potion prepared by adding powders of *kāsīsa*, *saindhava*, *kiṇva*, *vacā* and both the varieties of *rajanī* is useful for cleansing ulcers.

सालसारादि सारेषु पटोली त्रिफलासु च ।

**रसक्रिया** विधातव्या शोधनं शोधनेषु च ॥ ८५ ॥

*Śodhana rasakriyā*

The *rasakriyā* prepared of the drugs belonging to *sāla-sārādi* group, *paṭolī* and *triphalā* is useful for cleansing ulcers.

कषायाणामनुष्णातिरूक्षाणां[22] त्वक्षु[23] साधितम् ।

श्रृतशीतं कषायं तु **रोपणार्थं** प्रशस्यते ॥ ८६ ॥

*Ropaṇa kaṣāya*

The boiled and cooled decoction of astringent barks

which are not very hot in potency and which are exceedingly unctuous is useful for healing ulcers.

सोमामृताश्वगन्धा च काकोल्यादौ गणे तथा ।
क्षीरिप्ररोहेष्वपि च **वर्तयो रोपणाः** स्मृताः ॥ ८७ ॥

*Ropaṇa varti*

The suppository prepared of *soma*, *amṛtā*, *aśva gandhā*, drugs belonging to *kākolyādi* group, *praroha* (adventitious root) of *kṣiri vṛkṣas* helps in the healing of ulcers.

समंगा सोमसरला सोमवल्का सचन्दना ।
काकोल्यादिश्च **कल्कः** स्यात्प्रशस्तो **व्रणरोपणे** ॥८८॥

*Ropaṇa kalka*

The paste prepared of *samaṅgā*, *soma*, *saralā*, *soma valkā*, *candana* and the drugs belonging to the *kākolyādi* group is useful in the healing of ulcers.

पृथक्पर्ण्यात्मगुप्ता च हरिद्रे मालती सिता ।
काकोल्यादिश्च योज्यः स्याद्भिषजा **रोपणे घृते** ॥८९॥

*Ropaṇa ghṛta*

The medicated ghee for healing of ulcers is prepared of *pṛthak parṇī*, *ātma guptā*, both the varieties of *haridrā*, *mālatī*, *sitā* and drugs belonging to *kākolyādi* group.

कालानुसार्यगुरुणि हरिद्रे भद्रदारु च ।
प्रियङ्गवश्च लोध्रं च **तैले** योज्यानि **रोपणे** ॥ ९० ॥

*Ropaṇa taila*

The medicated oil for healing of ulcers is prepared of *kālānusārī*, *aguru*, both the types of *haridrā*, *bhadra dāru*, *priyaṅgu* and *lodhra*.

किंशुका त्रिफला लोध्रं कासीसं श्रवणाह्वया ।

धवाश्वकर्णयोस्त्वक्च रोपणं चूर्णमिष्यते ।

रसक्रिया रोपणार्थे विदधीत यथाक्रमम् ॥ ६१ ॥

*Ropaṇa cūrṇa & Rasa kriyā*

The powder of *kiṁśukā*, *triphalā*, *lodhra*, *kāsīsa*, *śravaṇā* and the bark of *dhava* as well as *aśva karṇa* is useful in the healing of ulcers. *Rasa kriyā* of these drugs also helps in the healing of ulcers.

अपामार्गाश्वगन्धा च तालपत्री सुवर्चला ।

उत्सादने प्रशस्यन्ते काकोल्यादिश्च यो गणः ॥६२॥

*Utsādana*

*Apāmārga*, *aśva gandhā*, *tāla patrī*, *suvarcalā* and drugs of *kākolyādi gaṇa* help in the filling up of ulcers by granulation tissue.

कासीसं सैंधवं किष्कं [?] कुरुविन्दो मनःशिला ।

कुक्कुटाण्डकपालानि सुमनो मुकुलानि च ॥ ६३ ॥

फले सैरीषकारंजे धातुचूर्णानि यानि च ।

व्रणेषूत्सन्नमांसेषु प्रशस्तान्यवसादने ॥ ६४ ॥

*Avasādana*

When there is granulation tissue in excess, then to bring it to proper level, drugs like *kāsīsa*, *saindhava*, *kiṣka*, *kuruvinda*, *manaḥśilā*, *kukkuṭāṇḍa kapāla*, buds of *sumana*, fruits of *sirīṣa* and *karañja* and powder of metals are useful.

समस्तवर्गमर्धं वा यथालाभमथापि वा ।

प्रयुञ्जीतभिषक् प्रायो यथोद्दिष्टेषु कर्मसु ॥ ६५ ॥

**Selection of drugs**

The physician should select either the whole group or half of it or whatever is readily available out of these drugs and use them in therapy.

ग्रथ चिकित्साकलिकात:

'वटीवटोदुम्बरवेतसानामश्वत्थवृक्षेण समन्वितानाम् ।
24
त्वक्पंचकं पंचमहीरुहाणामिति व्रणघ्नं श्वयथुघ्नमेतत् ॥' ९६ ॥

॥ इति पञ्चवल्कलम् ॥

**According to *Cikitsā kalikā***

Barks of five trees viz., *vaṭī*, *vaṭa*, *udumbara*, *vetasa* and *aśvattha* cure ulcers and inflammation. These are called *pañca valkala*.

'द्वौ काकोल्यौ जीवकः सार्षभः स्या—
न्मेदायुग्मं सार्द्धि [?] ऋद्धिश्च वृद्ध्या ।

इत्युद्दिष्टैरष्टवर्गः प्रदिष्टः
पित्तघ्नोऽयं गर्भदो बृंहणश्च ॥ ९७ ॥

॥ अष्टवर्गः ॥

*Aṣṭa varga*

Two varieties of *kākolī*, *jīvaka*, *ṛṣabhaka*, both the varieties of *medā*, *ṛddhi* and *vṛddhi*—these eight drugs taken together are called *aṣṭa varga*. It alleviates *pitta*, promotes conception and nourishment.

रसोनकन्दवत्कन्दं निःसारं सूक्ष्मपत्रकम् ।

जीवकर्षभकावेतौ हेमाद्रिशिखरोद्भवौ ॥ ९८ ॥

॥ इत्यष्टवर्गलक्षणम् ॥

**Description**

*Jīvaka* and *ṛṣabhaka* grow in the peaks of the Himalayas.

Its *kanda* (underground stem) is like that of the garlic. Its leaves are thin and fine.

**ग्रन्थान्तरात्**

जीवकः कूर्चकाकारो ऋषभो वृषशृङ्गवत् ।

**According to another text**

*Jivaka* has the shape of a *kūrcaka* (brush). *Ṛṣabhaka* is like the horn of a bull in shape.

श्वेतलोमान्वितं कन्दं लताजातं सरं ध्रुवम् ।

ऋद्धि वृद्धीति विज्ञेया विख्याता कौशयामले ॥९९॥

*Ṛddhi* and *vṛddhi* which are well known in *koṣayāmala* are the roots of creepers. These roots are covered with white hairs. They are certainly laxative.

मूलग्रन्थिसमं ऋद्धिर्वामावर्त्तफला तथा ।

'वृद्धिस्तु दीक्षणावर्त्तफलालक्ष्मकियत्क्तं ॥ १०० ॥

*Ṛddhi* is like a knot in the root and its fruit takes an anti-clock wise turn. On the other hand, *vṛddhi* has fruits which take a clock-wise turn.

25

शुष्कार्द्रकनिभं कंदं स्निग्धं मधुरशीतलं ।"

महामेदेति विख्यातो दुर्गन्धो मेद उच्यते ॥१०१॥

*Mahā medā*, which is a root, looks like a piece of dried ginger. It is unctuous, sweet and cooling. It has a foul smell of fat.

मेदा शुक्ला नखछेद्या मेदोधातुवदादिशेत् ।

*Medā* is white. It can be cut with the help of finger nail. It looks like fat tissue.

पीवरीव[?]निभस्कंदः सक्षीरं ससुगन्धिकम् ॥१०२॥

काकोली क्षीरकाकोली अधोर्ध्वं तं विनिर्दिशेत् ।

*Kākolī* and *kṣīra kākolī* have roots like those of *pīvarī*. They contains milky latex and they are fragrant. The lower part of it is known as *kākolī* where as the upper part is called *kṣīra kākolī*.

26

ईषच्छुक्ला तु काकोली क्षीरवत्पाण्डुराऽपरा ॥१०३॥

॥ इत्यष्टवर्गलक्षणम् ॥

*Kākolī* is slightly white in colour where as *kṣīra kākolī* is yellowish white like milk.

Thus ends the description of drugs belonging the group of *aṣṭavarga*.

ग्रन्थान्तरात्

कुष्ठमांसी हरिद्राभिर्मु राशैलेयचंपकैः ।
वचा कर्पूरमुस्तैश्च सर्वौषधिकमुच्यते ॥ १०४ ॥
भूतप्रेतग्रहहरा ज्वरघ्नी श्रीप्रदायिनी ।
सर्वौषधिस्तु विज्ञेया पामाप्रस्वेदनाशिनी ॥१०५॥

॥ इति सर्वौषधी ॥

*Sarvauṣadhi*

**From another Text**

*Kuṣṭha*, *māṁsī*, *haridrā*, *murā*, *saileya*, *campaka*, *vacā*, *karpūra* and *mustā*—these drugs taken together are called *sarvauṣadhi*. It alleviates the afflictions of *bhūta* (evil spirits), *pretas* and *graha*. It cures *jvara* (fever). It endows the person with auspiciousness. It also cures *pāmā* (eczema) and *prasveda* (excessive sweating).

सर्वौषधिक संमिश्रा संशुष्कामलकत्वचा ।

**सुगन्धामलकानीति** पित्तकृद्रुग्जयेत्तथा ॥ १०६ ॥

॥ इति सुगन्धामलकम् ॥

*Sugandhāmalaka*

If the fruit pulp of *āmalakī* is added to the group of drugs called *sarvauṣadhi* then it is called *sugandhāmalaka*. It cures diseases caused by the vitiation of *pitta*.

**धूर्जटितः**

शालूकतुत्थश्रीपुष्पैस्त्रि**सुगन्धि**भवेत्तथा ।

शालूकपत्री संयुक्तं **चातुर्जातक**मीरितम् ॥ १०७ ॥

कफपित्तास्यगन्धघ्नं सूदविज्ञैः प्रपूजितम् ।

*Tri sugandhi & Cātur jātaka*

**According to** *Dhūrjaṭi*

*Śāluka, tuttha* and *śrī puṣpa*—these three drugs taken together are called *tri sugandhi*. If *śāluka patrī* is added to it then it is called *cātur jātaka*. It alleviates *kapha* as well as *pitta* and removes foul smell of mouth. It is highly praised by persons who are well versed in the science of cooking.

**अन्यच्च**

त्वगेलापत्रकैस्तुल्यं त्रिसुगन्धि त्रिजातकम् ॥ १०८ ॥

नागकेशरसंयुक्तं चातुर्जातकमीरितम् ।

हृल्लासविषदुर्गन्धिवातश्लेष्महरे मते ॥ १०९ ॥

॥ इति त्रिसुगन्धिचातुर्जातके ॥

**Another view**

*Tvak, elā* and *patra*—these three drugs taken in equal quantity are called *tri sugandhi* or *tri jātaka*. If *nāga keśara* is added to it, then it is called *cātur jātaka*. Both of them cure *hṛllāsa* (nausea), *viṣa* (poisoning), *durgandhi* (foul smell) and vitiation of *vāyu* and *kapha*.

कंकोलकं पूगफलं लवङ्गकुसुमानि च ।
जातिफलानि कर्चूरमेतत्पञ्चसुगन्धिकम् ॥ ११० ॥

[योगरत्नाकरः पृष्ठ ६९]

*Pañca sugandhi*

*Kaṅkola*, *pūga phala*, *lavaṅga*, *jāti phala* and *karcūra*—these five drugs taken together are called *pañca sugandhika*.

चन्दनं कुंकुमं तुल्ये वरार्धमभिधीयते ।
त्रिभागं कुंकुमं यत्र तदुक्तं चाद्यपुष्पकम् ॥ १११ ॥

*Varārdha & Ādya puṣpaka*

*Candana* and *kuṁkuma* taken together in equal quantity are called *varārdha*. If three parts of *kuṁkuma* is added then it is called *ādya puṣpaka*.

कुंकुमागुरुकर्पूरकस्तूरीचन्दनानि च ।
महासुगन्धिमित्युक्तं नामतो यक्षकर्दमम् ॥ ११२ ॥

[योगरत्नाकरः पृष्ठ ६९]

*Mahā sugandhi*

*Kuṁkuma*, *aguru*, *karpūra*, *kastūrī* and *candana*—these drugs taken together are called *mahā sugandhi* and named as *yakṣa kardama*.

द्राक्षादाडिमखर्जूरमृदितं स्यात्सशर्करम् ।
27
लाजाचूर्णं समध्वाज्य सतर्पणमुदाहृतम् ॥ ११३ ॥

[योगरत्नाकरः पृष्ठ ६८]

*Saṁtarpaṇa*

The potion prepared of *drākṣā*, *dāḍima* and *kharjūra* mixed with sugar and powder of *lājā* along with honey and ghee is called *saṁtarpaṇa* or refreshing drink.

**अथ षड्रसानि द्रव्याण्युपदेक्ष्यामः**

घृतक्षीरवसामज्जा शालिगोधूमषष्टिकाः ।
कशेरुकं च शृङ्गाट गिलोड्यर्वारुमूत्रलाः ॥ ११४ ॥
काकोल्यादिर्गणोऽलाबुकालकं कतकाश्मरी ।
भक्षखर्जूरकद्राक्षापद्मकर्कटिका तथा ॥ ११५ ॥
मधूकेक्षुविकाराणि राजादनबलात्रयम् ।
पयस्विनी तालजया पयस्या गोक्षुरस्तथा ॥ ११६ ॥
कूष्मांडं कदलीमांसं मौक्तिकं क्षीरमोरटः ।
प्रियालमज्जावातामैर्वर्गोऽयं **मधुरो** मतः ॥ ११७ ॥
जया कपिकच्छू ।

**Classification of drugs according to their taste**

**Group of Sweet Drugs**

Ghee, milk, muscle fat, marrow, *śāli*, *godhūma*, *ṣaṣṭika*, *kaśeruka*, *śṛṅgāṭa*, *gilodya*, *ervāru*, *mūtrala* drugs, drugs belonging to *kākolyādi* group, *alābu*, *kālaka*, *kataka*, *kāśmarī*, *bhakṣa*, *kharjūraka*, *drākṣā*, *padma*, *karkaṭikā*, *madhūka*, sugar cane products, *rājādana*, three varieties of *balā*, *payasvinī*, *tāla*, *jayā*, *payasyā*, *gokṣura*, *kūṣmāṇḍa*, *kadalī*, meat, *muktā*, *kṣira moraṭa*, *priyāla majjā* and *vātāma*—these belong to the group of sweet drugs.

*Jayā* is popularly called *kapi kacchū*.

दाडिमं मातुलुंगं च प्रार्चानामलकं तथा ।
दधित्थामलकं चिंचा नीपकोशाम्रनिंबुकम् ॥ ११८ ॥
भव्यपालेवतं कोललकुचं वेत्रजं फलम् ।
बदरं चाथ जंबीरं करुणं चाम्लवेतसम् ॥ ११९ ॥
रजताम्रातकं चैव चणकाम्लं सकांजिकम् ।

चांगेरीतक्रदध्यम्लं सुरासौवीरशुक्तकम् ॥ १२० ॥

तुषोदकं च धान्याम्लं प्रभृतिश्**चाम्लवर्गकः** ।

**Group of sour drugs**

*Dāḍima, mātuluṅga, prācīnāmalaka, dadhittha, āmalaka, ciñcā, nīpa, kośāmra, nimbuka, bhavya, pālevata, kola, lakuca,* fruit of *vetra, badara, jambīra, karuṇa, amla vetasa, rajata, āmrātaka, caṇakāmla, kāñjika, cāṅgerī, takra, dadhyamla, surā, sauvīra. śuktaka, tuṣodaka, dhānyāmla* etc., belong to the group of sour drugs.

सैन्धवाक्षविडंपांक्यं रोमकं सागरोद्भवम् ॥ १२१ ॥

यवक्षारो खप्रसूतं स्वर्जिका नवसारकः ।

एवं **लवणवर्गः** स्यात्,

**Group of saline drugs**

*Saindhava, akṣa, viḍa, pākya, romaka, sāmudra, yava kṣāra, kha prasūta, svarjikā* and *navasāraka*—these belong to the group of saline drugs.

कटुवर्गमथो श्रृणु ॥ १२२ ॥

शिग्रुश्च सुरसादिश्च पिप्पल्यादिस्तथागणः ।

व्योषाभयरसोनं च चंडा सुमुखमूलकम् ॥ १२३ ॥

सुराह्वाबल्गुजफलं कालनिर्यासलाङ्गली ।

पीलूकशुकनासाह्वलवगादिभिरुत्तमः ।

28

ज्ञेयः **कटुकवर्गोऽयं** कर्पूरेणसमन्वितः ॥ १२४ ॥

व्योषा शतपुष्पी ।

**Group of pungent drugs**

*Śigru*, drugs of *surasādi* and *pippalyādi* groups, *vyoṣā, āmaya, rasona, caṇḍā, sumukha, mūlaka, surāhvā,* fruit of *abalguja*, extract of *kāla, lāṅgalī, pīluka, śuka nasāhva, lavaṅga* etc.,—these belong to the group of pungent drugs.

*Vyoṣā* is popularly called *śata puṣpī*.

व्याधिघ्नादि गुडूच्यादि माण्डूकी वैजयन्तिका ।
हरिद्राद्वयशक्राह्ववरुणेक्षुरशंखिनी ॥ १२५ ॥
दन्तीद्रवन्ती बृहतीश्यामासप्तच्छदस्तथा ।
व्याघ्री कोशफला तिक्ता कर्कोटी कारवेल्लिका ॥१२६॥
वार्ताकुकारवीगोपाकटभीशशिवाटिका ।
तथा वेत्रकरीराणि सुमना करवीरकौ ॥ १२७ ॥
त्रायमाणा वृश्चिकाली कुमारी पाटिका वृषा ।
शंखपुष्पी मेषशृङ्गी तथा मर्कटपिप्पली ॥ १२८ ॥
स्वादुकंटककस्तूरी बिंबनिर्गुण्डिका तथा ।
द्रव्यैरेवंविधैश्चान्यैस्तिक्तवर्ग उदाहृतः ॥ १२९ ॥
स्वादुकंटको विकंकतवृक्षः । शंखिनी यवतिक्ता ॥१३०॥

**Group of bitter drugs**

Drugs of *vyādhighnādi* and *guḍūcyādi* groups, *māṇḍūkī*, *vaijayantikā*, both the varieties of *haridrā*, *śakrāhva*, *varuṇa*, *ikṣura*, *śaṁkhinī*, *dantī*, *dravantī*, *bṛhatī*, *śyāmā*, *saptacchada*, *vyāghrī*, *kośaphalā*, *tiktā*, *karkoṭī*, *kāravellikā*, *vārtāku*, *kāravī*, *gopā*, *kaṭabhī*, *śaśī*, *vāṭikā*, *vetra*, *karīra*, *sumanā*, *karavīra*, *trāyamāṇā*, *vṛścikālī*, *kumārī*, *paṭikā*, *vṛṣā*, *śaṁkha puṣpī*, *meṣa-śṛṅgī*, *markaṭa*, *pippalī*, *svādu kaṇṭaka*, *kastūrī*, *bimba*, *nirguṇḍi*—these and such other drugs belong to the group of bitter drugs.

*Svādu kaṇṭaka*, is called *vikaṅkata vṛkṣa*. *Śaṅkhinī* is known as *yava tiktā*.

न्यग्रोधादिः प्रियंग्वादिः काककोलादिकस्तथा ।
अम्बष्ठादिश्च त्रिफला जम्बाम्रवकुलोद्भवः ।
स्फूर्जनागवधूशाकवनस्पतिफलानि च ॥ १३१ ॥



"सालसारादिकं चैव कतकस्य फलानि च ॥१३२॥"

झिण्टो सुकुण्डली चिल्ली जीवन्ती सुनिषण्णकः।
कलंवुषा निपालंकीप्रभृतीनि तथैव च ।
मूद्गनीवारकाद्याश्च कषायो वर्गसंज्ञितः ॥ १३३ ॥
काककोलादिकः लोध्रादिकः ॥ कुंडली कांचनारः ॥
स्फूर्जस्तिन्दुकः ॥ नागवधू सल्लकीत्यर्थः ॥ १३४ ॥

**Group of astringent drugs**

Drugs of *nyagrodhādi*, *priyaṅgvādi*, *kākakolādi*, and *ambaṣṭhādi* groups, fruits of *triphalā*, *jambu*, *āmra*, *vakula*, *sphūrja*, *nāga vadhū*, *śāka* and *vanaspati*, drugs of *sālasārādi* group, fruits of *kataka*, *jhinṭa*, *sukuṇḍalī*, *cillī*, *jīvantī*, *suniṣaṇṇaka*, *kalambuṣā*, *nipālaṅkī* etc., *mudga*, *nīvāra* etc.,—these belong to the group of astringent drugs.

*Kākakolādi* group is the same as *lodhrādi* group. *Kuṇḍalī* is called *kāñcanāra*. *Sphūrja* is called *tinduka*. *Nāga vadhu* is known as *sallakī*.

॥ इति षड्रसानि द्रव्याणि ॥

Thus ends the description of drugs classified according to their tastes.

मूर्वाम्लिकादहनसूरणसैन्धवानां योगो भवेत्पञ्चहुताशनाख्यः ।
दुर्नाममन्दाग्नियकृद्ग्रहामयं लीढ्वाढ्यवातदलनेष्वयमेवशस्तः ॥१३५॥
[पञ्चाग्निः]

*Pañcāgni*

*Mūrvā*, *amlikā*, *dahana*, *sūraṇa* and *saindhava*—these drugs taken together are called *pañca hutāśana*. It cures *durnāman* (piles), *mandāgni* (loss of the power of digestion), *yakṛdroga* (diseases of liver) and *grahāmaya* (diseases caused by the affliction of *grahas*). When taken in the form of a linctus, it cures *āḍhya vāta* (gout) successfully.

अथातः संप्रवक्ष्यामि द्रव्यं संशोधनादिकम् ।

यथा संशोधनादौ तु न मोहं गच्छति क्वचित् ॥ १३६॥

**Groups of drugs for** *saṁśodhana* **etc.,**

Now groups of drugs used for elimination of *doṣas* are being described so that no mistake is committed in the administration of therapies.

'मदनकुटजजीमूतकेक्ष्वाकुधामार्गवलोध्रकृवेतधनसर्षप-
विडङ्गपिप्पलीकरञ्जप्रपुन्नाटकोविदारकर्बुदारारिष्टा-
श्वगन्धामधूकसारविदुलबन्धुजीवकश्वेताशणपुष्पीबिंबी-
वचेन्द्रवारुणीद्वयं चेत्यूर्ध्वभागहराणि ॥ १३७ ॥

**Drugs for Emesis**

*Madana*, *kuṭaja*, *jīmūtaka*, *ikṣvāku*, *dhāmārgava*, *lodhra*, *kṛtavedhana*, *sarṣapa*, *viḍaṅga*, *pippalī*, *karañja*, *prapunnāṭa*, *kovidāra*, *karbudāra*, *ariṣṭa*, *aśva gandhā*, *madhūka sāra*, *vidula*, *bandhu jīvaka*, *śvetā*, *śaṇa puṣpī*, *bimbī*, *vaca* and both the varieties of *indra vāruṇī*—these drugs help in the elimination of *doṣas* through the upward tract.

30
त्रिवृद्दन्तीद्रवन्तीसप्तलाशंखिनीविषाणिकागवाक्षी-
छागलान्त्रीनीलिनीफलस्नुक्सुवर्णक्षीरीचित्रककिणिही-
तिल्वककंपिल्लकचंपकरम्यकपाटलापूगहरीतक्यामल-
विभीतकलिंगीकनकफलगुडैरण्डपूतीकमहावृक्ष-
सप्तच्छदार्कारग्वधपत्रज्योतिष्मतीचेत्यधोभागहराणि
॥ १३८ ॥

**Drugs for purgation**

*Trivṛt*, *dantī*, *dravantī*, *saptalā*, *śaṁkhinī*, *viṣāṇikā*, *gavākṣī*, *chāgalāntrī*, *nīlinī*, *phala*, *snuk*, *suvarṇa kṣīrī*, *citraka*, *kiṇihī*, *tilvaka*, *kampillaka*, *campaka*, *ramyaka*, *pāṭalā*, *pūga*, *harītakī*, *āmala*, *vibhītaka*, *liṅgī*, *kanaka phala*, *guḍa*, *eraṇḍa*, *pūtīka*, *mahā vṛkṣa*, *sapta cchada*, *arka*, *āragvadha*, *patra*, *jyotiṣmatī*—these drugs help in the elimination of *doṣas* through the downward tract.

अत्र[31] तिल्वकादीनां मूलानि ॥ पूगादीनामेरण्डान्तानां फलानि ॥ पूतीकारग्वधयोः पत्राणि ॥ क्षीरिणां[32] क्षीराणीति ॥ १३९ ॥

Of drugs from *tilvaka* upto *pāṭalā*, roots are to be used, from *pūga* upto *eraṇḍa*, fruits are to be used; of *pūtīka* and *āragvadha*, leaves are to be used and of other milky plants the latex is to be used.

कोशातकी – सप्तला — शङ्खिनी — देवदाली — हेमाह्वा — कारवेल्लीत्युभयतोभागहराणि ॥ एषां स्वरसा इति ॥१४०॥

**Drugs which are both Emetic & Purgative**

*Kośātākī, saptalā, śaṁkhinī, devadālī, hemāhvā and kāravelli*—these drugs help in the elimination of *doṣas* through both the upward and downward tracts.

The juice of these plants is to be used.

पिप्पलीमरिचविडङ्गमधुशिग्रुसिद्धार्थकशिरीषकरवीर-
बिंबीगिरिकर्णीकिणिहीवचाज्योतिष्मतीकरंजार्कालर्क-
लशुनातिविषाश्रृंगवेरतालीसतमालसुरसार्जकेङ्गुदीमे-
षश्रृङ्गीमातुलुंगीमुरङ्गीपीलुतिनिशशालतालमधूकला-
क्षाहिंगुलवणमद्यशकृद्रसमूत्राणीति **शिरोविरेचनानीति** ॥१४१॥

**Errhines**

*Pippalī, marica, viḍaṅga, madhu śigru, siddhārthaka, śirīṣa, karavīra, bimbī, girikarṇī, kiṇihī, vacā, jyotismatī, karañja, arka, alarka, laśuna, ativiṣā, sṛṅgavera, tālīsa, tamāla, surasā, arjaka, iṅgudī, meṣa sṛṅgī, mātuluṅgī, pīlu, tiniśa, śāla, tāla, madhūka, lākṣā, hiṅgu, lavaṇa, madya, śakṛt rasa* and urine—these help in the elimination of *doṣas* from the head.

करवीरादीनामर्कान्तानां मूलानि मातुलुङ्गीमुरङ्गीपी-
लुजातीनां पुष्पाणि ॥ १४२ ॥

Of the drugs from *karavīra* upto *arka*, roots are to be used and the flowers of *mātuluṅgī*, *muraṅgī*, *pīlu* and *jātī* are to be used.

भद्रदारुकुष्ठनिशामेषलशृङ्गी बातिबलार्तगलकालकक-
च्छूराशल्लकीकुबेराक्षीवीरतरुसहचराग्निमन्थवत्सादनी
श्वदंष्ट्रैरंडाश्मभेदकार्कालर्कशतावरीपुनर्नवावसुकव-
शिरकर्चूरभार्गीकार्पासीवृश्चिकालीधत्तूरबदरयवकोल-
कुलत्थप्रभृतीनि विदारिगन्धादिश्च द्वे पञ्चमूल्यौ-
समासेन **वातसंशमनो वर्गः** ॥ १४३ ॥

**Group of drugs for alleviation of** *vāyu*

*Bhadra dāru, kuṣṭha, niśā, meṣa śṛṅgī, balā, atibalā, ārtagala, kālaka, kacchura, śallakī, kuberakṣī, vīrataru, sahacara, agni mantha, vatsādanī, śvadaṁṣṭrā, eraṇḍa, aśma bhedaka, arka, alarka, śatāvarī, punarnavā, vasuka, vaśira, karcūra, bhārgī, kārpāsī, vṛścikali, dhattūra, badara, yava, kola, kulattha* etc., drugs belonging to the *vidārigandhādi* group and both the varieties of *pañca mūla*—these, in brief, are the alleviators of *vāyu*.

चन्दनकुचन्दनह्रीबेरोशीरमंजिष्ठापयस्याविदारिका-
शतावरीगुन्द्राशैवालककल्हारकोकन्दोत्पलकदलीमूर्वा-
प्रभृतीनिकाकोल्यादिसारिवादिन्यग्रोधादिरुत्पलादितृण-
पञ्चमूलमिति समासेन **पित्तसंशमनो वर्गः** ॥ १४४ ॥

**Group of drugs for alleviation of** *pitta*.

*Candana, kucandana, hrībera, uśīra. mañjiṣṭhā, payasyā, vidārikā, śatāvarī, gundrā, śaivālaka, kalhāra, kokanda, utpala, kadalī, mūrvā* etc. and drugs of *kākolyādi, sārivādi, nyagrodhādi, utpalādi* and *triṇa pañca mūla* groups these, in brief, are the alleviators of *pitta*.

कालेयकागरुतिलपर्णीकुष्ठहरिद्राशीतशिवशतपुष्पासर-
लरास्नाप्रकीर्योदकीर्येङ्गुदीसुमनसःकाकादनीलाङ्गल-
कीहस्तिकर्णमुंजातकलामज्जकप्रभृतीनि वल्लीकण्टक-
पञ्चमूल्यौ पिप्पल्यादिर्मुष्ककादिर्वचादिः
सुरतादिरारग्वधादिरिति समासेन **श्लेष्मसंशमनो
वर्गः** ॥ १४५ ॥

**Group of drugs for alleviation of** *kapha*

*Kāleyaka, agaru, tila parṇī, kuṣṭha, haridrā, śīta, śiva, śata-*

*puṣpā, sarala, rāsnā, prakīryā, udakīryā, iṅgudī, sumanas, kākādanī, lāṅgalakī, hasti karṇa, muñjātaka, lāmajjaka* etc. and drugs belonging to *valli pañca mūla, kaṇṭaka pañca mūla, pippalyādi, muṣkakādi, vacādi, surasādi, āragvadhādi* groups—these, in brief, are the alleviators of *kapha.*

तत्र सर्वाण्योषधानि व्याधिबलादधिकमौषधमुपयुक्तं
तमुपशम्यव्याधिमन्यमावहन्ति । अग्निबलादधिकमजीर्णं
विष्टभ्य वा पच्यते । पुरुषबलादधिकं ग्लानिमूर्छाम-
दानावहति । तस्मात्सममेव विदध्यात् ॥ १४६ ॥'

[सुश्रुतः सूत्र ३९ : ३-१०]

**Proper dosage**

If all these drugs are used in excess of the strength of the disease, then after curing the disease, they produce other ailments. If these are used in excess of the digestive power then they, being undigested, cause flatulence. If they are used in excess of the strength of the individual then they cause mental fatigue, fainting and intoxication. Therefore, these should be administered in appropriate dosage.

नवधान्यमाषतिलकुल्माषकुलत्थनिष्पावहरितशाका-
म्ललवणकटुगुडपिष्टविकृतिवल्लूरशुष्कशाकाजाविका-
नुपोदकमांसवसाशीतोदककृशरापायसदधिदुग्धतक्रमद्य-
प्रभृतीनि परिहरेत् ॥ १४७ ॥

**Unwholesome food for a patient**

Freshly harvested corns, *māṣa, tila, kulmāṣa, kulattha, niṣpāva*, green vegetables, ingredients having sour, saline and pungent tastes, pastries, dried fish, dry vegetables, meat as well as musale fat of goat, sheep and animals inhabiting marshy land and water, cold water, *kṛśarā, pāyasa*, curd, milk, butter milk, alcoholic drinks etc., should be avoided by a patient.

तक्रान्तो नवधान्यादिर्योऽयं वर्ग उदाहृतः ।

दोषसंजननो ह्येष विज्ञेयः पूयवर्धनः ॥ १४८ ॥

कुठेरकशिग्रुसुरससुमुखासुचिभूस्तृणाः ।

शुक्तं च चुक्रिकं चेति वर्गं हरितकं विदुः ॥ १४९ ॥

Ingredients enumerated above from freshly harvested corns upto butter milk aggravate *doṣas* and they cause pus formation. *Kuṭheraka, śigru, surasā, sumukha, suci, bhūstṛṇa, śukta* and *cukrika*—these are called *haritaka.*

**अतः सर्वप्राणिनामाहारार्थं वर्गं उपदिश्यते ।**

रक्तशालिषष्टिककंगुककुमुदकपाण्डुककरमर्दकसुगन्धककलमशात्तपुटी कुमोदकनीवारकोद्रवोद्दालकश्यामाकनन्दीमुखीवेणुयवाः, एणहरिणमृगकुरङ्गमातृकाः श्वदंष्ट्राकरालविष्किरहारीततित्तिरलावकाः कपिंजलवर्तीरकाश्च, मुद्गमकुष्ठवर्तुकलायमसूरमङ्गल्याचणकाढ़कीसतीनमाषाश्च, चिल्लीवास्तुकनिषण्णकजीवन्तीतण्डुलीयकमण्डूकपर्ण्यः, गव्यं घृतं सैन्धवं दाडिमामलकतंडुलवर्गः [?], ब्रह्मचर्यनिर्वातशयनोष्णोदकनिद्रास्वप्नः [?] व्यायामश्चैष वर्गः सर्वप्राणिनां **सामान्यतः पथ्यतमः** ॥ १५० ॥

**Wholesome food & regimens**

(*a*) *Rakta śāli, ṣaṣṭika, kaṅguka, kumudaka, pāṇḍuka, karamardaka, sugandhaka, kalama, śāttapuṭṭi, kumodaka, nīvāra, kodrava, uddālaka, śyāmāka, nandīmukhī veṇuyava,* (b) *eṇa, hariṇa, mṛga, kuraṅga, mātṛkā, śvadaṁṣṭra, karāla, viṣkira, hārīta, tittira, lāvaka, kapiñjala, vartiraka,* (c) *mudga, makuṣṭha, vartula kalāya, masūra, maṅgalyā, caṇaka, āḍḍhakī, satīna, māṣa* (d) *cillī, vāstuka, niṣaṇṇaka, jīvantī, taṇḍulīyaka, maṇḍūka parṇī,* (e) cow's milk, ghee, rock salt, *dāḍima, āmalaka,* (e) celibacy, sleep in a non-airy place, hot water, sleep and exercise—these are, in general, most wholesome for all living creatures.

**कृष्णात्रेयः**

त्रपुटं विद्यमानेषु भ्रमः कोपं पतञ्जलेः । [?]

शमी धान्येषु माषान्नमपथ्यत्वं प्रभाषते ॥ १५१ ॥

वातव्याधिप्रशमना शूलाध्मानविकृन्तनाः ।

बल्या वाजीकरा माषाः स्युरपथ्यतमाः कथम् ॥१५२॥

Among the *śamī dhānyas* (grains), *māṣa* is considered to be the most unwholesome. This view is not correct because *māṣa* cures diseases caused by the vitiation of *vāyu, śūla* (colic pain) and *ādhmāna* (flatulence). It promotes strength as well as virility. Why should it be treated as unwholesome ?

अवस्थान्तरबाहुल्याद्रोगादीनां व्यवस्थितम् ।
द्रव्यं नेच्छन्ति भिषजद्रष्टरि स्वस्थरक्षणम् ॥१५३॥
द्वयोरन्यतरादाने वदन्ति विषदुग्धयोः ।
दुग्धस्यैकान्ततो हितं विषस्यैकान्ततोऽहितं ॥१५४॥
33
स्वस्थरोगिणाम् ।

Disease have different varieties and stages. Therefore, physicians who aim at preservation of health do not fix a particular drug for a particular ailment. There are however things which are extremely good or extremely bad. For example, milk is always useful whereas poison is always harmful both for healthy persons as well as patients.

## NOTES AND REFERENCES

1. This is the 12th Chapter of *Ayurveda Saukhyaṁ* in Toḍarānanda and the opening invocation reads below :—

"गोपालिकानां करताडनेन कलंसनृत्यं प्रचकार बालः ।
सामस्वरो विश्वविनर्तको यस्तनोतु शं टोडरमल्लभूपे ॥"

2. 'कियद्भिरौप्यौषधसंग्रहैर्गणैर्निगद्यते' इति पंचमपुस्तके पाठः ।
3. 'स्यात्सप्तत्रिंशदमांभिर्गणैर्वीक्ष्यवातपित्तकफात्' इति प्रथमपुस्तके पाठः ।
4. 'भिषजः' इति द्वितीयपुस्तके पाठः ।
5. 'भिन्नान् मिश्रान् प्रयोजयेत्' इति आकरे पाठः ।

6. 'द्वय' इति प्रथमद्वितीयपुस्तकयोः पाठः ।
7. 'चिरविल्व' इति प्रथमपंचमपुस्तकयोः पाठः ।
8. 'त्रय' इति प्रथमपंचमपुस्तकयोः पाठः ।
9. 'वातरुजापहः इति प्रथमपंचमपुस्तकयोः पाठः ।
10. 'लोध्र' इति प्रथमपंचमपुस्तकयोः पाठः ।
11. द्रष्टव्यम् सुश्रुतः सूत्रः ३८ : २२-२३ ।
12. 'मूत्रदोषहरो·······रुचिप्रदः' पाठोऽयं प्रथमपंचमपुस्तकयोः नोपलभ्यते ।
13. द्रष्टव्यम् सुश्रुतः सूत्र ३८ : ५०-५१ ।
14. द्रष्टव्यम् सुश्रुतः सूत्र ३८ : ५४-५५ ।
15. द्रष्टव्यम् सुश्रुतः सूत्र ३८ : ५३ ।
16. द्रष्टव्यम् सुश्रुतः सूत्र ३८ : ५६, योगरत्नाकरः पृष्ठ ६७ ।
17. द्रष्टव्यम् सुश्रुतः सूत्र ३८ : ५८ ।
18. द्रष्टव्यम् सुश्रुतः सूत्र ३८ : ६०-६१ ।
19. द्रष्टव्यम् सुश्रुतः सूत्र ३८ : ६६-७० ।
20. द्रष्टव्यम् सुश्रुतः सूत्र ३८ : ७२-७६ ।
21. 'तृवृता' इति प्रथमपंचमपुस्तकयोः पाठः ।
22. 'वृष्याणां इति द्वितीयपुस्तके पाठः ।
वृक्षाणां इति प्रथमपंचमपुस्तकयोः पाठः ।
23. 'यत्तु' इति द्वितीयपुस्तके पाठः ।
24. द्रष्टव्यम् योगरत्नाकरः पृष्ठ ६८ ।
25. ''वृद्धिस्तु·······मधुरशीतलं'' इति प्रथमपंचमपुस्तकयोः पाठः ।
26. द्रष्टव्यम् भावप्रकाशः हरीतक्यादिवर्गः १२२ ।
27. 'सुगन्धवाढ्य'' इति आकरे पाठः ।
28. तद्यनेन इति द्वियीयतृतीयचतुर्थपुस्तकेषु पाठः ।
29. ''सालसारादिकं·······फलानिच'' इति प्रथमद्वितीयपुस्तकयोः पाठः ।
30. 'त्रिवृत्श्यामादन्ती' इति प्रथमपंचमपुस्तकयोः पाठः ।
'विवृताश्यामदन्ती' इति आकरे पाठः ।
31. 'त्रिवृत्तादीनां' इति द्वितीयपुस्तके पाठः ।
32. 'शेषाणां' इति आकरे पाठः ।

33. This is the end of the 12th chapter in *Ayurveda Saukhyaṁ* of Toḍarānanda and the colophon reads as below :

    इति श्रीमहाराजाधिराजटोडरमल्लविरचिते टोडरानन्दे आयुर्वेदसौख्ये गणोद्देशकथनं नाम द्वादशो हर्षः ।

# CHAPTER 31

द्रव्यनामगुणान् ज्ञात्वा भिषजः कर्म्म कुर्व्वते ।
तस्मादगदनामानि[1] वक्ष्यन्ते कर्म्मसिद्धये ॥ १ ॥

Physicians resort to therapeutic measures only after obtaining the knowledge of the names and properties of medicinal substances. Therefore, for successful accomplishment of the treatment of diseases names (synonyms) of therapeutically useful substances are being described.

**हरीतकी**

शिवा हरीतकी पथ्या चेतकी विजया जया ।
प्रपथ्या[2] प्रमथामोघा कायस्था प्राणदामृता[3] ॥ २ ॥
जीवनीया हैमवती पूतनामृतलाभया ।
वयस्था नंदि विज्ञेया श्रेयसी रोहिणी तथा ॥ ३ ॥

*Harītakī*

*Śivā, harītakī, pathyā, cetakī, vijayā, jayā, prapathyā,*

*pramathā*, *amoghā*, *kāyasthā*, *prāṇadā*, *amṛtā*, *jīvanīyā*, *haimavatī*, *pūtanā*, *amṛtalā*, *abhayā*, *vayasthā*, *nandi*, *śreyasī* and *rohiṇī*—these are synonymous.

**आमलक**

[4]धात्रीफलामृतफलामलकं श्रीफलं शिवम् ।

*Āmalaka*

*Dhatrī phala*, *amṛta phala*, *āmalaka*, *śrī phala* and *śiva*—these are synonymous.

**विभीतक**

विभीतकः कर्षफलो भूतवासः कलिद्रूमः ॥ ४ ॥

वासंतोऽक्षो विंध्यजातः संवर्त्तस्तिलपुष्पकः ।

*Vibhītaka*

*Vibhītaka*, *karṣa phala*, *bhūta vāsa*, *kali druma*, *vāsanta*, *akṣa*, *vindhya jāta*, *saṁvarta* and *tila puṣpaka*—these are synonymous.

**त्रिफला**

त्रिफला तत्त्रयेण स्याद्वरा श्रेष्ठा फलोत्तमा ॥५॥

*Triphalā*

*Harītakī*, *āmalaka* and *vibhītaka* are called *triphalā*, when taken together. *Varā*, *śreṣṭhā* and *phalottamā*—these are the synonyms of *triphalā*.

**भूम्यामलकी**

[5]भूधात्री वहुपत्रा स्याज्जटा तामलकी शिवा ।

*Bhūmyāmalakī*

*Bhū dhātrī*, *vahu patrā*, *jaṭā*, *tāmalakī* and *śivā*—these are the synonyms of *bhūmyāmalakī*.

**प्राचीनामलक**

प्राचीनामलकं प्राचीनागरं रक्तकं मतम् ॥ ६ ॥

*Prācīnāmalaka*

*Prācīnāmalaka, prācī nāgara* and *raktaka*—these are synonymous.

**वासा**

वासा वृषः सिंहमुखी भिषङ्मातारूषकः ।
शुक्ल हैमवती चैव सिंहास्यो वाजिदंतकः ॥ ७ ॥

*Vāsā*

*Vāsā, vṛṣa, siṁha mukhī, bhiṣaṅmātā, āṭaruṣaka, śukla, haimavatī, siṁhāsya* and *vāji dantaka*—these are synonymous.

**गुडूची**

गुडूची कुंडली छिन्ना वयस्थामृतवल्लरी ।
छिन्नोद्भवा छिन्नरुहामृता ज्वरविनाशिनी ॥ ८ ॥
वत्सादनी चंद्रहासा जीवंती चक्रलक्ष्यणा ।

*Guḍūcī*

*Guḍūcī, kuṇḍalī, chinnā, vayasthā, amṛta vallarī, chinnodbhavā, chinna ruhā amṛtā, jvara vināśinī, vatsādanī, candra hāsā, jīvantī, cakra lakṣaṇā*—these are synonymous.

**बिल्व**

बिल्वः शलाटु शैलूषो मालूरश्च सदाफलः ॥ ९ ॥
लक्ष्मीफलो गंधगर्भः शांडिल्यः कंटकी मतः ।

***Bilva***

***Bilva, śalāṭu,*** *śailūṣa, mālūra, sadā phala,* ***lakṣmī phala, gandha garbha, śāṅdilya,*** *kaṇṭakī*—these are synonymous.

**अरणि**

अग्निमंथो जयः केशी अरणिर्वैजयंतिका ॥ १० ॥

***Araṇī***

***Agni*** *mantha, jaya, keśī, araṇi* and *vaijayantikā*—these are synonymous.

**पाटलाकाष्ठपाटला**

पाटला कामदूती स्यात् कुम्भिका कालवृंतिका ।

स्थाल्यामोघा मधोर्दूती ताम्रपुष्पांबुवासिनी ।

अन्या फलेरुहा श्वेतकुंभीका काष्ठपाटला ॥११॥

*Paṭalā & Kāṣṭhapāṭālā*

*Paṭalā, kāma dūtī, kumbhikā, kālavṛntikā, sthālyā, amoghā, madhordūtī, tāmra puṣpā* and *ambu vāsinī*—these are the synonyms of *pāṭalā*. Another variety of it which is called *kāṣṭhapāṭalā* has two synonyms viz., *phale ruhā* and *śveta kuṁbhīkā*.

**गंभारि**

कास्मरी सर्वतोभद्रा श्रीपर्णी कृष्णवृंतिका ।

कंभारी काश्मरी हीराकाश्मरी भद्रपर्णिका ॥ १२ ॥

*Gaṁbhāri*

*Kāsmasī, sarvatobhadrā, śrī parṇī, kṛṣṇa vṛntikā, kaṁbhārī, kāśmarī, hīrā kāśmarī* and *bhadra parṇikā*—these are synonymous.

**स्योनाक**

स्योनाकः पृथुशिंवः[6] स्यात् शुकनासः कुटंनटः ।

भूतवृक्षश्च खट्वांगः टुंटुकः सल्लकोरलुः[7] ।

मयूरजंघो शालूकः प्रियंजीवः कटंभरः ॥ १३ ॥

*Śyonāka*

*Syonāka, pṛthu śimba, śuka nāsa, kutaṁnaṭa, bhūta vṛkṣa, khaṭvāṅga, ṭunṭuka, sallaka, aralu, mayūra jaṅgha, śāluka priyaṁjīva* and *kaṭaṁbhaka*—these are synonymous.

**महत्पंचमूल**

विल्वादिभिः पंचभिरेव यत्स्यात् तत्पंचमूलं महदग्निकारिः ॥ १४॥

*Mahat pañca mūla*

*Bilva, araṇi, pāṭalā, gambhārī* and *śyonāka*—these five drugs, taken together, are known as *mahat pañca mūla*. They are the promoters of digestion and metabolism.

**गोक्षुर**

गोक्षुरस्त्रिकटः कंदफलः स्यात्स्वादुकंटकः ।
गोकंटको भद्रकंटस्त्रिकंटो व्यालदंष्ट्रकः ।
श्वदंष्ट्रः स्थलश्रृंगाटः षडंगः क्षुरकस्त्रिकः ॥ १५ ॥

*Gokṣura*

*Gokṣura, trikaṭa, kaṇṭa phala, svādu kaṇṭaka, go kaṇṭaka, bhadra kaṇṭa, brikaṇṭa, vyāla daṁṣṭraka, śvadaṁṣṭra, sthala śṛṅgāṭa, ṣaḍaṅga, kṣuraka* and *trika*—these are synonymous.

**शालिपर्णी**

शालिपर्णी ध्रुवा सौम्या त्रिपर्णी पीतनी स्थिरा ।
विदारिगंधातिगुहा दीर्घमूलांशुमत्यपि ॥ १६ ॥

*Śali parṇī*

*Śāli parṇī, dhruvā, saumyā, tri parṇī, pītaṇī, sthirā, vidārigandhā, ati guhā, dīrgha mūlā* and *aṁśumati*—these are synonymous.

**पृश्निपर्णी**

पृश्निपर्णी क्रोष्टुपुच्छा धावनी कलशी गुहा ।
शृगालविट् वृत्तलता पृथक्पर्णी च पर्णिका ॥ १७ ॥

*Pṛśni parṇī*

*Pṛśni parṇī, kroṣṭu pucchā, dhāvanī, kalaśī, guhā, śṛgāla viṭ, vṛtta laṭā, pṛthak parṇī* and *parṇikā*—these are synonymous.

**बृहत्कंटकारी**

बृहती स्थूलभंटाकी विशदा च महोटिका ।

वृंताकी महती सिंही कंटकी राष्ट्रनाकुली ॥ १८ ॥

*Bṛhat kaṇṭakārī*

*Bṛhatī*, *sthūla bhaṇṭāki*, *viśadā*, *mahoṭikā vṛntākī*, *mahatī*, *siṁhī*, *kaṇṭakī* and *rāṣṭra nākulī*—these are the synonyms of *bṛhat kaṇṭakārī*.

**लघुकंटकारी**

कंटारिका कंटकिनी कंटकारी निदिग्धिका ।
दुःस्पर्शा धावनी क्षुद्रा स्याद्व्याघ्री दुःप्रधर्षिणी ॥१९॥

*Laghu kaṇṭakārī*

*Kaṇṭārikā*, *kaṇṭakinī*, *kaṇṭakārī*, *nidigdhikā*, *duḥsparśā*, *dhāvanī*, *kṣudrā*, *vyāghrī* and *duḥpradharṣiṇī*—these are the synonyms of *laghu kaṇṭakārī*.

**श्वेत कंटकारी**

सितक्षुद्रा चंद्रहास्या लक्ष्मणा क्षेत्रदूतिका[8] ।

*Śveta kaṇṭakārī*

*Sita kṣudrā*, *candra hāsyā*, *lakṣmaṇā* and *kṣetra dūtikā*—these are the synonyms of *śveta kaṇṭakārī*.

**लघुपंचमूल**

ह्रस्वाख्यं पंचमूलं स्यात्पंचभिर्गोक्षुरादिभिः ॥ २० ॥

*Laghu pāñca mūla*

*Gokṣura*, *śāli parṇī*, *pṛśni parṇī*, *bṛhat kaṇṭakārī* and *laghu kaṇṭakārī*—these five drugs, taken together, are known as *laghu pañca mūla*.

**दशमूल**

एताभ्यां पंचमूलाभ्यां दशमूलमुदाहृतम् ।

*Daśamūla*

The ten drugs, included in these two groups viz., *mahat*

*pañca mūla* and *laghu pañcamūla*, taken together are called *daśa mūla*.

**ऋद्धि वृद्धि**

ऋद्धि सुखं[9] युगं लक्ष्मीः सिद्धिः सर्वजनप्रिया ॥ २१ ॥

*Ṛddhi and vṛddhi*

Both *Ṛddhi* and *vṛddhi* (*sukha*) are called *lakṣmī*, *siddhi* and *sarva jana priyā*.

**काकोली**

काकोली मधुरा वीरा कायस्था वीरशुक्लिका ।
ध्वांक्षकोली[10] वायशोली स्वादुमांसी पयस्विनी ॥२२॥

*Kākolī*

*Kākolī, madhurā, virā, kāyasthā, vīra śuklikā, dhvāṅkṣa kolī, vāyaśolī, svādu māṁsī* and *payasvinī*—these are synonymous.

**क्षीरकाकोली**

द्वितीया क्षीरकाकोली शताह्वा क्षीरिणी मता ।

*Kṣīra kākolī*

The second variety of *kākolī*, which is known as *ksīra kākolī* has two synonyms viz., *śatāhvā* and *ksīriṇī*.

**मेदा**

मेदा ज्ञेया शाल्यपर्णी मणिछिद्राऽभयाधरा ॥ २३ ॥

*Medā*

*Medā, śālya parṇī, maṇi chidrā, abhayā* and *adharā*—these are synonymous.

**महामेदा**

महामेदा वसुछिद्रा त्रिदंता देवतामणिः[11] ।

*Mahāmedā*

*Mahā meda, vasu chidrā, tri dantā, devatā* and *mani*—these are synonymous.

**जीवक**

जीवको मधुरः श्रृंगी ह्रस्वांगः कूर्च्चशीर्षकः ।।२४।।

*Jivaka*

*Jīvaka, madhura, śṛṅgī, hrasvāṅga* and *kūrca śīrṣaka*—these are synonymous,

**ऋषभक**

ऋषभो धीर इंद्राक्ष विषाणी दुर्द्धरो वृषः ।

*Ṛṣabhaka*

*Ṛṣabha, dhīra, indrākṣa, viṣāṇī, durdhara* and *vṛṣa*—these are synonymous.

**अष्टवर्ग**

अष्टवर्गोष्टभिर्द्रव्यैरेतैः शीतोतिशुक्रलः ।। २५ ।।

*Aṣṭa varga*

*Ṛddhi, vṛddhi, kākolī, kṣīra kākolī, medā, mahā medā, jīvaka* and *ṛṣabhaka*—these eight drugs taken together are called *aṣṭa varga*. They are cooling and exceedingly spermatopoetic.

**जीवंती**

जीवंती जीवनी जीवा जीवनीया यशस्करी ।

शाकश्रेष्ठा जीवभद्रा मंगल्या जीववर्द्धनी ।। २६ ।।

*Jivantī*

*Jīvantī, jīvanī, jīvā, jīvanīyā, yaśaskarī, śāka śreṣṭhā, jīva bhadrā, maṅgalyā* and *jīva varḍhinī*—these are synonymous.

**मधुयष्टी**

मधुयष्टी क्लीतनकं यष्टीमधु मधूलिका ।

यष्ट्याह्वं मधुकं यष्टीमधुकं जलजं मधु ।। २७ ।।

*Madhu yaṣṭi*

*Madhu yaṣṭi, klītanaka, yasti madhu, madhūlikā, yaṣṭyāhva, madhuka, yaṣṭī madhuka, jalaja* and *madhu*—these are synonymous.

**माषपर्णी**

माषपर्णी कृष्णवृन्ता कांबोजी हयपुच्छिका ।
12
मांसमाषा सिंहमुखी स्वादुमाषा महासहा ॥ २८ ॥

*Māṣa parṇī*

*Māṣa parṇī, kṛṣṇa vṛntā, kāṁbojī, haya pucchikā, māṁsamāsā, siṁha mukhī, svādu māṣā* and *mahā sahā*—these are synonymous.

**मुद्गपर्णी**

मुद्गपर्णी क्षुद्रसहा सूर्यपर्णी कुरंगिनी ।
13
वनजा रंगिणी शिंवी सिंही मार्जारगंधिका ॥ २९ ॥

*Mudga parṇī*

*Mudga parṇī, kṣudra sahā, sūrya parṇī, kuraṅginī, vanajā, raṅgiṇī, śiṁbī, siṁhī* and *mārjāra gandhikā*—these are synonymous.

**जीवनीयगण**

जीवंती सूप्यपर्णीयुक् काकोल्यौ जीवकर्षभौ ।

मेदे ऽयष्टीति मधुरो जीवनीयगणो गुरुः ॥ ३० ॥

*Jīvanīya gaṇa*

*Jīvantī, māṣa parṇī, mudga parṇī, kākolī, kṣīra kākolī, jīvaka, ṛṣabhaka, medā, mahā medā* and *yaṣṭi madhu*—taken together, they are called *madhura gaṇa* (group of drugs having sweet taste) or *jīvanīya gaṇa* (group of drugs promoting vitality). They are heavy (*guru*).

**एरण्ड**

एरंडो दीर्घदंडः स्यात् वरुणो वर्द्धमानकः ।

चित्रः पंचागुलो व्याघ्रपुच्छो गंधर्व्वहस्तकः ॥ ३१ ॥

*Eaṇḍa*

*Eraṇḍa, dīrgha daṇḍa, varuṇa, vardhamāṇaka, citra, pañcāṅgula, vyāghra puccha* and *gandharva hastaka*—these are synonymous.

**रक्त एरंड**

रक्तदंडो हस्तिकर्णो व्याघ्रो व्याघ्रतरो रुबुः ।

उत्तानपत्रो दुर्व्वातः[14] आमवैरी वंचचुलः[15] ॥ ३२ ॥

*Rakta eraṇḍa*

*Rakta daṇḍa, hasti karṇa, vyāghra, vyāghratara, rubu, uttāna patra, durvāta, āma vairī* and *vacaṁcula*—these are the synonyms of the red variety of *eraṇḍa*.

**सारिवायुग्म**

सारिवा शारदास्फोता गोपकन्या प्रतानिका ।

गोपांगना गोपवल्ली लताह्वा काष्ठसारिवा ।

सारिवान्या कृष्णमूला भद्रचंदनसारिवा ॥ ३३ ॥

*Two varieties of Sārivā*

*Sārivā, śāradā, āsphotā, gopa kanyā, pratānikā, gopāṅganā, gopa vallī, latāhvā* and *kāṣṭha sārivā*—these are the synonyms of *sārivā*.

There is another variety of *sārivā* whose synonyms are *kṛṣṇa mūlā, bhadra candana* and *sārivā*.

**यवासा**

यासो मरुद्भवानंता दीर्घमूलो यवासकः ।

वालपत्रः समुद्रांतो दूरमूलोऽतिकंटकः ॥ ३४ ॥

धन्वयासस्ताम्रमूली दुःस्पर्शा स्याद्दुरालभा ।

दुरालंभा यासकश्च कच्छुरा धन्वयासकः ॥ ३५ ॥

*Yavāsā*

*Yāsa*, *marudbhavā*, *anantā*, *dīrgha mūla*, *yavāsaka*, *vāla patra*, *samudrānta*, *dūra mūla*, *ati kaṇṭaka*, *dhanva yāsa*, *tāmramūlī*, *duḥsparśā*, *durālabhā*, *durālambhā*, *yāsaka*, *kacchurā* and *dhanva yāsaka*—these are synonymous.

**महामुंडी**

महामुंडी लोभनीया छिन्नग्रंथिनिका स्मृता ।

भूतवृक्षः कुलहलो[16] लंबु[17] शालूककंटकः ।

कदंबपुष्पी मुंडी च गुणैः भुमिकदंबकः ॥ ३६ ॥

*Mahā muṇḍī*

*Mahā muṇḍī*, *lobhanīyā*, *chinna granthinikā*, *bhūta vṛkṣa*, *kulahala*, *lambu*, *śāluka kaṇṭaka*, *kadamba puṣpī*, *muṇḍī* and *bhūmi kadambaka*—these are synonymous.

**अपामार्ग**

अपामार्गस्तु शिखरी किणिही खरमंजरी ।

अधःशल्यः शैखरिकः प्रत्यक्पुष्पी मयूरकः ॥ ३७ ॥

*Apāmārga*

*Apāmārga*, *śikharī*, *kiṇihī*, *khara mañjarī*, *adhaḥ śalya*, *śaikharika*, *pratyak puṣpī* and *mayūraka*—these are synonymous.

**रक्तापामार्ग**

अन्यो रक्तो रक्तफलो वसिरः[18] कपिपिप्पली ।

*Rakta apāmārga*

*Rakta phala*, *vasira* and *kapi pippalī*—these are the synonyms of red variety of *apāmārga*.

**कंपिल्लक**

कंपिलो रेचनो रक्तश्चूर्णको व्रणशोधनः ।
19
रोहीतो रक्तशमनो रेची रंजनको मतः ॥ ३८ ॥

*Kampillaka*

*Kampila, recana, rakta cūrṇaka, vraṇa śodhana, rohita, rakta śamana, recī* and *rañjanaka*—these are the synonyms of *kampillaka*.

**दंती**

दंती घुणप्रिया नागदंती शीघ्रमुकूलकः ।
उपचित्रा निकुंभ स्याद्विशल्योदुंबरछदा ॥ ३९ ॥
आखुकर्णी वृषैरंडा द्रवंती संवरी मता ।
20
मूषिकाह्वा सुतश्रेणी प्रत्यक्श्रेणी कफंजिका ॥४०॥

*Dantī*

*Dantī, ghuṇa priyā, nāga dantī, śighra mukūlaka, upacitrā, nikumbha, viśalyā, udumbara cchadā, ākhu karṇī, vṛṣā, eraṇḍā, dravantī, saṁvarī, muṣikāhvā, suta śreṇī, pratyak śreṇī* and *kaphañjikā*—these are synonymous.

**जयपाल**

जयपालो दंतिबीजं ख्यातं तच्चिंचिणीफलं ।

*Jayapāla*

*Jayapāla, danti bīja* and *ciñciṇī phala*--these are synonymous.

**श्वेतनिशोथ**

21
त्रिवृत्कुंभोऽरुणा त्र्यस्रा भंडी कूटरवाहिनी ।
22
सर्वानुभूतिस्त्रिवृता त्रिपुटा सरलासिता ॥ ४१ ॥

*Śveta niśotha*

*Trivṛt, kumbha, aruṇā, tryasrā, bhaṇḍī, kuṭara vāhinī,*

*sarvānubhuti*, *trivṛtā*, *tripuṭā*, *saralā* and *sitā*—these are the synonyms of the white variety of *trivṛt*.

**श्यामनिशोथ**

त्रिवृत्काला कालमेषी कालपर्ण्यर्द्धचंद्रिका ।

सुषेणा स्यान्मालविका मसूरा विदला मता ॥ ४२ ॥

*Śyāma niśotha*

*Trivṛt*, *kālā*, *kāla meṣī*, *kāla parṇī*, *ardha candrikā*, *suṣeṇā*, *mālavikā*, *masūrā* and *vidalā*—these are the synonyms of black variety of *trivṛt*.

**इन्द्रवारुणी द्वय**

इंद्रवारुण्यथें द्राह्वा वृषभाक्षी[23] गवादनी[24] ।

इंद्रैर्वारुः क्षुद्रफला विशालेंद्री[25] विषादिनी ॥ ४३ ॥

अन्येद्रंवारुणी चित्रफला चित्रा महाफला ।

आत्मरक्षा नागदंती त्रपुंसी गजचिर्भिटा ॥ ४४ ॥

*Indra vāruṇī — two varieties*

*Indra vāruṇī*, *indrāhvā*, *vṛṣabhākṣī*, *gavādanī*, *indrairvāru*, *kṣudra phalā*, *viśālā*, *aindrī* and *viṣādanī*—these are the synonyms of *indra vāruṇī*.

There is another variety of *indra vāruṇī* whose synonyms are *citra phalā*, *citrā*, *mahā phalā*, *ātma rakṣā*, *nāga dantī*, *trapusī* and *gaja cirbhiṭā*.

**आरग्वध**

आरग्वधो राजवृक्षः शम्पाकः कृतमालकः ।

व्याधिघातः कर्णिकारः प्रग्रहश्चतुरंगुलः ।

आरोग्यशिबी स्वर्णद्रुः[26] कर्णी दीर्घफलो मतः ॥ ४५ ॥

*Āragvadha*

*Āragvadha*, *rājavṛkṣa*, *sampāka*, *kṛta mālaka*, *vyādhi ghāta*, *karṇikāra, pragraha, caturaṅgula, ārogya śiṁbi, svarṇadru, karṇī* and *dīrgha phala*—these are synonymous.

**नीलिनी**

नीलिनी नीलिका ग्राम्या श्रीफला भारवाहिनी ।

रंजनी कालिका मेला तुनी तुत्था विशोधनी ।।४६।।

*Nīlinī*

*Nīlinī, nīlīkā, grāmyā, śrī phalā, bhāra vāhinī, rañjanī, kālikā, melā, tunī, tutthā* and *viśodhanī*—these are synonymous.

**कटुकी**

कटुका रोहिणी तिक्ता चक्रांगी कटुरोहिणी ।

मत्स्यपित्ता कांडरुहा वष्णभद्रा द्विजांगिका ।। ४७ ।।

*Kaṭukī*

*Kaṭukā, rohiṇī, tiktā, cakrāṅgī, kaṭurohiṇī, matsya pittā, kāṇḍa ruhā, vṛṣṇa bhadrā* and *dvijāṅgikā*—these are synonymous.

**अंकोल**

अंकोलकस्ताम्रफलः पीतसारो निकोचकः ।

गुप्तस्नेहो विरेचीस्याद्भूसिता दीर्घकीलकः ।। ४८ ।।

*Aṅkola*

*Aṅkolaka, tāmra phala, pīta sāra, nikocaka, gupta sneha, virecī, bhūsitā, dīrgha kīlaka*—these are synonymous.

**सेहुंड**

सेहुंडो वज्रतुंडस्तु गंडीरो वज्रतुंडकः ।

स्नुही सामंतदुग्धासिपत्रा वज्री महातरुः ।। ४९ ।।

*Sehuṇḍa*

*Sehuṇḍa, vajra tuṇḍa, gaṇḍīra, vajra tuṇḍaka, snuhī, sāmanta dugdhā, asi patrā, vajrī* and *mahā taru*--these are synonymous.

**निंब**

निंबो नियमनो नेतारिष्टः स्यात्पारिभद्रकः ।

27

सुतिक्तः सर्वतोभद्रः पिचुमर्दः प्रभद्रकः ॥ ५० ॥

*Nimba*

*Nimba, niyamana, netā, ariṣṭa, pāribhadraka, sutikta, sarvatobhadra, picu marda* and *prabhadraka*—these are synonymous.

**महानिंब**

28

महानिंबो निंबरकः कार्म्मुको विषमुष्टिकः ।

रम्यको गिरिकोद्रेको क्षीरः स्यात्केशमुष्टिकः ॥५१॥

*Mahā nimba*

*Mahā nimba, nimbaraka, kārmuka, viṣa muṣṭika, ramyaka, girika, udreka, kṣīra* and *keśa muṣṭika*—these are synonymous.

**किराततिक्त**

29

किराततिक्तः कैरातो भूनिंबः रामसेनकः ।

किरातकोन्यो नैपालो नारीतिक्तो ज्वरांतकः ।

कांडतिक्तोर्ध्वतिक्तः स्यान्निद्रारिः सन्निपातहा ॥५२॥

*Kirāta tikta*

*Kirāta tikta, kairāta, bhūnimba* and *rāmasenaka*—these are the synonyms of *kirāta tikta*.

There is another variety of *kirāta tikta* whose synonyms are *naipāla, nārī tikta, jvarāntaka, kāṇḍa tikta, urdhva tikta, nidrāri* and *sannipātahā*.

**कुटज**

कुटजो मल्लिकापुष्पः कलिंगो गिरिमल्लिका ।

वत्सकः कुटजः कोटीवृक्षकः शक्रभूरुहः ॥ ५३ ॥

*Kuṭaja*

*Kutaja, mallikā puṣpa, kaliṅga, giri mallikā, vatsaka, koṭī vṛkṣaka* and *śakra bhūruha*—these are synonymous.

**इन्द्रयव**

ऐन्द्रयवस्तस्य फलं कालिंगः कौटजो मतः ।
शक्राह्वः पुरुहुतश्च प्रोक्तो भद्रयवस्तथा ॥ ५४ ॥

*Indra yava*

The fruit of *kuṭaja* is called *indra yava*. Its synonyms are *kāliṅga, kauṭaja, śakrāhva, puruhuta* and *bhadra yava.*

**मदनफल**

मदनः छर्द्नः पिंडी राठः पिंडीतकः फलम् ।
करहाटश्च तगरः शल्यको विषपुष्पकः ॥ ५५ ॥

*Madana phala*

*Madana, chardana, piṇḍī, rāṭha, piṇḍītaka phala, karahāṭa, tagara, śalyaka* and *viṣa puṣpaka*—these are synonymous.

**कंकुष्ठ**

कंकुष्ठकं काककुष्ठं रेचनं रंगुनायकम् ।
शोभनं चुलकं[30] रासं[31] वरांगं किंनुबालकम् ॥ ५६ ॥

*Kaṁkuṣṭha*

*Kaṁkuṣṭhaka, kāka kuṣṭha, recana, raṅga nāyaka, śobhana, culaka, rāsa, varāṅga* and *kiṁnubālaka*—these are synonymous.

**स्वर्णक्षीरी**

हेमाह्वा कनकक्षीरी हेमदुग्धा हिमावती ।
क्षीरिनी कांचनक्षीरी कटुपर्णी च कर्षिणी ॥ ५७ ॥

*Svarṇakṣīrī*

*Hemahvā, kanaka kṣīrī, hema dugdhā, himāvatī, kṣīrinī, kāñcana kṣīrī, kaṭu parṇī* and *karṣiṇī*—these are synonymous.

**सातला**

सातला विमला सारी[32] सप्तला वहुफेनिका ।

चर्मसाह्वा चर्म्मकसा फेना दीप्ता च नालिका[33] ॥५८॥

*Sātalā*

*Sātalā*, *vimalā*, *sārī*, *saptalā*, *vahu phenikā*, *carmasāhvā*, *carma kasā*, *phenā*, *dīptā* and *nālika*—these are synonymous.

**अश्मंतो**

अश्मंतो मालुकापत्रो युग्मपत्रोऽम्लपत्रकः ।

श्लक्ष्णत्वगश्मयोनिः स्यात्कुशली पापनाशनः ॥५९॥

*Aśmanta*

*Aśmanta*, *mālukā patra*, *yugma patra*, *amla patraka*, *ślakṣṇa tvak*, *aśma yoni*, *kuśalī* and *pāpa nāśana*—these are synonymous.

**कांचनार**

कांचनारः कांचनकः पाकारी रक्तपुष्पकः ।

कोविदारोऽस्यभेदः स्यात्कुद्दालः कुंडली कुली ।

आस्फोतोद्यलकः स्वल्पः[34] केशरी श्रीमरी हितः ॥६०॥

*Kāñcanāra*

*Kāñcanāra*, *kāñcanaka*, *pākārī* and *rakta puṣpaka*—these are the synonyms of *kāñcanāra*. A variety of this plant is called *kovidāra*. Its synonyms are *kuddāla*, *kuṇḍalī*, *kulī*, *āsphotā*, *udyalaka*, *svalpa*, *keśarī*, *śrīmarī* and *hita*.

**निगुंडी**

निगुंडी श्वेतकुसुमः सिंदुकः सिंदुवारकः[35] ।

*Nirguṇḍī*

*Nirguṇḍī*, *śveta kusuma*, *sinduka* and *sindu vāraka*—these are synonymous.

**सेफालिका**

36

भूतकेश्यपरो नीलसिंदुको नीलपुष्पकः ।

शेफालिका शीतभीरु धनको नीलमंजरी ॥ ६१ ॥

*Sephālikā*

The blue variety of *nirguṇḍī* is called *bhūta keśī*, *nīla sinduka*, *nīla puṣpaka*, *śephālikā*, *śīta bhīru*, *dhanaka* and *nīla mañjarī*.

**मेषशृंगी**

मेषश्रृंगी मेषवल्ली सर्पदंष्ट्राजश्रृंगिका ।

अन्या च दक्षिणावर्ति वृश्चिकाली विषाणिका ॥६२॥

*Meṣa śṛṅgī*

*Meṣa śṛṅgī*, *meṣa vallī*, *sarpa daṁṣṭrā* and *aja śṛṅgikā*—these are the synonyms of *meṣa śṛṅgī*. There is another variety of it whose synonyms are *dakṣiṇāvarti*, *vṛścikālī* and *viṣāṇikā*.

**श्वेतपुनर्नवा**

पुनर्नवा श्वेतमूला पृथ्वीको दीर्घपत्रकः ।

विशाखो दीर्घवर्षाभूः पुनर्भूर्म्मंडलच्छदः ॥ ६३ ॥

*Sveta punarnavā*

*Punarnavā*, *sveta mūlā*, *pṛthvīka*, *dīrgha patraka*, *viśākha*, *dīrgha varṣābhū*, *punarbhū* and *maṇḍala chada*—these are synonymous.

**रक्त पुनर्नवा**

पुनर्नवाऽपरारक्ता रक्तपुष्पः कठील्लकः ।

*Rakta punarnavā*

Synonyms of the red variety of *punarnavā* are *rakta puṣpa* and *kaṭhīllaka*.

**क्षुद्रवर्षाभुः**

क्रूरकः क्षुद्रवर्षाभूः वर्षकेतुः शिवाटिका ॥ ६४ ॥

*Kṣudra varṣābhū*

*Kruraka, kṣudra varṣā bhū, varṣa ketu* and *śivāṭikā*—these are the synonyms of the small variety of *punarnavā*.

**रास्ना**

रास्ना रस्या युक्तरसा रसना गंधनाकुली ।
सुगन्धमूलातिरसा श्रेयसी सुवहा रसा ॥ ६५ ॥

***Rāsnā***

***Rāsnā, rasyā, yukta rasā, rasanā, gandha nākulī, sugandha mūlā, atirasā, śreyasī, suvahā*** and ***rasā***—these are synonymous.

**अश्वगन्धा**

अश्वगन्धा तुरङ्गाह्वा गोकर्णाश्वावरोहकः ।
वराहकर्णी वरदा बल्या वाजीकरी वृषा ॥ ६६ ॥

*Aśva gandhā*

*Aśva gandhā, turaṅgāhvā, gokarṇā, aśvāvarohaka, varāha karṇī, varadā, balyā, vājikarī* and *vṛṣā*—these are synonymous.

**प्रसारणी**

प्रसारणी राजबला चारुपर्णी प्रतानिका ।
सरणी सारणी भद्रपर्णी सुप्रसरा सरा ॥ ६७ ॥

***Prasāraṇī***

***Prasāraṇī, rāja balā, cāru parṇī, pratānikā; saraṇī, sāraṇī, bhadra parṇī, suprasarā*** and ***sarā***—these are synonymous.

**शतावरी**

शतावरी भीरुपत्री द्वीपिकाधरकंटकी ।
नारायणी शतपदी शताह्वा वहुपुत्रिका ॥ ६८ ॥

*Śatāvarī*

*Śatāvarī, bhīru patrī, dvīpīkā, adhara kaṇṭakī, nārāyaṇī, śata padī, śatāhvā* and *vahu pūtrikā*—these are synonymous.

**महाशतावरी**

शतावर्य्याश्चकठोन्या पीवरी दीवरी वरी ।
अभीरुर्वहुपुत्रा च महापुरुषदंतिका ।
सहस्रवीर्य्या केशी स्यात्तुंगिनी सूक्ष्मपत्रिका ।।६६।।

*Mahā śatāvarī*

*Pīvarī, dīvarī, varī, abhīru, vahu putrā, mahā puruṣa dantikā, sahasra vīryā, keśī, tūṅginī* and *sūkṣma patrikā*—these are the synonyms of *mahā śatāvarī* (bigger variety of *śatāvarī*).

**बला**

बला वाट्यालकः शीतपाकी पाद्योदनाह्वयः ।
भद्रौदनी सभंगा स्यात्समांसा खरयष्टिका ।। ७० ।।

*Balā*

*Balā, vāṭyālaka, śīta pākī, pādyodana, bhadraudanī, sabhaṅgā, samāṁsā* and *khara yaṣṭikā*—these are synonymous.

**महाबला**

महाबला वीरपुष्पा सहदेवा वृहद्बला ।
वाट्यायनी देवसहा वाट्यास्यात्पीतपुष्पकः ।। ७१ ।।

*Mahā balā*

*Mahā balā, vīra puṣpā, sahadevā, bṛhadbalā, vāṭyāyanī, deva sahā, vaṭyā* and *pīta puṣpaka*—these are synonymous.

**अतिबला**

वलिकातिबला भारद्वाजी स्याद्वृक्षगंधिनी ।
गांगेरुकी नागबला विश्वदेवा गवेधुका ।। ७२ ।।

*Ati balā*

*Vālikā, ati balā, bhāradvājī, vṛkṣa gandhinī, gāṅgerukī, nāga balā, viśva devā* and *gavedhukā*—these are synonymous.

**तेजवती**

तेजस्विनी तेजवती तेजन्यश्च कवल्कला ।

महौजसी पारिजाता शीता [38]तेजातितेजिनी ।। ७३ ।।

*Tejavatī*

*Tejasvinī, tejavatī, tejanya, kavalkalā, mahaujasī, pārijātā, sītā, tejā* and *ati tejinī*—these are synonymous.

**ज्योतिष्मति**

ज्योतिष्मती वह्निरुचिः कंगुणी कटुभी तथा ।

*Jyotiśmati*

*Jyotiṣmati, vahni ruci, kaṅguṇī* and *kaṭubhī*—these are synonymous.

**देवदारु**

देवदारु सुराह्वा स्याद्भद्रदारुः सुरद्रुमः ।

भद्रकाष्ठं स्नेहवृक्षः किलिमं शक्रदारु च ।। ७४ ।।

*Deva dāru*

*Deva dāru, surāhvā, bhadra dāru, sura druma, bhadra kāṣṭha, sneha vṛkṣa, kilīma* and *śakra dāru*—these are synonymous.

**सरल**

सरलो [39]नंदनश्चीत्रानमेरुर्दीपवृक्षकः ।

पूतिदारुः पूतिवृक्षो [40]महादीर्घः कीलद्रुमः ।। ७५ ।।

*Sarala*

*Sarala, nandana, cītrā, nameru, dīpa vṛkṣaka, pūti dāru, pūti vṛkṣa, mahā dīrgha* and *kīla druma*—these are synonymous.

**पुष्कर मूल**

पौष्कराह्वं पद्मपत्रं पौष्करं पौष्करांघ्रिका ।

काश्मीरं पुष्करजटा मूलं वीरं सुगंधिकम् ॥ ७६ ॥

*Puṣkara mūla*

*Pauṣkarāhva*, *padma patra*, *pauṣkara*, *pauṣkarāṅghrikā*, *kāśmīra*, *puṣkara jaṭā*, *mūla*, *vīra* and *sugandhika*—these are synonymous.

**कुष्ठ**

कुष्ठं रोगाह्वयं वाप्यं कौवेरं पारिभद्रकम् ।
पारिहार्य्यं पारिभाव्यमुत्पलं हरिभद्रकम् ॥ ७७ ॥

*Kuṣṭha*

*Kuṣṭha*, *rogāhvaya*, *vāpya*, *kauvera*, *pāribhadraka*, *pārihārya*, *pāribhāvya*, *utpala* and *hari bhadraka*—these are synonymous.

**कर्कटशृंगी**

शृंगी कुलिरशृंगी स्याद्वक्रा कर्कटशृंगिका ।
कर्क्कटाख्या महाघोरा[41] शृंगीनाम्नी नतांग्यपि ॥७८॥

*Karkaṭa śṛṅgī*

*Śṛṅgī*. *kulira śṛṅgī*, *vakrā*, *karkaṭa śṛngikā*, *karkaṭākhyā*, *mahā ghorā*, *śṛṅgīnamnī* and *natāṅgī*—these are synonymous.

**रोहिषतृण**

भूतं रोहिषकं भूतीर्भूतीकं सरलं तृणम् ।
श्लामकं युगलं पौरं व्यामकं देवगंधकम् ॥ ७९ ॥

*Rohiṣa tṛṇa*

*Bhūta*, *rohiṣaka*, *bhūtī*, *bhūtīka*, *sarala*, *tṛṇa*, *śyāmaka*, *yugala*, *paura*, *vyāmaka* and *deva gandhaka*—these are synonymous.

**कट्फल**

कट्फलं कुमुदा कुंभी[42] श्रीपर्णी सोमपादपः ।
सोमवल्को महाकुंभी[43] भद्रा भद्रवती शिवा ॥ ८० ॥

*Kaṭphala*

*Kaṭphala, kumudā, kuṁbhī, śrīparṇī, soma pādapa, somavalka, mahā kuṁbhī, bhadrā, bhadravatī* and *śivā*—these are synonymous.

**भार्गी**

भार्गी भृगुभवा[44] वासा काशघ्नी भार्गपर्व्वणी ।
खरशाकं शुक्रमाता[45] फंजी ब्राह्मणयष्टिका ॥ ८१ ॥

*Bhārgī*

*Bhārgī, bhṛgu bhavā, vāsā, kāśaghnī, bhārga parvaṇī, khara śaka, śukra mātā, phañjī* and *brāhmaṇa yaṣṭikā*—these are synonymous.

**पाषाणभेद**

पाषाणभेदः पाषाणोऽश्मरीभेदोश्मभेदकः ।
शिलाभेदो दृषद्भेदो नगभिन्नगभेदनः ॥ ८२ ॥

*Pāṣāṇa bheda*

*Pāṣāṇa bheda, paṣāṇa, aśmarī bheda, aśma bhedaka, śilā bheda, dṛṣad bhedu, naga bhid* and *naga bhedana*—these are synonymous.

**मुस्ता**

मुस्तं वारिधरो मुस्ता मेघाख्यः कुरुविंदकः ।
वराहोऽव्यो घनो भद्रमुस्तं राजकसेरुकः[46] ।
पिण्डमुस्तं विषध्वंसी नागरोन्यः प्रकीर्त्तितः ॥ ८३ ॥

*Mustā*

*Musta, vāri dhara, mustā, meghākhya, kuru vindaka, varāha, avya, ghana, bhadra musta, rāja kaseruka, piṇḍa musta, viṣa dhvaṁsī*.—these are the synonyms of *mustā*. Another variety of it is called *nāgara*.

**धातकी**

धातकी कुंजरी सिन्धुपुष्पा प्रमोदिनी मता ।

पार्वतीया ताम्रपुष्पी सुराख्या मद्यवासिनी ॥ ८४ ॥

*Dhātakī*

*Dhātakī, kuñjarī, sindhu puṣpā, pramodinī, pārvatīyā, tāmra puṣpī, surākhyā* and *madya vāsinī*—these are synonymous.

**विदारीकंद**

विदारिका वृक्षवल्ली वृक्षकं दाविडालिका[47] ।

शृंगालिका कंदवल्ली स्वादुकं पापनाशकः ॥ ८५ ॥

अन्या शुक्ला क्षीरशुक्ला क्षीरवल्ली पयस्विनी ।

इक्षुवल्ली महाश्वेता क्षीरगंधेक्षुगंधिका ॥ ८६ ॥

*Vidārī kanda*

*Vidārikā, vṛkṣa vallī, vṛkṣaka, dāvīḍālikā, śṛgālikā, kaṅda vallī, svāduka, pāpa nāśaka*—these are the synonyms of *vidāri-kanda*. It has another variety whose synonyms are *śuklā, kṣīra śuklā, kṣīra vallī, payasvinī, ikṣu vallī, mahā śvetā, kṣīra gandhā* and *ikṣu gandhikā.*

**मायिका**

मायिका[48] वालिका[49] दष्टा[50] शचीदंत[51] सठंविका ।

अंवष्टकी सूचिमुखी कषाया शाकटमुखम् ॥ ८७ ॥

*Māyikā*

*Māyikā, vālikā, duṣṭā, śacī danta, saṭhaṁvikā, aṁvaṣṭhakī, sūcī mukhī, kaṣāyā* and *śākaṭa mukha*—these are synonymous.

**वाराही कंद**

वाराही माधवी गृष्टिः शौकरी वनमालिका ।

तस्याः कंदः कटिक्रोडनाम संवरनामकः ॥ ८- ॥

*Vārāhī kanda*

*Vārāhī, mādhavī, gṛṣṭi, śaukarī* and *vana mālikā*—these are the synonyms of the plant *vārāhī kanda.*

Its root (tuber) is called *kaṭi kroḍa* and *saṁvara.*

**पाठा**

पाठांवष्ठा वृहत्तिक्ता प्राचीनांवष्ठकी रसा ।

वरतिक्ता पापचेली श्रेयसी विद्धकर्णिका ॥ ८९ ॥

*Pāṭhā*

*Pāṭhā, aṁvaṣṭhā, vṛhattiktā, prācīnāmbaṣṭhakī, rasā, vara tiktā, pāpa celī, śreyasī* and *viddha karṇikā*—these are synonymous.

**मूर्वा**

मूर्व्वा देवी मधुरसा देवश्रेणी मधुस्रवा।

स्निग्धपर्णी पृथक्पर्णी मोरटा पीलुपर्णिका ॥ ९० ॥

*Mūrvā*

*Mūrvā, devī, madhu rasā, deva śreṇī, madhu sravā, snigdha parṇī, pṛthak parṇī, moraṭā* and *pīlu parṇikā*—these are synonymous.

**मंजिष्ठा**

मंजिष्ठा विजयरक्ता रक्तांगी कालमेषिका ।

रक्तयष्टिस्ताम्रवल्ली समंगा वस्त्रभूषणा ।

मंजुला विकसा भंडी छद्मिका ज्वरनाशिनी ॥ ९१ ॥

*Mañjiṣṭhā*

*Mañjiṣṭhā, vijaya raktā, raktāṅgī, kāla meṣikā, rakta yaṣṭi, tāmra vallī, samaṅgā, vastra bhūṣaṇā, mañjulā, vikasā, bhaṇḍī, chadmikā* and *jvara nāśinī*—these are synonymous.

**हरिद्रा**

हरिद्रा रंजनी[52] गौरी[53] रजनी वरवर्णिनी ।

पिंडी पीता वर्णवती निशा वर्णविनाशिनी ॥ ९२ ॥

*Haridrā*

*Haridrā, rañjanī, gaurī, rajanī, vara varṇinī, piṇḍī, pītā, varṇa vatī, niśā* and *varṇa vināśinī*-- these are synonymous.

**दारुहरिद्रा**

दार्वी दारुहरिद्रान्या पीतदारु पचंपचा ।
कटंकटेरी पीतद्रु: स्वर्णवर्णा कटंकटि: ॥ ६३ ॥

*Dāruharidrā*

Another variety of *haridrā* is called *dāru haridrā* and its synonyms are *dārvī, pīta dāru, pacaṁpacā, kaṭaṅkaṭerī, pītadru, svarṇa varṇā* and *kaṭaṅkaṭi.*

**चक्रमर्द**

प्रपुन्नाटस्त्वेडगजश्चक्रमर्द: प्रपुन्नट: ।
दद्रुघ्नो मर्दको मेषकुसुम: कुष्ठकृंतन: ॥ ६४ ॥

*Cakra marda*

*Prapunnāḍa, eḍagaja, cakra marda, prapunnaṭa, dadrughna, mardaka, meṣa kusuma* and *kuṣṭha kṛntana*—these are synonymous.

**वाकुची**

वाकुची चंद्रिका सोमवल्ली· पूतीफलांबरा ।
सोमराजी कृष्णफलावल्गुज: कालमेषिका ॥ ६५ ॥

*Vākucī*

*Vākucī, candrikā, soma vallī, pūtī phalā, ambarā, somarājī, kṛṣṇa phalā, avalguja* and *kāla meṣikā*—these are synonymous.

**भृंगराज**

भृंगराजो भेकराजो मार्क्कव: केशरंजन: ।

54

भृंगारको भृंगराजो भृंगाह्व: सूर्यवल्लभ: ॥ ६६ ॥

*Bhṛṅga rāja*

*Bhṛṅga rāja*, *bheka rāja*, *mārkava*, *keśa reñjana*, *aṅgāraka*, *bhṛṅgāhva* and *sūrya vallabha*—these are synonymous.

**पर्पट**

पर्प्पटः कवचो रेणुः पित्रहा [55] यवकंटकः ।
वरतिक्तः पर्प्पटकः [56] स्पृष्टीकश्चर्म्मकंटकः ॥ ९७ ॥

*Parpaṭa*

*Parpaṭa*, *kavaca*, *reṇu*, *pitrahā*, *yava kaṇṭaka*, *vara tikta*, *parpaṭaka*, *spṛṣṭīka* and *carma kaṇṭaka*—these are synonymous.

**शणपुष्पी**

[57] शणपुष्पी माल्यपुष्पी धावनी सणघंटिका ।
वृहत्पुष्पी स्वल्पघंटा घंटाशब्दोरुपुष्पिका ॥ ९८ ॥

*Śaṇa puṣpī*

*Śaṇa puṣpī*, *mālya puṣpī*, *dhāvanī*, *saṇa ghaṇṭikā*, *vṛhat puṣpī*, *svalpa ghaṇṭā*, *ghaṇṭā śabda* and *uru puṣpikā*—these are synonymous.

**त्रायमाणा**

त्रायमाणा सुहृत्त्राणा त्रायंती गिरीशानुजा ।
बलभद्रा कृतत्राणा वार्षिकं त्रायमानकम् ॥ ९९ ॥

*Trāya māṇā*

*Trāya māṇā*, *suhṛt trāṇā*, *trāyantī*, *girī śānujā*, *bala bhadrā*, *kṛta trāṇā*, *vārṣika* and *trāya mānaka*—these are synonymous.

**महाजालिनी**

महाजालिनीका चर्म्मरंगा स्यात्पीतकलिका ।
[58] आवर्त्तकी तिंदुकिनी विभांड रिक्तपुष्पिका ॥ १०० ॥

*Mahā jālinī*

*Mahā jālinīkā*, *carma raṅgā*, *pīta kalikā*, *avarttakī*, *tindu-*

*kinī, vibhāṇḍa* and *rikta puṣpikā*—these are synonymous.

**अतिविषा**

अतिविषा शुक्लकंदा विषा प्रतिविषाऽपरा ।
श्यामकंदा सिताश्रृंगी भंगुरोपविषाणिका ॥ १०१ ॥

*Ati viṣā*

*Ati viṣā, śukla kandā, viṣā* and *prati viṣā*—these are synonyms of *ativiṣā.*

There is another variety of it whose synonyms are *śyāma kandā, sitā śṛṅgī, bhaṅgurā* and *upa viṣānikā.*

**काकमाची**

काकमाची ध्वांक्षमाची कामबीज घनेफला ।
रसायनवरा सर्व्वतिक्ता स्यात्काकिनी कटुः ॥१०२॥

*Kākamācī*

*Kākamācī, dhvāṅkṣa mācī, kāma bīja, ghane phalā, rasāyana varā, sarva tiktā, kākinī* and *kaṭu*—these are synonymous.

**काकजंघा**

काकजंघा नदीकांता काकतिक्ता सुलोमशा ।
पारावतपदी काका मद[59]ध्मा[60]कर्म्मणी तथा ॥ १०३ ॥

*Kāka jaṅghā*

*Kāka jaṅghā, nadī kāntā, kākatiktā, sulomaśā, pārāvata padī, kākā* and *madadhmā-karmaṇī*—these are synonymous.

**लोध्र**

लोध्रस्तिरीटः कामीनस्तिल[61]वकः संतरोद्भवः ।
अन्यो घनस्त्वक्सारश्चेतरोलोध्राक्षिभेषजम् ॥ १०४ ॥

***Lodhra***

*Lodhra, tiriṭa, kānīna, tilvaka* and *santarodbhava*—these are the synonyms of *lodhra.*

It has another variety whose synonyms are *ghana tvaksāra* and *akṣi bheṣaja.*

**वृद्धदारु**

वृद्धदारुर्म्महाश्यामा जांगलो जीर्णवालुकः ।
अंतःकोटरपुष्पी स्यादावेगी छागलो[62] अपि ॥ १०५ ॥

*Vṛddha dāru*

*Vṛddha dāru, mahā śyāmā, jāṅgala, jīrṇa vāluka, antaḥ koṭara puṣpī, āvegī* and *chāgala*—these are synonymous.

**देवदाली**

देवदाली वृंतकोशो देवतांगो गरागरी[63] ।
जीमूतो[64] तारकी वेणी जालिन्याखुविषापहः ॥१०६॥

*Devadālī*

*Deva dālī, vṛnta kośa, devatāṅga, garāgarī, jīmūta, tārakī, veṇī, jālinī* and *ākhu viṣāpaha*—these are synonymous.

**हंसपदी**

हंसपादी हंसपदी रक्तपादी ·त्रिपादिका ।
प्रह्लादिनी[65] कीटमारी कीटनामा मधुस्रवा ॥ १०७ ॥

*Haṁsa padī*

*Haṁsa pādī, haṁsa padī, rakta pādī, tri pādikā, prahlādiṇī, kīṭa mārī, kīṭa nāmā* and *madhu sravā*—these are synonymous.

**सोमवल्ली**

सोमवल्ली यज्ञनेता सोमक्षीरी[66] द्विजप्रिया ।

***Somavallī***

*Soma vallī, yajña netā, soma kṣīrī* and *dvija priyā*—these

**are synonymous.**

**नाकुली**

[67]नाकुली सुवहा सर्प्पगंधिनी गंधनाकुली ।

नकुलेष्टा मता सर्प्पनेत्रा चीरितपत्रिका ॥ १०८ ॥

*Nākulī*

*Nākulī, suvahā, sarpa gandhinī, gandha nākulī, nakuleṣṭā, sarpa netrā* and *cīrita patrikā*—these are synonymous.

**वटपत्री**

वटपत्री [68]मोह्नी स्यात् दीपनी रैवती मता ।

*Vaṭa patrī*

*Vaṭa patrī, mohanī, dīpanī* and *raivatī*—these are synonymous.

**लज्जालु**

लज्जालुर्म्मोह्निनी स्पृक्का [69]खदिरा गंधकारिणी ।

नमस्कारी शमीपत्रा समंगा रक्तपादिका ॥ १०९ ॥

*Lajjālu*

*Lajjālu, mohinī, spṛkkā, khadirā, gandha kāriṇī, namaskarī, śamīpatrā, samaṅgā* and *rakta pādikā*—these are synonymous.

**मशली**

मुशली खलिनी तालपत्रीका चनपुष्पिका ।

महावृषा [70]वृष्यकंदा खर्जूरी तालमूलिका ॥ ११० ॥

*Muśalī*

*Muśalī, khalinī, tāla patrikā, cana puṣpikā, mahā vṛṣā, vṛṣya kandā, kharjūrī* and *tāla mūlikā*—these are synonymous.

**कपिकच्छू**

कपिकच्छू: स्वयंगप्ता [71]कंदला दुरवग्रहा ।

चंडात्मगुप्ता लांगूली[72] मर्क्कटी स्याच्च[73] हर्षणी ।

*Kapi kacchū*

*Kapi kacchū, svayaṁ guptā, kandalā, duravagrahā, caṇḍā, ātma guptā, lāṅgūlī, markaṭī* and *harṣaṇī*—these are synonymous.

**पुत्रंजीव**

पुत्रंजीवो गर्भंकरो यष्टिपुष्पोर्थसाधनः ॥ १११ ॥

*Putrañjīva*

*Putrañjīva, garbha kara, yaṣṭi puṣpa* and *artha sādhana*—these are synonymous.

**वंध्याकर्कोटी**

वंध्याकक्कोंटकी देवी कुमारी विषनाशिनी ।

मनोज्ञा नागदमनी वंध्यायोगेश्वरी मता ॥ ११२ ॥

*Vandhyā Karkoṭī*

*Vandhyā karkoṭakī, devī, kumārī, viṣa nāśinī, manojñā, nāga damanī* and *vandyā yogeśvarī*—these are synonymous.

**विष्णुक्रांता**

विष्णुक्रांता नीलपुष्पी जया[74] वश्यापराजिता ।

*Viṣṇu krāntā*

*Viṣṇu krāntā, nīla puṣpī, jayā, vaśyā* and *aparājitā*—these are synonymous.

**शंखपुष्पी**

शंखपुष्पी शंखनाम्नी किरीटी कंबुमालिनी ।

कंबुपुष्पी स्मृतिहिता मेघ्या वनविलासिनी ॥११३॥

*Śaṁkha puṣpī*

*Śaṁkha puṣpī, śaṁkha nāmnī, kirīṭī, kaṁbu mālinī, kaṁbu*

*puṣpī, smṛti hitā, medhyā* and *vana vilāsinī*—these are synonymous.

**दुग्धि**

दूग्धिका मधुपर्णी स्यात्क्षीरिणी स्वादुपुष्पिका ।।१२२।।

*Dugdhi*

*Dugdhikā, madhu parṇī, kṣīriṇī* and *svādu puṣpikā*—these are synonymous.

**अर्कपुष्पी**

अर्कपुष्पी क्रूरकर्म्मा जलकामा भिरिंडिका ।

*Arka puṣpī*

*Arka puṣpī, krūra karmā, jala kāmā* and *bhiriṇḍikā*—these are synonymous.

**भल्लातक**

भल्लातकोऽनलो भल्ली वीरवृक्षोग्निवक्त्रक:[75] ।

अरुष्करस्तथारुष्क: तपनोऽग्निमुखी धनु: ।। १२३ ।।

*Bhallātaka*

*Bhallātaka, anala, bhallī, vīra vṛkṣa, agni vaktraka, aruṣkara, āruṣka, tapana, agni mukhi* and *dhanu*—these are synonymous.

**चेरपोटी**

चेरपोटी[76] दीर्घपत्री कुंतली[77] तिक्तका मता ।। १२४ ।।

*Cerapoṭī*

*Cerapoṭī, dīrgha patrī, kuntalī* and *tiktakā*—these are synonymous.

**द्रोणपुष्पी**

द्रोणपुष्पी श्वसनक: पालिंदी कुंभयोनिका ।

छत्रातिछत्रिका द्रोणा कौंडिन्यो वृक्षसारक: ।।१२५।।

*Droṇa puṣpī*

*Droṇa puṣpī, śvasanaka, pālindī, kumbha yonikā, chatrā, atichatrikā, droṇā, kauṇḍinya* and *vṛkṣa sāraka*—these are synonymous.

**ब्राह्मी**

ब्राह्मी सरस्वती सोमा सत्याह्वा ब्रह्मचारिणी ।
मण्डूकपर्णी [78] मांडूकी त्वष्टी दिव्या महौषधी ।
कपोतवंका मुनिका लावण्या सोमवल्लरी ।। १२६ ।।

*Brāhmī*

*Brāhmī, sarasvatī, somā, satyāhvā, brahma cāriṇī, maṇḍūka parṇī, māṇḍūkī, tvaṣṭī, divyā, mahauṣadhī, kapota vaṅkā, munikā, lāvaṇyā* and *soma vallarī*—these are synonymous.

**सुवर्चला**

सुवर्च्चलार्क्ककांता स्यात् सूर्य्यभक्ता सुखोद्भवा ।
सूर्य्यावर्त्ता रविप्रीया त्वन्या ब्रह्मसुवर्च्चला ।।१२७।।

*Suvarcalā*

*Suvarcalā, arka kāntā, sūrya bhaktā, skuhodbhavā, sūryāvartā* and *rati priyā*—these are the synonyms of *suvarcalā*. Another variety of this plant is called *brahma suvarcalā.*

**मत्स्याक्षी**

मत्स्याक्षी वह्लिका [79] मत्स्यगंधिर्मत्स्यादनी तथा ।
तोयपिप्पल्यंबुवल्ली पत्तूरं [80] कचटं तथा ।
गोजिह्वा गोजिका गोभी दीर्घिका खरपर्णिनी ।।१२८।।

*Matsyākṣī*

*Matsyākṣī, vahlikā, matsya gandhi, matsyādanī, toya pippalī, ambu vallī, pattūra, kacaṭa, gojihvā, gojikā, gobhi, dīrghikā* and *khara parṇinī*—these are synonymous.

**नागदमनी**

नागाह्वा दमनी नागगंधा भुजगपर्णिनी ।।१२९।।

*Nāga damanī*

*Nāgāhvā*, *damanī*, *nāga gandhā* and *bhujaga parṇinī*—these are synonymous.

**गुंजा**

गुंजा शिखंडिका[81] ताम्रा रक्तिका काकणंतिका ।

श्वेतान्या चक्रिका चूडा दुर्म्माषा काकपीलुका ।।१३०।।

*Guñjā*

*Guñjā*, *śikhaṇḍikā*, *tāmrā*, *raktikā* and *kākaṇantikā*—these are the synonyms of red variety of *guñjā*. Synonyms of the white variety of *guñjā* are *cakrikā*, *cūḍā*, *durmāṣā* and *kāka pīlukā*.

**वेल्लंतर**

वेल्लंतरो दीर्घपत्रो[82] वीरद्रुर्वहुपत्रकः[83] ।। १३१ ।।

*Vellantara*

*Vellantara*, *dīrgha patra*, *vīradru* and *vahu patraka*—these are synonymous.

**वंदाक**

वंदाक स्याद्वृक्षरुहा शेखरी कामवृक्षकः ।

वृक्षादनी कामतरुः कामिन्यापदरोहिणी[84] ।। १३२ ।।

*Vandāka*

*Vandāka*, *vṛkṣa ruhā*, *śekharī*, *kāma vṛkṣaka*, *vṛkṣādanī* *kāma taru*, *kāminī* and *āpada rohiṇī*—these are synonymous.

**पिंडालू**

पिंडारः[85] करहाटः स्यात् तीक्ष्णकीलः कुरंगकः[86] ।

*Piṇḍālū*

*Piṇḍāra*, *karahāṭa*, *tīkṣṇa kīla* and *kuraṅgaka*—these are synonymous.

**छिक्किरणी**

छिक्किका क्षवकः क्रूरो नासासंवेदनः पटुः ॥ १३३ ॥

*Chikkiṇī*

*Chikkikā, kṣavaka*, *krūra*, *nāsā saṁvedana* and *paṭu*—these are synonymous.

**रोहितक**

रोहितो दाडिमीपुष्पो रुहितो कुटशाल्मलिः[87] ।

प्लीहारी रोहिणो रोही रक्तघ्नः पारिजातकः ॥१३४॥

*Rohitaka*

*Rohita*, *dāḍimī puṣpa*, *ruhita*, *kuṭa śālmali*, *plīhārī*, *rohiṇa*, *rohī*, *raktaghna* and *pārijātaka*—these are synonymous.

**मोचरस**

मोचकः स्यान्मोचरसः शाल्मलीवेष्टकः[88] स्मृतः ।

मोचनिर्य्यासकः पिच्छा मोचास्रावी च पिच्छकः ॥१३५॥

*Moca rasa*

*Mocaka*, *moca rasa*, *śālmalī veṣṭaka*, *moca niryāsaka*, *picchā*, *mocāsrāvī* and *picchaka*—these are synonymous.

**अजगंधी**

अजगंधी वत्सगंधा कवरी पूतिवर्व्वरः ।

*Aja gandhī*

*Aja gandhī*, *vatsa gandhā*, *kavarī* and *pūti varvara*—these are synonymous.

**सैरेयक**

सैरेयकः सहचरः सैरेयः किंकिरातकः ॥१३६ ॥

दासी सहचरो पिंडी सैर्य्यको मृदुकंटकः ।

रक्तपुष्पः कुरवकः पीतो ज्ञेयः कुरंटकः ।

नीलार्त्तगलकः प्रोक्तो वाणउँदानवाक्यपि ॥ १३७ ॥

*Saireyaka*

*Saireyaka*, *sahacara*, *saireya*, *kiṁkirātaka*, *dāsī*, *piṇḍī*, *sairyaka* and *mṛdu kaṇṭaka*—these are the synonyms of *saireyaka*. This plant with red flowers is called *kuravaka*, with yellow flowers is called *kuraṇṭaka* and with blue flowers is called *ārta galaka* as well as *vāṇa uṅdāna vāki*.

**गिरिकर्णिका**

89 श्वेतस्यंदा श्वेतपुष्पा कटभी गिरिकर्णिका ।

सितापराजिता श्वेता विषघ्नी मोहनाशिनी ।

नीलस्यंदाव्यक्तगंधा नीलपुष्पा गवादिनी ॥ १३८ ॥

*Giri karṇikā*

*Śveta syandā*, *śveta puṣpā*, *kaṭabhī*, *giri karṇikā*, *sitā aparājitā*, *śvetā*, *viṣaghnī* and *moha nāśinī*—these are the synonyms of the white variety of *giri karṇikā*. Its blue variety is called *nīla syandā*, *avyakta gandhā*, *nīla puṣpā* and *gavādinī*.

**कोकिलाक्ष**

इक्षुरः क्षुरको ध्वंडः कोकिलाक्षः क्षुरः स्मृतः ।

90 तैलकंटोऽतिक्षुरक्षः वालिका च सुगंधिका ॥ १३९ ॥

*Kokilākṣa*

*Ikṣura*, *kṣuraka*, *dhvaṇḍa*, *kokilākṣa*, *kṣura*, *taila kaṇṭa*, *ati kṣurakṣa*, *vālikā* and *sugandhikā*—these are synonymous.

**कार्प्पास**

91 कार्प्पासः पटदस्तूलः छादनो वादरः पिचुः ।

*Kārpāsa*

*Kārpāsa, paṭada, tūla, chādana, vādara* and *picu*—these are synonymous.

**आराम शीतला**

आरामशीतला देवगंधा कुक्कुटमर्द्दकः[92] ॥ १४० ॥

*Ārāma śītalā*

*Ārāma śītalā, deva gandhā* and *kukkuṭa mardaka*—these are synonymous.

**ताम्रचूडः**

कुक्कुरद्रुस्ताम्रचूडः[93] सूक्ष्मपत्रो मृदुच्छदः ।

*Tāmra cūḍa*

*Kukkura dru, tāmra cūḍa, sūkṣma patra*, and *mṛdu chada*—these are synonymous.

**वामी**

वामी[94] शंखधरा वारि ब्राह्मी च हिममोचिका ॥१४१॥

*Vāmī*

*Vāmī, śaṁkha dharā, vāri, brāhmī* and *hima mocikā*—these are synonymous.

**वलामोटा**

वलामोटा जया सूक्ष्मपत्रा ज्ञेयापराजिता ।

*Valā moṭā*

*Valā moṭā, jayā, sūkṣma patrā* and *aparājitā*—these are synonymous.

**शरपुंखा**

शरपुंखा कालशाकं प्लीहारि कालिका मता ॥१४२॥

*Śara puṁkhā*

*Śara puṁkhā, kāla śāka, plīhāri* and *kālikā*—these are synonymous.

**मयूर शिखा**

मयूराह्वशिखा ज्ञेया साहस्रमधुकच्छदा ।

*Mayūra śikhā*

*Mayūrāhva śikhā* and *sāhasra madhuka chadā*—these are synonymous.

**लक्ष्मणा**

लक्ष्मणा पुत्रदा रक्ता विदुपत्रा[95] च नागिनी ।। १४३ ।।

*Lakṣmaṇā*

*Lakṣmaṇā, putradā, raktā, vindu patrā* and *nāginī*—these are synonymous.

**मांसरोहिणी**

मांसरोहिण्यतिरुहा वृन्ता[96] चर्म्मकशा[97] कशा ।

*Māṁsa rohiṇī*

*Māṁsa rohiṇī, atiruhā, vṛntā, carma kaśā* and *kaśā*—these are synonymous.

**अस्थिसंहार**

अस्थिसंहारको वज्रवल्लरी क्रोष्टुघंटिका[98] ।। १४४ ।।

*Asthi saṁhāra*

*Asthi saṁhāraka, vajra vallarī* and *kroṣṭu ghaṇṭikā*—these are synonymous.

**अर्क्क**

अर्क्कः सूर्य्याह्वयः क्षीरी सदापुष्पा विकीरणः[99] ।

मंदारो वसुकोन्[100]यार्क्कोः राजार्हो दीर्घपुष्पकः ।। १४५ ।।

*Arka*

*Arka, sūryāhvaya, kṣīrī, sadā puṣpā, vikīraṇa, mandāra* and *vasuka*—these are the synonyms of *arka*. It has another variety which is called *rājārha* and *dīrgha puṣpaka*.

**करवीर**

करवीरोऽश्वहा श्वेतपुष्पा स्यात् शतकुंभकः ।

रक्तपुष्पोऽपरश्चंडो लगुडः करवीरकः ॥ १४६ ॥

***Karavīra***

*Karavīra, aśvahā, śveta puṣpā* and *śata kumbhaka*—these are the synonyms of *karavīra* having white flower. The other variety having red flower has synonyms like *caṇḍa, laguḍa* and *karavīraka*.

**धत्तूर**

धत्तूरः कितवो धूर्त्तो देवता मदनः शठः[101] ।

उन्मत्तो मातुलस्तुरी तरलः कनकाह्वयः ॥ १४७ ॥

***Dhattūra***

*Dhattūra, kitava, dhūrta, devatā, madana, śaṭha, unmatta, mātula, turī, tarala* and *kanaka*—these are synonymous.

**कलिहारी**

कलिहारी वह्निमुखी लांगली[102] गर्भपातनी ।

विशल्या हलिनी सीरीक्रमा वा शुक्रपुष्पिका[103] ॥१४८॥

***Kalihārī***

*Kalihārī, vahni mukhī, lāṅgalī, garbha pātanī, viśalyā, halinī, sīrīkramā* and *śukra puṣpikā*—these are synonymous.

**कुमारी**

कुमारी मंडला माता गृहकन्या सपिच्छला ॥ १४९ ॥

***Kumārī***

*Kumārī, maṇḍalā, mātā, gṛha kanyā* and *sapicchalā*—these are synonymous.

**भंगा**

भंगा गंजा मातुलानी मोहिनी विजया जया ।

***Bhaṅgā***

*Bhaṅgā, gañjā, mātulānī, mohinī, vijayā and jayā*—these are synonymous.

**कांचनी**

[104] कांचनी शोणफलिनी काकायुः काकवल्लरी ॥ १५० ॥

*Kāñcanī*

*Kāñcanī, śoṇa phalinī, kākāyu,* and *kāka vallarī*—these are synonymous.

**दूर्वा**

दूर्वा शिष्टा शीतकरी गोलोमी [105] शतपर्व्विका ।

अन्या श्वेता श्वेतदंडा भार्गवी दुर्म्मना रुहा ॥ १५१ ॥

*Dūrvā*

*Dūrvā, śiṣṭā, śīta karī, golomī* and *śata parvikā*—these are the synonyms of one variety of *dūrvā.* Synonyms of the other variety are *śveta, śveta daṇḍā, bhārgavī, durmanā* and *ruhā.*

**गंडदूर्व्वा**

गंडदूर्व्वा मत्स्यगंधा मत्स्याक्षी शकुलादनी ।

*Gaṇḍa dūrvā*

*Gaṇḍa dūrvā, matsya gandhā, matsyākṣī* and *śakulādanī*—these are synonymous.

**कास**

कासः सुकांडः [106] कासेक्षुरिषकः श्वेतचामरः ॥ १५२ ॥

*Kāsa*

*Kāsa, sukāṇḍa, kāsekṣu, iṣaka* and *śveta cāmara*—these are synonymous.

**दर्भ**

दर्भो बर्हिः कुशस्तीक्ष्णः [107] सूच्यग्रो यज्ञभूषणः ।

*Darbha*

*Darbha, barhi, kuśa, tīkṣṇa, sūcyagra* and *yajña bhūṣaṇa*—these are synonymous.

**मुंज**

मुंज क्षुर स्थूलगर्भो[108] वानाह्वो[109] ब्रह्ममेखलः ॥ १५३ ॥

*Muñja*

*Muñja, kṣura, sthūla garbha, vānāhva,* and *brahma mekhala*—these are synonymous.

**नल**

नलो[110] रंध्री[111] पुष्पमृत्युर्द्धमनो नर्त्तकः नटः[112] ।

*Nala*

*Nala, randhrī, puṣpa mṛtyu, dhamana, nartıaka* and *naṭa*—these are synonymous.

**वंश**

वंशो वेणु कीचकः[118] स्यात्कर्म्मारस्त्वचिसारकः[114] ॥१५४॥

*Vaṁśa*

*Vaṁśa, veṇu, kīcaka, karmāra* and *tvaci sāraka*—these are synonymous.

**खुरासानी यवानी**

यवानी यावनी[115] तीव्रा तुरुष्का मदकारिणी ।

*Khurāsāni yavāni*

*Yavānī, yāvanī, tīvra, turuṣkā* and *mada kāriṇi*—these are synonymous.

**खसखस**

तिलभेदः खसतिलः शुक्रपुष्पो लतत्फलः[116] ॥ १५५ ॥

*Khasa Khasa*

*Tila bheda, khasa tila, śukra puṣpa* and *latatphala*—these are the synonyms of *khasa khasa.*

**आफू**

आफुकं तद्रसोद्भूतं अहिफेनमफेनकं

*Āphū*

*Āphūka*, *ahiphena* and *aphenaka*—these are the synonyms of the drug prepared out of the juice of *khasa khasa*.

**पातालगरुड**

चिलहटो[117] महामूलः[118] पातालगरुडाह्वयः[119] ॥ १५६ ॥

*Pātāla garuḍa*

*Cilahaṭa*, *mahā mūla* and *pātāla garuḍa*—these are synonymous.

## NOTES AND REFERENCES

This is the 90th chapter of *Ayurveda Śaukhyaṁ* in *Toḍarānanda* and the opening invocation reads as below :

यस्यानुरागातिशयेन पूर्णा गोपांगना उद्धवमूचुरुःक्तै ।

प्राणप्रियैष्टोडरमल्लसज्ञं सर्वार्थपूर्णं कुरुतात् सभूपम् ॥

1. 'तस्मात् द्रव्यस्य' इति षष्ठपुस्तके पाठः ।
2. 'प्रमथ्या' इति षष्ठपुस्तके पाठः ।
3. 'प्राणदास्मृता' इति षष्ठपुस्तके पाठः
4. 'धात्रि' इति षष्ठपुस्तके पाठः ।
5. 'स्याच्चटा' इति षष्ठपुस्तके पाठः ।
6. 'श्योनाकः' इति षष्ठपुस्तके पाठः ।
7. 'शल्यकारलू' इति षष्ठपुस्तके पाठः ।
8. 'दूबिका' इति षष्ठपुस्तके पाठः ।
9. 'पुगं' इति षष्ठपुस्तके पाठः ।
10. 'सोली' इति पंचमषष्ठपुस्तकयोः पाठः ।

11. 'देवतामणी' इति प्रथमपुस्तके पाठा ।
12. 'स्वादु दुर्मुखी च' इति षष्ठपुस्तके पाठः ।
13. 'वनसा' इति षष्ठपुस्तके पाठः ।
14. 'उरुवुवातवैरीति चंचलः' इति पञ्चमपुस्तके पाठः ।
15. 'विवंवुल' इति षष्ठपुस्तके पाठः ।
16. 'चूतफलो' इति षष्ठपुस्तके पाठः।
17. 'लम्बा' इति पञ्चमपुस्तके पाठः ।
18. 'वशिरः' इति षष्ठपुस्तके पाठः ।
19. 'रेचि' इति षष्ठपुस्तके पाठः ।
20. 'सूत' इति प्रथमपुस्तके पाठः ।
21. 'अस्त्रा' इति प्रथमपुस्तके पाठः ।
22. 'त्रिपुरा' इति षष्ठपुस्तके पाठः ।
23. 'वृषभाख्या' इति षष्ठपुस्तके पाठः ।
24. 'गवादिनी' इति षष्ठपुस्तके पाठः ।
25. 'विषादनी' इति प्रथमपुस्तके पाठः ।
26. 'कर्णी' इति प्रथमपुस्तके पाठः ।
27. 'पचुमन्दः' इति पञ्चमषष्ठपुस्तकयोः पाठः ।
28. 'निंवकरः' इति षष्ठपुस्तके पाठः ।
29. 'समसेनकः' इति प्रथमपुस्तके पाठः ।
30. 'पुलकं' इति पञ्चमषष्ठपुस्तकयोः पाठः ।
31. 'हासं' इति पञ्चमषष्ठपुस्तकयोः पाठः ।
32. 'सीरी' इति प्रथमपुस्तके पाठः ।
33. 'नाडिका' इति पञ्चमपुस्तके पाठः ।
'नोलिका' इति षष्ठपुस्तके पाठः ।
34. 'केसरीश्रीमरी' इति प्रथमपुस्तके पाठः ।
35. 'सिंधुवारकः' इति पञ्चमपुस्तके पाठः ।
36. 'सिंधुको' इति पञ्चमपुस्तके पाठः ।
37. 'शतपाद्' इति प्रथमपुस्तके पाठः ।
38. 'तिक्तातितेजिनी' इति प्रथमपुस्तके पाठः ।
39. 'नंदनष्चीढानमेरुर्दीपवृक्षकः' इति पञ्चमपुस्तके पाठः ।
'नंदनश्चीडानमेरुर्दीपवृक्षकः' इति प्रथमपुस्तके पाठः ।

40. 'महावृक्ष:' इति षष्ठपुस्तके पाठः ।
41. 'महाघोषा' इति षष्ठपुस्तके पाठः ।
42. 'कुभिका' इति षष्ठपुस्तके पाठः ।
43. 'मह्रा' इति षष्ठपुस्तके पाठः ।
44. 'भृगुद्भवा' इति षष्ठपुस्तके पाठः ।
45. 'शुष्क' इति षष्ठपुस्तके पाठः ।
46. 'कशेरुक:' इति पञ्चमपुस्तके पाठः ।
47. 'दाविदालिका' इति षष्ठपुस्तके पाठः ।
48. 'माचिका' इति पञ्चमपुस्तके पाठः ।
'माविका' इति प्रथमपुस्तके पाठः ।
49. 'चालिका' इति षष्ठपुस्तके पाठः ।
50. 'वष्टा' इति प्रथमपुस्तके पाठः ।
51. 'शटीदंत' इति षष्ठपुस्तके पाठः ।
52. 'रंजिनी' इति षष्ठपुस्तके पाठः ।
53. 'गौरि' इति षष्ठपुस्तके पाठः ।
54. 'अंकारको' इति षष्ठपुस्तके पाठः ।
55. 'वयकंटक:' इति षष्ठपुस्तके पाठः ।
56. 'स्पष्टी' इति षष्ठपुस्तके पाठः ।
57. 'सनपुष्पी' इति षष्ठपुस्तके पाठः ।
58. 'आवर्त्तिका' इति षष्ठपुस्तके पाठः ।
59. 'मदध्या' इति षष्ठपुस्तके पाठः ।
60. 'कर्म्माणी' इति षष्ठपुस्तके पाठः ।
61. 'संतसोद्भव:' इति पञ्चमपुस्तके पाठ ।
62. 'छागलां' इति प्रथमपुस्तके पाठः ।
63. 'स्वरागरी' इति षष्ठपुस्तके पाठः ।
64. 'जालिन्यास्तुविषापह' इति प्रथमपुस्तके पाठः ।
65. 'कोटमादी' इति प्रथमपुस्तके पाठः ।
66. 'सोमक्षीरि' इति षष्ठपुस्तके पाठः
67. 'वाङ्ली' इति प्रथमपुस्तके पाठः ।
68. 'मोहि' इति षष्ठपुस्तके पाठः ।
69. 'खदिरी' इति षष्ठपुस्तके पाठः ।
70. 'वृषकंदा' इति षष्ठपुस्तके पाठः ।

71. 'कंदली' इति षष्ठपुस्तके पाठः ।
72. 'लांगुली' इति षष्ठपुस्तके पाठः ।
73. 'स्याच्चहर्षभी' इति प्रथमपुस्तके पाठः ।
74. 'नया' इति षष्ठपुस्तके पाठः ।
75. 'विरवृक्षोग्निवक्त्रकः' इति षष्ठपुस्तके पाठः ।
76. 'चिरपोटी' इति पंचमपुस्तके पाठः ।
चिरपोटी' इति षष्ठपुस्तके पाठः ।
77. 'कुंतला' इति षष्ठपुस्तके पाठः ।
78. 'लष्टी' इति षष्ठपुस्तके पाठः ।
79. 'मत्स्यगंधिर्मत्स्यादिनी' इति षष्ठपुस्तके पाठः ।
80. 'खरपर्णिका' इति षष्ठपुस्तके पाठः ।
81. 'शिखिडिनी' इति षष्ठपुस्तके पाठः ।
82. 'दीर्घपत्री' इति षष्ठपुस्तके पाठः ।
83. 'वीरद्रुर्बहुपुत्रकाः इति षष्ठपुस्तके पाठः ।
85. 'पिंडाकः' इति षष्ठपुस्तके पाठः ।
86. 'कुलंगकः इति षष्ठपुस्तके पाठः ।
87. 'कुटशालमली' इति पञ्चमपुस्तके पाठः।
88. 'शालमलीचेष्टकः' इति प्रथमपुस्तके पाठः ।
89. 'कटसी' इति प्रथमपुस्तके पाठः ।
'कटली' इति षष्ठपुस्तके पाठः ।
90. 'तैलकंटोतिक्षुरिक्षः' इति षष्ठपुस्तके पाठः ।
91. 'वोदनः' इति षष्ठपुस्तके पाठः ।
92. 'कुक्कुरमर्द्दकः इति षष्ठपुस्तके पाठः ।
93. 'कुक्कुटद्रुस्ताम्रचूडः' इति षष्ठपुस्तके पाठः ।
94. 'वासी' इति षष्ठपुस्तके पाठः ।
95. 'पुत्रा' इति प्रथमपुस्तके पाठः ।
96. 'चर्म्मकसा' इति प्रथमपुस्तके पाठः।
97. 'कसा' इति प्रथमपुस्तके पाठः ।
98. 'क्रोष्टुघंडिका' इति पंचमपुस्तके पाठः ।
99. 'वकीरणः' इति प्रथमपुस्तके पाठः ।
100. 'वसुकान्योर्क्को' इति प्रथमपुस्तके पाठः ।

101. 'वाठः' इति प्रथमपुस्तके पाठः ।
102. 'गर्भघातनी' इति षष्ठपुस्तके पाठः ।
103. 'शुक्तिपुष्पिका' इति पञ्चमपुस्तके पाठः ।
104. 'कावोनी' इति प्रथमपुस्तके पाठः ।
105. 'शतपर्व्वका' इति पंचमपुस्तके पाठः ।
106. 'श्वेतवामरः' इति षष्ठपुस्तके पाठः ।
107. 'सून्यग्रो' इति षष्ठपुस्तके पाठः ।
108. स्थूलदर्भो' इति पञ्चमपुस्तके पाठः ।
स्थूलगर्भा' इति षष्ठपुस्तके पाठः ।
109. 'वाताह्वो' इति षष्ठपुस्तके पाठः ।
110. 'तलो' इति प्रथमपुस्तके पाठः ।
111. 'गध्री' इति प्रथमपुस्तके पाठः ।
112. 'विटः' इति प्रथमपुस्तके पाठः ।
113. 'किचकः' इति पञ्चमपुस्तके पाठ ।
114. 'स्यात्कर्म्मारम्भस्त्वविसारकः' इति षष्ठपुस्तके पाठः ।
115. 'यवानी' इति प्रथमपुस्तके पाठः ।
116. 'लमफलः' इति पञ्चमपुस्तके पाठः ।
117. 'छिलहटो' इति पञ्चमपुस्तके पाठः ।
118. 'महीमूलः इति षष्ठपुस्तके पाठः ।

This is the end of the 90th chapter of *Ayurveda Saukhyaṁ* in *Toḍarānanda* and colophon reads as below:

इति श्री महाराजाधिराज श्री टोडरमल्लविरचिते श्री टोडरानन्दे ग्रायुर्वेदसौख्ये निघण्टौ ग्रभयादिको हर्षो चतुरशीतितमः (?) ।

## CHAPTER 32

**शुण्ठी**

शुण्ठी विश्वौषधं विश्वं कटुभद्रं कटूत्कटम् ।
महौषधं शृंगवेरं नागरं विश्वभेषजम् ॥ १ ॥

*Śuṇṭhī*

*Śuṇṭhī*, *viśauṣadha*, *viśva*, *kaṭu bhadra*, *kaṭūtkaṭa*, *mahauṣadha*, *sṛṅgavera*, *nāgara* and *viśva bheṣaja*—these are synonymous.

**आर्द्रकं**

आर्द्रक शृंगवेरं तु कंदौषधमुदाहृतम् ।

*Ardraka*

*Ārdraka*, *śṛṅgavera* and *kandauṣadha*—these are synonymous.

**मरिच**

मरिचं वल्लिजं तीक्ष्णं मलिनं श्यामभूषणं ॥ २ ॥

*Marica*

*Marica, vallija, tīkṣṇa, malina* and *śyāma bhuṣana*—these are synonymous.

**पिप्पली**

पिप्पली चपला कृष्णा मागधी मगधा कणा ।

कृष्णोपकुल्या वैदेही शौंडी स्यात्तीक्ष्णतंडुला ॥ ३ ॥

*Pippalī*

*Pippali, capalā, kṛṣṇā, māgadhī, magadhā, kaṇā, kṛṣṇā, upakulyā, vaidehī, śauṇḍī* and *tīkṣṇa taṇḍulā*—these are synonymous.

**त्र्यूषण, चतुरुषण**

विश्वोपकुल्यामरिचैस्त्र्यूषणं कटुकं कटु ।

व्योषं कटुत्रयं तत्स्यात्सग्रंथिः चतुरुषणम् ॥ ४ ॥

*Tryūṣaṇa and Caturuṣaṇa*

*Viśva, upakulyā* and *marica*, taken together, are called *tryūṣaṇa* and its synonyms are *kaṭuka, kaṭu, vyoṣa* and *kaṭutraya*. Along with *granthi*, they are called *caturuṣaṇa*.

**पिप्पली मूल**

कणामूलं कटुग्रंथि पिप्पलीमूल भूषणम् ।

षड्ग्रंथि ग्रंथिकमूलं मागधं वटिकाशिरः ॥ ५ ॥

*Pippalī mūla*

*Kaṇā mūla, kaṭu granthi, pippalī mūla, bhūṣaṇa, ṣaḍgranthi, granthika mūla, māgadha* and *vaṭikā śira*—these are synonymous.

**चव्य**

चव्यं चव्यनमुद्दिष्टं चविका कोलवल्लिका ।

*Cavya*

*Cavya, cavyana, cavikā* and *kola vallikā*—these are synonymous.

**गजपिप्पली**

तत्फलं श्रेयसी हस्तिमगधा गजपिप्पली ॥ ६ ॥

*Gaja pippalī*

The fruit of *cavya* is called *śreyasī*, *hasti magadhā* and *gaja pippalī*.

**चित्रक**

चित्रको हुतभुग्[1]व्यालः दारुणो दहनोऽरुणः ।
अग्निपाली[2] हविः पाठी वह्निनामा विशेषतः ॥ ७ ॥

*Citraka*

*Citraka*, *hutabhuk*, *vyāla*, *dāruṇa*, *dahana*, *aruṇa*, *agni pālī*, *havis*, *pāṭhī* and *vahnināma*—these are synonymous.

**पंचकोल, षडूषण**

पिप्पली मगधामूलं चव्यनागरचित्रकैः ।
पंचकोलं समरिचं षडूषणमुदाहृतम् ॥ ८ ॥

*Pañcakola & Ṣaḍūṣaṇa*

*Pippalī*, *magadhā mūla*, *cavya*, *nāgara*, and *citra*, taken together, they are called *pañca kola*. Along with *marica*, they are called *ṣaḍūṣaṇa*.

**शतपुष्पा**

शतपुष्पा शिफा[3] घोषा[4] शताह्व कारवी मिशी[5] ।
अवाक्पुष्पी त्वचिछत्रा[6] सेविका मगधी परा ॥ ९ ॥

*Śatapuṣpā*

*Śatapuṣpā*, *śiphā*, *ghoṣā*, *śatāhva*, *kārav̄ī*, *misī*, *avāk puṣpī*, *tvaci chatrā*, *sevikā* and *māgadhi*—these are synonymous.

**मिश्रेया**

मिश्रेया मिश्रा शालीनो[7] शाली शीतशिवा मता ।

*Miśreyā*

*Misreyā, miśra. śālīna, śalī* and *śita śivā*—these are synonymous.

**मेथी**

मेथिका वस्तिका सेलुराहित्थो वनमेथिका ।

अहित्थोल्पगुणस्तस्माद्वाजिनां स तु पूजितः ॥ १० ॥

*Methī*

*Vastikā* and *selu* are the synonyms of *methikā*. *Vana methikā* (wild variety) is called *āhittha.* The latter is inferior in quality but it is very useful for horses.

**अजमोदा**

अजमोदात्युग्रगंधा मोदा हस्तिमयूरकः ।

खराह्वा कारवी वल्ली वस्तिमोदा च मर्कटी ॥११॥

*Ajamodā*

*Ajamodā, atyugra gandhā, modā, hasti mayūraka, kharāhvā, kāravī, vallī, vasti modā* and *markaṭī*—these are synonymous.

**जीरा (श्वेत)**

जीरकं दीर्घकं शुक्लमजाजी कणजीरकम् ।

*Jīraka (śveta)*

*Jīraka, dīrghaka, śukla, ajājī* and *kaṇa jīraka*—these are synonymous.

**जीरा (कृष्ण)**

जीरकं जारणं कृष्णं वर्षाकालसुगंधिका ॥ १२ ॥

*Jīrā (kṛṣṇa)*

*Jīraka, jāraṇa, kṛṣṇa* and *varṣākāla sugandhikā*—these are synonymous.

**उपकुंचिका**

कालिका वापिका कुंची कारवी चोपकुंचिका ।
पृथ्वीका[10] सुषवी पृथ्वी स्थूलाजाज्युपकालिका ॥१३॥

*Upakuñcikā*

*Kālikā, vāpikā, kuñcī, kāravī, upa kuñcikā, pṛthvīkā, suṣavī, pṛthvī, sthūlājāji* and *upa kālikā*—these are synonymous.

**यवानी**

यवानी[11] दीप्यको दीप्यो दीपनीया यवानिका ।
जवसाह्वोग्रगंधिः स्यात् जवह्वा[12] भूकदंबकः ॥ १४ ॥

*Yavānī*

*Yavānī. dīpyaka, dīpya, dīpanīyā, yavānikā, javasāhvā, ugra gahdhi, javahvā* and *bhūkadambaka*—these are synonymous.

**चौहारी यवानी**

जवानीया[13] जवानी स्याच्चौहारी जंतुनाशनः ॥ १५ ॥

*Cauhārī yavānī*

*Javānīyā, javānī, cauhārī* and *jantu nāśana*—these are synonymous.

**अजगंधा**

अजगंधा पूति कीटी वर्व्वरी पूतिवर्द्धनः ।
कारवी खरपुष्पा च तुंगी पूतिमयूरकः ॥ १६ ॥

*Ajagandhā*

*Ajagandhā, pūti, kīṭī, varvarī, pūti vardhana, kāravī, khara puṣpā, tuṅgī, pūti mayūraka*—these are synonymous.

**वचा**

वचोग्रगंधा गोलोमी षड्ग्रंथा जटिला तथा ।
जटिला शतपर्व्वाख्या लोमशा हैमवत्यपि ॥ १७ ॥

*Vacā*

*Vacā, ugra gandhā, golomī, ṣaḍgranthā* and *jaṭilā*—these are the synonyms of *vacā*. There is another variety of *vacā* whose synonyms are *jaṭilā, śata parvā, lomaśā* and *haimavatī.*

**हपुषा**

हपुषा बपुषा विस्रा विगन्धा विश्वगंधिका ।
अन्या स्वच्छफला ध्वांक्षनाशिनी[14] मत्स्यगंधिका ।।१८।।

*Hapuṣā*

*Hapuṣā, vapuṣā, visrā, vigandhā* and *viśva gandhikā*—these are the synonyms of *hapuṣā.*

Another variety of *hapuṣā* is called *svaccha phalā, dhvāṁkṣa nāśinī* and *matsya gandhikā.*

**विडंग**

विडंगं जंतुहननं कृमिघ्नं क्षुद्रतंडुलम् ।
भूतघ्नी तंडुला घोषा करालं[15] भृङ्गमालिका[16] ।। १९ ।।

*Viḍaṅga*

*Viḍaṅga, jantu hanana, kṛmighna, kṣudra taṇḍula, bhūtaghnī, taṇḍulā, ghoṣā, karāla* and *bhṛṅga mālikā*—these are synonymous.

**धान्यक**

धान्यकं धान्यका धान्यं धानेयं चतुरन्नकम्[17] ।
कुस्तुंबुरुस्तदाद्रं[18] तु धाने धानेय कालिका ।। २० ।।

*Dhānyaka*

*Dhānyaka, dhānyakā, dhānya, dhāneya, caturannaka* and *kustumburu*—these are the synonyms of the dried variety of *dhānyaka.* When green, this is called *dhāne, dhāneya* and *kālikā.*

**हिंगुपत्री**

हिंगुपत्री पृथुस्तन्वी पृथ्वीका चारुपत्रिका ।

वाष्पिका कारवी तंद्री बिल्विका दीर्घिका तथा ॥२१॥

*Hingu patrī*

*Hiṇgu patrī, pṛthustanvī, pṛthvīkā, cāru patrikā, vāṣpikā, kāravī, tandrī, bilvikā* and *dīrghikā*—these are synonymous.

**हिंगु**

हिंगु वाह्लीकमत्युग्रं रामठं भूतनाशनम् ।

आरुटगंधं जरणं जंतुकं सूपधूपनम् ॥ २२ ॥

*Hingu*

*Hingu, vāhlīka, atyugra, rāmaṭha, bhūta nāśana, āruṭa gandha, jaraṇa, jantuka* and *sūpadhūpana*—these are synonymous.

**वंशरोचना**

वंशजा वैणवीक्षीरी त्वक्क्षीरी वंशरोचना ।

तुगाक्षीरी तुगात्वंशी वंशक्षीरी शुभा सिता ॥ २३ ॥

*Vaṁśa rocanā*

*Vaṁśajā, vaiṇavī kṣīrī, tvak kṣirī, vaṁśa rocanā, tugā kṣiri, tugā vaṁśī, vaṁśa kṣīrī śubhā* and *sitā*—these are synonymous.

**सैन्धव**

सैन्धवं सिंधुजं शुद्धं मणिमंथं 19 पटूत्तमम् ।

*Saindhava*

*Saindhava, sindhūja, śuddha, maṇi mantha* and *patūttama*—these are synonymous.

**सौवर्चल**

सौवर्च्चलं सुगंधाक्षं रुचकं हृद्यगंधकम् ॥ २४ ॥

*Sauvarcala*

*Sauvarcala*, *sugandhākṣa*, *rucaka* and *hṛdya gandhaka*—these are synonymous.

**विड**

विडं कृत्रिमकं पाक्यं धूर्त्तं [20]द्राविडमासुरम् ।

*Viḍa*

*Viḍa*, *kṛtrimaka*, *pākya*, *dhūrtta*, *drāviḍa* and *āsura*—these are synonymous.

**सामुद्र लवण**

सामुद्रं [21]वारिसंभूतमक्षीवं वशिरं तथा ॥ २५ ॥

*Sāmudra lavaṇa*

*Sāmudra*, *vārisaṁbhūta*, *akṣīva* and *vaśira*—these are synonymous.

**औद्भिदलवण**

औद्भिदं भूमिजं भौमं पार्थिवं पृथिवीभवम् ।

*Audbhida lavaṇa*

*Audbhida*, *bhūmija*, *bhauma*, *pārthiva* and *pṛthivī bhava*—these are synonymous.

**रोमकलवण**

गंडाख्यं रोमलवणं रोमसाकंभरीभवम् ॥ २६ ॥

*Romaka lavaṇa*

*Gaṇḍākhya*, *roma lavaṇa* and *roma sākambharī bhava*—these are synonymous.

**पांशुलवण**

क्षारं पांशुभवं त्वोषमौषं पाशवनं वसु ।

*Pāṁśu lavaṇa*

*Kṣāra*, *pāṁśu bhava*, *oṣa*, *auṣa*, *pāśavana* and *vasu*—these are synonymous.

**काच लवण**

काचं त्रिकूटं पाक्याह्वं लवणं काचसंभवम् ॥ २७ ॥

*Kāca lavaṇa*

*Kāca, trikūṭa, pākyāhva, lavaṇa* and *kāca saṁbhava*—these are synonymous.

**यवक्षार**

यवक्षारः सूक्ष्मणको यावशूको यवाग्रजः ।

*Yava kṣāra*

*Yava kṣāra, sūkṣmaṇaka, yāvaśūka* and *yavāgraja*—these are synonymous.

**स्वर्जिक्षार**

स्वर्जिका स्वर्ज्जिकः पाक्यः सुखवर्च्चःसुवर्च्चिका ॥ २८ ॥

*Svarji kṣāra*

*Svarjikā, svarjika, pākya, sukhavarca* and *suvarcikā*—these are synonymous.

**टंकण**

टंकणो मालतीजातो[22] द्राविलोह विशुद्धिदः ।

*Taṅkaṇa*

*Taṅkaṇa, mālatī jāta, drāviloha* and *viśuddhida*—these are synonymous.

**सुधाक्षार**

सुधामृताह्वयः शौधः भूषणं कटुशर्क्करा ॥ २९ ॥

*Sudhā kṣāra*

*Sudhā, amṛtā, śaudha, bhūṣaṇa* and *kaṭu śarkarā*—these are synonymous.

**सर्वक्षार**

पलाशतिलनालश्वदंष्ट्रकः कदलीभवः ।

अपामार्गोऽर्क्क सेहुंड मोक्षकादिसमुद्भवः ।।
23
क्षारा वह्निसमा सर्व्वे पाचना भेदि दारणाः ।। ३०।।

*Kṣāras in general*

*Kṣāras* collected from *palāśa*, *tila nāla*, *śvadaṁṣṭrā*, *kadalī*, *apāmārga*, *arka*, *sehuṇḍa* and *mokṣaka* are all like fire. They promote digestion. They have the property of penetrating and scraping.

## NOTES AND REFERENCES

1. This is the 91st chapter of *Ayurveda Saukhyaṁ* in *Toḍarānanda*, and the opening invocation read as below :

मनोरथान् माथुरसज्जनानां यो माधवो पूरयदब्जनेत्रः ।
कर्त्ता तथा टोडरमल्लभूपे भूयात्कृपालुर्जनताहितार्थे ।।

2. 'हुतभुकालो' इति षष्ठपुस्तके पाठः ।
3. 'पाली' इति षष्ठपुस्तके पाठः ।
4. 'शफा' इति प्रथमपुस्तके पाठः ।
5. 'व्योषा' इति षष्ठपुस्तके पाठः ।
6. 'मिसि' इति प्रथमपुस्तके पाठः ।
7. 'त्वविछिन्ना' इति षष्ठपुस्तके पाठः ।
8. 'शितशिवा' इति प्रथमपुस्तके पाठः ।
9. 'सेलुर इथो' इति प्रथमपुस्तके पाठः ।
10. 'वर्षाकालीसुगंधिका' इति प्रथमपुस्तके पाठः ।
'वर्षाकालसुगंधिकम्' इति षष्ठपुस्तके पाठः ।
11. 'सुखटी' इति षष्ठपुस्तके पाठः ।
12. 'जवानी' इति प्रथमपुस्तके पाठः ।
13. 'स्यात् द्यवल्ला' इति षष्ठपुस्तके पाठः ।

14. 'यवानीया' इति पंचमपुस्तके पाठः ।
15. 'ध्वांक्षनाशनी' इति प्रथमपुस्तके पाठः ।
16. 'कमलं' इति प्रथमपुस्तके पाठः ।
17. 'मृगमालिनी' इति प्रथमपुस्तके पाठः ।
18. 'च वितुन्नकं' इति पंचमपुस्तके पाठः ।
    'चतुस्रकं' षष्ठपुस्तके पाठः ।
19. 'धानी' इति षष्ठपुस्तके पाठः ।
20. 'लवणोत्तमम्' इति प्रथमपुस्तके पाठः ।
21. 'द्राविडमासिरम्' इति प्रथमपुस्तके पाठः ।
22. 'वारिजं' इति प्रथमपुस्तके पाठः ।
23. 'भारती' इनि षष्ठपुस्तके पाठः ।
24. This is the end of 91st chapter *Ayurveda Saukhyaṁ Toḍarānanda* and the colophon reads as below :

    इति श्रीमहाराजाधिराज श्रीटोडरमल्लविरचिते टोडरानंदे आयुर्वेदसौख्ये निघंटौ सुपादिकोहर्षः पंचाशीतितमः (?) ।

# CHAPTER 33

**कर्प्पूरः**

कर्प्पूर स्फटिकश्चद्रः सिताभ्रो हिमवालुका

हिमोपलः शीतरजो भूतिकस्तु[1] सिताह्वयः ॥ १ ॥

*Karpūra*

*Karpūra*, *sphaṭika*, *candra*, *sitābhra*, *hima valukā*, *himopala*, *sīta raja*, *bhutika* and *sitāhvaya*—these are synonymous.

**कस्तूरी**

कस्तूरिका मृगमदो वेघ्येमुख्या[2] मृगांडजा ।

मृगनाभिरथान्या स्याल्लताकस्तूरिकामदः ।

मार्ज्जारी प्रीतिका[3] पूतीवासः[4] स्याद्गंधिवेलिका[5] ॥२॥

***Kastūrī***

*Kastūrikā*, *mṛga mada*, *vedhye mukhyā*, *mṛgāṇḍaja* and *mṛga nābhi*—these are the synonyms of *kastūrī*.

Another variety of it (which is derived from a plant) is called *latā kastūrikā-mada*, *mārjārī*, *prītikā*, *pūtīvāsa* and *gandhi velikā*.

**चंदन**

चंदन तिलपर्णं स्यान्महार्हं श्वेतचंदनम् ।
भद्रश्रीयं मलयजं गोशीर्षं गंधसारकम् ॥ ३ ॥

*Candana*

*Candana*, *tila parṇa*, *mahārha*, *śveta candana*, *bhadra śrīya*, *malayaja*, *gośīrṣa* and *gandha sāraka*—these are synonymous.

**रक्तचंदन**

रक्त चंदनमुद्दिष्टं लोहितं क्षुद्रचंदनम् ।
ताम्रसारं रक्तसारं ज्योतिसोमं च रंजनम् ॥ ४ ॥

*Rakta candana*

*Rakta candana*, *lohita*, *kṣudra candana*, *tāmra sāra*, *rakta sāra*, *jyoti soma* and *rañjana*—these are synonymous.

**पीतचन्दन**

कालीयकं पीतसारं पीतं नारायणप्रियम्[6] ॥ ५ ॥

*Pīta candana*

*Kālīyaka*, *pīta sāra*, *pīta* and *nārāyaṇa priya*—these are synonymous.

**कृष्णागुरु**

कृष्णागुरुः स्वादुगुरु राजार्हं विश्वरुपकम् ।
जांगलं शीतनलिनं कृमिघ्नममलार्यकम् ॥ ६ ॥

*Kṛsṇāguru*

*Kṛṣṇāguru*, *svādvaguru*, *rājārha*, *viśva rūpaka*, *jāṅgala*, *śīta nalina*, *kṛmighna* and *amalāryaka*—these are synonymous.

**कुंकुम**

कुंकुमं चारुवाह्लीकं वर्ण्यमग्निशिखं वरम् ।
काश्मीरं पीतवस्त्राह्वं[7] संकोचं पिशुनं[8] शठम् ॥ ७ ॥

*Kuṁkuma*

*Kuṁkuma, cāru vāhlīka, varṇya, agni śikha, vara, kāśmīra, pīta vastrāhva saṁkoca, piśuna* and *śoṭha*—these are synonymous.

**शीलारस**

सिल्हकः कपिलो धूम्रः तुरुष्कः[9] पिण्डितः कपिः ।

*Śilārasa*

*Silhaka, kapila, dhūmra, turuṣka, piṇḍita* and *kapi*—these are synonymous.

**एलवालुक**

एवालुकमेलवालु[10] वालुकं हरिवालुकम् ॥ ८ ॥

*Ela vāluka*

*Evāluka, elavālu, vāluka* and *hari-vāluka*—these are synonymous.

**जातीफल**

जातीफलं जातिसुतं[11] शालूकं[12] मालतीसुतम् ।

*Jātī phala*

*Jātī phala, jāti suta, śālūka* and *mālatī suta*—these are synonymous.

**जातीपत्री**

जातीपत्री[13] जातिकोशो मालतीपत्रिका तथा ॥ ९ ॥

*Jātī patrī*

*Jātī patrī, jāti kośa* and *mālati patrikā*—these are synonymous.

**लवंग**

लवंगं शिखिरं डिठ्यं लवं[14] चंदनपुष्पकम् ।

श्रीपुष्पं देवकुसुमं श्रृंगारं वारिसंभवम् ॥ १० ॥

*Lavaṅga*

*Lavaṅga, śikhira, ḍiṭhya, lava, candana puṣpaka, śrīpuṣpa, deva kusuma, śṛṅgāra* and *vāri saṁbhava*—these are synonymous.

**कंकोल**

कंकोलं कटुकंकोलं मारीचं[15] माधवोचितम्[16] ।

*Kaṁkola*

*Kaṁkola, kaṭu kaṁkola, mārīca* and *mādhavocita*—these are synonymous.

**सूक्ष्मैला**

एला त्रुटिश्चंद्रवाला बहुला निष्कुटी द्विजा ।
कपोतवर्णा सूक्ष्मैला वरटी द्राविडी सखी ॥ ११ ॥

*Sūkṣmailā*

*Elā, truṭi, candra vālā, vahulā, niṣkuṭi, dvijā, kapota varṇā sūkṣmailā, varaṭi, drāviḍī* and *sakhī*—these are synonymous.

**स्थूलैला**

स्थूलैला त्रिपुटा कन्या भद्रैला त्रिदिवोद्भवा[17] ॥१२॥

*Sthūlailā*

*Sthūlailā, tripuṭā, kanyā, bhadrailā* and *tridivodbhavā*—these are synonymous.

**त्वक्**

त्वचं वरांगं सकलं त्वकोचं तनुकं वरम् ।
लाटपर्ण्यं[18] घनं भृंगं गुडत्वक् स्वर्णभूमिकम् ॥ १३ ॥

*Tvak*

*Tvak, varāṅga, sakala, tvakoca, tanuka, vara, lāṭa parṇya, ghana, bhṛṅga, guḍa tvak* and *svarṇa bhūmika*—these are synonymous.

**तेजपत्र**

पत्रं दलाह्वं तापसं तमालं रोम रोमशम्[19] ।

*Teja patra*

*Patra*, *dalāhva*, *tāpasa*, *tamāla*, *roma* and *romaśa*—these are synonymous.

**नागकेसर**

नागकेसरकं[20] नागं[21] चांपेयं केशरंजनम् ॥ १४ ॥

नागपुष्पं नागकिंजल्कं कनकं हेम कांचनम् ।

मारुह्यं हाटकं चैव जांबूनंद प्रकीर्त्तितम् ॥ १५ ॥

*Nāga kesara*

*Nāga kesaraka*, *nāga*, *cāmpeya*, *keśa rañjana*, *nāga puṣpa*, *nāga kiñjalka*, *kanaka*, *hema*, *kāñcana*, *māruhya*, *hāṭaka* and *jāmbūnada*—these are synonymous.

**त्रिसुगंधि, चतुर्ज्जातक**

एलादित्रिभिरुद्दिष्टं त्रिजातं त्रिसुगंधिकम् ।

चतुर्ज्जातं सनागं च द्वयं वातकफापहम् ॥ १६ ॥

*Trisugandhi and caturjāta*

*Elā*, *tvak* and *patra*—these three taken together are known as *trijāta* and also *trisugandhi*. Along with *nāga*, they are called *caturjāta*. Both of them alleviate *vāta* and *kapha*.

**तालीस**

तालीसपत्रं तालीसं धात्रीपर्ण्यं शुकोदरम् ।

अपरं ग्रंथिकापत्रं पत्राढ्यं[22] तुलसीच्छदः ॥ १७ ॥

*Tālīsa*

*Tālīsa patra*, *tālisa*, *dhatrī parṇī* and *śukodara*—these are the synonyms of *tālisa*.

It has another variety which is called *granthikā patra*, *patrāḍhya* and *tulasī chada.*

**सरल**

सरलो नंदनः[23] खेडो[24] नमेरुः पीतवृक्षकः ।

*Sarala*

*Sarala*, *nandana*, *kheḍa*, *nameru* and *pīta vṛkṣaka*—these are synonymous.

**श्रीवास**

श्रीवासो वेष्टको दासी श्रीनिवासः कपिद्रुमः ।।१८।।

*Śrīvāsa*

*Śrīvasa*, *veṣṭaka*, *dāsī*, *śrīnivāsa* and *kapi druma*—these are synonymous,

**बाला**

बालकं वारि ह्रीवेरं पिंगमानं[25] मनः[26] कचम् ।

उदीच्यं वज्रमंथाह्वं वरिष्ठं गंधमूलकम् ।। १९ ।।

*Bālā*

*Bālaka*, *vāri*, *hrīvera*, *piṅgamāna*, *mana*, *kaca*, *udīcya*, *vajra manthāhva*, *variṣṭha* and *gandha mūlaka*—these are synonymous.

**जटामांसी**

मांसी जटा भूतकेशी क्रव्यादी नलदं शिखा ।

कृष्णान्या पूतनाकेशी गंधमांसी पिशाचिका ।। २० ।।

*Jaṭā māṁsī*

*Māṁsī*, *jaṭā*, *bhūta keśī*, *kravyādi*, *nalada*, *śikhā*—these are the synonyms of *jaṭā māṁśī.*

There is another variety of it which is called *pūtanā*, *keśī*, *gandha māṁsī* and *piśācikā.*

**उशीर**

उशीरमभयं[27] सेव्यं वीरं वीरणमूलकम् ।

*Uśīra*

*Uśīra*, *abhaya*, *sevya*, *vīra* and *vīraṇa mūlaka*—these are synonymous.

**रेणुका**

रेणुका कपिला कौंती पांडुपुत्री हरेणुका ॥ २१ ॥

*Reṇukā*

*Reṇukā*, *kapilā*, *kauntī*, *pāṇḍu putrī* and *hareṇukā*.

**प्रियंगु**

प्रियंगु: फलिनी श्यामा कांताह्वा नंदिनी लता ।

*Priyaṅgu*

*Priyaṅgu*, *phalinī*, *śyāmā*, *kāntāhvā*, *nandinī* and *latā*—these are synonymous.

**पारिपेल**

पारिपेलं पुटं[28] वान्यं[29] शुकाह्वं पारिपेलवम्[30] ॥ २२ ॥

*Pāripela*

*Pāripela*, *puṭa*, *vānya*, *śukāhva* and *pāripelava*—these are synonymous.

**शैलेय**

शैलेयं[31] स्थविरं वृद्धं शिलापुष्पं शिलोद्भवम् ।

*Śaileya*

*Śaileya*, *sthavira*, *vṛddha*, *śilā puṣpa* and *śilodbhava*—these are synonymous.

**कुंदुरु**

कुंदुरुर्म्मेचक:[32] कंडू: खर्जूरो भीषणो बली ॥ २३ ॥

*Kunduru*

*Kunduru*, *mecaka*, *kaṇḍū*, *kharjara*, *bhiṣaṇa* and *balī*—these are synonymous.

**गुग्गुलु**

गुग्गुलुः सालनिर्यासो माहिषाक्षः पलंकषा ।
जटायु कौशिकोदुर्गः देवधूपः शिवः पुरः ॥ २४ ॥

*Guggulu*

*Guggulu*, *sāla niryāsa*, *mahiṣākṣa*, *palaṅkaṣā*, *jaṭāyu*, *kauśika*, *durga*, *deva dhūpa*, *śiva* and *pura*—these are synonymous.

**राल**

रालः सर्ज्जरसो यक्षधूपः सर्ज्जोग्निवल्लभः ।
क्षणकः शालनिर्य्यासो[33] लाख्यास्यललनो[34] वरः[35] ॥ २५ ॥

*Rāla*

*Rāla*, *sarja rasa*, *yakṣa dhūpa*, *sarja*, *agni vallabha*, *kṣaṇaka*, *śāla niryāsa*, *lākhyā*, *āsya lalana* and *vara*—these are synonymous.

**स्थौणेयक**

स्थौणेयकं बर्हचूडं शुकपर्णं शुकच्छदः ।

*Sthauṇeyaka*

*Sauṇeyaka*, *barha cūḍa*, *śuka parṇa* and *śuka chada*—these are synonymous.

**चोरक**

चोरकः कितवश्चंडो दुःपुत्रः शंकनो रिपुः ॥ २६ ॥

*Coraka*

*Coraka*, *kitava*, *caṇḍa*, *duḥputra*, *śaṁkana* and *ripu*—these are synonymous.

**एकांगी**

मुरा गंधवती दैत्या गंधाढ्या सुरभिः कुटिः ।

*Ekāṅgī*

*Murā*, *gandhavatī*, *daityā*, *gandhāḍhyā*, *surabhi* and *kuṭī*—these are synonymous.

**कर्चूर**

कर्चूरो द्रविडो गंधमूलको दुर्ल्लभः शटी[36] ॥ २७ ॥

*Karcūra*

*Karcūra*, *draviḍa*, *gandha mūlaka*, *durlabha* and *śaṭi*—these are synonymous.

**शटी**

शठी[37] पलाशी षडंग्रथा सुव्रता गंधमूलिनी ।

*Śaṭī*

*Śaṭhī*, *palāśī*, *ṣaḍgranthā*, *suvratā* and *gandha mūlinī*—these are synonymous.

**स्पृक्का**

स्पृक्का सृक् ब्राह्मणी देवी निर्म्माल्या कूलिला[38] वधूः ॥ २८ ॥

*Spṛkkā*

*Spṛkkā*, *sṛk*, *brāhmaṇī*, *devī*, *nirmālyā*, *kūlilā* and *vadhu*—these are synonymous.

**ग्रंथिपर्णी**

ग्रथिपर्णो नीलपुष्प[39] शुकपुष्पं विवर्णकम्[40] ।

*Granthi parṇī*

*Granthi parṇa*, *nīla puṣpa*, *śuka puṣpa* and *vivarṇaka*—these are synonymous.

**नली**

नलिका नर्त्तकी शून्या निर्मध्या धमनी नटी ॥ २९ ॥

*Nalī*

*Nalikā, nartakī, śūnyā, nīrmedhyā, dhamanī* and *naṭī*—these are synonymous.

**पद्मक**

पद्मकं मलयश्चारुः पीतरक्तश्च सुप्रभः ।

*Padmaka*

*Padmaka, malaya, cāru, pīta rakta* and *suprabha*—these are synonymous.

**पुंडरीक**

प्रपौंडरीकं पौंड्राह्वं शतपुष्पं सुपुष्पकम् ।। ३० ।।

*Puṇḍarīka*

*Prapauṇḍarīka, paundrāhva, śatapuṣpa* and *supuṣpaka*—these are synonymous.

**तगर**

तगरं वर्हिणं जिह्मं चक्राह्वं नहुषं नतम् ।
41
अपरं पिंडितगरं दीनं कटुमहोरगम् ।। ३१ ।।

*Tagara*

*Tagara, varhiṇa, jihma, cakrāhva, nahuṣa,* and *nata*—these are the synonyms of *tagara.*

There is another variety of it which is known as *piṇḍi tagara* and its synonyms are *dīna, kaṭn* and *mahoraga.*

**गोरोचना**

गोरोचना रुचिर्गौरी रोचना पिंगला मता ।

मंगल्या गौतभी मेध्या वंध्या गोपित्तसंभवा ।। ३२ ।।

*Gorocanā*

*Gorocanā, ruci, gaurī, rocanā, piṅgalā, maṅgalyā, gautamī, medhyā, vandhyā* and go *pitta sambhavā*—these are synonymous.

**नख**

नखांको नखरः शिल्पी हनुर्न्नागःहनुः खुरः ।
शुक्ति शंखो[42] व्याघ्रनखमन्याह्याह्यतलं पादम् ।। ३३ ।।

*Nakha*

*Nakhāṅka*, *nakhara*, *śilpī*, *hanurnāga*, *hanu*, *khura*, *śukti*, *śaṅkha* and *vyāghra nakha*—these are the synonyms of *nakha*.

There is another variety (of it) which is known as *hyāhya tala* and *pāda*.

**पतंग**

पत्तंगं पटरागं स्याद्रक्तकाष्ठं कुचंदनम् ।
सुरंगकं जगत्याह्वं[43] पत्तूरं पटरंजनम् ।। ३४ ।।

*Pataṅga*

*Pataṅga*, *paṭa rāga*, *rakta kāṣṭha*, *kucandana*, *suraṅgaka*, *jagatyāhva*, *pattūra* and *paṭa rañjana*—these are synonymous.

**लाक्षा**

लाक्षा निर्भत्सनो[44] रक्तद्रुम व्याधिः पलंकषा[45] ।
कृमिजा जन्तुदास्याह्वा[46] यावको रक्तको[47] मलः ।। ३५ ।।

*Lākṣā*

*Lākṣā*, *nirbharsana*, *rakta druma*, *vyādhi*, *palaṁkaṣā*, *kṛmijā*, *jantudā*, *āsyāhvā*, *yāvaka*, *raktaka* and *mala*—thrse are synonymous.

**पर्पटी**

पर्पटी रंजनी कृष्णा यतुका[48] जननी जनी ।

*Parpaṭī*

*Parpaṭī*, *rañjanī*, *kṛsṇā*, *yatukā*, *jananī* and *janī*—these are synonymous.

**पद्म**

पद्मिनी विशिनी ज्ञेया नलिनी सूर्य्यवल्लभा ।।३६।।

कुमुद्वती कैरविणी कुमुद्युडुपतिप्रिया ।

*Padma*

*Padminī*, *viśinī*, *nalinī*, *sūrya vallabhā*, *kumudvatī kairaviṇī kumudi* and *uḍupati priyā*—these are synonymous.

**पद्मचारिणी**

पद्मचारिण्यतिचरा पद्माह्वा चारटी मता ।। ३७ ।।

*Padma cāriṇī*

*Padma cāriṇī*, *aticarā*, *padmāhvā* and *cāraṭī*—these are synonymous.

**श्वेतकमल**

कमलं श्वेतमंभोजं सारसं सरसीरुहम् ।

सहस्रपत्रं श्रीगेहं शतपत्रं कुशेशयम् ।। ३८ ।।

पंकेरुहं तामरसं राजीवं पुष्करे रुहम् ।

अच्छमंभोरुहं पद्मं पुंडरीकं च पंकजम् ।। ३९ ।।

सरोजं नलिनी नीलमरविंदं महोत्पलम् ।

*Śveta kamala*

*Kamala*, *śvetamaṁbhoja*, *sārasa*, *sarasī ruha*, *sahasra patra*, *śrīgeha*, *śata patra*, *kuśeśaya*, *paṅkeruha*, *tāmarasa*, *rajīva*, *puṣkareruha*, *accha*, *aṁbhoruha*, *padma*, *puṇḍarīka*, *paṅkaja*, *saroja*, *nalinī*, *nīla*, *aravinda* and *mahotpala*—these are synonymous.

**रक्तोत्पल**

तेपलरक्तं कोकनदं हल्लक रक्तगंधिकम् ।। ४० ।।

*Raktotpala*

*Raktotpala, kokanada, hallaka* and *rakta gandhika*—these are synonymous.

**नीलोत्पल**

नीलोत्पलं कुवलयं भद्रमिंदीवरं मतम् ।

एतदेव सितंकिंचित्कुमुदं कैरवं कुमुत् ॥ ४१ ॥

*Nīlotpala*

*Nīlotpala, kuvalaya, bhadra* and *indīvara*—these are the synonyms of *nilotgala.*

It has another variety which is slightly wh te and its synonyms are *kumuda, kairava* and *kumut.*

**कल्हार**

कह्लारं ह्रस्वपाथोजं सौम्यं सौगंधिकं मतम् ।

*Kalhāra*

*Kalhāra, hrasva pāthoja, saumya* and *saugandhika*—these are synonymous.

**कमल केशर**

49

किंजल्कः केसरं गौरमापीतं कांचनाह्वयम् ॥ ४२ ॥

*Kamala keśara*

*Kiñjalka, kesara, gaura, āpīta* and *kāñcanāhvaya*—these are synonymous.

**पद्मबीज**

पद्मबीजं तु गालोढं पद्माह्वं पद्मकर्कटी ।

*Padma bīja*

*Padma bīja, gāloḍha, padmāhva* and *padma karkaṭi*—these are synonymous.

**मृणाल**

50
मृणालं विसमंभोजं नालं च नलिनीरुहम् ॥ ४३ ॥

*Mṛṇāla*

*Mṛṇāla, visa, ambhoja, nāla* and *nalinī ruha*—these are synonymous.

**शालूक**

51
पद्मादिमूलं शालूक शालीनं करहाटकः ।

*Śālūka*

*Śālūka, śālīna* and *karahāṭaka*—these are synonymous of the rhizome (*mūla*).of *padma* etc.

**जाती**

जाती प्रियंवदा राजी मालती सुमना मता ॥ ४४ ॥

पीतजात्यपरा पीतपुष्पा काञ्चनपुष्पिका ।

श्वेतजाती स्वर्णजाती वंधनामा जयंतिका ॥ ४५ ॥

*Jātī*

*Jātī, priyambadā, rājī, mālati* and *sumanā*—these are the synonyms of *jātī*.

There is another variety of it which is yellow in colour and it is called *pīta puṣpā* and *kāñcana puṣpikā*.

The white variety of it is called *śveta jātī, svarṇa jāti, vandha nāmā* and *jayantikā*.

**मालती**

52 53
मल्लिका मेदिनी मुक्ता बंधिनी मदयंतिका ।

*Mālatī*

*Mallikā, medinī, muktā, bandhinī* and *madayantika*—these sare ynonymous.

**यूथिका**

यूथिका हरिणी[54] बाला पुष्पगंधा शिखंडिनी[55] ॥ ४६ ॥

स्वर्णयूथी परापीता गणिका स्वर्णपुष्पिका[56] ।

*Yūthikā*

*Yūthikā, hariṇī, bālā, puṣpa gandhā, śikhaṇḍinī, svarṇa yūthī, parā pītā, gaṇikā* and *svarṇa puṣpikā*—thess are synonymous.

**सेवती**

कुब्जको भद्रतरणि बृहत्पुष्पा महासहा ॥ ४७ ॥

शतपुष्पा तरुण्युक्ता कर्णिका चारुकेसरा[57] ।

रक्तापरा रक्तपुष्पा लाक्षापुष्पातिमंजुला ॥ ४८ ॥

*Sevatī*

*Kubjaka, bhadra taraṇi, bṛhat puṣpā, mahā sahā, śata puṣpā, taruṇī, karṇikā* and *cāru kesarā*—these are the synonyms of *sevati.*

It has another variety having red flower and its synonyms are *rakta puṣpā, lākṣā puṣpā* and *atimañjulā.*

**केतकी**

केतकी सूचिका[58] पुष्पा जंबुकः कर्कशछदः ।

सुवर्णकेतकी चान्या लघुपुष्पा सुगंधिनी[59] ॥ ४९ ॥

*Ketakī*

*Ketakī, sūcikā puṣpā, jambuka* and *karkaśa chada*—these are the synonyms of *ketakī.*

It has another variety which is known as *suvarṇa ketakī, laghu puṣpā* and *sugandhinī.*

**वासंती**

वासंती सरला कुंदा प्रहसंती वसंतजा ।

*Vāsantī*

*Vasantī, saralā, kundā, prahasantī* and *vasantajā*—these are synonymous.

**माधवी**

नेपाली ग्रीष्मका लूता म्लायिनी वनमालिका ।।५०।।

वार्षिकी त्रिपुटा धन्या श्रीमती षड्पदप्रिया ।

माधवी मंडपः कामी पुष्पेंद्राभीष्टगंधकः ।। ५१ ।।

*Mādhavī*

*Nepālī, grīṣmakā, lūtā, mlāyinī, vana mālikā, vārṣikī, tripuṭā, dhanyā, śrimatī, ṣaḍpada priyā, mādhavī, maṇḍapa kāmī, puṣpendra* and *abhiṣṭa gandhaka*—these are synonymous.

**पुन्नाग**

चंपकः कांचनो रम्यश्चांपेयः सुरभिश्चलः[60] ।

पुन्नागः पाटलीपुष्पः केशरः[61] षट्पदालयः ।। ५२ ।।

*Punnāga*

*Campaka, kāñcana, ramya, cāmpeya, surabhi, cala, punnāga, pāṭalī puṣpa, keśara* and *ṣaṭpadālaya*—these are synonymous.

**वकुल**

वकुलः केसरी[62] मद्यगंध सिंहो विशारदः ।

वुकोवंक्र[63] स्थूलपुष्पो वसुकः शिवशेखरः ।। ५३ ।।

*Vakula*

*Vakula, kesara, madyagandha, simha* and *viśārada, vūkovaka, sthūla puṣpa, vasuka* and *śiva śekhara*—these are synonymous.

**कुंद**

कुंदः शुल्कः सदापुष्पो भृंगबंधुर्म्मनोरमः ।

***Kunda***

*Kunda, śukla, sadā puṣpa, bhṛnga bandhu* and *manorama*—these are synonymous.

**मुचकुन्दः**

मुचकुंदः क्षत्रवृक्षः चिवुकं प्रतिविष्णुकः ॥ ५४ ॥

*Muca kunda*

*Mucu kunda, ksatra vṛkṣa, civuka* and *prati visṇuka*—these are synonymous.

**वेला**

भूमंडली बिंबकिलो[64] द्विपदाष्टपदी तथा ।

तिलका क्षुरकः श्रीमान् विचित्रो मुखमंडनः ॥ ५५ ॥

गणेरुका कर्णिकारिः कर्णिश्च गणिकारिका ।

*Velā*

*Bhū maṇḍalī, bimba kila, dvipadā, aṣṭapadī, tilakā, kṣuraka, śrīmān, vicitra, mukha maṇḍana, gaṇerukā, karṇikāra, karṇi* and *gaṇikārikā*—these are synonymous.

**बंधुजीव**

बंधुजीवः शरत्पुष्पो वंधवंधूक[65] रक्तकः ॥ ५६ ॥

***Bandhu jīva***

*Bandhu jīva, śarat puṣpa, bandha bandhuka* and *raktaka*—these are synonymous.

**जपा**

जपापुष्पं जपारक्तं त्रिसंध्या वरुणाऽसिता ।

*Japā*

*Japā puṣpa, japā rakta, tri sandhyā, varuṇā* and *asitā*—these are synonymous.

**सिंदूरी**

सिंदूरी रक्तबीजा स्याद्रक्तपुष्पा सुकोमला ॥ ५७ ॥

***Sindūrī***

*Śindūrī, rakta **bījā, rakta puṣpā*** and *sukomala*—these are synonymous.

**तुलशी**

[66]तुलशी सुरसा गौरी भूतघ्नी वहुमंजरी ।

अपेतराक्षसी ग्राम्या सुलला[67] देवदुंदुभिः ॥ ५८ ॥

*Tulaśī*

*Tulaśī, surasā, gaurī, bhūtaghnī, vahu mañjarī, apeta rākṣasī, grāmyā, sulalā, deva dundubhi*—these are synonymous.

**मरुवक**

[68]मरुवन् मरुकस्तीक्ष्णः खरपत्रः फणिज्जकः ।

*Maruvaka*

*Maruvan, maruka, tīkṣṇa, khara patra, phaṇijjaka*—these are synonymous.

**दमन**

दमनो मदनो दांतः दमो मुनिसुतो मुनिः ॥ ५९ ॥

गंधोत्कटो दमनको विनीतः कुलपुत्रकः ।

***Damana***

*Damana, madana, dānta, dama, muni suta, muni, gandhotkaṭa, damanaka, vinīta* and *kula putraka*—these are synonymous.

**कुठेरक**

वर्व्वरी त्वर्ज्जकः कुंठो वैकुंठः स्यात्कुठेरकः ॥ ६० ॥

कपित्थार्ज्जक इत्यन्यो वटपत्रः कैटिजरः ।

[69]कृष्णार्ज्जकः कालमाता करालः कृष्णमल्लिका ॥६१॥

***Kuṭheraka***

***Varvarī,*** *arjaka, kuṇṭha, vaikuṇṭha, kuṭheraka* and

*kapitthārjaka*—there are the synonyms of *kuṭheraka.*

There is another variety of it which is known as *vaṭa patra, katijara, kṛṣṇārjaka, kāla mātā, karāla* and *kṛṣṇa mallikā.*

## NOTES AND REFERENCES

1. This is the 92nd chapter of *Ayurveda saukhyaṁ* in *Toḍarānanda* and the opening invocation reads as below ;

ब्रह्मांडनाथो वसुदेवसूनुर्व्रजांगनावाक्यवशो मुकुंदः ।

वसुंधरायाः प्रभुतां समस्तां श्रीटोडरे सर्वसुखं विधत्ताम् ॥

2. 'भूतिकरक्त' इति षष्ठपुस्तके पाठः ।
3. 'वेध्य' इति षष्ठपुस्तके पाठः ।
4. 'पूतिका' इति पंचमपुस्तके पाठः ।
   'भूतिका' इति षष्ठपुस्तके पाठः ।
5. 'पूतिकर' इति षष्ठपुस्तके पाठः ।
   'प्रीतिकचः' इति प्रथमपुस्तके पाठः ।
6. 'स्यङ्गधवेलिका' इति षष्ठपुस्तके पाठः ।
   'गंधवेलिका' इति पंचमपुस्तके पाठः ।
7. 'नारायंणलयं' इति प्रथमपुस्तके पाठः ।
8. 'पीतम' श्राह्वम् इति प्रथमपुस्तके पाठः ।
9. 'शकं' इति प्रथमपुस्तके पाठः ।
10. 'सुरुष्क' इति प्रथमपुस्तके पाठः ।
11. 'एवालुकम्' श्रनर्वालु इति प्रथमपुस्तके पाठः ।
12. 'सूतं' इति पंचमपुस्तके पाठः ।
13. 'शालुकं' इति पष्ठपुस्तके पाठः ।
14. 'जातिपत्री' इति प्रथमपुस्तके पाठः ।
15. 'लवंगं' इति प्रथमपुस्तके पाठः ।

16. 'मारिचं' इति षष्ठपुस्तके पाठः ।
17. 'माधवोषितं' इति पंचमपुस्तके पाठः ।
18. 'त्रिदिवाद्भिदा' इति षष्ठपुस्तके पाठः ।
19. 'ललाटपर्ण्यं' इति प्रथमपुस्तके पाठः ।
20. 'रोमसं' इति प्रथमपुस्तके पाठः ।
21. 'नागकेशरकं' इति पंचमपुस्तके पाठः ।
22. 'नामं' इति प्रथमपुस्तके पाठः ।
23. 'तुलसीछदः' इति पंचमपुस्तके पाठः ।
24. 'मदन' इति पंचमपुस्तके पाठः ।
25. 'पीडा' इति षष्ठपुस्तके पाठः ।
26. 'पिगलं' इति पंचमपुस्तके पाठः ।
27. 'मनं' इति पंचमपुस्तके पाठः ।
28. 'उसीरमभयं' इति प्रथमपुस्तके पाठः ।
29. 'वारिपेलं' इति प्रथमपुस्तके पाठः ।
30. 'चाण्यं' इति प्रथमपुस्तके पाठः ।
31. 'परिपेलनं' इति षष्ठपस्तके पाठः ।
32. 'शिलेयं' इति षष्ठपुस्तके पाठः ।
33. 'कंटु' इति षष्ठपुस्तके पाठः ।
34. 'सालनिर्य्यासो' इति प्रथमपुस्तके पाठः ।
35. 'ललवनो' इति प्रथमपुस्तके पाठः ।
36. 'चरः' इति प्रथमपुस्तके पाठः ।
37. 'सटी' इति प्रथमपुस्तंके पाठः ।
38. 'शटी' इति पंचमपुस्तके पाठः ।
'सटी' इति प्रथमपुस्तके पाठः ।
39. 'कुटिला' इति पंचमपुस्तके पाठः ।
40. 'नालपुष्पं' इति पंचमपुस्तके पाठः ।
41. 'विकर्णकं' इति पष्ठपुस्तके पाठः ।
42. 'पिंडतगरं' इति पंचमषष्ठपुस्तकयोः पाठः ।

43. 'संखो' इति प्रथमपुस्तके पाठः ।
44. 'जगन्याह्वं' इति षष्ठपुस्तके पाठः ।
45. 'निर्भत्स्वरा' इति पंचमपुस्तके पाठः ।
'निर्भत्सरा' इति षष्ठपुस्तके पाठः ।
46. 'फलम्' इति प्रथमपुस्तके पाठः ।
47. 'नालको' इति पंचमपुस्तके पाठः ।
48. 'नलः' इति षष्ठपुस्तके पाठः ।
49. 'जतुका' इति षष्ठपुस्तके पाठः ।
50. 'केशरं' इति पंचमपुस्तके पाठः ।
51. 'विषमंभोजम्' इति प्रथमपुस्तके पाठः ।
52. 'शालीनी' इति षष्ठपुस्तके पाठः ।
53. 'मेदनी' इति पंचमपुस्तके पाठः ।
'नंदनी' इति षष्ठपुस्तके पाठः ।
54. 'वंधनं' इति प्रथमपुस्तके पाठः ।
55. 'हरणी' इति प्रथमपुस्तके पाठः ।
56. 'सिखंडिनी' इति प्रथमपुस्तके पाठः ।
57. 'स्वर्णयूथिका' इति प्रथमपुस्तके पाठः ।
58. 'केशरा' इति षष्ठपुस्तके पाठः ।
59. 'सूतिका' इति पंचमपुस्तके पाठः ।
'सूविका' इति षष्ठपुस्तके पाठः ।
60. 'सुगंधिका' इति पंचमपुस्तके पाठः
61. 'सुरभीश्चलः' इति षष्ठपुस्तके पाठः ।
62. 'केसरः' इति प्रथमपुस्तके पाठः ।
63. 'केशरो' इति पंचमपुस्तके पाठः ।
64. 'चूकोवक' इति षष्ठपुस्तके पाठः ।
65. 'विचकिलो' इति पंचमपुस्तके पाठः ।
66. 'वंधवंधुक' इति षष्ठपुस्तके पाठः ।
67. 'तुलसी' इति षष्ठपुस्तके पाठः ।

68. 'सुरला' इति षष्ठपुस्तके पाठः ।
'सुलभा' इवि पंचमपुस्तके पाठः ।

69. 'मखन्' इति षष्ठपुस्तके पाठः ।

70. 'कालभाला' इति पंचमपुस्तके पाठः ।
'कालभाना' इति षष्ठपुस्तके पाठः ।

71. This is the end of 92nd chapter of *Ayurveda Saukhyaṁ* in Toḍarānanda and the Colophon reads as below ;

इति श्रीमहाराजाधिराजटोडरमल्लविरचिते टोडरानंदे श्रायुर्वेदसौख्ये कर्पूरादिवर्गे निघंटौ षडशीतितमो (?) हर्षः ।

# CHAPTER 34

**सुवर्ण**[1]

सुवर्ण कनकं हेम हाटकं ब्रह्मकांचनम्[2] ।
चामीकरं शतकुंभं तपनीयं च रुक्मकम् ।
जांबूनदं हिरण्यं च सुरत्नं[3] जातरुपकम् ॥ १ ॥

*Suvarṇa*

*Suvarṇa, kanaka, hema, hāṭaka, brahma kāñcana, cāmikara, śata kumbha, tapanīya, rukmaka, jāmbū nada, hiraṇya, suratna* and *jāta rūpaka*—these are synonymous.

**रुप्यक**

रुप्यकं रजतं कुष्ठं[4] तारं श्वेतं वसूत्तमम् ।

*Rupyaka*

*Rupyaka, rajata, kuṣṭha, tāra, śveta* and *vasūttama*—these are synonymous.

**ताम्र**

ताम्रं म्लेछमुख शुल्वं नैपालं रविनामकम् ॥ २ ॥

*Tāmra*

*Tāmra, mlecha mukha. śulva. naipāla* and *ravi nāmaka*—these are synonymous.

**कांस्य**

कांस्यं लोहं निजघोषं पंचलोहं प्रकाशनम् ।। ३ ।।

*Kāṁsya*

*Kāṁsya, loha, nija ghoṣa, pañca loha* and *prakāśana*—these are synonymous.

**पित्तल**

पीतलोहं कपिलोहं[5] कपिलं सौख्यमारकम् ।

वर्त्तलोहं नृलोहं च रजनी निर्म्महेश्वरी ।। ४ ।।

*Pittala*

*Pīta loha, kapi loha, kapila, saukhya māraka, varta loha, nṛloha, rajanī* and *nirmaheśvarī*—these are synonymous.

**वंग**

रंगस्तु[6] खुरकं वंगं त्रपुस्यात्करटी घनम् ।

*Vaṅga*

*Raṅga, khuraka, vaṅga. trapu, karaṭī* and *ghana*—these are synonymous.

**नाग**

सीसं धातुभवं नागमुरगं परिपिष्टकम् ।। ५ ।।

*Nāga*

*Sīsa, dhātu bhava, nāga, uraga* and *pari piṣṭaka*—these are synonymous.

**लौह**

लोहं[7] शस्त्रमयः कुष्टं खंडं पारावतं घनम् ।

*Lauha*

*Loha*, *śastra*, *ayaḥ*, *kuṣṭha*, *khaṇḍa*, *pārāvata* and *ghana*—these are synonymous.

**मंडूर**

कृष्णायस्तन्मलं किट्टं मंडूरं लोहजं रजः ॥ ६ ॥

*Maṇḍūra*

*Kṛṣṇāyaḥ mala*, *kiṭṭa*, *maṇḍūra*, *lohaja* and *rajas*—these are synonymous.

**पारद**

पारदश्चपलो हेमनिधिः सूतो रसोत्तमः ।

त्रिनेत्रो रोषणः स्वामी हरबीजं रसः प्रभुः ॥ ७ ॥

*Pārada*

*Pārada*, *capala*, *hema nidhi*, *sūta*, *rasottama*, *trinetra*, *roṣaṇa*, *svāmīn*, *hara bīja*, *rasa* and *prabhu*—these are synonymous.

**अभ्र**

अभ्रकं स्वच्छमाकाशं पटलं वरपीतकम् ।

*Abhra*

*Abhraka*, *svaccha*, *ākāśa*, *paṭala* and *vara pītaka*—these are synonymous.

**गंधक**

गंधः सौगंधिको लेली गंधास्मा गंधपीतक ॥ ८ ॥

*Gandhaka*

*Gandha*, *saugandhika*, *lelī*, *gandhāsma* and *gandha pītaka*—these are synonymous.

**माक्षीक**

माक्षीकं धातुमाक्षीकं ताप्यं तापीजमुच्यते ।

*Mākṣīka*

*Mākṣīka, dhātu mākṣīka, tāpya* and *tāpīja*—these are synonymous.

**मनःशिला**

मनःशिला शिला गोला नैपाली[8] कुनटी कुला ।

दिव्यौषधिर्न्नागमाता मनोगुप्ता मनोह्विका ॥ ९ ॥

*Manaḥśilā*

*Manaḥ śilā, śilā, golā, naipālī, kunaṭī. kulā, divyauṣadhi, nāga mātā, mano guptā* and *manohvikā*—these are synonymous.

**हरिताल**

हरितालं मल्लं तालं गोदंतं नटभूषणम् ॥ १० ॥

*Haritāla*

*Haritāla, malla, tāla, godanta* and *naṭa bhūṣaṇa*—these are synonymous.

**गैरिक**

गैरिकं रक्तपाषाणां गिरिमृच्च गवेरुकम् ।

स्वर्णवर्णं परंवर्णं[9] मंडनं स्वर्णगैरिकम् ॥ ११ ॥

*Gairika*

*Gairika, rakta pāṣāṇa, giri mṛt, gaveruka, svarṇa varṇa, paraṁ varṇa, maṇḍana* and *svarṇa gairika*—these are synonymous.

**तुत्थ**

तुत्थं खर्प्परिकातुत्थममृतासंगमुच्यते ।

मयूरग्रीवकं चान्यत् शिखिकंठं च तुत्थकम् ॥ १२ ॥

*Tuttha*

*Tuttha, kharparikā tuttha* and *amṛtā saṅga*—these are synonyms of *tuttha*.

Another variety of it is called *mayūra grīvaka* and its synonyms are *śikhi kaṇṭha* and *tutthaka.*

**कासीस**

कासीसं धातुकासीसं खेचरं तप्तलोमशम् ।

*Kāsīsa*

*Kāsīsa, dhātu kasīsa, khecara* and *tapta lomaśa.*

**पुष्प कासीस**

अपरं पुष्पकासीसं तुवरं वस्त्रागहृत्[10] ॥ १३ ॥

*Puṣpa kāsīsa*

Another variety of *kāsīsa* is called *puṣpa kāsīsa* and its synonyms are *tuvara* and *vastra rāga hṛt.*

**हिंगुल**

हिंगुलं दरदं म्लेछं[11] सौकतं चूर्णपारदम् ।

*Hiṅgula*

*Hiṅgula, darada, mlecha, saukata* and *cūrṇa pārada*—these are synonymous.

**सिंदूर**

सिंदूरं नागजं रक्तं श्रीमत् शृंगारभूषणम् ।
वसंतमंडनं[12] नागगर्भं रक्तरजस्तथा ॥ १४ ॥

*Sindūra*

*Sindūra, nāgaja, rakta, śrīmat, sṛṅgāra bhūṣaṇa, vasanta. maṇḍana, nāga garbha* and *rakta raja*—these are synonymous.

**सौवीर अंजन**

सौवीरमंजनं कृष्णं कालं नीलं सुवीरजम् ।

*Sauvīra añjana*

*Sauvīra, añjana, kṛṣṇa, kāla, nīla* and *suvīraja*—these are synonymous.

**स्रोतोऽञ्जन**

13

स्रोतोंजनं तु स्रोतोजं नदीजं यामुनं वरम् ।। १५ ।।

*Srotoñjana*

*Srotañjana*, *srotoja*, *nadīja*, *jāmuna* and *vara*—these are synonymous.

**रसाञ्जन**

रसांजनं रसोद्भूतं तार्क्ष्शैलं च वार्षिकम् ।

रसाग्र्यं कृत्रिमं तार्क्ष्यं दिव्यं दार्व्या रसोद्भवम् ।।१६।।

*Rasāñjana*

*Rasāñjana*, *rasodbhūta*, *tārkṣa śaila*, *vārṣika* and *rasāgrya*—these are the synonyms of *rasāñjana*.

It is also prepared artificially which is known as *tārksya*, *divya* and *dārvī rasodbhava*.

**पुष्पांजन**

14

पुष्पांजनं पुष्पकेतु रीतिजं कुसुमांजनम् ।। १७ ।।

*Puṣpāñjana*

*Puṣpāñjana*, *puṣpa ketu*, *rītija* and *kusumāñjana*—these are synonymous.

**शिलाजतु**

शिलाजत्वश्मजं शैलनिर्यासो गिरिसाह्वयम् ।

शिलाह्वं गिरिजं शैलं गैरेयं गिरिजत्वपि ।। १८ ।।

*Silājatu*

*Śilājatu*, *asmaja*, *śaila niryāsa*, *girisāhvaya*, *śilāhva*, *girija*, *śaila*, *gaireya* and *giri jatu*—these are synonymous.

**बोल**

15

बोलं गंधरसं पौरं निल्लोंहं वार्व्वरं बलम् ।

*Bola*

*Bola, gandha rasa, paura, nirloha, vārvara* and *bala*—these are synonymous.

**स्फटिका**

स्फटिकाख्यामृता [16]वंध्या कांक्षी सौराष्ट्रसंभवा ।
[17]आढकी तुवरी त्वन्या मृत्तिका सुरमृत्तिका ।। १९ ।।

*Sphaṭikā*

*Sphaṭikā, amṛtā, vandhyā, kāṁkṣī, saurāṣṭra saṁbhavā, āḍhakī* and *tuvarī*—these are the synonyms of *sphaṭikā*.

It has another variety whose synonyms are *mṛttikā* and *sura mṛttikā*.

**समुद्रफेन**

समुद्रफेनो डिंडरिः फेनो वारिकफोब्धिजः ।। २० ।।

*Samudra phena*

*Samudra phena, ḍiṇḍari, phena, vari kapha* and *abdhija*—these are synonymous.

**प्रवाल**

प्रवालं विद्रूमं सिंधुलताग्रं रक्तवर्णकम् ।

*Pravāla*

*Pravāla, vidrūma, sindhu latāgra* and *rakta varṇaka*—these are synonymous.

**मुक्ता**

मौक्तिकं [18]मोतिक मुक्ताफलं मुक्ता [19]च शुक्तिजम् ।।२१।।

*Muktā*

*Mauktika, motika, muktā phala, muktā* and *śuktija*—these are synonymous.

**माणिक्य**

माणिक्यं पद्मरागं स्याद्वसुरत्नं सुरत्नकम् ।

*Māṇikya*

*Māṇikya. padma rāga, vasu ratna* and *suratnaka*—these are synonymous.

**सूर्यकांत**

सूर्यकांतः सूर्यमणिः सूर्याख्यो दहनोपलः ॥ २२ ॥

*Sūrya kānta*

*Sūrya kānta, sūrya maṇi, sūryākhya* and *dahanopala*—these are synonymous.

**चन्द्रकांत**

चंद्रकांतश्चद्रमणिः[20] स्फटिकः स्फटिकोमलः ।

*Candra kānta*

*Candra kānta, candra maṇi, sphaṭika* and *sphaṭikomala*—these are synonymous.

**गोमेद**

गोमेदः सुन्दरं पीतं रक्तं तृणचरं तथा ॥ २३ ॥

*Gomeda*

*Gomeda, sundara, pīta, rakta* and *tṛṇa cara*—these are synonymous.

**हीरा**

हीरकं विदुरं वज्रं स्वारिचक्रं[21] च तारकम् ।

*Hīrā*

*Hīraka, vidura, vajra, svāricakra* and *tāraka*—these are synonymous.

**वैडूर्य**

नीलरत्नं नीलमणिः वैडूर्यं[22] वालवज्जंनम्[23] ॥ २४ ॥

*Vaidūrya*

*Nīla ratna, nīla maṇi, vaidūrya* and *vāla varjana*—these are synonymous.

**मरकत**

गुरुत्मतं मरकतं दृषद्गर्भो हरिन्मणिः । 24

*Marakata*

*Garut mat, marakata, dṛṣadgarbha* and *harin maṇi*—these are synonymous.

**शुक्ति**

मुक्तास्फोटोब्धिमंडूकी शुक्तिमौक्तिकमंदिरम् ।। २५ ।।

*Śukti*

*Muktā sphoṭa, abdhi maṇḍukī, śukti* and *mauktika mandira*-these are synonymous.

**शंख**

शंखं कंबुर्ज्जलचरो वारिजो दीर्घनिस्वनः ।

*Śaṁkha*

*Saṁkha, kaṁbu, jala cara, vārija* and *dīrgha nisvana*—these are synonymous.

**लघुशंख**

शंखो लघुः शंखनकः शंबूको वारिशुक्तयः ।। २६ ।।

*Laghu śaṁkha*

*Laghu saṁkha, śaṁkhanaka, śambūka* and *vāri śukti*—these are synonymous.

**कर्पादका**

कपर्दा क्षुरका ज्ञेया खरा च खरवाटिका ।

*Kapardikā*

*Kapardā, kṣurakā, kharā* and *khara vātikā*—these are synonymous.

**खटिका**

खटीमकोलः[25] खटिनी[26] श्वेतानाडी तरंगकः ॥ २७ ॥

*Khaṭikā*

*Khaṭī, makola, khaṭinī, śvetā nāḍī* and *taraṅgaka*—these are synonymous.

**गौडपाषाण**

तद्भेदो गौडपाषाणः क्षीरपाक उदाहृतः ।

*Gauḍa pāṣāṇa*

A variety of *khaṭī* is called *gauḍa pāṣāṇa* and its synonym is *kṣīra pāka*.

**पंक, वालुका**

पंक कर्दमको ज्ञेयो वालुकाः सिकतास्तथा ॥ २८ ॥

*Paṅka and Vālukā*

*Paṅka* is called *kardamaka* and *vālukā* is called *sikatā*.

**चुंबकपाषाण**

चुंबकः[27] कांतपाषाणोऽयस्कांतो लोहकर्षकः ।

*Cuṁbaka pāṣāṇa*

***Cumbaka***, *kānta pāṣāṇa, ayaskānta* and *loha karṣaka*—these are synonymous.

**काच**

काचः कृत्रिमरत्नं स्यात् पिंगणः काचभाजनम् ॥२९॥

*Kāca*

***Kāca***, *kṛtrima ratna, piṅgaṇa* and *kāca bhājana*—these are synonymous.

## NOTES AND REFERENCES

1. This is the 93rd chapter of *Ayurveda Saukhyaṁ in Toḍarānanda* and the opening invocation reads as below :

पद्मालया कृष्णहृदालया सती पादांवुजं कामयतेन्यसेवितम् ।

समत्सरा सा तुलसीपदे सदा श्री टोडरेतेलयुतास्तु संस्थिता ।

2. भर्म्मकांचनं इति पंचमपुस्तके पाठः ।
3. सुरत्नं इति प्रथमपुस्तके पाठः ।
4. सुर्य्यं इति षष्ठपुस्तके पाठः ।
5. सहिद्रनकं इति प्रथमपुस्तके पाठः ।
6. वंगकंतीरकं इति प्रथमपुस्तके पाठः ।
7. रोध्रं इति प्रथमपुस्तके पाठः ।
8. नेपाली इति प्रथमपुस्तके पाठः ।
9. मंडलं इति षष्ठपुस्तके पाठः ।
10. वस्त्ररागदृक् इति प्रथमपुस्तके पाठः ।
11. सौकंदं इति प्रथमपुस्तके पाठः ।
12. वसंतमंडलं इति षष्ठपुस्तके पाठः ।
13. चरं इति षष्ठपुस्तके पाठः ।
14. रीभिजं इति प्रथमपुस्तके पाठः ।
15. वर्वरश्चरं इति षष्ठपुस्तके पाठः ।
16. वष्पी इति प्रथमपुस्तके पाठः ।
17. श्राटकी इति षष्ठपुस्तके पाठः ।
18. मौलिकं इति पंचमपुस्तके पाठः । शौक्तिकं इति षष्ठपुस्तके पाठः ।
19. सुक्तिजं इति प्रथमपुस्तके पाठः । शौक्तिकं षष्ठपुस्तके पाठः ।
20. चंद्रकांतभद्रमणिः इति षष्ठपुस्तके पाठः ।
21. स्वरि इति षष्ठपुस्तके पाठः ।
22. वैदूर्यं इति षष्ठपुस्तके पाठः ।

23. वालवह्वहं इति षष्ठपुस्तके पाठः ।

24. इषग्दंभं इति प्रथमपुस्तके पाठः ।

55. खटिमकालः इति षष्ठपुस्तके पाठः ।

26. नरंगतः इति षष्ठपुस्तके पाठः ।

27. कंवुकः इति षष्ठपुस्तके पाठः ।

This is the end of the 93rd chapter in *Ayurveda Saukhyaṁ* in *Toḍarānanda* and the colophon reads as below :

इति श्रीमहाराजाधिराजटोडरमल्लविरचिते टोडरानंदे आयुर्वेदसौख्ये निघंटौ स्वर्णादिवर्गः सप्ताशीतितमोहर्षः (?) ।

# CHAPTER 35

**वट**[1]

वटो रक्तफलः[2] क्षीरी वहुपादो वनस्पतिः ।

यक्षवासः प दरोहि[3] न्यग्रोधः स्कंदपा[4] ध्रुवः ॥ १ ॥

*Vaṭa*

*Vaṭa*, *rakta phala*, *kṣīrī*, *vahu pāda*, *vanaspati*, *yakṣa vāsa*, *pāda rohi*, *nyagrodha*, *skandapa* and *dhruva*—these are synonymous.

**अश्वत्थ**

पिप्पलः श्यामलोऽश्वत्थः क्षीरवृक्षो गजाशनः ।

हरिवासश्चलदलो मंगल्यो वोधिपादयः ॥ २ ॥

*Aśvattha*

*Pippala*, *śyāmala*, *aśvattha*, *ksīra vṛkṣa*, *gajāśana*, *hari vāsa*, *cala dala*, *maṅgalya* and *vodhi pādapa*—these are synonymous.

**उदुंबर**

उदुंबरः क्षीरवृक्षो जंतुवृक्षः सदाफलः ।

हेमदुग्धः कृमिफलो यज्ञांगः शीतवल्कलः ॥ ३ ॥

*Udumbara*

*Udumbara*, *kṣīra vṛkṣa*, *jantu vṛkṣa*, *sadā phala*, *hema dugdha*, *kṛmi phala*, *yajñāṅga* and *śīta vālkala*—these are synonymous.

**काष्ठोदुम्बर**

काकोदुंबरिका फल्गुर्म्मलयूः[5][6] श्वित्रभेषजम् ।

*Kāṣṭhodumbara*

*Kākodumbarikā*, *phalgu*, *malayu* and *śvitra bheṣaja*—these are synonymous.

**प्लक्ष**

प्लक्षः पृयश्चारुवृक्षः[7] स्वपार्श्वो गर्द्दभांडकः ॥ ४ ॥

वटी[8] कमंडलुः ।

*Plakṣa*

*Plakṣa*, *pṛya*, *cāru vṛkṣa*, *svapārśva*, *gardhabhāṇḍaka*, *vaṭi* and *kamaṇḍalu*—these are synonymous.

**नंदी**

नंदी वृक्षोऽश्वत्थभेदः प्ररोही गजपादपः ।

*Nandī*

A variety of *aśvattha* is called *nandī vṛkṣa*. Its synonyms are *prarohī* and *gaja pādapa*.

**कदम्ब**

कदम्बो गंधमत्पुष्पः प्रावृषेण्यो महोन्नतिः ।

अन्यो धूलिकदंबः स्यान्नीपो राजकदंबकः ॥ ५ ॥

*Kadamba*

*Kadamba, gandhamat puṣpa, prāvṛṣeṇya,* and *mahonnati*—these are the synonyms of *kadmaba.*

A variety of it is called *dhuli kadamba.* Its synonyms are *nīpa* and *rāja kadamba.*

**अर्जुन**

ककुभोर्ज्जुननामस्यान्नंदी सर्ज्जः शठद्रुमः ॥ ६ ॥

*Arjuna*

*Kakubha, arjuna, nandī, sarja* and *śaṭha druma*—these are synonymous.

**शिरीष**

शिरीषः प्लवगोविप्रः शुकवृक्षः कपीतनः ।

मृदुपुष्पः श्यामवर्णो भंडीरनीफलस्तथा ॥ ७ ॥

*Śirīṣa*

*Śirīṣa, plavaga, vipra, śuka vṛkṣa, kapītana, mṛdu puṣpa, syāma varṇa* and *bhaṇḍīranī phala*—these are synonymous.

**आर्तगल**

अर्गटः[9] स्यादार्त्तगलो वहुकंटः प्रतर्षणः ।

*Ārtagala*

*Argaṭa, ārta gala, vahu kaṇṭa* and *pratarṣaṇa*—these are synonymous.

**वेतस**

वेतसो वंजुलो नम्रो[10] वानीरो दीर्घपत्रकः ।

नादेयो मेघपुष्पो[11]न्यस्तोयकामो निकुंजकः ॥ ८ ॥

*Vetasa*

*Vetasa, vañjula, namra, vānīra, dīrgha patraka, nādeya* and *megha puṣpa*—these are the synonyms of *vetasa.*

There is another variety of it which is called *toya kāma* and *nikuñjaka*.

**जलवेतस**

जलौकासंवृतोंऽभोजो निचुलो जलवेतसः ।

*Jala vetasa*

*Jalaukā saṁvṛta*, *ambhoja*, *nicula* and *jala vetasa*—these are synonymous.

**समुद्रफल**

इज्जलो हिज्जलो गुछाफलः स्यात्कछपालिका[12] ॥ ९ ॥

*Samudra phala*

*Ijjala*, *hijjala*, *gucchā phala* and *kaccha pālikā*—these are synonymous.

**श्लेष्मातक**

श्लेष्मातकः कर्व्वुदारः पिच्छिलो भूतपादपः ।

शेलुः शैलश्च शैलुकः शैलूको द्विजकुत्सकः[13] ॥ १० ॥

*Śleṣmātaka*

*Śleṣmātaka*, *karvudāra*, *picchila*, *bhūta pādapa*, *śelu*, *śaila*, *śailuka*, *śailūka* and *dvija kutsaka*—these are synonymous.

**पीलु**

पीलुः शीत सहस्राक्षी तीक्ष्णद्रुः करभप्रियः ॥ ११ ॥

सहस्रांगी गुडफला[14] तत्फलं पीलु पीलुजम् ।

*Pīlu*

*Pīlu*, *śīta*, *sahasrākṣī*, *tīkṣṇadru*, *karabha priya*, *sahasrāṅgī* and *guḍa phalā*—these are the synonyms of *pīlu tree*.

Its fruits are called *pīlu* and *pīluja*.

**साक**

साकः[15] करछदो भूमीसहो दीर्घछदो मतः ॥ १२ ॥

*Śāka*

*Sāka, kara chada, bhūmī saha* and *dīrgha chada*—these are synonymous.

**शाल**

शालः सर्जरसः सर्ज्जः श्रीकृन्मारीचपत्रकः । 16

*Śāla*

*Śāla, sarja rasa, sarja, śrīkṛt* and *mārica patraka*—these are synonymous.

**तमाल**

तमाल उक्तस्तापिच्छः कालस्कंधोऽसितद्रुमः ॥ १३ ॥

*Tamāla*

*Tamāla, tāpiñcha, kāla skandha* and *asita druma*—these are synonymous.

**खदिर**

खदिरो रक्तसारं स्याद्गायत्री बालपत्रिका । 17

खदिरः श्वेतसारोन्यः कार्म्मुकः कुब्जकंटकः ॥ १४ ॥

*Khadira*

*Khadira, rakta sāra, gāyatrī* and *vāla patrikā*—these are the synonyms of *khadira*.

It has another variety which is known as *śveta sāra, kārmuka* and *kubja kaṇṭaka*.

**विट्खदिर**

इरिमेदो विट्खदिरो गोधास्कंधोऽरिमेदकः ।

*Viṭ khadira*

*Irimeda, viṭ khadira, godhā skandha* and *arimedaka*—these are synonymous.

**बब्बूल**

बब्बूलः किंकिरात स्यात् शीतकः पीतपुष्पकः ।।१५।।

*Babbula*

*Babbula*, *kiṁ kirāta*, *śītaka* and *pīta puṣpaka*—these are synonymous.

**विजय सार**

वीजकः सनकः सौरीप्रियः काम्पोलकप्रियः ।

*Vijaya sāra*

*Vījaka*, *sanaka*, *saurī priya* and *kāmpolaka priya*—these are synonymous.

**तिनिस**

तिनिसः स्यंदनो नेमी सर्व्वसारोश्मगर्भकः[18] ।। १६ ।।

*Tīnisa*

*Tinisa*, *syandana*, *nemī*, *sarva sāra* and *aśma garbhaka*—these are synonymous.

**भूर्ज्ज**

भूर्जोभूयो वहुपुटो मृदुत्वक्[19] सूक्ष्मपत्रकः[20] ।

*Bhūrja*

*Bhūrja*, *bhūyas*, *vahu puṭa*, *mṛdu tvak* and *sūkṣma patraka*—these are synonymous.

**पलाश**

पलाशः किंशुकः किर्म्मी यज्ञको ब्रह्मपादपः ।
क्षारश्रेष्ठो रक्तपुष्पस्तृवृतः[21] समिदुत्तमः ।। १७ ।।

*Palāśa*

*Palāśa*, *kiṁśuka*, *kirmī*, *yajñaka*, *brahma pādapa*, *kṣāra śreṣṭha*, *rakta puṣpa*, *tṛvṛta* and *samiduttama*—these are synonymous.

**धव**

धवो नंदितरुर्गौरः शकटाख्यो[22] धुरंधरः ॥ १८ ॥

*Dhava*

*Dhava*, *nandi taru*, *gaura*, *śakaṭākhya* and *dhurandhara*—these are synonymous.

**धन्वन**

धन्वनो गोत्रविटपी धर्म्मानो[23] गोत्रपुष्पकः ।

*Dhanvana*

*Dhanvana*, *gotra viṭapī*, *dharmāna* and *gotra puṣpaka*—these are synonymous.

**अजकर्ण**

सर्ज्जोऽजकर्णो स्वेदघ्नो लतावृक्षः कुदेहकम् ॥ १९ ॥

*Aja karṇa*

*Sarja*, *ajakarṇa*, *svedaghna*, *latā vṛkṣa* and *kudehaka*—these are synonymous.

**वरुण**

वरुणो वारुणः सेतुः शाकवृक्षः कुमारकः ।

*Varuṇa*

*Varuṇa*, *vāruṇa*, *setu*, *śāka vṛkṣa* and *kumāraka*—these are synonymous.

**जिंगिणि**

जिंगिणी[24] जांगिणी[25] जिंगा[26] सुनिर्ज्जासा च मोदकी[27] ॥२०॥

*Jiṅgiṇi*

*Jiṅgiṇī*, *jāṅgiṇī*, *jiṅgā*, *sunirjāsā*, and *modakī*—these are synonymous.

**शल्लकी**

शल्लकी वल्लकी मोचा गजभक्ष्या महेरुणा[28] ।

गंधवीरा[29] कुंदुरुकी सुस्रावा वनकर्णिका ।। २१ ।।

*Śallakī*

*Śallakī*, *vallakī*, *mocā*, *gaja bhakṣyā*, *maheruṇā*, *gandha vīrā*, *kundurukī*, *susrāvā* and *vana karṇikā*—these are synonymous.

**इंगुदी**

इंगुदी भिल्लकोवृक्षः कंटकस्तापसद्रुमः ।

*Iṅgudī*

*Iṅgudī*, *bhillaka vṛkṣa*, *kaṇṭaka* and *tāpasa druma*—these are synonymous.

**करहारी**

करंवरश्च[30] शुण्डीक[31] कटभी तृणशौंडिकः ।। २२ ।।

*Karahārī*

*Karaṁvara*, *śuṇḍīka*, *kaṭabhī* and *tṛṇa śauṇḍika*—these are synonymous.

**मुष्कक**

मुष्कको मोषको[32] घंटा शिखरी क्षुद्रपाटलिः ।

*Muṣkaka*

*Muṣkaka*, *moṣaka*, *ghaṇṭā*, *śikharī* and *kṣudra pāṭalī*—these are synonymous.

**पारिभद्र**

पारिभद्रो निंबवृक्षो रक्तपुष्पः प्रभद्रकः ।

कंटकीपारिजातः स्यात् मंदारः कंटकिंशुकः ।।२३।।

*Pāribhadra*

*Pāribhadra*, *nimba vṛkṣa*, *rakta puṣpa*, *prabhadraka*, *kaṇṭakī*, *pārijāta*, *mandāra* and *kaṇṭa kiṁśuka*—these are synonymous.

**शाल्मली**

33

शाल्मली तूलिनी मोचा कुक्कुटी रक्तपुष्पिका ।

कंटकाढ्या स्थूलफला पिच्छिला चिरजीविनी ॥२४॥

*Śālmalī*

*Śālmalī, tūlinī, mocā, kukkuṭī, rakta puṣpikā, kaṇṭakāḍhyā, sthūla phalā, pichilā* and *cirajīvinī*—these are synonymous.

**तुणि**

गणेरुक श्रीपतिस्तु नकोन नन्दिपादपः ॥ २५ ॥

*Tuṇi*

*Gaṇeruka, śrīpatī, nakona* and *nandi pādapa*—these are synonymous.

**सप्तपर्ण**

34

सप्तपर्णो गुच्छपुष्पो छत्री शाल्मलिपत्रिका ।

*Sapta parṇa*

*Sapta parṇa, gucha puṣpa, chatrī* and *śālmali patrikā*—these are synonymous.

**हरिद्रा**

हारिद्रकः पीतवर्णः श्रीमान् गौरद्रुमोवरः ॥ २६ ॥

*Haridrā*

*Hāridraka, pīta varṇa, śrīmān, gaura druma* and *vara*—these are synonymous.

**करंज**

करंजो नक्तमालः स्यात् नक्ताह्वो घृतवर्णकः ।

पूतिकोन्यः पूतिपर्णः प्रकीर्णश्चिरबिल्वकः ॥ २७ ॥

*Karañja*

*Karañja, nakta māla, naktāhva* and *ghṛta varṇaka*—these are the synonyms of *karañja*.

Another variety of it is called *pūtika*, *pūti parṇa*, *prakīrṇa* and *cira bilvaka*.

**करंजी**

करंजिः काकतिक्ता च वयस्यांगारवल्लरी[35] ।
तिरिणिक्षि[36]र्गजः[37]कंटः कंरजीश्चीरिणी द्विपा ॥ २८ ॥

*Karañjī*

*Karañji*, *kākạ tiktā*, *vayasyā*, *aṅgāra vallarī*, *tiriṇikṣi*, *gaja kaṇṭa*, *karañjī*, *cīriṇī* and *dvipā*—these are synonymous.

**शमी**

शमी तुंगा शंकुफला पवित्रा केशहृत्फला ।
लक्ष्मी शिवा व्याधिशमी भूशमी शंकराह्वया ॥ २९ ॥

*Śamī*

*Śamī*, *tuṅgā*, *śaṅku phalā*, *pavitrā*, *keśa hṛt phalā*, *lakṣmī*, *śivā*, *vyādhi śamī*, *bhūśamī* and *śaṅkarāhvayā*—these are synonymous.

**शिरीषिका**

शिरीषिका डिंडिणिका दुर्वाला[38]म्बुशिरीषिकाः ।

*Śirīṣikā*

*Śirīṣikā*, *ḍiṇḍiṇikā*, *durbāḷā* and *ambu śirīṣikā*—these are synonymous.

**अरिष्टक**

अरिष्टको गर्भपाती कुंभवीर्य्यश्च फेनिलः ।
रक्षाबीजो रक्तबीजः पीतफेनार्थसाधनः ॥ ३० ॥

*Ariṣṭaka*

*Ariṣṭaka*, *garbha pātī*, *kumbha vīrya*, *phenila*, *rakṣā bīja*, *pīta phena* and *artha sādhana*—these are synonymous.

**सिसपा**

सिंसिपा कपिला कृष्णा सरा मंडलपत्रिका ।

अन्या कुसिंसिपा भस्मपिंगला स्याद्विशोधिनी ।

*Siṁsapā*

*Siṁsipā*, *kapilā*, *kṛṣṇā*, *sarā* and *maṇḍala patrikā*—these are the synonyms of *siṁsapā*.

It has another variety whose synonyms are *kusiṁsipā*, *bhasma piṅgalā* and *viśodhinī*.

**अगस्त्य**

अगस्त्याह्वो वंगसेनो मधुशिग्रुर्मुनिद्रुमः[39] ।। ३१ ।।

*Agastya*

*Agastyāhva*, *vaṅga sena*, *madhu śigru* and *muni druma*—these are synonymous.

## NOTES AND REFERENCES

1. This is the 94th chapter of *Ayurveda Saukhyaṁ* in *Toḍarānanda* and the opening invocation reads as below :

यमादिभिर्योगिगणैर यो सम्यग्गृहीतुं व्रजकामिनीभिः ।

सुप्रेमवद्धः सगृहं सपुत्रं श्रीटोडरं सर्वं सुखं प्रकुर्यात् ।

2. 'पदः' इति प्रथमपुस्तके पाठः ।
3. 'पटारोहि' इति प्रथमपुस्तके पाठः ।
4. 'स्कंदयोध्र्वः' इति प्रथमपुस्तके पाठः ।
5. 'फल्गू' इति षष्ठपुस्तके पाठः ।
6. 'र्म्मलपू' इति षष्ठपुस्तके पाठः ।

7. 'प्लवश्चारुवृक्षः' इति षष्ठपुस्तके पाठः ।
8. 'हृत्चगो' इति षष्ठपुस्तके पाठः ।
9. 'श्रागंटः' इति पंचमपुस्तके पाठः ।
10. नम्रो इति प्रथमपुस्तके पाठः ।
11. 'मेदापुष्पोन्यस्तोयकामो' इति षष्ठपुस्तके पाठः ।
12. 'स्यात्कछपाब्धिका' इति पंचमपुस्तके पाठः ।
13. 'द्विजकुत्सितः' इति पंचमपुस्तके पाठः ।
14. 'गुडपला' इति प्रथमपुस्तके पाठः ।
15. 'शाकः' इति पंचमपुस्तके पाठः ।
16. 'श्रीकृन्मारीचिपत्रकः' इति प्रथमपुस्तके पाठः ।
17. 'दंतधावनः' इति षष्ठपुस्तके पाठः ।
18. 'सर्व्वसारोग्यनामकः' इति षष्ठपुस्तके पाठः ।
19. 'मृदुलः' इति प्रथमपुस्तके पाठः ।
20. 'श्लेष्मपत्रकः' इति प्रथमपुस्तके पाठः ।
21. 'शमिदुत्तमः इति प्रथमपुस्तके पाठः ।
22. 'शकटाख्योदु' इति षष्ठपुस्तके पाठः ।
23. 'वर्म्मानो' इति षष्ठपुस्तके पाठः ।
24. 'जिंगिनी' इति षष्ठपुस्तके पाठः ।
25. 'जंगिंनी' इति षष्ठपुस्तके पाठः ।
26. 'जंगा' इति षष्ठपुस्तके पाठः ।
27. 'मोदिका' इति पंचमपुस्तके पाठः ।
28. 'महारुहा' इति पंचमपुस्तके पाठः ।
29. 'कुंदुरकी' इति षष्ठपुस्तके पाठः ।
30. 'कंटभर' इति षष्ठपुस्तके पाठः ।
31. 'श्वासकुली' इति षष्ठपुस्तके पाठः
32. 'मोखको' इति प्रथमपुस्तके पाठः ।
33. 'तुलनि' इति षष्ठपुस्तके पाठः ।

34. 'शाल्मलिपात्रका' इति पंचमपुस्तके पाठः ।

35. 'वयस्थांगारवल्लरी' इति पंचमपुस्तके पाठः ।

36. 'तिरिणिछ' इति प्रथमपुस्तके पाठः ।

37. 'गजकरंज' इति पंचमपुस्तके पाठः ।

38. 'डिंडिनि' इति षष्ठपुस्तके पाठः ।

39. This is the end of 94th chapter of *Ayurveda Saukhyaṁ* in *Toḍarānanda* and the colophon reads as below:

इति श्री महाराजाधिराजटोडरमल्लविरचिते टोडरानंदे आयुर्व्वेद-सौख्ये निघंटौ वनस्पतिवर्गो अष्टाशीतितमोहर्षः (?)।

# CHAPTER 36

**द्राक्षा**[1]

द्राक्षा मधुफला स्वाद्वी हारहूरा फलोत्तमा ।[2]

मृद्वीका मधुयोनिश्च रसाला गोस्तनी गुडा ॥ १ ॥

द्राक्षा पक्वा सरा शीता चक्षुष्या बृंहणी गुरुः ।

हंति तृष्णाज्वरश्वासवातवातास्रकामलाः ॥ २ ॥

कृच्छ्रास्रपित्तसंमोहदाह—शोफमदात्ययान् ।

आमा स्वल्पगुणा गुर्व्वी सैवाम्ला रक्तपित्तजित् ॥ ३ ॥

निर्व्वीजान्या लघ द्राक्षा गोस्तनी सदृशं गुणैः ।

द्राक्षा पर्व्वतजा लघ्वी साम्लाश्लेष्मास्रपित्तजित् ॥४॥

***Drākṣā***

*Drākṣā*, *madhu phalā*, *svādvī*, *hāra hūrā*, *phalottamā*, *mṛdvīkā*, *madhu yoni*, *rasālā*, *gostanī* and *guḍā*—these are synonymous.

Ripe *drākṣā* is *sara* (laxative), *śīta* (cooling), *cakṣuṣya* (promoter of eye sight), *bṛmhaṇa* (nourishing) and guru (heavy). It cures *tṛṣṇā* (morbid thirst), *jvara* (fever), *śvāsa* (asthma), *vāta* (diseases of nervous system), *vātāsra* (gout), *kāmalā* (jaundice), *kṛcchra* (dysuria), *asra pitta* (a condition characterised by bleeding from different parts of the body), *saṁmoha* (unconsciousness), *dāha* (burning syndrome), *śopha* (oedema) and *madātyaya* (alcoholism).

*Unripe drākṣā* is inferior in quality and heavy.

The sour variety of *drākṣā* cures *rakta pitta* (a condition characterised by bleeding from different parts of the body).

A variety of *drākṣā* is without seed and is similar to *gostanī* variety in its properties.

The variety of *drākṣā* which grows in the mountains is light and sour. It cures *asra pitta*.

**आम्र**

आम्रो वनोत्सवश्चूतः सहकारोतिसौरभः ।
माकंदः पिकबंधुः स्याद्रसालः कामवल्लभ ॥ ५ ॥
आम्रो ग्राही प्रमेहास्रकफपित्तव्रणान् जयेत् ।
तत्फलं आममत्युष्णं रुक्षं[3] दोषत्रयास्रकृत् ॥ ६ ॥
पक्वं तु मधुरं वृष्यं स्निग्धं हृद्यं बलप्रदम् ।
गुरुर्वातहरं रुच्यं वर्ण्यं शीतमपित्तलम् ॥ ७ ॥
रसस्तस्य सरः स्निग्धो[4] पाचनो बलवर्णकृत् ।

*Āmra*

*Āmra*, *vanotsava*, *cūta*, *sahakāra*, *ati saurabha*, *mākanda*, *pika baudhu*, *rasāla* and *kāma vallabha*—these are synonymous.

*Āmra* is *grāhī* (constipative) and it *cures prameha* (obstinate urinary disorders including diabetes) as well as diseases caused by vitiated blood, *kapha* and *pitta* and ulcers.

Unripe fruits of *āmra* is exceedingly hot and ununctuous it vitiates all the three *doṣas* as well blood.

Ripe fruits of *āmra* is sweet, *vṛṣya* (aphrodisiac), *unctuous*, *hṛdya* (cardiac tonic), *bala prada* (promoter of strength), heavy *vāta hara* (alleviator of vāta), *rucya* (relishing), *varṇya* (promoter of complexion), *śīta* (cooling) and *apittala* (which does not vitiate *pitta*).

Juice of *āmra* is *sara* (laxative), unctuous, *pācana* (carminative) and promoter of strength as well as complexion.

**जम्बु**

महाजंबू राजजंबू महास्कंधो बृहत्फलः ॥ ८ ॥
क्षुद्रजंबूश्चीरपत्रा मेघाभा काकबल्लभाः ।
जंबू संग्राहिणी रूक्षा कफपित्तव्रणास्रजित् ॥ ९ ॥
राजजंबूफलं स्वादु विष्टंभि गुरु रोचनम् ।
क्षुद्रजंबूफलं तद्वद्विशेषाद्दाहनाशनम् ॥ १० ॥

***Jambu***

*Mahā jaṁbū*, *rāja jaṁbū*, *mahā skandha* and *bṛhat phala*—these are the synonyms of bigger variety of *jaṁbū*.

The smaller variety of *jaṁbū* is called *kṣudra jaṁbū*, *cīra patrā*, *meghābhā* and *kāka ballabhā*.

*Jaṁbū* is *saṁgrāhiṇī* (constipative) and *ununctuous*. It cures vitiated *kapha*, *pitta*, *ulcer* and blood.

*Rāja jaṁbū* fruit is sweet, *viṣṭaṁbhi* (causing wind formation in abdomen), heavy and *rocana* (appetiser).

The fruit of *kṣudra jaṁbū* is like *rāja jaṁbū* in property but its special action is to cure *dāha* (burning syndrome).

**नारिकेल**

नालिकेरस्तुंगवृक्षो लतावृक्षो महाफलः ।

तृणराजस्त्वक्षफल लांगली दृढबीजकम् ।। ११ ।।

नालिकेरफलं शीतं दुर्जरं बस्तिशोधनम् ।

विष्टंभि बृंहणं बल्यं वातपित्तास्रदाहजित् ।। १२ ।।

तस्यांभः शीतलं हृद्यं दीपनं शुक्रलं लघु ।

तस्मादपि शिरोमज्जा शुक्रला वातपित्तजित् ।।१३।।

*Nārikela*

*Nālikera*, *tuṅga vṛkṣa*, *latā vṛkṣa*, *mahā phala*, *tṛṇa rāja*, *akṣa phala*, *lāṅgalī* and *dṛḍha bījaka*—these are synonymous.

The fruit of *nārikera* is *śīta* (cooling), *durjara* (difficult of digestion), *basti śodhana* (purifier of urinary bladder), *viṣṭambhi* (causing wind formation in abdomen), *bṛṁhaṇa* (nourishing) and *balya* (promoter of strength), It cures vitiated *vāta*, *pitta* and blood. It also cures *dāha* (burning syndrome).

Water of *nārikela* is cooling, *hṛdya* (cardiac tonic), *dīpana* (stimulant of digestion), *śukrala* (promoter of semen) and *laghu* (light).

Its *śiro majjā* (pith at the top of the tree) of *nārikela* is promoter of semen and it cures both *vāta* and *pitta*.

**खर्ज्जूरिका**

बृहत्खर्जुरिका श्रेणी सफला द्वीपसंभवा ।

पिंडखर्जुरिका[6] खर्जुः दुःप्रहर्षास्तु कंटकी ।। १४ ।।

अन्या स्कंधफला स्वाद्वी दुरारोहा मृदुछदा ।

भूमिखर्ज्जुरिका काको कर्क्कटी[7] राजकर्क्कटी ।।१५।।

खर्जुरिका[8] फलं शीतं स्वादु स्निग्धं क्षतास्रजित् ।

बल्यं हंति मरुत्पित्तं मदमूर्छामदात्ययान् ।। १६ ।।

तस्मादल्पगुणं ज्ञेयमन्यत्खर्ज्जुरिका फलम् ।

तन्मज्जामूर्द्धजा शीता वृष्या पित्तास्रदाहजित ।। १७ ।।

*Kharjūrikā*

*Bṛhat kharjūrikā*, *śreṇī*, *saphalā* and *dvīpa saṁbhavā*—these are the synonyms of bigger variety of *kharjūra*.

Another variety of it is called *piṇḍa kharjūrikā*, *kharju*, *duḥ praharṣā* and *kaṇṭaki*.

The third variety of it is called *skandha phalā*, *svādvī*, *durārohā* and *mṛdu chadā*.

The fourth variety of it is called *bhūmi kharjūrikā*, *kāka*, *karkaṭī* and *rāja karkaṭī*.

The fruit of *kharjūrikā* is cooling, sweet and unctuous. It cures consumption and diseases caused by the vitiation of blood. It is promoter of strength. It cures vitiation of *vāyu* and *pitta*, *mada* (intoxication), *mūrchā* (fainting) and *madātyaya* (alcoholism)..

Fruits of other varieties of *kharjūrikā* are inferior in quality.

Its *mūrdhaja majjā* (pith at the top of the tree is cooling and *vṛṣya* (aphrodisiac). It cures vitiated *pitta* as well as blood and *dāha* (burning syndrome).

**सिलेमानी खर्जूर**

[9]

सिलेमान्यपरा लोके मृदुला निर्ब्बलीफला ।

सिलेमानी श्रमभ्रांतिदाहमूर्छास्रपित्तनुत् ।। १८ ।।

*Silemāni kharjūra*

Another variety of *kharjūra* is called *silemāni* and its synonyms are *mṛdula* and *nirbalī phalā*.

*Silemāni* cures *śrama* (exhaustion), *bhrānti* (giddiness), *dāha* (burning syndrome), *mūrchā* (fainting) and *asra pitta* (a condition characterised by bleeding from different parts of the body).

**कदली**

कदली ग्रंथिनी मोचा रंभा वीरा यतछदा[10] ।

कदली योनिदोषास्ररक्तपित्तहरा हिमा ।। १९ ।।

तत्कंदः शीतलो बल्यः केश्यः पित्तकफास्रजित् ।

तत्फलं मधुरं शीतं विष्टंभि कफकृद्गुरु ।। २० ।।

स्निग्धपित्तास्रतृट्दाह — क्षतक्षयसमीरजित् ।

*Kadalī*

*Kadalī*, *granthinī*, *mocā*, *rambhā*, *vīrā* and *yata chadā*--these are synonymous.

*Kaladī* cures *yoni doṣa* (ailments of female genital tract), *asra* (vitiated blood) and *rakta pitta* (a disease characterised by bleeding from various parts of the body). It is cooling.

The *kanda* (rhizome) of this plant is *śītala* (cooling), *balya* (strength promoting), and *keśya* (good for hair growth). It cures vitiated *pitta*, *kapha* and blood.

The fruit of *kadalī* is sweet, cooling and *viṣṭambhi* (which produces gas in the abdomen). It produces *kapha*. It is heavy and unctuous. It alleviates vitiated *pitta* and blood. It cures *dāha* (burning syndrome), *kṣata* (consumption), *kṣaya* (emaciation) and *vitiated vāyu*.

**दाडिम**

दाडिमी रक्तकुसुमा दंतबीजा शुकप्रिया ।। २१ ।।

दाडिमं दीपनं हृद्यं रोचनं नातिपित्तलम् ।

कषायानुरसं ग्राहि द्विधा स्वाद्वम्लभेदतः ।। २२ ।।

तयोः स्वादु त्रिदोषघ्नंमम्लं वातवलासहृत् ।

शुष्काम्लो दाडिमीसारः कुट्टितो वातपित्तहृत् ॥२३॥

*Dāḍima*

*Dāḍimī, rakta kusumā, danta bījā* and *śuka priyā*—these are synonymous.

*Dāḍima* is *dīpana* (digestive stimulant), *hṛdya* (cardiac tonic) and *rocana* (appetiser), It does not vitiate *pitta* in excess. Its subsidiary taste (anurasa) is astringent and it is constipative.

It is of two types viz., sweet and sour. The sweet variety alleviates all the three *doṣas* where as the sour variety alleviates only *vāta* and *kapha.*

The dried and pounded extract of the sour variety of *dāḍima* alleviates *vāta* and *pitta.*

**बदर**

बदरी कर्क्कटी घोंटा करटी युग्मकंटिका ।

अन्या स्निग्धछदा कोशफला[11] सौवीरिकापरा ॥ २४ ॥

हस्तिकोलिः[12] परास्वाद्वी लघ्वी कर्क्कंधुबांधवा ।

वदर्य्या शीतलास्तिक्ता रूक्ष्या पित्तकफापहा ॥ २५ ॥

बदरं त्ववरं कौलं फेनिलं कुवलं[13] कुहम्[14] ।

कर्क्कंधु ह्रस्वबदरं संकटं कंधु कंधुकम् ॥ २६ ॥

पक्वमामं च मधुरं मतं सौवीरकं महत् ।

*Badara*

*Badarī, karkaṭī, ghoṇṭā, karaṭī* and *yugma kaṇṭikā*—these are synonymous. Another variety of it is called *snigdha chadā* and *kośa phalā.* The thirst variety is called *sauvīrikā.* The fourth variety of it is called *hasti koli, parāsvādvī, laghvī* and *karkandhu bāndhavā.*

All these types of *vadarī* are cooling, bitter and ununctuous. They alleviate *pitta* and *kapha*.

The fifth variety of it is called *badara, avara kola, phenila, kuvala* and *kuca.* Synonyms of the sixth variety are *karkandhu, hrasva badara, saṁkaṭa, kandhu* and *kandhuka.*

Both the ripe and unripe types of *sauvīraka* (bigger variety) are sweet in taste.

**लघु बदर**

बदरं लघु संग्राहि[15] रुच्यमुष्णं समीरजित् ॥ २७ ॥
कफपित्तकरं[16] तद्वत्कोलं गुरु सरं[17] स्मृतम् ।
सौवीरं बदरं शीतं भेदनं गुरु शुक्रलम्[18] ॥ २८ ॥
बृंहणं पित्तदाहास्रक्षयतृष्णानिलापहम् ।
कर्कंधु मधुरं स्निग्धं गुरु पित्तानिलापहम् ॥ २९ ॥
शुष्कं मेदाग्निकृत्सर्वं लघुतृष्णाक्लमास्रजित् ।
मरुत्पित्तहरं तस्य मज्जा वृष्यो बलप्रदः ॥ ३० ॥

*Laghu badara*

*Badara* is light, constipative, appetiser and hot. It alleviates *vāyu. Kola* aggravates *kapha* and *piatt.* It is heavy and laxative.

*Sauvīra* type of *badara* is cooling, *bhedana* (purgative), *guru* (heavy), *śukrala* (promoter of semen) and *bṛmhaṇa* (nourishing). It alleviates vitiated *pitta, dāha* (burning syndrome), vitiated blood, *kṣaya* (emaciation), *tṛṣṇā* (morbid thirst) and vitiated *vāyu.*

*Karkandhu* is sweet, unctuous and heavy. It alleviates *pitta* and *vāyu.*

Dry fruits of all these varieties promote *medas* (fat) and *agni* (digestive power). These are light and they cure *tṛṣṇā* (morbid thirst), *klama* (mental fatigue) and vitiation of blood.

The pulp of this fruit alleviates *vāyu* and *pitta*. It is *vṛṣya* (aphrodisiac) and promoter of strength.

**क्षीरी**

क्षीरी क्षत्रिया राजाह्वा राजादन फलासिनी ।
राजन्यस्तस्य भेदोन्यश्चिवुको मुचिलिंदकः[19] ।। ३१ ।।
क्षीरिवृक्षफलं शीतं स्निग्धं गुरु बलप्रदम् ।
तृष्णामूर्छामदभ्रांतिक्षयदोषत्रयास्रजित् ।। ३२ ।।

*Kṣīrī*

*Kṣīrī, kṣatriyā, rājāhvā, rājādana, phalāsinī* and *rājanya*—these are synonymous.

It has another variety which is called *civuka* and *muci lindaka*.

The fruit of *kṣīri vṛkṣa* is cooling, unctuous, heavy and promoter of strength. It cures *tṛṣṇā* (morbid thirst), *mūrchā* (fainting), *mada* (intoxication), *bhrānti* (giddiness), *kṣaya* (emaciation) and all the three vitiated *doṣas* as well as blood.

**प्रियाल**

चारो धनः पटः शालः[20] प्रियालो[21] मुनिवल्लभः ।
चारः पित्तकफास्रघ्नः तत्फलं मधुरं गुरु ।। ३३ ।।
स्निग्धं सरं मरुत्पित्तदाहतृष्णाक्षतापहम्[22] ।
तन्मज्जा मधुरो वृष्यः शुक्रलः त्तवातजित् ।।३४ ।।

*Priyāla*

*Cāra, dhana, paṭa, śāla, priyāla* and *muni vallabha*—these are synonymous.

*Cāra* cures vitiated *pitta, kapha* and blood.

Its fruit is sweet, heavy, unctuous and laxative. It cures vitiated *vāta* and *pitta, dāha* (burning syndrome), *tṛṣṇā* (morbid thirst) and *kṣata* (consumption).

The pulp of the fruit of *priyāla* is sweet, *vṛṣya* (aphrodisiac) and *śukrala* (spermatopoetic.) It cures vitiated *pitta* and *vāta*.

**परुषक**

परुषको मृदुफलो परुषो शोषणः[23] परः ।
परूषकं कषायाम्लमामं पित्तकरं लघु ॥ ३५ ॥
पक्वं तु मधुरं पाके शीतं विष्टंभि बृंहणम् ।
हृद्यं तृट्पित्तदाहास्रक्षतक्षयसमीरजित् ॥ ३६ ॥

*Paruṣaka*

*Paruṣaka*, *mṛdu phala*, *paruṣa* and *śoṣaṇa*—these are synonymous.

Unripe *Paruṣaka* is astringent and sour in taste. It vitiates *pitta* and is light.

Ripe variety of *paruṣaka* is sweet in *vipāka* (taste that emerges after digestion), cooling, *viṣṭambhi* (produces gas in abdomen), *bṛmhaṇa* (nourishing) and *hṛdya* (cardiac tonic). It cures *tṛṭ* (morbid thirst), vitiated *pitta*, *dāha* (burning syndrome), vitiated blood, *kṣata* (consumption), *kṣaya* (emaciation) and vitiated *vāyu*.

**तिंदुक**

तिंदुकः स्यंदनः स्फोर्यः[24] कालसारश्च रावणः ।
काकपीलु स्यादपरो ग्रन्यच्च विषतिंदुका ॥ ३७ ॥
तिंदुको व्रणवातघ्नः तत्सारः पित्तरोगजित् ।
आममस्य फलं ग्राहि वातलं शीतलं लघु ॥ ३८ ॥
पक्वं पित्तप्रमेहास्रश्लेष्मघ्नं विशदं गुरु ।
विषतिंदुकमप्येवं[25] विशेषाद्ग्राहि शीतलम् ॥ ३९ ॥

*Tinduka*

*Tinduka, syandana, sphaurya, kāla sāra, rāvaṇa* and *ḳāka pīlu*—these are the synonyms of *tinduka*.

There is another variety (which is different) which is called *viṣa tindukā*.

*Tinduka* cures ulcers and vitiated *vāta*. Its pulp (*sāra*) cures diseases caused by *pitta*.

The unripe fruit of it is constipative, *vātala* (vitiater of *vāta*), cooling and light.

The ripe fruit alleviates vitiated *pitta*, *prameha* (obstinate urinary disorders including diabetes), vitiated blood & *kapha*, *viśada* (non slimy) and heavy.

*Viṣa tinduka* is specially constipative (*grāhi*) and cooling.

**किंकिरणी**

किंकिणी ग्रंथिका व्याघ्री पादो देवतरूर्व्वरः ।

किंकिणी तुवरा तिक्ता पित्तश्लेष्महरा हिमा ॥४०॥

तत्फलं वातलं त्वामं पक्वं स्वादु त्रिदोषजित् ।

***Kiṁkiṇī***

*Kiṁkiṇī, granthikā, vyāghrī, pāda, deva taru* and *vara*—these are synonymous.

*Kiṁkiṇī* is pungent and bitter. It alleviates *pitta* and *śleṣman*. It is cooling.

Unripe fruit of *kiṁkiṇī* aggravates *vāyu*. The ripe fruit is sweet and it cures all the three vitiated *doṣas*.

**आरु**

आरुष्कं वीरसेनं च जातिभेदाच्चतुर्व्विधम् ॥ ४१ ॥

26

आरुष्कं जारणं वातमेहार्शःकफनाशनम् ।

*Āru*

*Āruṣka* and *vīra sena*—these are synonymous. It is of four types.

*Āruṣka* promotes digestion (*jāraṇa*) and it cures vitiated ***vāta***, *meha* (obstinate urinary disorders including diabetes), ***arśas*** (piles) and vitiated *kapha*.

**मधूक**

मधूको मधुकस्तीक्ष्णसारः स्याद्गूढपुष्पकः ॥ ४२ ॥
जेलाफलो मधुष्टीलो मधुकोष्ठो महाद्रुमः ।
मधूकोन्यो ह्रस्वफलो मध्वगो दीर्घपत्रकः ॥ ४३ ॥
मधूकः कफवातघ्नः कषायो व्रणरोपणः ।
तत्पुष्पं मधुरं बल्यं शीतलं गुरु बृंहणम् ॥ ४४ ॥
फलं शीतं गुरुस्वादुशुक्रलं वातपित्तजित् ।
अहृद्यं हंति तृष्णास्रदाहश्वासक्षतक्षयान् ॥ ४५ ॥

*Madhūka*

*Madhūka*, *madhuka*, *tīkṣṇa sāra*, *gūḍha puṣpaka*, *jelā phala*, *madhuṣṭīla*, *madhu koṣṭha* and *mahā druma*—these are synonymous.

Another variety of *madhūka* is called *hrasva phala*, *madhvaga* and *dīrgha patraka*.

*Madhūka* alleviates *kapha* and *vāta*. It is astringent and it helps in the healing of ulcers.

The flower of *madhūka* is sweet, *balya* (promoter of strength), cooling, heavy and *bṛṁhaṇa* (nourishing).

Its fruit is cooling, heavy, sweet and *śukrala* (spermatopoetic). It alleviates *vāta* and *pitta*. It is *ahṛdya* (not good for heart). It cures *tṛṣṇā* (morbid thirst), vitiated blood, *dāha* (burning syndrome), *śvāsa* (asthma), *kṣata* (consumption) and *kṣaya* (emaciation).

**पनस**

पनसः [27]कंटकिफल[28]स्त्वांशपो गर्भकंटकः ।
पनसं शीतलं पक्वं स्निग्धं पित्तानिलापहम् ॥ ४६ ॥
बलशुक्रप्रदं हंति रक्तपित्तक्षतक्षयान् ।
आमं तदेव विष्टंभि वातलं तुवरं गुरु ॥ ४७ ॥

*Panasa*

*Panasa*, *kaṇṭaki phala*, *āṁśapa* and *garbha kaṇṭaka*—these are synonymous.

Ripe *panasa* is cooling and unctuous. It alleviates *pitta* and *vāyu.* It promotes strength and semen. It cures *rakta pitta* (a condition characterised by bleeding from different parts of the body), *kṣata* (consumption) and *kṣaya* (emaciation).

Unripe panasa is *viṣṭaṁbhi* (wind forming). It aggravates *vāyu* and it is astringent a well as heavy.

**लकुच**

लकुचं क्षुद्रपनसो लकुचोग्रंथि[29]मत्फलः ।
लकुचं गुरु विष्टंभि स्वाद्वम्लं रक्तपित्तजित् ॥ ४८ ॥
श्लेष्मकारि समीरघ्नमुष्णं शुक्राग्निनाशनम् ।

*Lakuca*

*Lakuca*, *kṣudra panasa* and *granthimat phala*—these are synonymous.

*Lakuca* is heavy, *viṣṭaṁbhi* (wind forming) and sweet and sour in taste. It cures *rakta pitta* (a disease characterised by bleeding from different parts of the body). It aggravates *kapha* and alleviates *vāta*. It is hot. It reduces the semen as well as the power of digestion.

**ताल**

तालो ध्वजो दुरारोहस्तृणराजो महाद्रुमः ॥ ४९ ॥

तालवृक्षो मरुत्पित्तव्रणजित् मदशुक्रकृत् ।
तत्फलं शीतलं बल्यं स्निग्धं स्वादुरसं गुरु ॥ ५० ॥
विष्टंभि वातपित्तास्राक्षतदाहक्षयापहम् ।
बीजं मूत्रकरं विष्टं वातपित्तहरं हिम ॥ ५१ ॥

*Tāla*

*Tāla, dhvaja, durāroha, tṛṇa rāja* and *mahā druma*—these are synonymous.

*Tāla* cures vitiated *vāta, pitta* and ulcer. It produces *mada* (intoxication) and *śukra* (semen).

Its fruit is cooling, strength promoting, unctuous, sweet, heavy and *viṣṭambhi* (wind forming). It cures vitiated *vāta, pitta* and blood. It also cures *kṣata* (consumption), *dāha* (burning syndrome) and *kṣaya* (emaciation).

Its seed is diuretic and wind forming. It alleviates *vāta* and *pitta*. It is cooling.

**खर्बूज**

खर्बूजं फलराजं स्यादमृताह्वं दशांगुलम् ।
खर्बूजं मूत्रलं बल्यं कोष्ठशुद्धिकरं गुरु ॥ ५२ ॥
स्निग्धं[30] स्वादुकरं शीतं वृष्यं पित्तानिलापहम् ।

*Kharbūja*

*Kharbūja, phala rāja, amṛtāhva* and *daśāṅgula*—these are synonymous.

*Kharbūja* is diuretic, strength promoting, laxatixe, heavy, unctuous, sweet, cooling and *vṛṣya* (aphrodisiac). It alleviates *pitta* and *vāta*.

**सेव**

मुष्टिप्रमाणं[31] वरुदं सेवं सिविति काफलम् ॥ ५३ ॥

फलं सिंवितिकापूर्व्वं वातपित्तहरं गुरु ।

बृंहणं कफकृद्वृष्यं स्वादुपाकं सरं हिमम् ॥ ५४ ॥

अन्यदंभफलं चापो महासिंविर्तिका फलम् ।

तत्फलं सेव्यगुणकृद्विशेषात्तुवरं हिमम् ॥ ५५ ॥

*Seva*

*Muṣti pramāṇa*, *varuda*, *seva* and *simbitikā phala*—these are synonymous.

The fruit of *simbitikā* alleviates *vāyu* and *pitta*. It is heavy, *bṛmhaṇa* (nourishing), *kaphakṛt* (aggravater of *kapha*), *vṛṣya* (aphrodisiac), *svādu pāka* (sweet in taste after digestion), laxative and cooling.

Another variety of it is called *ambha phala*, *āpa* and *mahā simbitikā phala*. Its properties are similar to those of *seva*. It is specially cooling.

**अमृत**

अमृताह्वं रुचिफलं लघुबिल्वफलाकृतिः ।

अमृतं गुरुवातघ्नं स्वाद्वम्लं रुचिशुक्रकृत् ॥ ५६ ॥

*Amṛta*

*Amṛtāhva*, *ruci phala* and *laghu bilva phalākṛti*—these are synonymous.

*Amṛta* is heavy, alleviator of *vāta*, sweet, sour and appetiser. It is spermatopoetic.

**बादाम**

बादामं सुफलं वातवैरि नेत्रोपमं फलम् ।

बादाममुष्णं सुस्निग्धं वातघ्नं बलशुक्रकृत् ॥ ५७ ॥

*Bādāma*

*Bādāma*, *suphala*, *vāta vairi* and *netropama phala*—these are synonymous.

*Bādāma* is hot and exceedingly unctuous. It alleviates *vāyu*. It promotes strength and semen.

**निकोचक, पिस्ता**

निकोचकं दारुफलं मकोष्ठं जलगोजकम् ।
पिस्तं मुकूलकं ज्ञेयं दंतीफलसमाकृतिः ॥ ५८ ॥

निकोचकं गुरुस्निग्धं वृष्योष्णं स्वादु बृंहणम् ।
रक्तप्रसादनं बल्यं वातघ्नं कफपित्तकृत् ॥ ५९ ॥

तद्वत् मुकुलकं ज्ञेयं विशेषात् गुरु दुर्ज्जरम् ।

*Nikocaka, Pistā*

*Nikocaka*, *dāru phala*, *makoṣṭha* and *jala gojaka*—these are the synonyms of *nikocaka*.

*Pista*, *mukūḷaka* and *dantī phala samākṛti*—these are the synonyms of *pistā*.

*Nikocaka* is heavy, unctuous, *vṛṣya* (aphrodisiac), *hot*, sweet and *bṛṁhaṇa* (nourishing). It is hemopoetic and strength promoting. It alleviates *vāta* and aggravates *kapha* as well as *pitta*.

*Mukulaka* has similar properties. It is especially heavy and difficult for digestion.

**केला**

केलानामामवातघ्नमम्लोष्णं रेचनं गुरु ।
पक्वं स्वादु हिमं बल्यं वातपित्तविनाशनम् ॥ ६० ॥

*Kelā*

Unripe *kelā* alleviates *vāyu*. It is sour, hot, purgative and heavy.

Ripe *kela* is sweet, cooling and strength promoting. It alleviates *vāyu* and *pitta.*

**आरु**

आलूकभल्लूभल्लूकं[34] भल्लूरक्तफलं तथा ।
आलूकं रसनं[35] शीतं स्वाद्वम्लवातपित्तहृत् ॥ ६१ ॥

*Āru*

*Ālūka, bhallū, bhallūka* and *bhallū rakta phala*—these are sy nymous.

*Ālūka* is juicy (*rasana*), cooling, sweet and sour. It alleviates *vāta* and *pitta.*

**अंजीर**

अंजीरं मंजुलं ज्ञेयं काकोदुंबरिका फलम् ।
अंजीरं शीतलं स्वादु गुरु पित्तास्रवातजित् ॥ ६२ ॥

*Añjīra*

*Añjīra, mañjula* and *kākodumbarikā phala*—these are synonymous.

*Añjīra* is cooling, sweet and heavy. It alleviates *pitta, rakta* and *vāta.*

**अक्षोट**

अक्षोडको वृंतफलो कंदरालः पृथुच्छदः ।
अक्षोटं[36] मधुरं बल्यं गुरूष्णं वातहृत्सरम् ॥ ६३ ॥

*Akṣoṭa*

*Akṣoḍaka, vṛnta phala, kandarāla* and *pṛthu chada*—these are synonymous.

*Akṣoṭa* is sweet, strength promoting, heavy, hot, alleviater of *vāta* and laxative.

**पालेवक, मालवक**

पालेवतं सितपुष्पं तिंदुकाभफलं मतम् ।

अन्यत् मालवकं ज्ञेयं महापालेवतं तथा ॥ ६४ ॥

पालेवतं हिमं स्वादु गुरुष्णं वह्निवातजित् ।

तद्वत् मालवक हृद्यं तृष्णाघ्नमिष्टमस्तकम् ॥ ६५ ॥

*Pālevaka & Mālavāaka*

*Pālevata, sita puṣpa* and *tindukābha phala*—these are sy nymous.

Another variety of it is called *mālavaka* and *mahā pālevata phala*.

*Pālevata* is cooling, sweet, heavy and hot. It suppresses digestive power and alleviates *vāyu*.

*Mālavaka* is *hṛdya* (cardiac tonic). It cures *tṛṣṇā* (morbid thirst). It is useful for brain (*mastaka*).

**तूत**

[37] तूदं भूदं ब्रह्मकाष्ठं ब्रह्मण्यं ब्रह्मदारु च ।

[39] तूदं गुरु हिमं पक्वं स्वादुपित्तानिलापहम् ॥ ६६ ॥

*Tūta*

*Tūda, bhūda, brahma kāṣtha, brahmaṇya* and *brhma dāru*—these are synonymous.

Ripe *tūda* is heavy, cooling and sweet. It alleviates *pitta* and *anila*.

**गांगेरुक, तोदन**

गांगेरुकं कर्क्कटकं कर्कटं मृगलेंडकम् ।

तोदनं क्रंदनं धान्यं मृगपिछदृशं तथा ॥ ६७ ॥

गांगेरु रेचनं पक्वं गुरु वातास्रपित्तजित् ॥ ६८ ॥

तोदनं ग्राहि मधुरं वातपित्तहरं लघु ।

तूतादि त्रितयं चाममम्लं गुरु तु पित्तलम् ॥ ६९ ॥

*Gāṅgerūka & Todana*

*Gāṅgeruka*, *karkaṭaka*, *karkaṭa* and *mṛga leṇḍaka*—these are the synonyms of *gāṅgeruka*.

*Todana*, *krandana*, *dhānya* and *mṛga picha dṛśa*—these are synonymous.

Ripe *gāṅgeru* is purgative and heavy. It alleviates *vāta*, blood and *pitta*.

*Todana* is constipative and sweet. It alleviates *vāta* and *pitta*. It is light.

Unripe *tūta*, *gāṅgeruka* and *todana* are sour and heavy. They aggravate *pitta*.

**तुवरक**

वृक्षस्तुवरको ज्ञेयोभल्लातकसमो गुणैः ।

कषायं तत्फलं पत्रैः केसराभः[40] समुद्रजः[41] ॥ ७० ॥

तौवरं कफजित्पाके कटूष्णं व्रणमेहजित् ।

*Tuvaraka*

*Tuvaraka* tree has properties like those of *bhallātaka*. Its fruit is astringent in taste. Its leaves are like *kesara* and it grows near sea.

The fruit of *tuvara* alleviates *kapha*. In *vipāka* (taste after digestion) it is pungent.

It is hot and it cures ulcer and *meha* (obstinate urinary disorders including diabetes).

**बीजपूरक**

42
बीजपूरो मातुलुंगः केसरी फलपूरकः ॥ ७१ ॥
बीजपूरफलं रुच्यं रसेऽम्लं दीपनं लघु ।
रक्तपित्तकरं कंठजिह्वाग्रशोधनं परम् ॥ ७२ ॥
त्वचोऽस्य तिक्तगुर्व्वम्लं कृमिवातकफापहम् ।
तन्मांसं बृंहणं शीतं गुरु पित्तसमीरजित् ॥ ७३ ॥
43
केसरं लघु संग्राहि शूलगुल्मोदरापहम् ।
बीजमुष्णं कृमिश्लेष्मवातजिद्गर्भदं गुरु ॥ ७४ ॥
तत्पुष्पं शीतलं ग्राहि रक्तपित्तहरं लघु ।

*Bīja pūraka*

*Bīja pūra*, *mātuluṅga*, *kesarī* and *phala pūraka*—these are synonymous.

The fruit of *bīja pūra* is appetiser. It is sour in taste. It stimulates digestion and is light. It causes *rakta pitta* (a disease characterised by bleeding from different parts of the body). It cleanses throat and tip of the tongue.

The skin of the fruit of *bīja pūraka* is bitter, heavy and sour. It cures *kṛmī* (intestinal parasites). It alleviates *vāta* and *kapha*.

The pulp (*māṁsa*) of *bija pūraka* is *bṛṁhaṇa* (nourishing), cooling and heavy. It alleviates *pitta* and *vāyu*.

Its *kesara* (pistil) is light and constipative. It cures *śūla* (colic pain), *gulma* (phantom tumour) and *udara* (obstinate diseases of abdomen including ascitis).

Its flower is cooling and constipative. It cures *rakta pitta* (a disease characterised by bleeding from different parts of the body) and it is light.

**मधुकर्कटिका**

मधुकर्कटिका स्वादुलुंगी घंटालिका घटा ।। ७५ ।।

मधुकर्कटिका शीता रक्तपित्तहरा गुरुः ।

*Madhu karkaṭikā*

*Madhu karkaṭikā, svādu, luṅgī, ghaṇṭālikā* and *ghaṭā*—these are synonymous.

*Madhu karkaṭikā* is cooling. It cures *rakta pitta* (a disease characterised by bleeding from different parts of the body). It is heavy.

**नारंगी**

44

नारंगको नागरंगो गोरक्षो योगसाधकः ।। ७६ ।।

नारंगमम्लं मधुरं रुच्यं वातहरं सरम् ।

स्वाद्वम्लमपरं हृद्यं दुर्ज्जरं वातनाशनम् ।। ७७ ।।

*Nāraṅgī*

*Nāraṅgaka, nāgaraṅga, gorakṣa* and *yoga sādhaka*—these are synonymous.

*Nāraṅga* is sour and sweet in taste. It is appetiser. It alleviates *vāta*. It is laxative.

Another variety of it which is also sweet and sour, is *hṛdya* (cardiac tonic) and *durjara* (difficult for digestion). It alleviates *vāta*.

**जंबीरक**

जंबीरको दंतशठो जंभीलो जंभलो मतः ।

जंबीरमुष्णं शूलघ्नं गुरुष्णं कफवातजित् ।। ७८ ।।

आस्यवैरस्य—हृत्पीडावह्निमांद्यकृमीन्जयेत् ।

*Jaṁbīraka*

*Jaṁbīraka*, *danta śaṭha*, *jambhīla* and *jambhala*—these are synonymous.

*Jambīra* is hot and it cures *śūla* (colic pain). It is heavy and hot. It alleviates *kapha* and *vāta*. It cures *āsya vairasya* (distaste in the mouth), *hṛt pīḍā* (pain in cardiac region), *agni māndya* (suppression of the power of digestion) and *kṛmi* (intestinal parasites).

**अम्लवेतस**

अम्लोऽम्लवेतसः चुक्रो[45] वेतसः[46] स्वरभेदकः[47] ॥ ७९ ॥

अम्लवेतसमत्युष्णं भेदनं लघु दीपनम् ।

हृद्रोगशूलगुल्मघ्नं पित्तास्रकफदूषणम्[48] ॥ ८० ॥

*Amla vetasa*

*Amla*, *amla vetasa*, *cukra*, *vetasa* and *svara bhedaka*—these are synonymous.

*Amla vetasa* is exceedingly hot, purgative, light and digestive stimulant. It cures *hṛd roga* (heart disease), *śūla* (colic pain) and *gulma* (phantom tumour). It vitiates *pitta*, blood and *kapha*.

**साराम्लक**

साराम्लकः सारफलो रसालः सारपादपः

साराम्लमम्लं वातघ्नं गुरु पित्तकफप्रदम् ॥ ८१ ॥

*ārāmlaka*

*Sārāmlaka*, *sāra phala*, *rasāla* and *sāra pādapa*—these are synonymous.

*Sārāmla* is sour. It alleviates *vāyu*. It is heavy and it aggravates *pitta* and *kapha*.

**निंबुक**

नम्रुक निबूक राजनिंबूकमपरं स्मृतम् ।

निबुकं पाचनं हृद्यं तीक्ष्णोष्णं कफवातजित् ।। ८२ ।।

निंबुकमम्लं वातघ्नं पाचनं दीपनं लघु ।

राजनिंबूफलं स्वादुगुरुपित्तसमीरजित् ।। ८३ ।।

निंबुकं कृमिसमूहनाशनं तीक्ष्णमाममुदरग्रहापहम् ।

वातपित्तकफशूलनाशनं [49] नष्टधातुरुचिशोधनं परम् ।। ८४ ।।

त्रिदोषसद्यज्वरपीडितानां दोषश्चितानां विषमज्वराणाम् ।

मलक्षये बद्धगुदे हितं च विषूचि[50]कानां मुनयो वदन्ति ।। ८५ ।।

*Nimbuka*

*Nimbuka* and *nibūka*—these are the synonyms of *nimbu*.

It has another variety which is called *rāja nimbūka*.

*Nibuka* is *pācana* (carminative), *hṛdya* (cardiac tonic), sharp and hot. It alleviates *kapha* and *vāta*.

*Nimbuka* is sour, *vātaghna* (alleviater of *vāta*), *pācana* (carminative), *dīpana* (digestive stimulant) and light.

The fruit of *rāja nimbu* is sweet and heavy. It alleviates *pitta* and *vāyu*.

*Nimbuka* destroys all types of *kṛmi* (parasites). It is sharp in action. It cures *āma* (product of improper digestion and metabolism), *udara* (obstinate abdominal disorders including ascitis) and *graha* (planetary afflictions). It cures the *vātika*, *paittika* and *ślaiṣmika* types of *śūla* (colic pain). It replenishes and cleanses the vitiated *dhātus*. It is useful for patients suffering from *acute* (*sadya*) fever caused by the vitiation of all the three *doṣas* and *viṣama jvara* (irregular fever) caused by the accumulation of vitiated *doṣas*. It is also useful when there is diminution of waste products (*mala*) and when there is obstruction in the anus. It cures *visūcikā* (choleric diarrhoea).

**कर्मरंग**

कर्म्मरंगं रामफलं भव्यं पिच्छिलबीजकम् ।

कर्म्मरंगं हिमं ग्राहि स्वाद्वम्लं कफपित्तजित् ॥ ८६ ॥

*Karma raṅga*

*Karma raṅga, rāma phala, bhavya,* and *picchila bījaka*—these are synonymous.

*Karma raṅga*, is cooling, constipative, sweet and sour. It cures *kapha* and *pitta.*

**अम्लिका**

अम्लिका चुक्रिका चिंचा तित्तिडी शुक्ति चंडिका ।

अम्लिकामा गुरुर्व्वातहरा पित्तकफास्रकृत् ॥ ८७ ॥

पक्वा तद्वत्सरा रुच्या वह्निवस्तिविशुद्धिकृत् ।

शुष्का हृद्या श्रमभ्रांतितृष्णाक्लमहरा लघुः ॥ ८८ ॥

*Amlikā*

*Amlikā, cukrikā, ciñcā, tittiḍī, śukti* and *caṇḍikā*—these are synonymous.

Unripe *amlikā* is heavy. It alleviates *vāta* and vitiates *pitta, kapha* and blood.

Ripe *amlikā* is laxative and appetiser. It is a digestive stimulant and it cleanses the urinary bladder.

Dried *amlikā* is *hṛdya* (cardiac tonic). It cures *śrama* (exhaustion), *bhrānti* (giddiness), *tṛṣṇā* (morbid thirst) and *klama* (mental fatigue). It is light.

**तित्तिडीक**

तित्तिडीकं तु वृक्षाम्लमम्लशाकोम्लपादपः ।

तित्तिडीक समीरघ्नमाममुष्णं परं गुरु ॥ ८९ ॥

तत्फलं लघु संग्राहि ग्रहणीकफवातजित् ।

*Tittiḍīka*

*Tittiḍīka*, *vṛkṣāmla*, *amla śāka* and *amla pādapa*—these are synonymous.

Unripe *tittiḍīka* alleviates *vāyu*. It is *uṣṇa* (hot) and exceedingly heavy.

Its fruit is light and constipative, It cures *grahaṇī* (sprue syndrome), *kapha* and *vāta*.

**करमर्द**

करमर्दः सुषेणस्याद्वन्याकृष्णफलापरा ॥ ६० ॥
करमर्दं गुरूष्णाम्लं रक्तपित्तकफप्रदम् ।
तत्पक्वं मधुरं रुच्यं लघु पित्तसमीरजित् ॥ ६१ ॥
शुष्कं पक्ववदस्यामंपक्वमप्यार्द्रमामवत ।

*Karamarda*

*Karamarda*, *suṣeṇa*, *vanyā* and *kṛṣṇa phalā*—these are synonymous.

*Karamarda* is heavy, hot and sour. It produces *rakta pitta* (a disease characterised by bleeding from different parts of the body) and *kapha*.

Ripe *karamarda* is sweet, appetiser and light. It alleviates *pitta* and *vāyu*.

Dried *karamarda* is like ripe *karamarda* in its properties.

Unripe but dried *karamarda* is like green unripe *karamarda* in property.

**कपित्थ**

कपित्थको दधिफलः कपित्थः सुरभिच्छदः ॥ ६२ ॥
कपित्थमामं संग्राहि लघु दोषत्रयापहम् ।
पक्वं गुरु तृषाहिक्काशमनं वातपित्तजित् ॥ ६३ ॥

स्वाद्वम्लं तु वरं कंठशोधनं ग्राहि दुर्जरम् ।

*Kapittha*

*Kapitthaka, dadhi phala, kapittha* and *surabhi chada*—these are synonymous.

Unripe variety of *kapittha* is constipative and light. It alleviates all the three *doṣas.*

Ripe *kapittha* is heavy. It cures *tṛṣā* (morbid thirst), *hikkā* (hiccup) and vitiated *vāta* as well as *pitta.* It is sweet and sour. It cleanses the throat. It is constipative and it is difficult of digestion.

**कपित्थपत्री**

कपित्थपत्री फणिजा कुलजा निंबपत्रिका ।। ९४ ।।

कपित्थपत्री तीक्ष्णोष्णा कफमेहविषापहा ।

*Kapittha patrī*

*Kapittha patrī, phaṇijā, kulajā* and *nimba patrikā*—these are synonymous.

*Kapittha patrī* is sharp and hot. It alleviates *kapha, meha* (obstinate urinary disorders including diabetes) and poisoning.

**आम्रातक**

51

आम्रातकश्चाम्रतटः पल्लीशो द्रुफलः कपिः ।। ९५ ।।

आम्रातमामं वातघ्नं गुरूष्णं रुचिकृत्सरम् ।

पक्वं स्वादु हिमं वृष्यं मरुत्पित्तकफास्रजित् ।।९६।।

*Āmrātaka*

*Āmrātaka, āmra taṭa, palliśa, druphala* and *kapi*—these are synonymous.

Unripe *āmrāta* alleviates *vāta.* It is heavy, hot, appetiser and laxative.

Ripe *āmrātaka* is sweet, cooling and *vṛṣya* (aphrodisiac).

It alleviates *vāyu*, *pitta*, *kapha* and blood.

राजाम्र

52

राजाम्रष्टक आम्रातः कामाह्वो राजपुत्रकः ।

राजाम्रं मधुरं शीतं ग्राहि पित्तकफापहम् ॥ ९७ ॥

*Rājāmra*

*Rājāmra ṣtaka*, *āmrāta*, *kāmāhva*, and *rāja putraka*—these are synonymous.

*Rājāmra* is sweet, cooling and constipative. It alleviates both *pitta* and *kapha*.

चतुरम्ल, पंचाम्ल

वृक्षाम्लसुषेणचिंचाकपित्थैश्चतुराम्लकम् ।

अम्लवेतसवृक्षाम्लदाडिमी बदरैः क्वचित् ॥ ९८ ॥

बीजपूरचुतैरेतैः पंचाम्लमुदितं बुधैः ।

*Caturamla*, *Pañcāmla*

*Vṛkṣāmla*, *suṣeṇa*, *ciñcā* and *kapittha*—these four taken together are known as *caturamla*.

According to some, *amla vetasa*, *vṛkṣāmla*, *dāḍimī* and *badara*—these four taken together are called *caturamlaka*.

Added with *bījapūra* or *cuta*, they are called *pañcāmla*.

कोशाम्र

कोशाम्रको घनस्कंधो जंतुवृक्षः सुकोशकः ॥ ९९ ॥

कोशाम्रः कुष्ठशोथास्रपित्तव्रणकफापहः ।

तत्फलं ग्राहि वातघ्नमम्लोष्णं गुरु पित्तलम् ॥१००॥

मज्जा पित्तसमीरघ्नः स्वादुर्बल्योऽग्निदीपनः ।

*Kośāmra*

*Kośāmra*, *ghana skandha*, *jantu vṛkṣa* and *sukośaka*—these are synonymous.

*Kośāmra* cures *kuṣṭha* (obstinate skin diseases including leprosy), *śotha* (oedema), *rakta pitta* (a disease characterised by bleeding from different parts of the body), *vraṇa* (ulcer) and vitiated *kapha*.

Its fruit is constipative, alleviater of *vāta*, sour, hot and heavy. It aggravates *pitta*.

Its fruit pulp alleviates *pitta* and *vāyu*. It is sweet and strength promoting. It stimulates the power of digestion.

सुपारी

क्रमुकं कृमिकं पूगं पूगीफलमुदाहृतम् ॥ १०१ ॥

पूगं गुरु हिमं रुक्षं कषायं कफपित्तजित् ।

53

मोहनं दीपनं रुच्यं आस्यवैरस्यनाशनम् ॥ १०२ ॥

आर्द्रं तद्गुर्वभिष्यंदि वह्निदृष्टिहरं परम् ।

स्विन्नं त्रिदोषहृत्सर्व्वं तद्भेदान् तद्वदादिशेत्॥१०३॥

*Supārī*

*Kramuka*, *kṛmika*, *pūga* and *pūgī phala*—these are synonymous.

*Pūga* is heavy, cooling, ununctuous and astringent. It alleviates *kapha* and *pitta*. It is *mohana* (intoxicating), *dīpana* (digestive stimulant), and *rucya* (appetiser). It cures *āsya vairasya* (distaste in mouth).

Wet *pūga* is heavy and *abhiṣyandi* (which obstructs the channels of circulation). It suppresses the power of digestion (*vahni*) and reduces eye sight (*dṛṣṭi*) in excess.

The boiled *pūga* alleviates all the three *doṣas*.

It has many varieties and all of them have similar properties.

**तांबूल**

[54]

तांबूल वल्ली तांबूली नागिनी नागवल्लरी ।
तांबूलं विशदं रुच्यं तीक्ष्णोष्णं तुवरं सरम् ॥ १०४ ॥
तिक्तं क्षारोषणं काम्यं रक्तपित्तहरं लघु ।

[55]

बल्यं श्लेष्मास्यदौर्गंध्यं मेहवातश्रमापहम् ॥ १०५ ॥

*Tāmbūla*

*Tāmbūla, vallī, tāmbūlī nāginī* and *nāga vallarī*—these are synonymous.

*Tāmbūla* is *viśada* (non slimy), appetiser, sharp, hot, pungent, laxative, bitter, *kṣāra* (alkaline) and *uṣaṇa* (saline and alkaline). It is *kāmya* (stimulant of passion). It alleviates *rakta pitta* (a disease characterised by bleeding from different parts of the body). It is light. It promotes strength. It cures vitiated *kapha, āsya daurgandhya* (foul smell from mouth), *meha* (obstinate urinary disorders including diabetes), vitiated *vāta* and *śrama* (exhaustion).

**लवली**

घनस्कंधं महत्प्रांशु प्रपुन्नाटः समंछदः ।
सुगंधमूला लवली पांडुकोमलवल्कला ॥ १०६ ॥
लवल्याः फलमुद्दिष्टं समं ज्योत्स्नाफलं तथा ।
लवलीफलमस्रार्शोवातपित्तहरं लघु ॥ १०७ ॥

*Lavalī*

*Ghana skandha, mahat prāṁśu, prapunnāṭa, samaṁ chada, sugandha mūlā, lavalī, pāṇḍu komala valkalā*—these are synonymous.

The fruit of *lavalī* is like that of *jyotsnā* in property.

The fruit of *lavalī* cures vitiated blood, *arśas* (piles), vitiated *vāta* and *pitta*. It is light.

फलतुल्यं गुणं सर्व्वं मज्जानमपि निर्द्दिशेत् ।
फलं हिमाग्निदुर्व्वातव्यालकीटादिदूषितम् ॥ १०८ ॥
अकालजातं नाश्नीयात् पाकातीतमभूषितम् ।
आमं दोषकरं प्रायः[56] फलं बिल्वं विनाऽखिलम् ॥१०९॥

*General description of fruits*

The pulp of the fruit has the property of the fruit itself.

Fruits which are afflicted by snow, fire, storm, wild animals, and insects and which are unseasonal should not be eaten. Similarly, excessively ripe fruits should not be eaten.

All fruits in general produce *āma doṣa* (a product of improper digestion and metabolism). The fruit of *bilva* is an exception to this general rule.

## NOTES AND REFERENCES

1. This is the 95th chapter of *Ayurveda Saukhyaṁ* in *Toḍarānanda*, and the opening invocation reads as below :

   हरिप्रिया प्रीतिमती प्रियेण प्रियान्विते टोडरमल्लभूपे ।
   भूयात्सदा श्रीहरिणा सपुत्रे यशोधिके ब्राह्मणधर्म्ममित्रे ।

2. 'हारहुरा' इति पंचमपुस्तके पाठः ।
3. 'दोषत्रयाहृत्' इति प्रथमपुस्तके पाठः ।
4. 'रोचनो' इति षष्ठपुस्तके पाठः ।
5. 'तद्वद्विशेषाद् वातनाशनम्' इति षष्ठपुस्तके पाठः ।

6. 'कंटका' इति पंचमपुस्तके पाठः ।
7. 'कक्कंरी' इति षष्ठपुस्तके पाठः ।
8. 'खर्जूरीका' इति षष्ठपुस्तके पाठः ।
9. 'लिंवसी' इति षष्ठपुस्तके पाठः ।
10. 'पीतछदा' इति पंचमपुस्तके पाठः ।
    'यत्वचा' इति षष्ठपुस्तके पाठः ।
11. 'काशपाला' इति पष्ठपुस्तके पाठः ।
    'कोशपाला' इति प्रथमपुस्तके पाठः ।
12. 'हस्तिकोलः इति षष्ठपुस्तके पाठः ।
13. 'वहुलं' इति षष्ठपुस्तके पाठः ।
14. 'कुलं' इति षष्ठपुस्तके पाठः ।
15. 'संग्राही' इति पंचमपुस्तके पाठः ।
16. 'कफपित्तहरं' इति षष्ठपुस्तके पाठः ।
17. 'त रं' इति षष्ठपुस्तके पाठः ।
18. 'शीतलम्' इति प्रथमपुस्तके पाठः ।
19. 'मुनितिंदुकः' इति षष्ठपुस्तके पाठः ।
20. 'शाली' इति षष्ठपुस्तके पाठः ।
21. 'पियालो' इति षष्ठपुस्तके पाठः ।
22. 'क्षुधापहं' इति षष्ठपुस्तके पाठः ।
23. 'परुषोऽशोधनः' इति षष्ठपुस्तके पाठः ।
24. 'स्फुर्यः' इति पंचमपुस्तके पाठः ।
25. 'विशतिंदुकमप्येवं' इति षष्ठपुस्तके पाठः ।
26. 'चारणं' इति षष्ठपुस्तके पाठः ।
27. 'कंटकी' इति पंचमपुस्तके पाठः ।
    'कंटपि' इति षष्ठपुस्तके पाठः
28. 'फलस्त्वांसपो' इति प्रथमपुस्तके पाठः ।

29. 'लकुचोग्रंथिमत्फला:' इति पंचमपुस्तके पाठः ।
30. 'स्वादुतरः' इति पंचमपुस्तके पाठः ।
31. 'वदरं' इति प्रथमपुस्तके पाठः ।
32. 'चिकोचकं' इति प्रथमपुस्तके पाठः ।
33. 'पिष्टं' इति षष्ठपुस्तके पाठः ।
34. 'अलूकमल्लूभल्लूकम्' इति प्रथमपुस्तके पाठः ।
35. 'रसतः' इति प्रथमपुस्तके पाठः ।
36. 'अक्षोडं' इति प्रथमपुस्तके पाठः ।
37. 'तूतं' इति पंचमपुस्तके पाठः ।
38. 'तूदं' इति पंचमपुस्तके पाठः ।
39. 'भूदं' इति षष्ठपुस्तके पाठः ।
    'तूतं' इति पंचमपुस्तके पाठः ।
40. 'केशराभः' इति पंचमपुस्तके पाठः ।
41. 'समुद्रजैः' इत्ति षष्ठपुस्तके पाठः ।
42. 'केशरी' इति पंचमपुस्तके पाठः ।
43. 'केशरं' इति पंचमपुस्तके पाठः ।
44. 'गोरक्षोयोगसारकः' इति षष्ठपुस्तके पाठः ।
45. 'शुक्रों' इति प्रथमपुस्तके पाठः ।
46. 'चेतनः' इति प्रथमपुस्तके पाठः ।
47. 'शतभेदकः' इति प्रथमपुस्तके पाठः ।
48. 'पित्तास्रकफदीपनम्' इति प्रथमपुस्तके पाठः ।
49. 'निहंतिनष्टधातुरुचिशोधनम्' इति प्रथमपुस्तके पाठः ।
50. 'विसूचिकानां' इति प्रथमपुस्तके पाठः ।
51. 'आम्रतकश्चाम्रवटः' इति पंचमपुस्तके पाठः ।
    'आम्रातकश्चाम्रतदः' इति षष्ठपुस्तके पाठः ।
52. 'राजपत्रकः' इति प्रथमपुस्तके पाठः ।

53. 'मेहनं' इति षष्ठपुस्तके पाठः ।

54. 'नागवल्लकी' इति षष्ठपुस्तके पाठः ।

55. 'मलवातश्रमापहम्' इति प्रथमपुस्तके पाठः ।

56. This is the end of 95th chapter of *Ayurveda Saukhyaṁ* in *Toḍarānanda* and the colophon reads as below :

इति श्रीमहाराजाधिराजटोडरमल्लविरचिते टोडरानंदे आयुर्वेदसौख्ये निघंटौ फलवर्गनाम एकोननवतितमोहर्षः (?) ॥

# CHAPTFR 37

कूष्मांड [1]

कूष्मांडकी [2] पुष्पफला सोमका च महाफला ।

कर्कारुरपरा लघ्वी स्वादु [3] भूराजकर्कटी ॥ १ ॥

*Kūṣmāṇḍa*

*Kuṣmāṇḍakī, puṣpa phalā, somakā* and *mahā phalā*—these are the synonyms of *kuṣmāṇḍaka*.

It has a smaller variety which is called *kàrkāru*. The sweet variety of *kuṣmāṇḍakī* is called *bhūrāja karkaṭī*.

कालिंग

कालिंगं कृष्णबीजं स्यात् कालिंदं [4] फलवर्त्तुलम् ।

*Kāliṅga*

*Kāliṅga, kṛṣṇa bīja, kālinda* and *phala varttula*—these are synonymous.

तुंबी

तुंबी मिष्टा महातुंबी [5] राजालाबुरलावुनी ॥ २ ॥

*Tumbī*

*Tumbī*, *miṣṭā*, *mahā tumbī*, *rājālābu*, *alāvunī*—these are synonymous.

**कटुतुंबी**

कटुतुंबी पिंडफला राजपुत्री[6] च दुग्धिनी ।

*Kaṭu tumbī*

*Kaṭu tumbī*, *piṇḍa phalā*, *rāja putrī* and *dugdhinī*—these are synonymous.

**कर्कटी**

कर्कटी लोमसी[7] व्याल[8] पत्रैर्वारु बृहत्फला ॥ ३ ॥

*Karkaṭī*

*Karkaṭi*, *lomasī*, *vyāla*, *patrairvāru* and *bṛhat phalā*—these are synonymous.

**त्रपुस**

त्रपुसी[9] कंटकिलता सुधावासो परंकिटः[10] ।
छर्द्यायनी[11] मूलफला[12] स्यात्तिक्ता हस्तिपर्णिनी ॥ ४ ॥

*Trapusa*

*Trapusī*, *kaṇṭaki latā*, *sudhāvāsa*, *paraṅkiṭa*, *chardyāyanī*, *mūla phalā*, *tiktā* and *hasti parṇinī*—these are synonymous.

**चिर्भटी**

चिर्भिटं धेनुदुग्धं तत् ज्ञेयं गोरक्षकर्कटी ।

*Cirbhaṭī*

*Cirbhiṭa*, *dhenu dugdha* and *gorakṣa karkaṭi*—these are synonymous.

**वालुक**

वालुकं कांडुकं वालु तत् शीतं मधुरं[13] गुरु ॥ ५ ॥

शीर्णवृन्तं चित्रफलं विचित्रं पीतवर्णकम् ।

*Vāluka*

*Vāluka*, *kāṇḍuka*, *vālu*, *śīrṇa vṛnta*, *citra phala*, *vicitra* and *pīta varṇaka*—these are synonymous.

*Vāluka* is cooling, sweet and heavy.

**कोशातकी**

कोशातकी कृतछिद्रा जालिनी कृतवेधना ॥ ६ ॥
मृदंगफलिनी क्षोडा घोंटाली कक्कर्शछदा ।

*Kośātakī*

*Kośātakī*, *kṛta chidrā*, *jālinī*, *kṛta vedhanā*, *mṛdaṅga phalinī*, *kṣoḍā*, *ghoṇṭālī* and *karkaśa chadā*—these are synonymous.

**राजकोशातकी**

राजकोशातकी मिष्टा महाजालिः प्रपीतकः ॥ ७ ॥

*Rāja kośātakī*

*Rāja kośātakī*, *miṣṭā*, *mahājāli* and *prapītaka*—these are synonymous.

**महाकोशातकी**

महाकोशातकी त्वन्या हस्तिघोषा महाफला ।

*Mahā kośātakī*

Another variety of *kośātakī* is called *mahā kośātakī*. Its synonyms are *hasti ghoṣā* and *mahā phalā*.

**वृंताकी**

वृंताकी वर्त्तिका वृंता भंटाकी भंटिका मता ॥ ८ ॥
अपरः श्वेतवार्त्ताकः कुकुटांडफलोपमा ।
तस्माद्धीनगुणं किंचिदर्शशां च हितः स्मृतः ॥ ९ ॥

*Vṛntākī*

*Vṛntākī*, *varttikā*, *vṛntā*, *bhanṭākī* and *bhanṭikā*—these are the synonyms of *vṛntākī*.

A variety of it is called *śveta vārtāka* and it looks like an egg of the hen. It is slightly inferior in quality and it is useful for *arśas* (piles).

**बिंबी**

बिंबी रक्तफला गोल्हा तुंडी दंतच्छदोपमा ।

*Bimbī*

*Bimbī, rakta phalā, golhā, tuṇḍī* and *dantachadopamā*—these are synonymous.

**कारवेल्लक**

कारवेल्लं कठिल्लं स्यादुग्रकांडं सुकांडकम् ।। १० ।।

करवेल्ली वारिवल्ली बृहद्वल्यपरा स्मृता ।

*Kāravellaka*

*Kāravella, kaṭhilla, ugra kāṇḍa,* and *sukāṇḍaka*—these are the synonyms of *kāravellaka.*

It has a variety which is called *kara vellī, vāri vallī* and *bṛhat vallī.*

**कर्कोटक**

[14] तद्वत्कर्कोटकं कुष्ठकिलासारुचिनाशनम् ।। ११ ।।

*Karkoṭaka*

*Karkoṭaka* cures *kuṣṭha* (obstinate skin disease including leprosy), *kilāsa* (leucoderma) and *aruci* (anorexia).

**वंध्याकर्क्कोटकी, डेंडिका**

वंध्याकर्क्कोटकी देवी नागारिर्विषकंटका[15] ।

डेंडिका विषमुष्टिः स्याद्विषमुष्टि समुष्टिका ।।१२।।

*Vandhyā karkoṭakī, Dendika*

*Vandhyā karkoṭakī, devī, nāgāri* and *viṣa kaṇṭakā*—these are the synonyms of *vandhyā karkoṭakī.*

*Deṇḍikā, viṣamuṣṭi* and *sumuṣṭikā*—these are the synonyms of *ḍeṇḍikā*.

**कोलसिंबी**

कोलसिंबी[16] कृष्णफला षट्का सूकरपालिका[17] ।

*Kola simbī*

*Kola simbī, kṛṣṇa phalā, ṣaṭkā* and *sūkara pālikā*—these are synonymous.

**डिंडिसा**

डिंडिसो रोमसफलो[18] तिंडिसो[19] मुनिनिर्मितः ॥ १३ ॥

*Diṇḍisā*

*Diṇḍisa, romasa phala, tiṇḍisa* and *muni nirmita*—these are synonymous.

**सिंबि**

सिंबि[20]. कुसिंबिः कुत्सास्रसिंबी पुस्तकसिंबिका ।

*Simbi*

*Simbi, kusimbi, kutsāsra simbī* and *pustaka simbika*—these are synonymous.

**वास्तूक**

वास्तूकः क्षारपत्रः स्यात् शाकवीरः प्रसादकः ॥१४॥

*Vāstūka*

*Vastūka, kṣāra patra, śāka vīra* and *prasādaka*—these are synonymous.

**जीवंतक**

जीवंतकः शाकवीरः रक्तनालः प्रनालकः[21] ।

*Jīvantaka*

*Jīvantaka, śāka vīra, raka nāḷa* and *pranāḷaka*—these are synonymous.

**चिल्ली**

चिल्ली महद्दला रक्ता चिल्लिका गौडवास्तुकः[22] ॥१५॥

*Cillī*

*Cillī, mahaddalā, raktā, cillikā* and *gauḍa vāstuka*—these are synonymous.

**कालशाक**

कालशाक कालिका स्याच्चुचुका चंचुको मतः ।

*Kāla śāka*

*Kāla śāka, kālikā, cucukā* and *cañcuka*—these are synonymous.

**तंदुलीयक**

तंदुलीयो मेघनादः[23] कांडीरस्तंदुलीयकः[24] ॥ १६ ॥

विषघ्नः कंदरोन्यः स्यान्मारिषो मार्षकस्तथा ।

*Tandulīyaka*

*Tandulīya, megha nāda, kāṇḍīra, tandulīyaka, viṣaghna* and *kandara*—these are the synonyms of *tandulīyaka.*

It has another variety which is known as *mārīṣa* and *mārṣaka.*

**फोगो**

फोगो मरूद्भवः शुंगी सूक्ष्मपुष्पः[25] शशादनः ॥ १७ ॥

*Phogo*

*Phogo, marūdbhava, śuṅgī, sūkṣma puṣpa* and *śaśādana*—these are synonymous.

**पटोल**

पटोलः पांडुको जाली कूलकः कर्कशछदः ।

राजीफलः पांडुफलः राजमानमृतफलः ॥ १८ ॥

तिक्तोत्तमा बीजगर्भापरा राजपटोलिका ।

*Paṭola*

*Paṭola, pāṇḍuka, jālī, kūlaka, karkaśa chada, rājī phala, pāṇḍu phala, rājamān, amṛta phala, tiktottamā* and *bīja garbhā*—these are the synonyms of *paṭola*.

It has another variety which is called *rāja paṭolikā*.

**चिच्चिड**

चिच्चिडो स्मीरकूलान्यः श्वेतराजी[26] बृहत्फलः[27] ।।१९।।

*Ciccinḍa*

*Ciccinḍa* and *smīra kūla*—these are the synonyms of *ciccinḍa*.

Another variety of it is known as *śveta rājī* and *bṛhat phala*.

**पालंक्या**

पालंक्या वास्तुकाकारा क्षारिका वीरतच्छदा ।

*Pālaṅkyā*

*Pālaṅkyā, vāstukākārā, kṣārikā* and *vīrata chadā*—these are synonymous.

**उपोदिका**

पोतक्युपोदिका प्रोक्ता मत्स्यकाली सुतुंगिका[28] ।।२०।।

*Upodikā*

*Potakī, upodikā, matsya kālī* and *sutuṅgikā*—these are synonymous.

**लोणिक**

लोणिकोष्ट्रा बृहत्कोटी कुटिरस्तु कुटिंजरः ।

गण्डरुकी[29] स्यात् गण्डरु[30] फंजी[31] फंजीतकस्तथा ।। २१ ।।

*Loṇika*

*Loṇika, uṣṭrā, bṛhat koṭī, kuṭira, kuṭiñjara, gaṇḍarukī, gaṇḍaru, phañjī* and *phañjītaka*—these are synonymous.

**सुनिषन्नक**

सुनिषणः स्वस्तिकः स्याद्वरा वस्तिकपर्णिकः ।

*Sunişannaka*

*Sunişaṇa*, *svastika*, *varā*, *vastika parṇika*—these are synonymous.

**सिरवार**

[32]
सिरवारः कुरंडीस्यान्नाडीतुन्नालिका मता ॥ २२ ॥

*Sira vāra*

*Sira vāra*, *kuraṇḍī*, *nāḍītun* and *nālikā*—these are synonymous.

**सर्षपशाक**

सार्षपं सर्षपोद्भूतं कौसुंभं तु कुसुंभजम् ।

*Sarşapa śāka*

*Sārṣapa*, *sarṣapodbhūta*, *kausumbha* and *kusumbhaja*—these are synonymous.

**चणकशाक**

[33]
चाणकं शाकमुद्दिष्टं दुर्ज्जरं कफवातजित् ॥ २३ ॥

*Caṇaka śāka*

*Caṇaka śāka* is difficult of digestion. It alleviates *kapha* and *vāta*.

**कलायशाक**

कलायशाकं भेदि स्याल्लघुपित्तकफापहम् ।

*Kalāya śāka*

*Kalāya śāka* is purgative. It is light and it alleviates *pitta* and *kapha*.

**चांगेरी**

[34]
चांगेरी त्वम्लिका चुक्रा छत्राम्लीका चतुःछदा ॥२४॥

*Cāṅgerī*

*Cāṅgerī, amlikā, cukrā, chatrāmlīkā* and *catuḥ chadā*—these are synonymous.

**कासमर्द, गृञ्जन**

35 कासमर्दः कर्कशः स्यात् गृंजनो गजरस्तथा ।

*Kāsa marda & Gṛñjana*

*Kāsa marda* and *karkaśa*—these are synonymous.

*Gṛñjana* and *gajara*—these are synonymous.

**लशुन**

मूलकं हस्तिकंदः तद्बालमूलकपोतिका ॥ २५ ॥

*Mūlaka*

*Mūlaka* and *hasti kanda*—these are the synonyms of *mūlaka*.

The tender variety of *mūlaka* is called *bāla mūlaka* and *potikā*.

**करीरक**

करीरको गूढपत्रो क्रकचो ग्रंथिलो मतः । 36

*Karīraka*

*Karīraka, gūḍha patra, krakaca* and *granthila*—these are synonymous.

**शिग्रु**

शिग्रु सौभांजनः कृष्णगंधः स्याद्बहुलच्छदः ॥ २६ ॥

रक्तोऽन्यो मधुशिग्रुस्तु श्वेतोऽन्यो हरितच्छदः ।

तद्बीजं श्वेतमरिचं तीक्ष्णोष्णं चक्षुषे हितम् ॥ २७ ॥

तत्पुष्पं मधुरं ग्राहि वातलं कफशोथजित् ।

*Śigru*

*Śigru, saubhāñjana, kṛṣṇa gandha* and *bahula chada*—these are the synonyms of *śigru.*

It has a red variety which is called *madhu sigru* and the white variety of it is called *harita chada.*

Its seed is called *śveta marica* which is sharp, hot and useful for eye.

The flower of *sigru* is sweet and constipative. It aggravates *vāyu* and cures vitiated *kapha* and oedema.

**लशुन**

लशुनः स्यादुग्रगंधो[37] यवनेष्टो[38] रसोनकः ॥ २८ ॥

गृंजनोऽन्योमहाकंदो जर्ज्जरो दीर्घपत्रकः ।

*Laśuna*

*Laśuna, ugra gandha, yavaneṣṭa* and *rasonaka*—these are synonymous.

Another variety of it is called *gṛñjana, mahā kanda, jarjjara* and *dīrgha patrāka.*

**पलांडु**

पलांडुर्यवनेष्टश्च दुर्गंधो मुखदूषकः ॥ २९ ॥

*Palāṇḍu*

*Palāṇḍu, yavaneṣṭa, durgandha* and *mukha dūṣaka*—these are synonymous.

**क्षीरपलांडु**

पलांडुकः क्षीरपलांडुरुक्तः सक्षीरवान् क्षौद्ररसो यदि स्यात् ।

*Kṣīra palāṇḍu*

*Palāṇḍuka* having a milky juice which tastes like honey is called *kṣīra palāṇḍu.*

**गृंजन**

गृंजनः पित्तलो ग्राही तीक्ष्णोष्णो रोगनाशनः ॥३०॥

गंधाकृतिरसैस्तुल्यः सूक्ष्मनालपलांडुवत् ।

स्वल्पः [39] मूलकसंकाशः कंदो गृंजनमुच्यते ॥ ३१ ॥

[40] ग्रंथिपर्णः समाकारः पत्रैः कैश्चिन्मनीषिभिः ।

*Gṛñjana*

*Gṛñjana* aggravates *pitta*. It is constipative, sharp and hot. It cures diseases (?). In smell, shape and taste, it is like *sūkṣma nāla palāṇḍu*.

Some scholars hold a plant like small radish as *gṛñjana*. Some others, however, call another plant having leaves like those of *granthi parṇa* as *gṛñjana*.

**सूरण**

सूरणः कंदलः कंदो गुदामयहरः परः ॥ ३२ ॥

वज्रकंदः सुरेंद्र स्याद्वन्योऽन्यश्चित्रदंडकः ।

*Sūraṇa*

*Sūraṇa*, *kandala*, *kanda*, *gudāmaya hara*, *vajra kanda* and *surendra*—these are the synonyms of *sūraṇa*.

Another wild variety of it is called *citra daṇḍa*.

**अस्थि संहार**

[41] ग्रस्थिशृंखलिको वज्री [42] ग्रंथिमानस्थिसंहृता ॥ ३३ ॥

*Asthi saṁhāra*

*Asthi śṛnkhalika*, *vajrī*, *granthimān* and *asthi saṁhṛtā*—these are synonymous.

**वाराही**

वाराही माधवी गृष्टिस्तत्कंदः सौकरः कीटः ।

*Vārāhī*

*Vārāhī, mādhavi* and *gṛṣṭi*—these are the synonyms of *vārāhī*.

Its *rhizome* (root ?) is called *śaukara* and *kīṭa*.

**मूशली**

43

मुशली तालपत्री स्यात्बलिनी तालमूलिका ।। ३४ ।।

*Mūśalī*

*Muśalī, tālapatri, balinī* and *tāla mūlikā* —these are synonymous.

**केयु**

केयुका फलुको पीलुकेयुका दलशालिनी ।

*Keyu*

*Keyukā, phaluka, pīlu keyukā* and *dala śālinī*—these are synonymous.

**भूछत्र**

भूछत्रं पृथिवीकंदः शिलींध्रं कंदकं मतम् ।। ३५ ।।

*Bhūchatra*

*Bhūchatra, pṛthivī kanda, śilindhra* and *kandaka*—these are synonymous.

**मानकंद**

स्थूलकंदो ग्रामकंदो मानकोऽन्यो महच्छदः

*Māṇa kanda*

*Sthūla kanda, grāma kanda* and *mānaka*– these are the synonyms of *māna kanda*.

It has another variety having bigger leaves.

**कसेरु**

44

कसेरुकं स्वल्पकंदं बृहद्राजकसेरुकम् ।। ३६।।

*Kaseru*

*Kaseruka* and *svalpa kanda*—these are the synonyms of *kaseru.*

It has a bigger variety which is called *rāja kaseruka.*

**शृङ्गाटक**

शृंगाटो जलकंदः स्यात्त्रिकोणस्त्रिकटस्त्रिकः ।

*Śṛṅgāṭaka*

*Śṛṅgāṭa, jala kanda, trikoṇa, trikaṭa* and *trika*—these are synonymous.

**पिंडालु**

पिंडालुकं[45] कच्छगंधं मध्वालु स्यात्तु रोमशम् ॥ ३७ ॥

शंखालु शंखसंकाशं काष्ठालु स्वल्पकोष्ठकम् ।

हस्तालुकं महाकाष्ठं रक्तालु रक्तकंदकम् ॥ ३८ ॥

अतिजीर्णमकालोत्थं रूक्षशीतमभूमिजम् ।

जठरं कोमलं वातिशीतं व्यालादिदूषितम् ।

शुष्कं शाकं च सकलं नाश्नीयान्मूलकं[46] विना ॥३९॥

*Piṇḍālu*

*Piṇḍālu, kacha gandha, madhvālu, romaśa, śaṅkhālu, śaṅkha saṁkāśa, kāṣṭhālu, svalpa koṣṭhaka, hastāluka, mahā kāṣṭha, raktālu* and *rakta kandaka*—these are synonymous.

All leafy vegetables which are *atijīrṇa* (very old), *akālottha* (unseasonal), *rūkṣa* (ununctuous), *śīta* (cold), *abhūmija* (not grown on ground), *jaṭhara* (preserved since long), *komala* (soft), *atiśīta* (excessively cold), *vyālādi dūṣita* (eaten by animals insects etc.) and *śuṣka* (dry) should not be used. *Mūlaka* is an exception to this rule.

## NOTES AND REFERENCES

1. This is the 96th chapter in *Ayurveda Saukhyaṁ* in *Toḍarānanda* and the opening invocation reads as below :

   यो हृद्रमोरामसुहृद्भिर्त्ता विश्वस्यकर्त्तानृपतौ सुखानाम् ।

   सुखायभूयाद्भुविटोडरेंद्रे भूदेव सद्धर्म्मिसुहृज्जनानाम् ।

2. 'कुष्मांडकी' इति षष्ठपुस्तके पाठः ।
3. 'रूराजकर्क्कटी' इति प्रथमपुस्तके पाठः ।
4. 'कालिंगं' इति पंचमपुस्तके पाठः ।
5. 'वुरसाम्वुनी' इति पंचमपुस्तके पाठः ।
   'पुरुलाविनी' इति षष्ठपुस्तके पाठः ।
6. 'तुंबी' इति षष्ठपुस्तके पाठः ।
7. 'लोमशा' इति पंचमपुस्तके पाठः ।
8. 'वालय' इति पंचमपुस्तके पाठः ।
9. 'त्रपुसं' इति पंचमपुस्तके पाठः ।
10. 'पलंकिटा' इति षष्ठपुस्तक पाठः ।
    'परंकटुः' इति पंचमपुस्तके पाठः ।
11. 'छर्द्यादिनी' इति षष्ठपुस्तके पाठः ।
12. 'मूत्रफला' इति प्रथमपुस्तके पाठः ।
13. 'श्लेष्मल' इति षष्ठपुस्तके पाठः ।
14. 'तद्वत्कुवटिकम् इति षष्ठपुस्तके पाठः ।
15. 'व्विषकंटिका' इति प्रथमपुस्तके पाठः ।
16. 'कोलशिंवी' इति षष्ठपुस्तके पाठः ।
17. 'सूकरपादिका' इति पंचमपुस्तके पाठः ।
18. 'तिंदिशो' इति पंचमपुस्तके पाठः ।
19. मुनिनिर्मिता' इति पंचमपुस्तके पाठः ।
20. सिंवीः' इति पंचमपुस्तके पाठः ।
21. 'प्रणालकः' इति षष्ठपुस्तके पाठः ।

22. 'गौर' इति पंचमपुस्तके पाठः ।
23. 'महानादः' इति षष्ठपुस्तके पाठः ।
24. 'कांडीयस्तंदुलीयकः' इति षष्ठपुस्तके पाठः ।
25. 'सूक्ष्मपत्रः' इति पंचमपुस्तके पाठः ।
26. 'श्चतगंधो' इति षष्ठपुस्तके पाठः ।
27. 'महाफला' इति षष्ठपुस्तके पाठः ।
28. 'सुरंगिका' इति पंचमपुस्तके पाठः ।
29-31. हृ॰ हृ॰रुः स्याछुंहृ हुकः' इति प्रथमपुस्तके पाठः ।
32. 'कुरंडीस्यान्नारीतुन्नालिका' इति षष्ठपुस्तके पाठः ।
33. 'चानाकं' इति षष्ठपुस्तके पाठः ।
34. 'क्षुद्रा' इति षष्ठपुस्तके पाठः ।
35. 'काशर्द्कः' इति पंचमपुस्तके पाठः ।
36. 'सस्थिलो' इति षष्ठपुस्तके पाठः ।
37. 'लसुनः' इति प्रथमपुस्तके पाठः ।
38. 'जवनेष्टो' इति प्रथमपुस्तके पाठः ।
39. 'शंकाशकं' इति षष्ठपुस्तके पाठः ।
'संकासः' इति पंचमपुस्तके पाठः ।
40. 'वर्णः' इति प्रथमपुस्तके पाठः ।
41. 'अस्थिश्रृंस्वरिका' इति षष्ठपुस्तके पाठः ।
42. 'ग्रंथिमानस्थिवृंहणः' इति षष्ठपुस्तके पाठः ।
43. 'स्यावंलि' इति षष्ठपुस्तके पाठः ।
44. 'बृहद्राजकशेरुकम्' इति पंचमपुस्तके पाठः ।
45. 'कत्थगन्ध' इति षष्ठपुस्तके पाठः ।

This is the end of 96th chapter of *Ayurveda Saukhyaṁ* not in *Toḍarānanda* and the colophon reads as below :

इति श्रीमहाराजाधिराजटोडरमल्लविरचिते टोडरानंदे ग्रायुर्वेद-सौख्ये निघंटौ शाकवर्गे नवतितमो हर्षः (?) ।

# CHAPTER 38

1
**जल**

पानीयं जीवनं नीरं कीलालममृतं जलम् ।
आपोंभस्तोयमुदकं पाथोंबुसलिलं पयः ॥ १ ॥

*Jala*

*Pānīya*, *jīvana*, *nīra*, *kīlāla*, *amṛta*, *jala*, *āpa*, *ambha*, *toya*, *udaka*, *pātha*, *ambu*, *salila* and *payas*—these are synonymous.

**दुग्ध**

दुग्धं प्रस्रवणं क्षीरं सौम्यं संजीवनं पयः ।

*Dugdha*

*Dugdha*, *prasravaṇa*, *kṣīra*, *saumya*, *sañjīvana* and *payas*—these are synonymous.

**दधि**

दधि स्त्यानंपयः सम्यक्स्त्यानमीषत्तु मंदकम् ॥ २ ॥

*Dadhi*

*Dadhi* and *styānaṁ payas*—these are the synonyms of well

fermented *dadhi*. If it is slightly fermented then it is called *mandaka*.

**तक्र**

दंडाहतं कालसेयं गोरसं च विलोडितम् ।
सरसं निर्ज्जलं घोलं मथितं सरवर्जितम् ॥ ३ ॥
समोदकं श्वेतमथमुदश्वित् ह्यर्द्धवारिकम् ।
पादोदकं भवेत्तक्रमूर्द्धभोन्योवभाषिते ॥ ४ ॥

*Takra*

*Daṇḍāhata, kālaseya, gorasa, viloḍita, sarasa, nirjala, ghola, mathita* and *sara varjita*—these are synonymous.

*Dadhi* mixed with equal quantity of water is known as *śveta*.

*Dadhi* mixed with half of water is called *udaśvit*.

*Dadhi* mixed with one fourth of water is called *takra*.

**नवनीत**

हैयंगवीनं सरजं नवनीतमनुमंथजम् ।

*Navanīta*

*Hayaṁgavīna, saraja, navaṇīta* and *anumanthaja*—these are synonymous.

**घृत**

घृतमाज्यं हविः सर्पिराज्यारममृताह्वयम् ॥ ५ ॥

*Ghṛta*

*Ghṛta, ājya, havis, sarpis, ājyāra* and *amṛtāhvaya*—these are synonymous.

**मद्य**

मद्यं हारा[2] सुरा मंदा[3] मदिरा वरुणात्मजा ।
सुधा गंधोत्तमा कल्पा देवसृष्टा च वारुणी ॥ ६ ॥

*Madya*

*Madya, hārā, surā, mandā, madirā, varuṇātmajā, sudhā, gandhottamā, kalpā, devaśṛṣṭā* and *vāruṇī*—these are synonymous.

**इक्षु**

इक्षुर्म्महारसो वेणुनिःसृतो गुडपत्रकः

तृणराजो मधुतृणो गंडीरी मृत्युपुष्पकः ॥ ७ ॥

*Ikṣu*

*Ikṣu, mahārasa, veṇu niḥsṛta, guḍa patraka, tṛṇa rāja, madhu tṛṇa, gaṇḍīrī* and *mṛtyu puṣpaka*—these are synonymous.

**इक्षुविकार**

सिता मत्स्यांडिका पल्ली मीनांडो घल्लकस्तथा ।

अन्या सितोपला शुद्धा सिकता छत्रिकामला ॥ ८ ॥

खंडमथ खंडसिता माधवी मधुशर्क्करा ।

फाणितं क्षुद्रगुडको गुडस्त्विक्षुरसोद्भवः ॥ ९ ॥

*Ikṣu vikāra*

*Sitā, matsyāṇḍikā, pallī, mīnāṇḍī* and *ghallaka*—these are the synonyms of *matsyāṇḍikā*.

Another variety of it is called *sitopalā*, *śuddhā*, *sikatā*, *chatrikā* and *amalā*.

*Khaṇḍa* and *sitā*—these are the synonyms of *khaṇḍa*.

*Mādhavī* is called *madhu śarkarā*. *Phāṇita, kṣudra guḍaka* and *guḍa*—these are prepared from sugar cane juice.

**मधु**

मधु पुष्पासवः पुष्परसो माक्षिकमीरितम् ।

माक्षिकं पैत्तिकं क्षौद्रं भ्रामरं मध्वविस्तरात् ॥१०॥

माक्षिकं तैलसंकाशं पैत्तिकं घृतवर्णकम् ।

क्षौद्रं कपिलवर्णं स्याद्भ्रामरं स्फटिकोपमम् ॥ ११ ॥

*Madhu*

*Madhu, puṣpāsava, puṣpa rasa,* and *mākṣika*—these are the synonyms of *madhu.*

*Mākṣika, paittika, kṣaudra* and *bhrāmara*—these are in brief the different varieties of *madhu.*

*Mākṣika* is like oil. *Paittika* has the colour of ghee. *Kṣaudra* is reddish brown in colour and *bhrāmara* is like a crystal.

**मधूच्छिष्ट**

मदनं मधुजं सिक्थं मधूच्छिष्टं मधूषितम् ।

*Madhūcchiṣṭa*

*Madana, madhuja, siktha, madhūcchiṣṭa* and *madhūṣita*—these are synonymous.

**धान्यवर्ग**

शालयो रक्तशल्याद्या ब्रीहयः षष्टिकादयः ॥ १२ ॥

मुद्गादिर्द्विदलं सौचकङ्ग्वादि तृणधान्यकम् ।

क्षुद्रधान्यं कुधान्यं तत्स्थूलधान्यं यवादिकम् ॥ १३ ॥

रक्तशालिर्लोहितः स्याद्गरुडः शकुनाहृतः ।

सुगंधिको महाशालिकमलस्तु कलामको ॥ १४ ॥

*Group of dhānya*

*Rakta śāli* etc., belong to *śāli* group. *ṣaṣṭika* etc., belong to *brihi* group. *Mudga* etc., belong to *dvidala* (dicotyleden) group, *Sauca kaṅgu* etc., belong to *tṛṇa dhānya* group. *Kṣudra dhānya* is called *kudhānya*. *Yava* etc., are called *sthūla dhānya*. *Rakta śāli* is called *lohita, garuḍa* is called *śakunāhṛta, sugandhika* is called *mahā śāli* and *kalama* is called *kalāmaka.*

क्षीरी

क्षीरेयं परमान्नं स्यात्पायसं क्षीरतंदुलैः ।

क्षीरिका दुर्ज्जरा बल्या धातुपुष्टिप्रदा गुरु ॥ १५ ॥

विष्टंभिनी हरेत्पित्तं रक्तपित्ताग्निमारुतान् ।

*Kṣīrī*

*Kṣīreya, paramānna* and *pāyasa*—these are synonyms of *kṣīrī* which is prepared of milk and rice.

*Kṣīrikā* is difficult of digestion and strength promoting. It provides nourishment to tissue elements. It is heavy and constipative. It alleviates *pitta, rakta pitta* (a disease characterised by bleeding from different parts of the body), *agni* (digestive power) and *vāyu.*

रागषाडव

गुडादिपक्वक्वथितमाममाम्रफलं पुनः ॥ १६ ॥

स्नेहैला नागरैर्युक्तं ज्ञातव्यो रागषाडवः ।

सितारुचकसिंधूत्थैः सवृक्षाम्लपरुषकैः ॥ १७ ॥

जंबूफलरसैर्युक्तो रागो राजिकया कृतः ।

षाडवा मधुरोष्णादिरससंयोगसंभवाः ॥ १८ ॥

दीपना बृंहणा रुच्या हृद्या स्तृष्णाश्रमापहाः ।

*Rāga ṣāḍava*

A preparation of green fruits of *āmra* fermented after boiling with *guḍa* etc.. and added with *sneha* (oil), *elā*, and *nāgara* is called *rāga ṣāḍava,*

A preparation of the juice of the fruit of *jambu* mixed with *sitā, rucaka, sindhuttha, vṛkṣāmla, paruṣaka* and *rājikā* is called *rāga.*

Various types of *ṣāḍavas*, prepared by the juices which are sweet & hot, are stimulant of digestion, nourishing and appetiser It is a cardiac tonic. It alleviates thirst & fatigue.

**खंडाम्र, खंडामलक**

> आम्रामलकलेह्याद्याः हृद्याः पुष्टिबलप्रदाः ॥ १६ ॥
>
> तर्प्पणा रोचनास्निग्धा मधुरा गुरवस्तथा ।

*Khaṇḍāmra and Khaṇḍāmalaka*

*Lehyas* prepared of *āmra* and *āmalaka* are cardiac tonic, promoter of plumpness and strength, nourishing, appetiser, unctuous, sweet and heavy.

**शिखरिणि**

> ससितं दधिमध्वाज्यमरिचैलादिसंस्कृतम् ॥ २० ॥
>
> मथितं कान्तकामिन्या कर्पूरपरिपाचितम् ।
>
> रसाला शिखरिण्युक्ता मार्जिता मार्जिका बुधैः ॥२१॥
>
> रसाला शुक्रला बल्या रोचनी वातपित्तजित् ।
>
> स्निग्धा गुरुः प्रतिश्यायं विशेषेण विनाशयेत् ॥ २२ ॥

*Śikhariṇi*

Sugar and *dadhi* mixed with *madhu*, *ājya* and *marica*, churned by a beautiful lady and mixed with *karpūra* is called *rasālā, śikhariṇi, mārjitā and mārjikā.*

*Rasālā* is *spermatopoetic*, strength promoting and appetiser. It alleviates aggravated *vāta* and *pitta*. It is unctuous and heavy. It specially cures *pratiśyāya* (cold).

**पानक**

> द्राक्षाश्रीकपरुषादि जलखंडादिमिश्रितम् ।
>
> मारिचार्द्रककर्प्पूरचातुर्जातादिसंस्कृतम् ॥ २३ ॥
>
> पानकं द्विविधं तत्स्यादम्लानम्लविभेदतः ।

द्राक्षा खजूरकाश्मर्य समधूकपरुषकैः ॥ २४ ॥
पंचसाराभिधानं च चंद्रपूर्णाभिवासितम् ।
पानकं मूत्रलं हृद्यं प्रीणनं तृट्श्रमापहम् ॥ २५ ॥
यथाद्रव्यं गुणं तत्तु गुरुलध्वादिनिर्दिशेत् ।
पंचसाराभिधं पित्ततृष्णादाहश्रमापहम् ॥ २६ ॥
माध्वीकं श्रमदाहास्रपित्तक्लमतृषापहम् ।
परूषकानां लोकानां(?)हृद्यं विष्टंभि पाचनम् ॥ २७ ॥
अम्लीकायाः सरं तृष्णाकृमिदाहश्रमापहम् ।

*Pānaka*

The potion prepared of *drākṣā*, *śrīka*, *paruṣa* etc., mixed with water and *khaṇḍa* (a type of sugar) and impregnated with *marica*, *ārdraka*, *karpūra*, *caturjātaka* (*tvak*, *elā*, *patra* and *nāga kesara*) etc., is called *pānaka*.

*Pānaka* is of two types—one is sour and the other is not sour.

The *pānaka* prepared of *drākṣā*, *kharjūra*, *kāśmarya*, *madhūka* and *paruṣaka* and mixed with *karpūra* is called *pañca sāra*.

*Pānaka* is diuretic, cardiac tonic and nourishing. It cures morbid thirst and exhaustion.

The heaviness and lightness of *pānaka* should be determined according to the property of its ingerdients.

*Pañca sāra* type of *pānaka* cures aggravated *pitta*, morbid thirst, burning syndrome and exhaustion.

*Mādhvika* type of *pānaka* cures exhaustion, burning syndrome, *asra pitta* (a disease characterised by bleeding from different parts of the body), *klama* (mental fatigue) and morbid thirst,

The *pānaka* prepared of *paruṣaka* and *loka* (?) is cardiac tonic, constipative and carminative.

The *pānaka* prepared of *amlikā* is laxative and it cures morbid thirst, intestinal warm infestation, burning syndrome and exhaustion.

**सट्टक**

सुस्नेहं दधि निर्म्मथ्य पटे शर्क्करयान्वितम् ॥ २८ ॥
सव्योषं दाडिमाजाजिसट्टकोऽयमुदाहृतः ।
सट्टको रोचनो स्वर्यः पित्तानिलहरो गुरुः ॥ २९ ॥
दीपनस्तर्प्पणो बल्यः श्रमक्लमतृषापहः ।

*Saṭṭaka*

On a piece of cloth, *dadhi* with lot of fat and sugar should be triturated well. To this *vyoṣa* (*śuṇṭhī*, *pippalī* and *marica*), *dāḍima* and *ajāji* should be added. This is called *saṭṭaka*.

*Saṭṭaka* is appetiser and promoter of good voice. It alleviates *pitta* and *vāyu*. It is heavy, digestive stimulant, nourshing and strength promoting. It cures exhaustion, mental fatigue and morbid thirst.

**मण्डक**

कुकूल कर्परभृष्टा कदांगारविपाचिता ॥ ३० ॥
मांडकाद्या यथापूर्व्वं गुरवो बृंहणा मता ।
मंडकः मिश्रितः सूक्ष्मो कर्प्परादिषु पाचितः ॥ ३१ ॥
स एव किंचित्स्थूलस्तु बुधैः पूपालिका मता ।
अंगारकर्क्करी सैव विज्ञेयागांरपाचिता ॥ ३२ ॥
अत्युष्णो मंडकः पथ्यः शीतः स गुरुरुच्यते ।
अंगारमंडक ग्राही लघु दोषत्रयापहः ॥ ३३ ॥

*Maṇḍaka*

*Maṇḍaka* is prepared over *kukula* (iron frying pan) or *kharpara* (earthen pan) in low charcoal heat. The former type (prepared over iron pan) is heavier and more nourishing than the latter (prepared over earthen pan).

*Maṇḍaka* which is fried over an earthen pan should be thin. The thicker one is called *pūpālikā*.

The *maṇḍaka* prepared over charcoal is called *aṅgāra karkarī*.

*Maṇḍaka* is very wholesome when it is very hot. The cold *maṇḍaka* is heavy.

*Aṅgāra maṇḍaka* is constipative and light. It alleviates all the three *doṣas*.

**पोलिका**

पोलिका कफकृद्बल्या पित्तला वातनुद्गुरु ।
अंगारकर्क[8]री बल्या बृंहणी शुक्रला लघुः ॥ ३४ ॥
दीपनी कफहृद्रोगपीनसश्[9]वासकासजित् ।

*Polikā*

*Polikā* aggravates *kapha*. It promotes strength. It aggravates *pitta* and alleviates *vāyu*.

*Aṅgāra karkarī* promotes strength, corpulence and semen. It is light and stimulant of digestion. It alleviates *kapha*, heart disease, *pīnasa* (chronic cold), asthma and cough.

**शालिपिष्ट**

शालिपिष्टकृताः भक्ष्याः नातिबल्याः विदाहिनः ॥३५॥
अवृष्या गुरवश्चोष्णाः[10] कफपित्तप्रकोपनाः[11] ।

*Śāli piṣṭa*

Eatables prepared of the paste of *śāli* do not promote strength adequately and they produce burning sensation. They are not aphrodisiac. They are heavy and hot. They aggravate *kapha* and *pitta*.

**गोधूमभक्ष**

गोधूमविहिताः भक्ष्याः बल्याः पित्तानिलापहाः ॥३६॥

*Godhūma bhakṣya*

Eatables prepared of wheat promote strength and they alleviate *pitta* as well as *vāyu*.

**वैदलभक्ष**

वैदला वातला भक्ष्या गुरवस्तु सरा हिमाः ।

*Vaidala bhakṣya*

Eatables prepared of *vaidala* (pulses) aggravate *vāyu*. They are heavy, laxative and cooling.

**माषभक्ष्य**

माषपिष्टकृता भक्ष्याः बल्याः पित्तकफप्रदाः ॥ ३७ ॥

*Māṣa bhakṣya*

Eatables prepared of the paste of *māṣa* promote strength. They aggravate *pitta* and *kapha*.

**अन्यभक्ष**

विचार्यान्नगुणान् भक्ष्यानन्यानपि विनिर्दिशेत् ।

*Other bhakṣyas in general*

Properties of other eatables should be determined by the properties of their ingredients.

**गुडयुक्तभक्ष्य**

गौडिका गुरवो भक्ष्याः वातघ्नाः कफशुक्रलाः ॥ ३८ ॥

*Guḍa yukta bhakṣya*

Eatables prepared by mixing *guḍa* alleviates *vāyu*. They produce more of *kapha* and *semen*.

**घृतपक्व भक्ष्य**

12

घृतपाचितभक्ष्यास्तु बल्याः पित्तानिलापहाः ।

*Ghṛta pakva bhakṣya*

Eatables fried with ghee promote strength. They alleviate *pitta* and *vāyu.*

**तैलपक्व भक्ष्य**

तैलजाः दृक्समीरघ्नास्तूष्णाः पित्तास्रदूषणाः ॥ ३९ ॥

*Taila pakva bhakṣya*

Eatables fried with oil reduce eye sight and *vāyu*. They are hot. They vitiate *pitta* and *rakta.*

**दुग्धभक्ष्य**

दुग्धालोडितगोधूमशालिपिष्टादिनिर्मिताः
वातपित्तहराभक्ष्याः हृद्याः शुक्रबलप्रदाः ॥ ४० ॥

*Dugdha bhakyṣa*

Eatables prepared by boiling the paste of *godhūma, śāli* etc., in milk alleviate *vāyu* and *pitta*. They are cardiac tonics and they promote *semen* as well as strength,

**घृतपूर**

क्षीरेण मर्दितं चूर्णं गोधूमानां सुगालितम् ।
विस्तार्य सर्पिषा पक्त्वा ततः सिताविमिश्रितम् ॥४१॥
घृतपुरोऽयमुद्दिष्टः कर्पूरमरिचान्वितः ।
संमितः मर्द्दितः क्षीरनालिकेररसादिभिः ॥ ४२ ॥
अवगाह्य घृते पक्त्वा घृतपूरो परिस्मृतः ।
घृतपूरो गुरुर्वृष्यो हृद्यः पित्तानिलापहा ॥ ४३ ॥
सद्यःप्राणप्रदो बल्यो क्षतजित् बृंहणः परः ।

*Ghṛta pūra*

The well filtered flour of wheat should be kneaded with milk and boiled with ghee. Thereafter, sugar should be added to it. Then *karpūra* and *marica* should be mixed. This is called *ghṛta pūra*.

Refined wheat flour should be mixed with milk and juice of *nārikera*. The dough should then be boiled in ghee. This is also called *ghṛta pūra*.

*Ghṛta pūra* is heavy, aphrodisiac and cardiac tonic. It alleviates *pitta* and *vāyu*. It is instantaneously life-giving.

It promotes strength and alleviates *kṣata* (consumption). It is extremely nourishing.

**संयाव**

संमिता सर्प्पिषा भृष्टं सितामरिचमिश्रितम् ॥ ४४ ॥
एलालवंगकर्प्पूरचूर्णादि परिसंस्कृतम् ।
13
क्षिप्त्वान्यसम्मितालम्बपुटेषु च घृते पचेत् ॥ ४५ ॥
खंडे न्यसेत्ततः पक्वे संयावोऽयमुदाहृतः ।
सम्मिता मधुदुग्धेनमर्दयित्वा सुशोभनम् ॥ ४६ ॥
पचेद् घृतोत्तरे खंडे न्यसेत्पक्वं नवे घटे ।
ततो मरिचचूर्णेन खंडचूर्णेन चूर्णितम् ॥ ४७ ॥
14
कुर्यात्कर्प्पूरसंयुक्तं संयोवममृतोपमम् ।

*Saṁyāva*

Refined wheat flour should be fried with ghee and mixed with sugar and *marica*. It should then be impregnated with the powder of *elā*, *lavaṅga* and *karpūra*. This should be pressed with the help of some unprocessed wheat flour over a wooden plate (*ālamba puṭa*) and then fried in ghee. Thereafter, it should be boiled in sugar syrup. This preparation is called ***saṁyāva***.

Refined wheat flour should be kneaded with honey and milk. It should then be fried in ghee and sugar syrup consecutively. This should be kept in a new jar and sprinkled with the powder of *marica*, sugar and camphor. This is called *saṁyāva* which is like *ambrosia*.

**मधुशीर्षक**

15

मर्द्दयित्वा सुसमितामपूपास्तनवः कृताः ॥ ४८ ॥
मातुलुंगत्वचाखंडपक्वमार्द्रकपूरितम् ।
विधाय पूपकं वृत्तं गंधाढ्यं केशरान्वितम् ॥ ४९ ॥
पक्त्वा सर्प्पिषि खण्डे च गाहितो मधुशीर्षकः ।

*Madhu śīrṣaka*

Thin *apūpas* should be prepared by kneading the refined wheat flour. These should be filled up with a mixture of boiled pieces of the skin of the fruit of *matuluṅga* and *ardraka*. In these rounded *apūpas*, fragrant things like *keśara* should be added and these should be boiled in ghee and sugar (syrup) consecutively. This preparation is called *madhu śīrṣaka*.

**मधुपूपक**

समितां गुडतोयेन मेलयित्वा सुगालितम् ॥ ५० ॥
घृते विस्तार्य विपचेत् सुघृतं मधुपूपकः ।

*Madhu pūpaka*

Refined wheat flour should be mixed with *guḍa toya* and filtered. This should he kneaded with ghee and then boiled in good quantity of ghee. This is called *madhu pūpaka*.

**दधिपूपक**

शालिपिष्टयुतं दध्ना मर्द्दयित्वा घृते पचेत् ॥ ५१ ॥
वेष्टयेत्पक्वखडन सुवृत्ता दधिपूपका ।
संयावा मधुशीर्षाद्याः पूपकाः दधिपूपकाः ॥ ५२ ॥

गुरवो बृंहणाः हृद्याः वृष्याः पित्तानिलापहाः ।

एते संस्कारभेदेन विविधास्तेऽपि तद्गुणाः ॥५३॥

*Dadhi pūpaka*

Paste of *śāli* should be kneaded with *dadhi* and fried in ghee. Rounded pieces of this dough should be smeared with sugar syrup. These are called *dadhi pūpaka*.

*Saṁyāva*, *madhu śīrṣa* etc., *pūpaka* and *dadhi pūpaka* are heavy, nourishing, cardiac tonic and aphrodisiac. They alleviate *pitta* and *vāyu*.

There are different types of these preparations and their properties vary depending upon their method of processing.

**विष्यन्दन**

दधि क्षीरे समे पक्त्वा अर्धभागावशेषयेत् ।

आवपेद्रक्तशालीनां तंडुलस्तिलसंयुताम् ॥ ५४ ॥

पियालपनसाब्जानां बीजं मुष्टि समापयेत् ।

क्षीरतुल्यंघृतं चैव शर्क्करामरिचान्विता ॥ ५५ ॥

सिद्धस्त्रिकटुकोपेतः कर्प्पूरेणाधिवासितः ।

एष विष्यंदनो नाम देवलोकेऽपि दुर्ल्लभः ॥ ५६ ॥

यस्मात्पक्वेऽपि घृतेन स्कंदते सर्व्वतोमुखम् ।

तस्मात्सूपविधानज्ञैः विष्यंदन इति स्मृतः ॥ ५७ ॥

विष्यंदो बृंहणो हृद्यः पित्तानिलहरो गुरुः ।

*Viṣyandana*

Curd and milk should be taken in equal quantity and boiled till half remains. To this, the rice of red variety of *śāli* and *tila* should be added. One *muṣṭi* of the seeds of each of *piyāla*, *panasa* and *abja* should then be mixed with it. Ghee should then be taken in the same quantity as that of milk and added to it with sugar and *marica*. After boiling, *trikaṭu* (*śuṇṭhi*, *pippalī* and *marica*) should be added along with fragrant things like *karpūra*. This preparation is called *viṣyandana* and it is rare even in the heaven.

When boiled in ghee, it gets condensed (*skandana*) from all sides for which it is called *viṣyandana* by the experts in the science of cooking.

*Viṣyandana* is *bṛmhaṇa* (nourishing) and cardiac tonic. It alleviates *pitta* and *vāyu*, and it is heavy.

**लप्सिका**

समितां भर्ज्जयेत्तप्ते घृते सितां ततो न्यसेत् ।। ५८ ।।

चारमज्जादिसंयुक्ता पयसा योजयेत्तदा ।

एलैलादियुता तज्ज्ञैर्लक्षिका[16] ललिता मता ।। ५९ ।।

[17]लप्सिका बृंहणी वृष्या वातपित्तहरा गुरुः ।

*Lapsikā*

In the hot ghee refined wheat flour should be added. To this sugar should be added thereafter. Milk boiled with the fruit pulp of *cāra* should then be added. It should then be mixed with *elā*. This is known as *lapsikā* or *lalitā*.

*Lapsikā* is nourishing and aphrodisiac. It alleviates *vāyu* and *pitta*. It is heavy.

**फेनिका**

फेनिका पुटिनी शुभ्रा वातपित्तहरा लघुः ।। ६० ।।

लक्षणं फेनिकादीनां सूपकारैः विचारयेत् ।

*Phenikā* etc.

*Phenikā*, *puṭinī* and *śubhrā*—these preparations alleviate *vāta* and *pitta*. They are light.

Their methods of preparation may be ascertained from expert cooks.

**मोदक**

मोदकाः लड्डुकाः प्रोक्तास्ते चानेकविधाः मताः॥६१॥
दधि क्षीरनष्टदुग्धं समिता माषपिष्टिका।
सूरणार्द्रककूष्माण्डशालूकामिषमत्स्यकाः ॥ ६२ ॥
इत्यादिभिर्बहुविधाः फलास्ते सूपशास्त्रतः ।
द्रव्यं विचार्य्य मतिमांस्तद्गुणानपि निर्दिशेत्॥ ६३ ॥
मोदकाः दुर्ज्जराः वृष्याः बल्याः पित्तानिलापहाः ।

*Modaka*

*Modaka* is called *la ḍḍuka.* It is of various types. *Dadhi,* milk, chease, refined wheat flour, paste of *māṣa*, *sūraṇa*, *ārdraka, kūṣmāṇḍa*, *śālūka*, meat, fish, various types of fruits—these, among others, are the ingredients of *modaka.* Their details may be obtained from *sūpa śāstra.* Their properties will be the same as those of their ingredients.

*Modakas* are difficult of digestion, aphrodisiac and strength promoting. They alleviate *pitta* and *vāyu.*

**वटक**

माषमुद्गादिपिष्टोक्ता वटिका वटकादयः ॥ ६४ ॥
तत्कारणगुणान् ज्ञात्वा तद्गुणानपि निर्दिशेत् ।
माषान्नवटको हृद्यो विदाहि पवनापहः ॥ ६५ ॥
सांडाकी वटको दृष्टिनाशनो दोषलो गुरुः ।
तुषांवुः वटको रुच्यः पित्तलः कफवातजित् ॥ ६६ ॥

*Vaṭaka*

Preparations of the paste of *māṣa* and *mudga* are called *vaṭaka* and *vaṭikā*. Their properties should be determined on the basis of the properties of their ingredients.

*Vaṭaka* prepared of *māṣa* is cardiac tonic. It cures burning sensation and it alleviates *vāyu.*

*Vaṭaka* prepared of *sāṇḍākī* is harmful for eye sight. It aggravates *doṣas* and it is heavy.

*Vaṭaka* prepared to *tuṣāmbu* is appetiser. It aggravates *pitta* and it alleviates *kapha* and *vāta*.

**इंडरी**

इंडरीशुक्रला रुक्षा विष्टंभिः कफवातकृत् ।

*Iṇḍarī*

*Iṇḍarī* promotes the quantity of semen. It is ununctuous and constipative. It aggravates *kapha* and *vāta*.

**सोमालिका**

सोमालिका गुरुर्वृष्या रोचनो दोषनाशिनी ॥ ६७ ॥

*Somālikā*

*Somālikā* is heavy, *aphrodisiac* and appetiser. It alleviates (all) *doṣas*.

**कुंडलिका (जलेबी)**

द्विप्रस्थं शुद्धसमितां प्रस्थं गोधूममिलितम् ।
विमर्द्य पयसा स्थाप्यं प्रयोज्या च यंदाम्लताम् ॥६८॥
सछिद्रे नालिकेरस्य पात्रे निक्षिप्य निर्म्मले ।
परिभ्राम्य परिभ्राम्य घृते तप्ते विपाचयेत् ॥ ६९ ॥
(कर्प्पूरवासितैर्धूपः) विज्ञेयो नृपवल्लभा ।
सुपक्त्वा कंकणाकारं सितालेहेविनिक्षिपेत् ॥ ७० ॥
सा तु कुंडलिका नाम पुष्टिकान्तिबलप्रदा ।

*Kuṇḍalikā*

Two *prasthas* of refined wheat flour and one *prastha* of

*godhūma* should be mixed with milk and kneaded. This dough should be kept till it becomes sour. Through a clean cup of coconut shell having a hole at the bottom, this dough should be poured in a whirling manner over hot ghee. When fully boiled it takes the shape of an armlet. It should then be dropped in sugar syrup. This preparation is called *kuṇḍalikā*.

*Kuṇḍalikā* promotes plumpness, complexion and strength.

**कुल्माष**

गोधूमाद्यास्तु कुल्माषा अर्द्धस्विन्ना मता क्वचित् ।।७१।।

कुल्माषा गुरवो रुक्षा वातला भिन्नवर्चसाम् ।

*Kulmāṣa*

According to some scholars half soaked *godhūma* etc., are called *kulmāṣa*.

*Kulmāṣa* is heavy and ununctuous. It aggravates *vāyu* and causes purgation.

**मंथ**

नविनस्तूषसंभृष्टः यवचूर्णं तु सक्तवः ।। ७२ ।।

सक्तवस्तु घृताभ्यक्ता शीतवारिविलोडिता ।

नातिद्रवा नातिसांद्रा मंथ सद्भिः प्रकीर्त्तिताः ।।७३।।

मंथो बलकरः सद्यः परिणामे बलापहः ।

गेहतृष्णाभयछर्दिकुष्ठदेहश्रमान् जयेत् ।। ७४ ।।

द्राक्षामधुयुतो बल्यः कफश्रममदापहः ।

वर्गत्रयसमायुक्तो दोषवर्च्चोनुलोमनः ।। ७५ ।।

*Mantha*

Freshly harvested barley should be fried with husk and then made to a powder. This is called *saktu*.

*Saktu* should be kneaded with ghee and then mixed with cold water. It should be neither very thick nor very thin. This preparation is called *mantha*.

*Mantha* immediately promotes strength, but in the long run, it reduces strength. It cures *meha* (obstinate urinary disorders including diabetes), *tṛṣṇā* (morbid thirst), *bhaya* (fear complex), *chardi* (vomiting), *kuṣṭha* (obstinate skin diseases including leprosy) and *deha śrama* (physical fatigue). Mixed with *drākṣā* and honey it promotes strength and alleviates aggravated *kapha*, fatigue and intoxicating conditions.

When mixed with three groups of medicines, it brings *dosas* and feces downwards.

सक्तु

सक्तवो यवजाः शीताः दीपनाः लघवः सराः ।
कफपित्तहरा रूक्षा लेखना पातनास्तु ते ॥ ७६ ॥
सद्योबलकराः पथ्या घर्म्मादिक्लांतदेहिनाम् ।
निस्तुषैर्भर्ज्जितैः पिष्टैश्चणकैः सूपवैकृताः ॥ ७७ ॥
सक्तवः शर्करसर्प्पिर्युक्ता ग्रीष्मेऽतिपूजिताः ।
पिंडी प्रोक्ता गुरुस्तेषां द्रवत्वाल्लेहिका लघुः ॥ ७८ ॥
नाभुक्त्वा न रदैश्छित्वा न निशायां न च वा बहु ।
न जलान्तरिता सद्भिः सक्तुनद्यान्न केवलम् ॥७९॥

*Saktu*

*Saktu* prepared of *yava* is cooling, stimulant of digestion, light and laxative. It alleviates *kapha* and *pitta*. It is ununctuous, *lekhana* (having scraping effect) and *pātana* (?) It promotes strength instantaneously & is wholesome for persons fatigued by the heat of the sun.

*Saktu* is also prepared by frying and pounding dehusked pulses like *caṇaka*.

Mixed with sugar and ghee *saktu* is exceedingly useful in summer season.

It is heavy when prepared in the form of a bolus (*piṇḍi*) and when prepared in the form of a thin linctus (*lehikā*) it is light.

*Saktu* should not be taken in empty stomach. It should not be chewed. It should not be taken at night. It should not be consumed in excess quantity. Eating of *saktu* should not be interrupted by drinking of water. *Saktu* should not be taken alone.

**लाजा**

भृष्टशाल्यादिजा लाजा धाना भृष्टयवोद्भवा ।
लाजा लघुतरा शीता बल्या पित्तकफप्रदा ॥ ८० ॥

छर्द्यतीसार ˚दाहास्रमेहमेदस्तृषापहा ।

*Lājā*

Fried *śāli* etc., are called *lājā* and fried *yava* etc., are called *dhānā*.

*Lājā* is lighter, cooling and strength promoting. It aggravates *pitta* and *kapha*. It cures *chardi* (vomiting), *atisāra* (diarrhoea), *dāha* (burning syndrome), *asra* (vitiation of blood), *meha* (obstinate urinary disorders including diabetes) and *tṛṣā* (morbid thirst).

**धाना**

धाना विष्टंभिनी रुक्षा कफमेदोपहा[18] लघुः ॥ ८१ ॥

*Dhānā*

*Dhānā* is constipative and ununctuous. It reduces *kapha* and *medas*. It is light.

**पृथुका**

पक्वार्द्रा व्रीह्यः सम्यक्पीडिताः पृथुकाः मताः ।

पृथुका गुरवो बल्या श्लेष्मलाः वातनाशनाः ॥ ८२ ॥

*Pṛthukā*

Boiled and wet *brīhi* etc., are pounded (pressed). These are called *pṛthukā*.

*Pṛthukā* is heavy and strength promoting. It aggravates *kapha* and alleviates *vāyu*.

**होलक**

सिबिधान्यैरर्धपक्वैः सुभृष्टो होलको मतः ।

होलकोऽल्पानिलोमेदकफदश्च स्वभावतः ॥ ८३ ॥

*Holaka*

*Holaka* is prepared by frying half boiled *simbi dhānya* By nature, *holaka* produces *vāyu, medas* and *kapha* in small quantity.

**उंवी**

अपक्व भृष्टगोधूमः उलुंवो लुंव उंविका ।

उंवी कफप्रदा बल्या लघुः पित्तानिलापहा ॥ ८४ ॥

*Uṁvī*

Immature wheat when fried is called *uluṁva, luṁva* and *uṁvikā*.

*Uṁvī* aggravates *kapha*. It is strength promoting and light. It alleviates *pitta* and *vāyu*.

## NOTES AND REFERENCES

1 This is the 97th chapter of *Ayurveda saukhyaṁ* in *Toḍarā-uvupv* vnd the opening invocation reads as below.

रमाधवो रामसमन्वितः सत्रसाधवं टोडरमल्लसंज्ञम् ।

सपुत्ररामं जगतो हिताय पूर्णं प्रकुर्याद्धनधर्मसोख्यैः ।

2. 'हाला' इति पंचमपुस्तके पाठः ।
3. 'मंडा' इति पंचमपुस्तके पाठः ।
4. 'वल्लकस्तथा' इति पंचमपुस्तके पाठः ।
5. 'कामिथा' इति प्रथमपुस्तके पाठः ।
6. 'सूचितः' इति पंचमपुस्तके पाठः ।
7. 'अंगारकर्क्कटी' इति पंचमपुस्तके पाठः ।
8. 'कर्क्कटी' इति पंचमपुस्तके पाठः ।
9. 'श्लेष्मा कफपित्तप्रकोपनाः' इति पंचमपुस्तके पाठः ।
10. In mss I & V, at the end of this verse it is written 'अस्त्र पिष्टा न भक्ष्याः' ।
11. 'वातघ्ना कफ शुक्ला' इति पंचमपुस्तके पाठः ।
12. 'पित्ताकफापहाः' इति पंचमपुस्तके पाठः ।
13. 'समितालम्बपुटेषु' इति पंचमपुस्तके पाठः ।
14. 'संजावममृतोपमम्' इति प्रथमपुस्तके पाठः ।
15. 'सुसमितामयूषास्तन्वः' इति प्रथमपुस्तके पाठः ।
16. 'युतानक्तैर्लप्सिका' इति पंचमपुस्तके पाठः ।
17. 'लप्सिका' इति पंचमपुस्तके पाठः ।
18. 'गुरुः' इति प्रथमपुस्तके पाठः ।

19. This is the end of 97th chapter of *Ayurveda Saukhyaṁ* in *Toḍarānanda* and the colophon reads as below :

पूर्णं सौख्यमिदं शिवं वितनुतां श्रीटोडरेंद्रे सदा ।

धन्यं वृत्तिकरं सुधर्म्माभिभवं प्राणिप्रियं शर्म्मदम् ।।८५।।

आयुर्वेदसमुद्रजं सुरतरो रूपं द्वितीयं परम् ।

भूमावंकुरितं प्रयोगसुदलं नैरुज्य भूयः फलम् ।। ८६ ।।

यो वेदार्थसमूहमौक्तिकगणैः श्रीटोडरानंदकः ।

पूर्णो वारिधिरेष सर्व्वजगतां वर्व्वत्ति धर्म्मार्थदः ॥८७॥

अंतर्वाणिविभूषणैरुपरितो गीर्व्वाणतुल्यैः शिवै ।

रालोड्यार्थतरंगवान् विरचितः शास्त्राणि राजाज्ञया ॥८८॥

विश्वेषां परमार्थदोऽखिलजनां ज्ञानांधकारे रविः ।

सद्धर्म्माब्जिसुबोधने च शशिवत्तापत्रये राजते ॥८९॥

श्रीगोविंदपदारविन्दे वसतामानंददो यः सतां—

मन्वर्थं भजते सुनामसकलं भूयान्मुदे सर्व्वदा ॥९०॥

इति श्रीमद्विविधविरुदावलीविराजमानदरघुमांधातृभरतादिसमयप्रवृत्तपदवीप्रवर्त्तकांत्ययुगाभिःकृतश्रीमूर्त्तिमहददरिद्रादिदुःखवद्धकाक्रांतः ब्राह्मणादिपक्षिगणाश्रयः कल्पपादपः समस्तशणपलतासंपोषणाद्दौर्दंडदुष्टप्रदमनातिविकटप्रोच्चदुर्गममित्रक्षपणक्षमकोपकटाक्षः हस्तिहयहीरहेमादिदानविस्मारितहरिश्चंद्रादिचक्रवर्त्तिवर्गो दुदन्वदंतरावर्त्तिविश्वंभराधिनाथप्रतापलीढा विप्लुष्टदिगंतस्थपरिपंथि सीमंतिनीहृद्गर्भ श्रीमदकवरसाहिपुरःसर भारोद्धरणक्षम प्रचंडदौर्दंडनिरंतरधर्म्मानुरक्तांतःकरणः द्वितीययुधिष्ठिर श्रीमद्गोविंदपादारविंदार्प्पितसमस्तमनोवृत्यंवरीषप्रह्लादादिसदाग्रहाखिलक्षत्रवंशावतंसमूर्द्धन्यललामकरुणाकूपारगरिमा चलप्रवरागाधांतःकरणातिप्रसिद्धटंडणवंशपारावारोद्भूत भूचंद्रमा महाराजाधिराज श्रीटोडरमल्लविरचिते टोडरानंदे आयुर्वेदसौख्ये एकनवतितमो हर्षः (?)॥ शुभमस्तु॥ मांगल्यं भूयात्॥ श्री श्री ॥ लिखितं कायस्थ माथुरमेवरि गोपाचलीठा हरिवंशुतत्पुत्रदयालदासलिखितम ॥ श्रीगोपीजनवल्लभाय ननः ॥

# INDEX

(*Glossary of Technical Words*)

# INDEX II

(*Drugs & Diet described in this Text*)

# INDEX III

(*Synonyms of Drugs*)